NMS
Psychiatry

NMS
Psychiatry

6th EDITION

Editor

Joshua T. Thornhill IV, MD

Professor of Clinical Psychiatry
Associate Dean for Medical Education and Academic Affairs
University of South Carolina School of Medicine
Department of Neuropsychiatry and Behavioral Science
Columbia, South Carolina

Wolters Kluwer | Lippincott Williams & Wilkins
Health
Philadelphia · Baltimore · New York · London
Buenos Aires · Hong Kong · Sydney · Tokyo

Acquisitions Editor: Susan Rhyner
Product Manager: Stacey Sebring
Marketing Manager: Joy Fisher-Williams
Manufacturing Coordinator: Margie Orzech
Designer: Holly Reid McLaughlin
Compositor: Aptara, Inc.

Sixth Edition

Library of Congress Cataloging-in-Publication Data

Psychiatry. – Sixth Edition / Editor, Joshua T. Thornhill IV, MD,
Professor of Clinical Psychiatry, Associate Dean for Medical Education
and Academic Affairs, University of South Carolina School of Medicine,
Department of Neuropsychiatry and Behavioral Science, Columbia, South
Carolina.
       p. ; cm. – (NMS)
 Includes bibliographical references and index.
 Summary: "In this sixth edition of NMS Psychiatry, each chapter as
well as the drug appendix has been updated to include the latest
medications and treatment protocols. New chapters have been added on the
emerging fields of emergency and geriatric psychiatry. In addition, we
have continued to revise, update, and add new questions to each chapter
and to the comprehensive examination to help students prepare for
National Board of Medical Examiners (NBME) Subject examinations as well
as the United States Medical Licensing Exam (USMLE) Step 2"–Provided by
publisher.
 ISBN 978-1-60831-574-1 (pbk. : alk. paper) 1. Psychiatry–Outlines,
syllabi, etc. 2. Psychiatry–Examinations, questions, etc. I.
Thornhill, Joshua T., IV, editor. II. Series: National medical series
for independent study.
 [DNLM: 1. Psychiatry–Examination Questions. 2. Mental
Disorders–Examination Questions. WM 18.2]
 RC457.2.P78 2012
 616.890076–dc22
                                              2010054470

DISCLAIMER

Care has been taken to confirm the accuracy of the information present and to describe generally accepted practices. However, the authors, editors, and publisher are not responsible for errors or omissions or for any consequences from application of the information in this book and make no warranty, expressed or implied, with respect to the currency, completeness, or accuracy of the contents of the publication. Application of this information in a particular situation remains the professional responsibility of the practitioner; the clinical treatments described and recommended may not be considered absolute and universal recommendations.

The authors, editors, and publisher have exerted every effort to ensure that drug selection and dosage set forth in this text are in accordance with the current recommendations and practice at the time of publication. However, in view of ongoing research, changes in government regulations, and the constant flow of information relating to drug therapy and drug reactions, the reader is urged to check the package insert for each drug for any change in indications and dosage and for added warnings and precautions. This is particularly important when the recommended agent is a new or infrequently employed drug.

Some drugs and medical devices presented in this publication have Food and Drug Administration (FDA) clearance for limited use in restricted research settings. It is the responsibility of the health care provider to ascertain the FDA status of each drug or device planned for use in their clinical practice.

To purchase additional copies of this book, call our customer service department at **(800) 638-3030** or fax orders to **(301) 223-2320**. International customers should call **(301) 223-2300**.

Visit Lippincott Williams & Wilkins on the Internet: http://www.lww.com. Lippincott Williams & Wilkins customer service representatives are available from 8:30 am to 6:00 pm, EST.

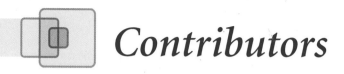

Contributors

James G. Bouknight, MD, PhD
Professor of Clinical Psychiatry
Department of Neuropsychiatry and Behavioral
  Science
University of South Carolina School of Medicine
Director, Geriatric Psychiatry Fellowship
Palmetto Health
Columbia, South Carolina

Robert J. Breen, MD
DMH Associate Professor of Clinical Psychiatry
Department of Neuropsychiatry and Behavioral
  Science
University of South Carolina School of Medicine
Medical Director, G. Werber Bryan Psychiatric
  Hospital
South Carolina Department of Mental Health
Columbia, South Carolina

William Burke, PhD, LPC
Clinical Assistant Professor of Behavioral
  Science
Department of Neuropsychiatry and Behavioral
  Science
University of South Carolina School of Medicine
President and Clinical Director of SEA
Columbia, South Carolina

Nioaka N. Campbell, MD
Associate Professor of Psychiatry
Department of Neuropsychiatry and Behavioral
  Science
University of South Carolina School of Medicine
Director, General Psychiatry Residency Training
  Program
Palmetto Health
Columbia, South Carolina

Harvey L. Causey III, MD
DMH Assistant Professor of Clinical Psychiatry
Department of Neuropsychiatry and Behavioral
  Science
University of South Carolina School of Medicine
Medical Director, Morris Village Alcohol and
  Drug Treatment Center
South Carolina Department of Mental Health
Columbia, South Carolina

R. Gregg Dwyer, MD, EdD
Associate Professor
Director, Forensic Psychiatry Program and
  Sexual Behaviors Clinic and Lab
Department of Psychiatry
Medical University of South Carolina
Charleston, South Carolina

Richard L. Frierson, MD
Professor of Clinical Psychiatry
Department of Neuropsychiatry and Behavioral
  Science
University of South Carolina School of Medicine
Director, Forensic Psychiatry Fellowship
Palmetto Health
Columbia, South Carolina

Leslie E. Frinks, MD
Assistant Professor of Clinical Psychiatry
Department of Neuropsychiatry and Behavioral
  Science
University of South Carolina
Assistant Director, General Psychiatry Residency
  Training Program
Palmetto Health
Columbia, South Carolina

Suzanne Garfinkle, MD, MSc
Fellow in Child and Adolescent Psychiatry
Department of Psychiatry
Mount Sinai School of Medicine
New York, New York

Angela D. Harper, MD
Clinical Assistant Professor of Psychiatry
Department of Neuropsychiatry and Behavioral
  Science
University of South Carolina School of Medicine
Private Practice, Comprehensive Behavioral
  Care, LLC
Columbia, South Carolina

Rachel A. Houchins, MD
Assistant Professor of Clinical Psychiatry
Department of Neuropsychiatry and Behavioral
    Science
University of South Carolina School of Medicine
Trauma Surgery Consult Liaison Psychiatry
Emergency Room Psychiatrist
Palmetto Health
Columbia, South Carolina

Meera Narasimhan, MD
Professor of Clinical Psychiatry
Interim Chair, Department of Neuropsychiatry
    and Behavioral Science
University of South Carolina School of
    Medicine
Columbia, South Carolina

Jeffrey D. Raynor, MD
PHA Assistant Professor of Clinical Psychiatry
Department of Neuropsychiatry and Behavioral
    Science
University of South Carolina School of Medicine
Psychiatric Hospitalist
Palmetto Health
Columbia, South Carolina

Kimberly Butterfly Rudd, MD
DMH Assistant Professor of Clinical Psychiatry
Department of Neuropsychiatry and Behavioral
    Science
University of South Carolina School of
    Medicine
Geriatric Psychiatrist, G. Werber Bryan
    Psychiatric Hospital
South Carolina Department of Mental Health
Columbia, South Carolina

James H. Scully Jr., MD
Medical Director/CEO
American Psychiatric Association
Arlington, Virginia
Clinical Professor of Psychiatry
Department of Neuropsychiatry and Behavioral
    Science
University of South Carolina School of Medicine
Columbia, South Carolina
Clinical Professor of Psychiatry and Behavioral
    Sciences
Department of Psychiatry and Behavioral
    Sciences
George Washington University School of
    Medicine and Health Sciences
Washington, DC

Shilpa Srinivasan, MD
Associate Professor of Clinical Psychiatry
Director, M-III Psychiatry Clerkship
Department of Neuropsychiatry and Behavioral
    Science
University of South Carolina School of Medicine
Assistant Director, Geriatric Psychiatry
    Fellowship
Palmetto Health
Columbia, South Carolina

Craig Stuck, MD
Assistant Professor of Clinical Psychiatry
Department of Neuropsychiatry and Behavioral
    Science
University of South Carolina School of Medicine
Director, Child and Adolescent Psychiatry
    Residency Training Program
Palmetto Health
Columbia, South Carolina

Joshua T. Thornhill IV, MD
Professor of Clinical Psychiatry
Associate Dean for Medical Education and
    Academic Affairs
Department of Neuropsychiatry and Behavioral
    Science
University of South Carolina School of Medicine
Columbia, South Carolina

Eric R. Williams, MD
Clinical Assistant Professor of Psychiatry
Department of Neuropsychiatry and Behavioral
    Science
University of South Carolina School of Medicine
Columbia, South Carolina

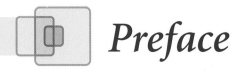

Preface

We are already a decade into the twenty-first century and the scientific basis of psychiatry continues to expand. New medications have been developed for the treatment of individuals with schizophrenia, mood disorders, and severe anxiety disorders. Focused psychotherapeutic techniques have been proven as effective treatments. Because of the importance of evidence-based medical practice, scientifically based practice guidelines developed by the American Psychiatric Association are now the norm instead of the exception. These guidelines, as well as the *Diagnostic and Statistical Manual of Mental Disorders,* 4th edition, text revision (*DSM-IV-TR*), have been used extensively in the preparation of this book.

In this sixth edition of *NMS Psychiatry,* each chapter as well as the drug appendix has been updated to include the latest medications and treatment protocols. New chapters have been added on the emerging fields of emergency and geriatric psychiatry. In addition, we have continued to revise, update, and add new questions to each chapter and to the comprehensive examination to help students prepare for National Board of Medical Examiners (NBME) subject examinations as well as the U.S. Medical Licensing Exam (USMLE) Step 2.

Finally, with this edition, we are fortunate to have added several new contributors: Drs. Bouknight, Burke, Causey, Dwyer, Frinks, Garfinkle, Houchins, Narasimhan, Raynor, Rudd, Srinivasan, Stuck, and Williams.

Joshua T. Thornhill IV, MD

Acknowledgments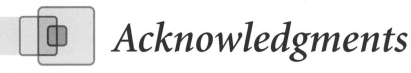

This edition is dedicated to Dr. Mark J. Corsale; words cannot describe my thanks and gratitude for all of your years of hard work with me. In addition, I am honored by the outstanding contributions to this edition by all of our authors; they are truly leaders in their field. Thank you.

Contents

chapter 1

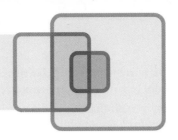

The Clinical Examination

JAMES H. SCULLY · JOSHUA T. THORNHILL IV

I OVERVIEW

A General psychiatric evaluation

1. The psychiatric evaluation differs from a routine medical examination in that it includes a **mental status examination** rather than a physical examination, although a physical examination may be included. The examiner asks the patient about **feelings and relationships,** not just historical facts. The psychiatric evaluation consists of:
   a. **Collecting data** from a careful history of the patient's problems
   b. **Conducting an examination**
   c. **Establishing a psychiatric diagnosis and developing a differential diagnosis** for further study
   d. **Constructing a treatment plan**

2. The primary method of obtaining data for a psychiatric evaluation is the face-to-face **interview.**
   a. **Sensitivity** is required because of the embarrassment many patients have about disclosing emotional problems. Special skills are necessary when taking psychiatric histories because many patients are embarrassed about disclosing their emotional problems. In general, people are less willing to discuss psychiatric symptoms than physical ones. Most patients are not psychotic, but many patients, especially those who are confused or disorganized, can be helped by the physician to give accurate details of their history.
   b. **Confidentiality** is important in all physician–patient interactions, especially when psychiatric issues are discussed. To maintain confidentiality, physicians should not discuss their patients in hallways or elevators. In teaching programs, case material must be presented, but it is important to maintain anonymity. Participants in any conference are bound by confidentiality.
   c. **Exceptions to the rule of confidentiality** are made when the need for safety is paramount such as in cases of child abuse or when threats are made to harm others.
   d. **Collateral sources,** such as record review and interviews of persons close to patients, may provide important additional information.

B Interview

1. **Verbal communication.** During the first few minutes of the interview, the physician should allow the patient to talk about any symptoms. The patient should feel comfortable enough to provide personal information.

2. **Nonverbal communication** such as facial expression and posture is equally important. It is also important to note how the story is told (e.g., tone of voice, feelings expressed).

C History of the present illness   Information should be obtained about the following:

1. **Onset, duration, or change of symptoms over time**

2. **Stressful events, especially losses,** including death of a loved one, job loss, or financial problems

3. **Patient perception of any change in her- or himself** or the perception of change in the patient by another individual (e.g., spouse, friend, supervisor at work)

4. **Previous psychiatric illness or treatment,** including medication, hospitalization, or other therapy, and responses to treatment (both positive and negative)

5. **Legal issues** with respect to the current illness (e.g., lawsuit, arrest, incarceration) or if the patient is a student, problems in school (e.g., truancy, suspension, expulsion)

6. **Secondary gain,** which is any benefit that the patient derives from the current problem (e.g., monetary compensation; relief from responsibilities at home, school, or work)

D **Personal history**

1. **Developmental milestones.** The physician should:
   a. Obtain information about the patient's **early development,** including details about the patient's mother's pregnancy and delivery. Information may be obtained from the patient, family members, or hospital records.
   b. Assess the patient's **temperament** as a child and determine any important family events (e.g., death, separation, divorce) that may have influenced the patient's temperament.
   c. Obtain information about the patient's **early experiences and relationships,** including school experiences (i.e., academic performance, delinquency), friends, family stability, early sexual experiences, and history of neglect or abuse. The patient's early relationships with parents, siblings, and friends can be important barometers of development.
   d. Assess important cultural and religious influences that affect the patient.

2. **Social history.** The physician should:
   a. Determine the breadth of the patient's **social life** (e.g., whether the patient is a loner, how difficult it is for the patient to establish friendships). The physician should assess both present and past levels of functioning in various social roles (e.g., marriage, parenting, work).
   b. Determine whether any **changes in personality** have been noted by the patient or by the patient's family or friends.
   c. Determine the patient's **marital status** or involvement in an intimate relationship, as well as the current level of **sexual functioning** and **sexual orientation.**
   d. Obtain the patient's **employment history,** including the number of jobs held and the reasons the jobs were terminated. Note any problems with alcoholism or antisocial behavior at work.
   e. Obtain the patient's **military service history** (if applicable), including the highest rank attained and a history of any disciplinary problems or combat experience.

3. **Family history.** The physician should:
   a. Ask the patient whether any **family members** have undergone **psychiatric hospitalization** or any other mental health treatment, attempted suicide, had problems with alcohol, or had other psychiatric problems. Families often deny significant psychiatric history.
   b. Determine **genetic risk factors** for mental disorders and **family attitudes** toward mental illness and treatment.
   c. Determine whether any family member is successfully using any **psychotropic medication** for the same illness. If so, there is a good chance that the medication will also help the patient.

4. **Previous psychiatric history**
   a. Note the **recurrence of an earlier problem** in the history of the current illness. List episodes of any **other psychiatric illness** chronologically.
   b. Note and record any **previous treatments in chronologic order,** including the name and address of the therapist, length of treatment, medications and dosages, and outcome of treatment.

5. **Substance use and abuse**
   a. Ask screening questions about **alcohol and drug problems,** including whether family or friends have ever objected to the patient's drinking or drug use and whether the patient has ever thought that he or she has had a problem with alcohol or drugs, either legal or illegal. Also, consider the use of **tobacco.**
   b. Note any negative consequences of substance use, including tolerance, withdrawal, or effect on the present illness. The interviewer should be nonjudgmental but should ask specific questions about the consequences of alcohol or drug use, such as driving under the influence.

II PSYCHIATRIC EXAMINATION

The assessment of a patient with a psychiatric disorder should always include the psychiatric interview and the mental status examination. It may also include a physical examination, laboratory studies, and psychological tests.

A Psychiatric interview

1. **Physician–patient relationship**

   a. **Patients are often anxious** about a psychiatric evaluation. Although they may be self-referred, many patients are referred by another health care professional and may be ambivalent about the psychiatric examination. The physician should be courteous and respectful and should acknowledge the patient's feelings about being interviewed.

   b. The **environment** may affect the difficulty of the evaluation. The setting may range from a quiet, private office to a busy, noisy emergency department in a general hospital.

   c. Family members or others may provide important information. However, the physician should always obtain the **patient's permission to question family members.**

   d. Interruptions should be minimized, and **sufficient time should be allowed for completion of the interview.** Traditionally, the interview is 50 to 60 minutes long, but 20 minutes may be enough.

   e. The physician should sit at **eye level** with the patient.

2. **Mental status.** The **informal mental status examination** that includes an evaluation of the following patient characteristics begins immediately:

   a. Appearance *ambulatory, well-kempt, no distress*

   b. Manner of relating *distant, polite, (demeanor)*

   c. Use of language *coherent, goal-oriented, organized*

   d. Mood and affect *Euthymic, Irritable, constricted (affect)*

   e. Content of discussion (e.g., family problems, work issues)

   f. Perceptions

   g. Abstracting ability

   h. Judgment

   i. Insight *know they're sick?*

3. **Interview technique.** The examiner should:

   a. Lead the interview with the use of both open-ended and direct questions.

      (1) **Open-ended questions** allow patients to use their own words (e.g., "Tell me about your home life," "Tell me about your hospital stay").

      (2) **Direct questions** are used to elicit specific information (e.g., "Have you ever consulted a mental health professional before?" "Are you thinking about killing yourself?").

   b. Clearly communicate that he or she is listening.

      (1) **Attentive silence.** Nonverbal cues such as nodding and leaning forward demonstrate attention. The physician should establish eye contact and convey the message that he or she is interested in what the patient is saying.

      (2) **Facilitation.** Use of encouraging comments (e.g., "Tell me more about it") helps the patient focus while relating the history.

      (3) **Summarization.** By summarizing the patient's words, the physician lets the patient know that he or she is listening and allows the patient to correct any misunderstanding. The interviewer should summarize portions of the patient's story (e.g., "So, you have been increasingly sad for 3 weeks, during which time you have lost 7 pounds and have been waking up at 4:00 AM?").

      (4) **Clarification.** The role of clarifying statements is similar to summary statements but also includes connections that the patient may not recognize. A clarifying statement allows the interviewer to confirm the accuracy of the information and the patient to correct it if necessary. For example, the physician might say, "Your difficulty sleeping and your crying spells began in mid-September. Was this after your youngest child left for college?"

B **Mental status examination**   In contrast to the psychiatric history, which is a record of a patient's entire life, the mental status examination is an evaluation of a patient at one point in time. During the interview, the physician observes the following characteristics:

1. **Appearance.** The patient's overall appearance, dress, grooming, and any unusual features or gestures are noteworthy.

2. **Attitude.** How the patient relates to the interviewer (e.g., hostile, cooperative, evasive) may be important.

3. **Behavior and psychomotor activity.** Such features as gait, position, and overall level of activity may include unusual mannerisms, agitation, or psychomotor retardation. Manic patients may be unable to sit still, and schizophrenic patients may adopt bizarre postures or move stiffly and awkwardly.

4. **Speech**
   a. **Rate of speech** (e.g., rapid, slow, halting)
   b. **Amount of speech** (e.g., taciturn, lacking spontaneity, grandiose)
   c. **Tone of speech** (e.g., monotone, singsong, slurred)
   d. **Speech impairment** (e.g., dysarthria, stuttering, echolalia), accent, dialect, or any other obvious speech pattern
   e. **Aphasia** (a disorder of speech and language that is caused by neurologic illness). The patient may be either unable to speak normally or unable to comprehend speech properly. Aphasia that is caused by disorders of speech and language should be differentiated from aphasia that is caused by psychiatric illness.

5. **Mood and affect.** The emotional state that the patient experiences internally is known as **mood,** and the outward expression of the patient's internal emotional state is known as **affect.**
   a. **Mood in relationship to affect.** The interviewer notes whether the patient's mood and affect are the same. For example, a patient who has a depressed mood is likely to appear sad and quiet and to speak softly and slowly. However, some depressed patients have an agitated and anxious affect. On the other hand, a schizophrenic individual may act silly or unconcerned while discussing a sad event such as the death of a loved one. This inappropriate division between affective feeling and thought content led to the use of the term "schizophrenia," which means "split mind," not "split personality."
   b. **Depth and range of emotional expression**
      (1) **Labile affect** describes sudden shifts in emotional state. The patient may laugh one minute and cry the next without a clear stimulus.
      (2) **Flat affect** describes a shallow and blunted emotional state. Facial expression and voice lack spontaneity.

6. **Perception.** The presence of a perceptual problem is noted in the mental status examination or in the history. Perceptual abnormalities involve the sensory nervous system and include the following:
   a. **Hallucinations** are false perceptions of a sensory stimulus. Any sensory modality can be involved.
      (1) **Auditory hallucinations** are seen in psychosis. The hallucinations involve voices, not just sounds, that criticize, comment, or command.
      (2) **Visual hallucinations** are often seen with organic psychosis, especially toxic or drug-related states.
      (3) **Gustatory (taste) and olfactory (smell) hallucinations** should alert the physician to a disorder of the temporal lobe.
      (4) **Tactile hallucinations** are also seen in organic states such as alcohol withdrawal or cocaine and amphetamine abuse. **Formication** is the tactile hallucination of insects crawling over the skin.
      (5) **Kinesthetic hallucinations** include feeling movement when none occurs. The "out-of-body" experiences described in near-death situations may be kinesthetic hallucinations. People usually describe this phenomenon as floating above their body and looking down on the scene.
      (6) **Hypnagogic hallucinations** (brief hallucinations of any type that occur while falling asleep) or **hypnopompic hallucinations** (brief hallucinations of any type that occur while awakening) occur in normal individuals and are not considered serious or pathologic.

b. **Illusions** are misinterpretations of an actual sensory stimulus. For example, a patient in the hospital may misperceive the movement of the bed curtain as a person and become frightened. Illusions occur in individuals with schizophrenia but are most common in delirium.

c. **Depersonalization and derealization** are alterations in an individual's perception of reality. With depersonalization, patients feel detached and view themselves as strange and unreal. Derealization involves a similar alteration in the patient's sense of reality of the outside world. Objects in the outside world may seem altered in size and shape, and people appear dead or mechanical.

7. **Thought process.** The pattern of a patient's speech allows the examiner to note the quality of the thought process, including its flow, logic, and associations. Abnormalities of the thinking process include the following:

a. **Loose associations.** This abnormality involves the shifting of ideas from one to another with no logical connection, accompanied by a lack of awareness on the part of the patient that these ideas are not connected. The patient's thoughts are difficult for the examiner to follow.

b. **Tangential thinking.** The patient wanders off the subject as new but related words are spoken. Usually it is possible to follow the patient's thoughts, but the patient often loses track of the interviewer's question.

c. **Circumstantiality.** As with tangential thinking, the patient loses the point of what he or she is saying but stays within the general topic area. Irrelevant details cause digressions in conversation. These digressions are mild if the patient is merely anxious, but they can be severe if he or she is delirious and distractible.

d. **Blocking.** This problem occurs when the thinking process stops altogether and the mind goes blank. It is found in individuals with acute anxiety and schizophrenia.

e. **Perseveration.** This repetition of the same words or phrases occurs despite the interviewer's direction to stop.

f. **Echolalia.** This problem is the direct repetition of the interviewer's words.

g. **Flight of ideas.** This process, which is seen in mania, is characterized by rapid speech with quick changes of ideas that may be associated in some way, such as by the sound of the words. It may also involve loose associations.

8. **Content of thought.** Disturbances in thought content include:

a. **Delusions** are fixed, false beliefs that are outside the patient's culture. For example, a belief that one's thoughts are being broadcast outside one's head is a delusion, but a belief in Santa Claus is not. Delusions may be paranoid (or persecutory), grandiose, nihilistic, somatic, or bizarre. **Delusions of reference** involve the belief that some person or object has special significance or power (e.g., a disc jockey is sending special commands to the patient).

   (1) Because delusions are fixed, false beliefs, they cannot be corrected by the physician. Contradiction of the patient's delusional belief may cause the patient to become angry and stop the interview.

   (2) The physician should not pretend to agree with the delusion but should take a neutral position and continue the examination.

b. **Obsessions** are persistent, intrusive thoughts, ideas, or impulses. The patient realizes that the ideas do not make sense and are not being imposed from outside (i.e., delusion). An example is a man who is always fighting an impulse to run down the hall of an office building through a plate glass window at the end. He knows that this action is potentially life threatening, and he does not want to hurt himself, but he cannot stop thinking about it and feeling anxious. Other common obsessions include fears of contamination and unrealistic fears about physical health, as seen in hypochondriasis (see Chapter 8).

c. Questions about **suicidal and homicidal thoughts** should be part of every mental status examination. It is important to exercise judgment and tact in discussing these issues. Assessment of **issues of safety** is one of the most important parts of the examination.

9. **Judgment.** By determining whether the patient understands the consequences of his or her actions, the clinician may assess the patient's social judgment. The physician may ask the patient a judgment question (e.g., "What would you do if you were stranded at Kennedy Airport with only $1.00 in your pocket?"). The examiner must recognize differences in cultural values when assessing judgment.

10. **Insight.** The physician should assess the patient's awareness of the problem, the cause of the problem, and what type of help is needed. Many people with serious mental illness such as bipolar disorder or schizophrenia lack insight and refuse necessary treatment.

11. **Cognition.** The mental status examination measures the ability of the brain to function. A formal mental status examination, a number of which are available, is necessary to adequately examine the patient's orientation, concentration, and memory. All mental status examinations are limited in scope compared with extensive neuropsychological tests, but the mini-mental state examination is a useful bedside clinical examination.

C Physical examination   Assessment of the general medical or neurologic condition of the patient is sometimes necessary. An examination should be conducted if there is concern that an undiagnosed medical illness is contributing to or causing psychiatric symptoms. The examiner should note the following:

1. General appearance

2. Vital signs

3. Neurologic status, including motor, sensory function, gait, coordination, muscle tone, and any involuntary movements

4. Skin, with attention to scars from self-injury or tattoos

5. Any other area that has been noted in the history of present illness. Examination of the head, neck, heart, lungs, abdomen, and extremities may be indicated.

D Clinical laboratory studies   The clinical laboratory is increasingly important in the diagnosis and treatment of psychiatric illness. The three functions of laboratory tests are screening for any underlying medical condition that might be causing the psychiatric symptoms, monitoring blood levels of psychotropic medications, and providing a baseline of biologic indicators as part of the diagnosis and treatment process. For example, obtaining an electrocardiogram (ECG) before giving tricyclic antidepressants (TCAs) may be appropriate.

1. **Screening tests for psychiatric illness caused by a general medical condition**
    a. **Nonselective studies**
        (1) Complete blood count (CBC)
        (2) Blood chemistry evaluation
            (a) Fasting blood glucose or hemoglobin A1c
            (b) Electrolyte levels, including calcium and phosphorus
            (c) Liver function tests
            (d) Renal function tests
        (3) Urinalysis and urine drug screen
        (4) Syphilis serology, lyme serology, and HIV test
        (5) ECG
        (6) Thyroid function tests
        (7) Chest radiograph
        (8) Vitamin B_{12} and folate levels
        (9) Lipid profile
        (10) Pregnancy test
    b. **Selective procedures** when clinically indicated (i.e., when results of routine laboratory studies are negative but a biologic cause is suspected)
        (1) Arterial blood gas analysis
        (2) Blood alcohol level
        (3) Monospot test for infectious mononucleosis
        (4) Lumbar puncture and examination of the cerebrospinal fluid (CSF)
        (5) Porphobilinogen and τ-aminolevulinic acid levels
        (6) Heavy metal screen
        (7) Antinuclear antibodies
        (8) Serum and urine copper levels

c. Electroencephalography (EEG)

   (1) The EEG is used to diagnose a variety of seizure disorders. The behavior associated with a temporal lobe seizure or partial complex seizure is sometimes difficult to distinguish from functional psychiatric disorders.

   (2) In delirium that is caused by metabolic problems, EEG results usually show high-voltage, slow-wave activity. These findings can be helpful in the differential diagnosis.

d. Neuroendocrine tests

   (1) Dexamethasone suppression test. Although the value of this test in diagnosing mental illness is limited, it can be used in a depressed patient to follow response to treatment. The patient is given 1 mg dexamethasone orally at 11:00 PM. Plasma cortisol levels are measured at 8:00 AM and 4:00 PM (rarely also at 11:00 PM). Dexamethasone ordinarily suppresses the patient's cortisol response. Plasma cortisol levels greater than 5 µg/dl are considered abnormal. Unfortunately, many conditions such as dehydration, alcohol abuse, hypertension, diabetes, and weight loss give a false-positive result. This test may help the patient accept diagnosis and treatment.

   (2) Thyrotropin-releasing hormone (TRH) stimulation test. Some depressed patients have a subclinical hypothyroid condition that causes depression. Other patients have lithium-induced hypothyroidism. The TRH stimulation test involves the intravenous injection of 500 µg TRH. Thyroid-stimulating hormone (TSH) is measured after 15, 30, and 90 minutes. Normally, plasma TSH levels increase sharply to 10 to 20 µg/ml above the baseline level. An increase of less than 7 µg/ml is considered suppressed. This finding may correlate with the diagnosis of depression or subclinical hypothyroidism.

e. Sleep studies: polysomnography. Several medical problems associated with psychiatric symptoms such as sleep apnea, seizure disorders, headaches, sexual dysfunction, and insomnia can be evaluated by the sleep laboratory. Patients with major depression also have abnormal sleep patterns. The sleep laboratory uses the EEG, ECG, and electromyogram (EMG) in addition to the penile tumescence plethysmograph, oxygen saturation, and movement-measuring devices. In depression, findings include:

   (1) Hyposomnia

   (2) Rapid eye movement (REM) latency, which is a shortened time between the onset of sleep and the onset of the first REM period (<65 minutes)

   (3) Greater proportion of REM sleep early in the night

2. Plasma levels of psychotropic drugs. The judgment of the clinician is the most important aspect of monitoring therapeutic efficiency of drugs. However, it is increasingly useful to monitor blood levels of certain psychotropic agents.

a. Lithium. Because of the potential toxicity of lithium at blood levels close to therapeutic levels, monitoring lithium levels is mandatory. Plasma samples should be drawn 10 to 12 hours after the last dose.

   (1) Therapeutic levels range from 0.6 to 1.5 mg/L.

   (2) Toxicity usually occurs at levels greater than 2.0 mg/L but may occur at lower levels.

b. Carbamazepine. A pretreatment CBC, reticulocyte count, and serum iron level should be performed. There is a small risk of agranulocytosis and aplastic anemia. During the first 3 months, weekly CBCs are indicated; thereafter, they can be performed monthly. Liver function tests are taken every 6 months.

c. Valproate. Serum levels may be useful in following treatment; 45 to 50 mg/ml is considered therapeutic. Liver function tests are performed every 6 to 12 months.

d. Cyclic antidepressants. Plasma levels of TCAs may be useful in adjusting dosages, assessing compliance, and minimizing toxic side effects.

   (1) Nortriptyline and amitriptyline have therapeutic windows (i.e., the therapeutic effect increases until an upper limit of the blood level is reached).

   (2) Imipramine and desipramine have a linear dose–response curve. Above certain levels, side effects outweigh therapeutic effects.

e. Neuroleptics. Therapeutic levels for antipsychotic medications are not as well established as those for antidepressants. Blood levels may be used to evaluate compliance or nonabsorption.

    f. Clozapine. Use of this antipsychotic agent requires a weekly white blood cell (WBC) count and differential for the first 6 months followed by every other week for an additional 6 months and then once a month until it is discontinued because of potential toxicity.

   3. Brain imaging for identifying biologic markers

[handwritten margin note: better for Calcification →]

    a. Computed tomography (CT). A CT scan can visualize lesions larger than 0.5 cm on cross-section. It also shows increased ventricle size associated with loss of brain cells. High ventricle:brain ratios (VBRs) are seen in patients with chronic schizophrenia and bipolar disorder.

[handwritten margin note: better for everything else →]

    b. Magnetic resonance imaging (MRI). MRI scanning is based on measuring radiofrequencies emitted by nuclei when a strong magnetic field is applied. Detailed anatomy can be seen. MRI shows white matter lesions that are not seen by CT scan such as those that occur with demyelinating diseases (e.g., multiple sclerosis [MS]). With the exception of calcification, MRI generally provides superior detail compared with CT; as a result, it has generally replaced CT scanning as an imaging technique. It should be noted that the closed tube in which the patient is placed while an MRI scan is being performed often precipitates a claustrophobic response.

    c. Functional magnetic resonance imaging (fMRI). Computer enhancement with fMRI allows the detection of different levels of oxygenated blood. Increased brain activity causes increased blood flow; therefore, the functional activity of the brain can be measured indirectly. No radioisotopes are used. fMRI has been used to study organization of language in the brain, including problems such as dyslexia.

    d. Single-photon emission computed tomography (SPECT). Single-photon–emitting radioisotopes such as xenon 133 or iodine 123 are used. Xenon is inhaled, the isotopes are distributed to areas of the brain by blood flow, and brain activity is measured indirectly by photon detectors around the head.

    e. Positron emission tomography (PET). A PET scan shows specific areas of brain activity. Organic compounds such as glucose are labeled by short-lived, positron-emitting elements of oxygen, carbon, and nitrogen. A cyclotron is required to produce the labeled glucose, which limits widespread use of this technique. The prepared compound can be localized in the brain, showing biochemical activity of specific brain areas. For example, decreased activity in the frontal cortex is seen in patients with schizophrenia. PET scans do not show detailed anatomy or lesions smaller than 0.5 cm.

E **Psychological tests** These tests provide a standardized objective measure of certain patient characteristics, such as intelligence and personality.

   1. Intelligence tests

    a. Most intelligence tests measure the **intelligence quotient (IQ),** which is arbitrarily defined as mental age divided by chronologic age multiplied by 100. An individual test score is compared with a standard or norm that is established by assigning the same tasks to a large group of people. These tests are influenced by culture and do not measure the entire intellectual capacity of the individual being tested. By definition, an average IQ is 100 (range, 90–110).

    b. The **Wechsler Adult Intelligence Scale (WAIS)** is the most widely used intelligence test for adults.

      (1) The WAIS has six verbal and five performance components, including information, comprehension, arithmetic, similarities, digit span, vocabulary, picture completion, block design, picture arrangement, object assembly, and digit symbol.

      (2) The WAIS generates a verbal IQ; a performance IQ; and a full-scale, or combined, IQ. A difference between the verbal and performance IQ scores of greater than 10 points suggests an organic brain syndrome.

   2. Personality tests

    a. Minnesota Multiphasic Personality Inventory (MMPI). The MMPI consists of 550 yes-or-no questions. The results are given as scores in 10 scales: hypochondriasis, paranoia, masculinity–femininity, psychopathy, depression, hysteria, psychasthenia, schizophrenia, hypomania, and social introversion. The pattern of scores is interpreted by comparing the patient's score and subscores against standardized data. Although the test is objective, a trained psychologist should interpret the results.

    b. Rorschach test. In this famous inkblot test, 10 standard ambiguous inkblots are shown to the patient in a predetermined order. The interviewer explores the patient's responses. This projective test shows the patient's thinking and association patterns.

    c. **Thematic apperception test (TAT).** This test is also projective and consists of 30 pictures, not all of which are shown. The psychologist chooses a specific picture, depending on the psychological area to be examined. For example, one picture shows a seated young woman looking up at an older man. The patient is asked to create a story about the picture. This process indirectly reveals the patient's fantasies, fears, and conflicts. The test is not useful in developing a descriptive diagnosis.

    d. **Sentence completion test.** This test is also used to elicit the patient's associations. It consists of a series of incomplete sentences that the patient is asked to complete (e.g., "I am afraid . . . ," "I feel guilty . . . ," "My mother is . . ."). The psychologist notes the themes and tone of the responses as well as any subject areas that the patient avoids.

    e. **Draw-a-person test.** This test was originally used only with children, but it can also be used with adults. The patient is asked to draw a picture of a person. Then the patient is asked to draw a person of the sex opposite from the person in the first drawing. This test assumes that the drawing represents to some degree the patient's view of him- or herself. The test can also be used to detect brain damage.

3. **Neuropsychological tests.** Specific aspects of brain function are tested by neuropsychological tests, which are usually given in a battery. Expertise is required to conduct these tests. Neuropsychological tests can detect subtle cognitive defects in patients who are not known to be demented and can assess strengths and weaknesses to aid in the rehabilitation of patients with brain damage.

    a. **The Halstead-Reitan Neuropsychological Test Battery** includes:

        (1) The **trail-making test,** in which the patient is asked to connect alternating numbers and letters. This test assesses the patient's visuomotor perception.

        (2) The **rhythm test,** in which the patient is asked to identify pairs of rhythmic beats. It assesses auditory perception, attention, and concentration.

        (3) Other subtests that allow the neuropsychologist to evaluate a variety of brain functions such as perception, sensation, concept formation, visuomotor integration, and abstract thought.

    b. The **Luria-Nebraska Neuropsychological Test Battery** and the **Bender-Gestalt Battery** are also used to diagnose brain damage.

III   CLASSIFICATION OF MENTAL DISORDERS

A   **Definitions**   Although the term **"mental disorder"** does not have a precise definition, the *Diagnostic and Statistical Manual of Mental Disorders,* 4th edition, text revision (*DSM-IV-TR*), defines it as a "clinically significant behavioral or psychological syndrome or pattern that occurs in an individual and that is associated with present distress or disability or with a significantly increased risk of suffering death, pain, disability, or an important loss of freedom." Historically, mental disorders were dealt with separately from physical disorders. This practice perpetuates the belief of mind–body dualism.

1. **Causes of mental illness** can be:
    a. Biologic
    b. Psychological
    c. Sociocultural–environmental

2. **Normal reactions to stressful events** such as the death of a loved one are not considered mental disorders.

3. **Socially unacceptable behavior** such as crime is not necessarily indicative of a mental disorder.

4. Few **diagnostic systems** consider mental disorders to involve both biologic and psychological factors, but this split impairs the development of a comprehensive, integrated understanding of mental disorders.

B   **Classification of mental disorders**   The *DSM-IV-TR* is based on empiric findings from literature reviews of data reanalysis and field trials. It uses a multiaxial assessment.

1. **Diagnostic axes**
    a. **Axis I: clinical syndromes.** These syndromes include organic mental disorders, schizophrenia, depression, substance abuse, and other conditions that may be a focus of clinical attention.

    b. Axis II: personality disorders and mental retardation. These disorders include prominent maladaptive personality features, defense mechanisms, and the diagnosis of mental retardation.

    c. Axis III: general medical disorders. These physical disorders are not necessarily causes of the psychiatric symptoms, but they are relevant to the treatment.

2. Other domains for assessment

    a. Axis IV: psychosocial and environmental problems. These problems include stresses that may affect the context in which the disorder developed. Generally, only psychosocial or environmental stresses that were present during the past year are listed. Stresses that occurred before the previous year are noted if they clearly contribute to the current disorder or treatment (i.e., history of trauma in a patient who is being treated for posttraumatic stress disorder [PTSD]). Common sources of stress include:

      (1) Change in marital status (e.g., engagement, marriage, separation)

      (2) Parenting stress (e.g., birth, illness of a child, problem with a child)

      (3) Interpersonal problems (e.g., disagreement with friends, dispute with neighbors)

      (4) Occupational problems (e.g., trouble at school or work, unemployment, retirement)

      (5) Change in living circumstances (e.g., moving)

      (6) Change in financial status, especially loss

      (7) Legal problems (e.g., arrest, lawsuit, trial)

      (8) Developmental milestones (e.g., puberty, menopause)

      (9) Physical illness or injury (when related to the development of an Axis I disorder, it is listed in Axis III)

      (10) Other stresses (e.g., natural disaster, rape, unwanted pregnancy, death of a close friend)

    b. Axis V: global assessment of functioning (GAF). The physician rates the patient's level of psychological, social, and occupational functioning at the time of the evaluation. The GAF may also be used to rate the highest level of functioning for at least a few months during the past year.

IV   PREVALENCE OF PSYCHIATRIC DISORDERS

The largest study of the prevalence of psychiatric disorders is the Epidemiologic Catchment Area (ECA) study. Fifteen diagnostic categories from the *Diagnostic and Statistical Manual of Mental Disorders,* 3rd edition, revised (*DSM-III-R*), were studied in five sites. More than 20,000 people—a cross-section of the general population—were involved.

A In any one year, a mental disorder or substance abuse disorder affects 28.1% of the American population older than 18 years of age (>52 million people). In comparison, nearly 50% of Americans have a respiratory illness, and more than 20% have a cardiovascular disease.

B Severe mental illness affects 2.8% of the American adult population, or approximately 5 million adults.

C Overall, the rates for men and women are approximately the same, but rates for men and women differ for specific disorders.

    1. Men have higher rates of substance abuse and antisocial personality disorder.

    2. Women have higher rates of depression, phobia, and dysthymic disorder.

D The **National Comorbidity Survey (NCS)** involved structured diagnostic interviews in more than 8,000 Americans.

    1. Of respondents 15 to 54 years of age, 48% reported at least one mental disorder some time during their life. Thirty percent of these individuals reported at least one mental disorder in the previous year; 10% experienced major depression, 7.2% alcohol dependence, 2.8% drug dependence, 2.3% panic disorder, and 0.3% schizophrenia.

    2. Fourteen percent of respondents reported three or more psychiatric disorders in their lifetime. This group reported 53.9% of all the lifetime disorders and 89.5% of the severe disorders in the past year.

3. Major depression was the most common disorder, with a lifetime incidence of 17.1%. It accounted for more "bed days"—people in bed and not at work—than any other disorder except for cardiovascular illness (National Institute of Mental Health [NIMH]). Alcohol dependence was associated with a lifetime history of 14.1%.

E Treatment

1. Only 42% of respondents with one or more disorders received any professional care. Only 26% received treatment in the mental health sector. Only one in 12 (8%) received treatment in substance abuse facilities.

2. Only 58.8% of respondents with three or more disorders (the most severely ill) received professional care. Of these patients, 41% received treatment in the mental health specialty sector and 14.8% received treatment in substance abuse facilities.

BIBLIOGRAPHY

American Psychiatric Association: *Diagnostic and Statistical Manual of Mental Disorders,* 4th ed., text revision. Washington, DC, American Psychiatric Association, 2000.

American Psychiatric Association: *Practice Guidelines for Psychiatric Evaluation of Adults.* Washington, DC, American Psychiatric Association, 2006.

Gaw A: *Culture, Ethnicity and Mental Illness.* Washington, DC, American Psychiatric Press, 1993.

Hales RE, Yudofsky SC, Talbott JA: *Textbook of Psychiatry,* 2nd ed. Washington, DC, American Psychiatric Press, 1994.

Kessler R, McGonagle KA, Zhao S, et al: Lifetime and 12-month prevalence of DSM-III-R psychiatric disorders in the United States: Results from the National Comorbidity Survey. *Arch Gen Psychiatry* 5:8–19, 1994.

Regier DA, Narrow WE, Rae DS, et al: The de facto US mental and addictive disorder service system: Epidemiologic catchment area prospective 1-year prevalence rates of disorders and services. *Arch Gen Psychiatry* 50:85–94, 1993.

Stoudemire A, Fogel BS: *Psychiatric Care of the Medical Patient.* New York, Oxford Press, 1993.

Winokur G, Clayton PJ: *The Medical Basis of Psychiatry,* 2nd ed. Philadelphia, WB Saunders, 1994.

Study Questions

Directions: *Each of the numbered questions is followed by answers. Select the ONE lettered answer that is BEST in each case.*

1. A 35-year-old lawyer has been evaluated in the emergency department for cardiac disease after an episode of palpitation and tightening of the chest. His medical condition is entirely normal, but he remains anxious. A psychiatric evaluation is considered. Special skills are required of the physician who conducts the examination for which of the following reasons?

- A The patient may be embarrassed about disclosing emotional problems.
- B The patient may threaten a lawsuit if psychiatric questions are asked.
- C A male patient is generally unwilling to discuss psychological issues.
- D The patient may still have cardiac disease that should be ruled out before a psychiatric evaluation is performed.
- E The patient will deny any psychiatric problems if he thinks he has heart disease.

2. A 38-year-old man is evaluated for psychiatric illness after being held hostage in a bank robbery in which he was a customer. He feels too upset to return to work, and he is on paid leave from his job. His request to remain on leave is an example of which of the following?

- A Counterphobic reaction
- B Malingering
- C Perceptual distortion
- D Psychotic distortion
- E Secondary gain

3. During psychiatric evaluation of a 19-year-old college student who has attempted suicide by overdose, the examiner asks the question: "Did you take the pills before or after you talked to your boyfriend?" This is an example of which of the following kinds of interview techniques?

- A Clarification
- B Confrontation
- C Facilitation
- D Open-ended question
- E Summarization

4. A 27-year-old man admits that he has persistent thoughts of curse words while attending church. Although he does not want to have the thoughts and is bothered by them, he cannot seem to stop them. He does not act on saying them aloud. Which of the following is the best description of this type of thinking?

- A Delusional
- B Derealization
- C Obsessional
- D Perseveration — verbal
- E Referential

5. A young woman with schizophrenia is undergoing a psychiatric evaluation. The physician asks her why she has missed her last two appointments. The woman says that she does not want to be put in the hospital again and that the clinic reminds her of the hospital. Which of the following areas of the mental status examination best describes the problem?

- A Association
- B Cognition
- C Delusion
- D Insight
- E Judgment

6. The dexamethasone suppression test is not used extensively in general psychiatric evaluations for which of the following reasons?

- A It is too expensive.
- B Its side effects include adrenal suppression.
- C It is contraindicated in pregnancy.
- D It has too many false-positive results.
- E It is associated with increased suicide.

7. A 40-year-old man with a history of chronic undifferentiated schizophrenia for more than 20 years is being evaluated. No medications have yet proved successful, and the man remains chronically psychotic. The best brain imaging method to demonstrate decreased activity in his frontal cortex is which of the following?

- A Computed tomography (CT) — *structure*
- B Magnetic resonance imaging (MRI) — *structure*
- C Positron emission tomography (PET) — *fxn*
- D Single-photon emission computed tomography (SPECT)

8. A 65-year-old woman is evaluated a few days after the death of her husband from a heart attack. She cries easily and says that she has difficulty sleeping, has trouble concentrating, and is not sure if life is worth living. Her condition is best described by which of the following?

- A Adjustment disorder
- B Major depression
- C Minor depression
- D Normal reaction to stress
- E Posttraumatic stress disorder (PTSD)

Directions: *Each set of matching questions in this section consists of a list of four to 26 lettered options (some of which may be in figures) followed by several numbered items. For each numbered item, select the ONE lettered option that is most closely associated with it. Each lettered option may be selected once, more than once, or not at all.*

QUESTIONS 9–11

Select the perceptual problem that most likely applies to each patient.

- A Depersonalization
- B Derealization
- C Formication
- D Illusion
- E Olfactory hallucination

9. A 44-year-old chronic cocaine abuser is treated for self-inflicted skin excoriations; the patient feels that there are "bugs crawling all over me." He has scratched himself repeatedly in the past. He appears confused and admits to using cocaine that day. *Formication (C)*

10. A 29-year-old woman who is being treated for anxiety describes an episode at work in which everyone appeared to be mechanical and unfeeling. At times like this, she becomes frightened and thinks she is going insane. She has had this experience before, and it always passes after a few minutes.

Derealization (B)

11. A 60-year-old man in the coronary care unit becomes agitated because he believes the orderly mopping the floor is going to attack him with a club. The patient has been unstable medically, and his Po_2 is below normal. *Illusion (D) → he is delirious*

QUESTIONS 12–15

Select the impairment in thought process that most likely applies to each patient.

[A] Blocking
[B] Circumstantiality
[C] Echolalia
[D] Flight of ideas
[E] Loose associations
[F] Perseveration
[G] Tangential thinking

12. A 50-year-old woman is asked during a psychiatric examination if she had ever been a patient in a psychiatric hospital. She responds, "That was the summer we were at the beach; it rained for 2 weeks. I was sad, but my sister Sarah did not help. She and I have never really gotten along."

Circumstantiality (B).

13. A 22-year-old man is brought to the emergency department for evaluation. He appears confused but gives his name. When asked his occupation, he says, "Jesus was a carpenter. I am the right hand of God. I don't offend anyone." *Loose Associations (E)*

14. A 30-year-old man who is being treated for bipolar illness has discontinued his medications for several months. He is brought to the clinic in an agitated state. When asked how he is feeling, he replies, "I am wonderful, the most wonderful in the universe. The universal gym is my invention, but Jim is just Dandy." *Flight of Ideas (D)*

15. A 29-year-old woman with chronic schizophrenia rocks in her chair and does not seem to respond to an examiner's questions except to say, "No hope, no hope, no hope."

Perseveration (F)

QUESTIONS 16–18

Select the Diagnostic and Statistical Manual of Mental Disorders, 4th edition, text revision (DSM-IV-TR), axis that is used to assess the situation described.

[A] Axis I
[B] Axis II
[C] Axis III
[D] Axis IV
[E] Axis V

16. A 32-year-old woman who has been treated for recurrent depression for 1 year has responded well to interpersonal psychotherapy and antidepressant medication. She tells her physician that her husband has just told her that he has been having an affair and wants a divorce.

Axis IV : psychosocial/environmental problems

17. A 58-year-old man is being treated for both recurrent depression and alcohol abuse. He has done well in treatment for both disorders, with an occasional slip in his drinking, and he has been sober for more than 1 year. He has just been told he has a liver mass that may be cancerous and is very upset.

Axis III : health

18. A 24-year-old man suffers a severe head injury from a motorcycle accident. After awakening from a coma, he seems to be a different person, with poor social skills, gross and disgusting behavior, and foul language. *Axis I : physical causes of mental disorders*

Answers and Explanations

1. The answer is A [*I A 2 a*]. Sensitivity is required in conducting a psychiatric evaluation because many people (not just men) find it difficult to discuss emotional issues. Malpractice suits may arise from failure to perform the appropriate examination when indicated. The examination should not be delayed until all other illnesses have been ruled out.

2. The answer is E [*I C 6*]. Secondary gain is any benefit that the patient derives from the current problem such as paid leave from work. The man may have an anxiety disorder such as posttraumatic stress disorder (PTSD), and he may not be faking or malingering. Perceptual and psychotic distortions have not been discussed. A counterphobic reaction would involve confronting the fear rather than avoiding it.

3. The answer is A [*II A 3 b (4)*]. Clarification statements may be similar to summary statements but also may include connections that the patient may not recognize (i.e., the relationship between the suicidal gesture and the phone call). The question, which is direct rather than open ended, does not need to be confrontational in tone.

4. The answer is C [*II B 8 b*]. The curse words are persistent and intrusive thoughts, which makes them obsessions. The patient is aware that the ideas make no sense, so the patient is not delusional. The ideas may be repetitive, but the patient does not perseverate in saying them.

5. The answer is D [*II B 10*]. The young woman shows a lack of insight into her illness, which can lead to a refusal of needed treatment. Although poor judgment may result, the problem is primarily caused by a lack of insight.

6. The answer is D [*II D 1 d (1)*]. The dexamethasone suppression test shows a lack of suppression of plasma cortisol levels not only in patients with depression but also in those with other conditions such as dehydration, alcohol abuse, and weight loss. This lack of specificity is the major reason why it is not widely used; it is not expensive, and it does not have any serious side effects.

7. The answer is C [*II D 3 e*]. Positron emission tomography (PET) shows specific areas of brain activity better than other scanning techniques. PET is more expensive than single-photon emission computed tomography (SPECT), which has limited its use. Computed tomography (CT) and magnetic resonance imaging (MRI) are used to visualize brain structure rather than function.

8. The answer is D [*III A 2*]. The death of a spouse is a highly stressful event, and strong responses do not constitute mental illness. There is a wide range of "normal" reactions to death of a spouse, and cultural influences may also be important.

9. The answer is C [*II B 6 a (4)*]. Tactile hallucinations are seen in organic states such as cocaine abuse. Formication is the hallucination of insects crawling over the skin.

10. The answer is B [*II B 6 c*]. The patient describes derealization. Derealization involves an alteration in the sense of reality of the outside world. Objects may seem altered in size and shape, and people may appear dead or mechanical.

11. The answer is D [*II B 6 b*]. Patients in coronary care units are susceptible to delirious states. Illusions are common in delirium. The patient misperceived an actual sensory stimulus (i.e., the mop in the hands of the orderly) as a weapon.

12. The answer is B [*II B 7 c*]. The patient has not responded to the question but is in the general topic area. The irrelevant details represent digressions.

13. The answer is E [*II B 7 a*]. Loose associations are difficult to follow. There is no logical connection between patient statements, and the patient does not appear to be aware that the ideas are not connected.

14. The answer is D [*II B 7 g*]. This man, who is in a manic state, exhibits flight of ideas, which is seen in mania. In this case, this thought process involves rapid changes of ideas that are associated by the sound of the words.

15. The answer is F [*II B 7 e*]. The repetition of the same words or phrases despite the interviewer's direction to stop is perseveration.

16. The answer is D [*III B 2 a*]. Axis IV is the domain of psychosocial and environmental problems, including interpersonal problems and change in marital status. These stresses may affect another axis such as the one that represents the disorder for which the patient is being treated.

17. The answer is C [*III B 1 c*]. The knowledge that the liver mass may be cancerous is likely to influence the man's treatment for depression. However, the tumor may also be a consequence of the alcohol abuse.

18. The answer is A [*III B 1 a*]. Although this may appear to be a personality disorder (Axis II), the disorder is a newly acquired clinical syndrome caused by brain injury. Physical causes of mental disorders are listed on Axis I.

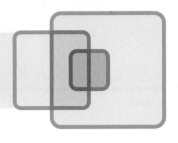

chapter 2

Psychotic Disorders

ROBERT BREEN

I INTRODUCTION

Psychosis may be defined as a loss of contact with reality and most often manifests itself as delusional thinking or hallucinations. Recent research suggests that there may be more similarities than differences between psychotic processes in different psychiatric disorders.

A **Schizophrenia,** the most costly psychotic disorder, is characterized by derangement of thought processes, affect, and behavior. The disorder involves expression of positive and negative symptoms and cognitive dysfunction.

1. **Positive symptoms** are those that are added to the presentation such as **delusions, hallucinations, catatonia,** and **agitation.**

2. **Negative symptoms** are patient characteristics that appear missing from the presentation. This may involve **affective flattening, apathy, social withdrawal, anhedonia,** and **poverty of thought** and **content of speech.**

B **Established biologic markers or pathognomonic clinical features that define schizophrenia do not exist.**

1. The *Diagnostic and Statistical Manual of Mental Disorders,* 4th edition, text revision (*DSM-IV-TR*), has been edited so that elements from previous diagnostic systems and from studies of the frequency of symptoms in different populations form the current diagnostic criteria for schizophrenia.

   a. The **diagnostic criteria** of the *DSM-IV-TR* represent a departure from trends established by the *Diagnostic and Statistical Manual of Mental Disorders,* third edition (*DSM-III*), and the *Diagnostic and Statistical Manual of Mental Disorders,* third edition, revision (*DSM-III-R*), in that they are **less specific concerning symptoms** of schizophrenia and oriented more toward the course of the disorder (Tables 2–1 and 2–2). Current criteria for the diagnosis of schizophrenia require that some symptoms be present for at least 6 months, with significant disturbance for at least 1 month of that time. The actual course varies widely among individuals.

   b. The newer criteria are **more inclusive.**

2. The **International Pilot Study of Schizophrenia,** a World Health Organization study, attempted to discover reliable methods of diagnosing schizophrenia across different cultures and national boundaries.

   a. Using psychiatric interviews and the Present State Examination (PSE), researchers noted the **most common symptoms** (Table 2–3). However, these frequently occurring symptoms are also common in other conditions such as organic mental disorders and mood disorders.

   b. This diagnostic approach is of limited use with individual patients because it does not propose minimal or threshold criteria for the diagnosis in individual cases. Rather, it has been a basis for other diagnostic systems such as the *DSM-III-R* and, to a lesser extent, the *DSM-IV.*

C Even in research studies of schizophrenia, when rigorous diagnostic criteria are applied, the prognosis is highly variable.

TABLE 2-1 *DSM-IV-TR* Diagnostic Criteria for Schizophrenia

A. Two of the following for most of 1 month:
  1. Delusions
  2. Hallucinations
  3. Disorganized speech
  4. Grossly disorganized or catatonic behavior
  5. Negative symptoms
  (Note: Only one of these is required if delusions are bizarre or if hallucinations consist of a voice keeping up a running commentary on the person's behavior or thoughts or if there are two or more voices conversing with each other.)
B. Marked social or occupational dysfunction
C. Duration of at least 6 months of persistent symptoms such as attenuated forms of group A symptoms (above) or negative symptoms. At least 1 month of this must include a group A symptom.
D. Symptoms of schizoaffective and mood disorder are ruled out.
E. Substance abuse and medical conditions are ruled out as etiologic.

[handwritten: ✳ no mood Δ's]

Reprinted with permission from the Diagnostic and Statistical Manual of Mental Disorders, Fourth Edition, Text Revision, (Copyright 2000). American Psychiatric Association.

II   **EPIDEMIOLOGY**

It is difficult to draw precise conclusions concerning the epidemiology of schizophrenia. Studies have often conflicted because of difficulty in defining diagnostic criteria, difficulty in sampling methods for such a disabling psychotic illness, and differences in expression and prognosis across different cultures.

TABLE 2-2 Schizophrenia Subtypes

In all of the following subtypes of schizophrenia, the diagnostic criteria for schizophrenia must be met first, particularly criterion A symptoms:

Paranoid Type

[handwritten: speech/behavior/affect okay →]

A. Preoccupation with one or more delusions or frequent auditory hallucinations
B. Does not have prominent disorganized speech, disorganized behavior, flat or inappropriate affect, or catatonic behavior

Disorganized Type

[handwritten: opposite ↘]

A. All of the following are prominent:
  1. Disorganized speech
  2. Disorganized behavior
  3. Flat or inappropriate affect
B. Does not meet criteria for catatonic type

Catatonic Type
The clinical picture is dominated by at least two of the following:
A. Motoric immobility as evidenced by catalepsy or stupor
B. Excessive motor activity (apparently purposeless and not influenced by external stimuli)
C. Extreme negativism or mutism
D. Peculiarities of voluntary movement such as posturing, stereotyped movements, prominent mannerisms, or prominent grimacing
E. Echolalia or echopraxia

Undifferentiated Type
Symptoms of schizophrenia criterion A are present, but the criteria are not met for paranoid, catatonic, or disorganized types.

Residual Type
A. Criterion A for schizophrenia is no longer met and criteria for other subtypes of schizophrenia are not met.
B. Evidence of the disturbance (evidenced by negative symptoms or two or more criterion A symptoms) is present in an attenuated form.

Reprinted with permission from the Diagnostic and Statistical Manual of Mental Disorders, Fourth Edition, Text Revision, (Copyright 2000). American Psychiatric Association.

TABLE 2–3 Symptoms of Schizophrenia

Most Frequently Found Symptoms*	Highest Reliability of Symptoms	Lowest Reliability of Symptoms
Lack of insight	Suicidal ideation	Negativism
Auditory hallucinations	Elated thoughts	Perseveration
Verbal hallucinations	Ideas of reference	Stereotyped behavior (e.g., lip
Ideas of reference	Delusions of grandeur	smacking, chewing)
Suspiciousness	Hearing thoughts aloud	
Flatness of affect	Derealization	
Voices speaking to the patient	Lack of concentration	
Delusional mood	Hopelessness	
Delusions of persecution	Delusions of persecution and reference	
Inadequate description of problems		
Thought alienation		
Thoughts spoken aloud		

*In descending order.

A **Incidence, prevalence, and cost**

1. **Incidence.** Reported values range between 0.11 and 0.70 per 1,000. The most recent studies indicate that the incidence of schizophrenia may have declined during the past 10 to 20 years. Problems with sampling and changes in diagnostic criteria may account for the decreased incidence.

2. **Prevalence.** As with the incidence of schizophrenia, developing countries generally have lower prevalence rates of schizophrenia, which reflects lower incidence rates and better prognostic expectations than in the industrialized world (e.g., schizophrenic patients in developing countries tend to recover from their illness at a higher rate than do schizophrenic patients in industrialized nations).

    a. **Point prevalence** (i.e., the number of cases at one moment in time) has been widely estimated to range between 0.6 and 8.3.

    b. **Lifetime prevalence** in the United States was estimated to be 1.1% in the Epidemiologic Catchment Area (ECA) study.

3. **Cost.** In the United States, the most recent cost estimate for schizophrenia is $63 billion annually.

B **Gender** Schizophrenia occurs in men and women at approximately equal rates; however, men tend to develop the disease earlier than do women. In developing countries, men appear to suffer from schizophrenia at a rate that may be several times that of women. Perhaps because of the difference in age of onset, whereas men with schizophrenia tend never to have been married, affected women tend to be divorced or separated.

C **Role of socioeconomic status** The prevalence and incidence of schizophrenia as well as disease course correlate with socioeconomic status.

1. **In the United States,** the highest rates are found in the **lower socioeconomic classes,** suggesting that either socioeconomic factors produce or precipitate schizophrenia or that schizophrenic patients tend to drift downward in socioeconomic status (i.e., **drift hypothesis**). According to the ECA studies, the risk of schizophrenia in people in the lowest socioeconomic quartile was eight times higher than in individuals in the highest quartile.

2. **In cities with populations of more than 100,000,** the incidence increases in proportion to the size of the city, although this relationship does not hold true in rural areas and smaller cities.

3. **Migration status increases the incidence** of schizophrenia, possibly accounting for some of the difference in rates between cities and rural settings.

III ETIOLOGY

Just as Eugen Bleuler felt the need to refer to the "group of schizophrenias," we must think in terms of the "etiologies" of schizophrenia. The etiology of schizophrenia is complex and yet undetermined. No one set of theories can account for the complicated onset and far-ranging symptoms of schizophrenia. Schizophrenia transmission in families does not fit any known pattern of pure genetic transmission, and current theories suggest a pattern that may be activated through as yet unknown biologic, social, and psychological factors. Proposed etiologies include the following:

A Genetic theories Genetic factors clearly play a role, but the actual manner of genetic transmission of schizophrenia is complicated. Various psychotic disorders, not just schizophrenia, are more common in families of persons with schizophrenia. (This association is also valid for adopted relatives.) Recent evidence suggests that genetic mutations are more prevalent in persons with schizophrenia

1. **Familial transmission.** Some studies show high rates of mental illness in relatives of patients with schizophrenia (not necessarily schizophrenia). Alternatively, positive traits such as creativity are found in some cases. The risk of disease in first-degree relatives of individuals with the illness is about 10%.
    a. **Twins**
        (1) A simple single gene transmission of schizophrenia is no longer plausible. Findings indicate that monozygotic twins have a 40% to 65% risk of developing schizophrenia, despite having identical genotypes.
        (2) According to one study, when monozygotic twins are raised together they have a concordance rate of 91%, but monozygotic twins raised apart have a concordance rate of 78%. Other studies of twins reveal a concordance rate of 40% to 50% for monozygotic twins and about 10% to 14% for dizygotic twins.
    b. **Parents.** If both parents are schizophrenic, a child's risk of developing schizophrenia ranges between 15% and 55%. Single gene transmission with variable penetrance is suggested by findings of increased risk in families with more than one schizophrenic member. The risk is 17% in persons with one sibling and one parent with schizophrenia and 47% in those with two parents with schizophrenia.

2. **Other genetic associations. Polygenic transmission** more easily accounts for some of the discord in genetic studies; it is consistent with the differences in severity of the disease and the variable rates of pathology in some families. To prove a polygenic basis of transmission will likely take more progress in efforts to map the entire human genome.
    a. **Schizotypal personality disorder** is more common in relatives of persons with schizophrenia. (This association is also valid for adopted relatives.)
    b. **Defects in smooth pursuit eye movements** have also been associated with some familial patterns of transmission. Although the association cannot explain all of the smooth pursuit ocular motor dysfunction in schizophrenia, it has proved useful in studies of the genetic transmission of schizophrenia.

B Developmental theories Rigorous research studies in the latter half of the twentieth century have suggested that developmental factors play a major role in the etiology of schizophrenia.

1. **Fetal exposure to risk factors**
    a. **Season of birth** appears to be correlated with the risk of developing schizophrenia. In both the Northern and Southern hemispheres, the risk for developing schizophrenia is greatest for individuals born in the late winter and early spring. **Prenatal exposure to a virus** such as influenza is implicated.
    b. **Prenatal malnutrition** has also been suggested. There was an increase in the risk of developing schizophrenia for persons born after the Dutch hardship winter (1945–1946) during World War II, when food was scarce in the Netherlands. This effect has also been demonstrated following the 1959–1961 famine in China. Low birth weight is also associated with an increased risk of developing schizophrenia.

2. **Obstetric complications. Fetal hypoxia** is known to cause such neurologic conditions as cerebral palsy and mental retardation. Up to a ninefold increase in risk of schizophrenia is associated

with preeclampsia. However, schizophrenia is much less common than obstetric complications, so fetal hypoxia is not the sole etiologic factor.

C **Psychological theories**

1. **Psychological testing** is clearly abnormal in persons with schizophrenia and also in some of their relatives without expression of the disease. Biologic differences more readily explain such testing abnormalities. Psychological testing does show:
   a. **Lack of creativity and imagination** on the Thematic Apperception Test and the Rorschach test in persons with schizophrenia. Test results indicate preservation of verbal intelligence but not performance intelligence quotient (IQ) on the Wechsler Adult Intelligence Scale (WAIS).
   b. **Attention deficits,** which are common on testing in both persons with schizophrenia and some of their relatives.
   c. **Loss of executive function,** which makes it difficult for persons with schizophrenia to make choices and decisions about simple things such as what to wear and when to eat. Clinical loss of executive function may be a factor in the development of negative symptoms.

2. At one time, theories involving **family interaction** were a credible etiologic basis for schizophrenia, but the rapidly increasing mass of biologic data concerning the development of schizophrenia has negated these hypotheses.
   a. The theory that the illness was caused by mistakes in mothering by a so-called **"schizophrenogenic mother"** has been discredited.
   b. **Double-bind communications** are no longer thought to play an etiologic role in schizophrenia. Double-bind communication has the following characteristics:
      (1) An **intense relationship** between those involved
      (2) Two messages expressed on different levels that **conflict with or deny each other**
      (3) A child who is forbidden from commenting on or clarifying messages, which results in frequent "no-win" situations in which the child cannot avoid conflict no matter the response
   c. **"Expressed emotions,"** with a high level of affect with criticism and overinvolvement, were once thought to cause schizophrenia. More recent research indicates that this style of communication does occur in some families but that it is more likely to cause later exacerbations of schizophrenia, not the first episode. Family education projects that attempt to change this style and make it more noncritical have had positive effects on outcome.

3. **Cultural causes** of schizophrenia have been investigated to explain differences in incidence between industrialized and rural areas. However, economic factors that affect access to nutrition, sanitation, and health care are more likely to account for any cultural differences.

D **Biologic mechanisms**   Modern scientific study has attempted to explain schizophrenia through chemical or biologic mechanisms. No one abnormality appears to account for the spectrum of symptoms in schizophrenia. Most likely, abnormal cell development or cell damage in multiple regions of the brain mediated by multiple chemical messenger systems cause the disease.

1. **Neurotransmitter system abnormalities**
   a. **Dopamine.** One of the oldest theories of the etiology of schizophrenia is that dopamine and dopaminergic neurons are the primary systems involved in the pathophysiology of schizophrenia.

      antipsychotics block DA receptors

      (1) Dopamine receptors, particularly D-2 receptors, are found in abnormal numbers in the brains of persons with schizophrenia. D-2 receptor blockade is the sine qua non of the antipsychotic effects of typical antipsychotics.

      +Sx ⇒ ↑DA in limbic

      (2) **Positron emission tomography** (PET) scans indicate increased activity of dopaminergic neurons in the limbic system, which is strongly correlated with hallucinations and other positive symptoms of schizophrenia.

      −Sx ⇒ ↓DA in frontal

      (3) PET scans also indicate decreased activity of dopaminergic neurons in the frontal lobes and prefrontal cortex, which is correlated with the negative symptoms of schizophrenia.
   b. **Serotonin.** Investigation into serotoninergic systems has been one of the most active areas of schizophrenia research and drug development from 1970 to 2000.

      ↑ Serotonin

      (1) Early investigation of some psychotomimetic compounds showed high levels of activity in serotoninergic systems of the brain.

(2) Serotoninergic neurons are known to project from the midbrain into the prefrontal cortex and frontal lobes and a variety of other brain regions that may inhibit the function of dopaminergic neurons.

(3) Abnormal levels of serotonin and its metabolite 5-hydroxyindoleacetic acid have been found in the cerebrospinal fluid (CSF) of persons with schizophrenia (and also in those who have committed suicide).

  c. **Glutamate.** An exciting new area of research into the biologic dysfunction of schizophrenia is centered on the neurotransmitter glutamate.

(1) Glutamate levels are reduced in the CSF of persons with schizophrenia. In addition, glutamate receptor antagonists such as phencyclidine can cause schizophrenia-like psychotic symptoms in normal research subjects.

(2) In vivo testing using magnetic resonance imaging (MRI) spectroscopy and postmortem pathologic studies have both demonstrated signs of decreased glutamate activity in the pyramidal neurons of the prefrontal cortex.

(3) Glutaminergic neurons interact with both serotonergic and dopaminergic systems.

(4) Glutaminergic neurotransmission is most likely linked to the cognitive deficits in schizophrenia.

  d. **γ-Aminobutyric acid (GABA).** Scientists also believe that GABA, a fast-acting neurotransmitter in the brain that plays a critical role in the expression of anxiety disorders, plays an inhibitory role with dopaminergic neurons. In this way, GABA may be responsible for terminating or controlling the activity within dopamine systems.

(1) Low levels of GABA are found early in the course of schizophrenia.

(2) Benzodiazepines, which work in part as GABA agonists, can relieve some symptoms of schizophrenia in some patients.

(3) Baclofen, a GABA receptor antagonist, can exacerbate schizophrenia.

2. **Structural abnormalities.** More than 100 years of scientific research have revealed a wide range of structural abnormalities in the brains of persons with schizophrenia. Unfortunately, such studies have tended to be small, sometimes lacking rigorous controls.

  a. **Enlargement of the lateral ventricles** is the most consistent finding. With loss of brain mass through developmental failure or neuron death, the CSF would expand to fill the space.

  b. Loss of brain gray matter appears to start in the parietal area and spreads to much of the brain as the disease progresses. It is hoped that early treatment may arrest or reverse some of this loss.

  c. **Abnormalities in the cell architecture** in the **prefrontal cortex** have been reported. This condition may impair the effective transmission of neuronal impulses from the limbic system as well as from higher-order association areas in the parietal and temporal regions.

3. **Functional abnormalities.** The development of **PET and MRI spectroscopy** allows viewing of the functioning brains of persons with schizophrenia with little risk of harm to the subjects.

  a. An **increase in activity in the limbic system** is closely correlated with the **positive symptoms** of schizophrenia. Administration of either a **typical** or a **first- or second-generation antipsychotic** can reverse this overactivity.

  b. **A decrease in activity in the frontal lobes** of persons with schizophrenia is closely correlated with the **negative symptoms** of schizophrenia. Administration of **a second-generation antipsychotic** can sometimes reverse this hypoactive state.

4. **Other abnormalities**

  a. Recent studies have found **abnormal levels of phospholipids** in some cell membranes of schizophrenia patients. Abnormal cell membrane function would disable normal neurotransmitter function.

  b. **G proteins,** another cell membrane constituent, may play a role in schizophrenia. G proteins have a key function: they relay messages from neurotransmitter receptors in the membrane to second messenger systems within the neuron. Activation of these second messenger systems can influence multiple intracellular processes, including genetic transcription within the nucleus.

IV CHARACTERISTIC FEATURES

Clinical expression of schizophrenia varies according to diagnostic criteria used to define the population and, to some extent, the etiologic models of the clinician or researcher. In general, features of schizophrenia reported by patients (e.g., hallucinations) tend to be more reliable than those observed by clinicians (e.g., poverty of thought content). Symptoms usually include disruptions in areas of psychological and social functioning. However, even in cases of severe disruption, some areas of functioning may be preserved (e.g., a hospitalized patient with chronic schizophrenia who exhibits bizarre behavior and severe disruptions of speech and thinking may retain the skills of a concert pianist). Symptoms of schizophrenia may change and become less severe over the course of the illness.

A **Form of thought** refers to the structure of thought as experienced by patients and displayed through verbal communication. Disturbances in the form of thought are defined as a **formal thought disorder,** which may manifest in the following ways:

1. **Loosening of associations** is observed in speech when connections among the patient's ideas are absent or obscure. Listeners may feel as if understanding of the patient's thought had been suddenly lost. (In contrast, in the tangentiality and flight of ideas typical of mania and anxiety disorders, patients may express coherent ideas but lose the point of a string of ideas.) Examples of loosening of associations are listed below.
   a. **Word use may be highly idiosyncratic and individualized.** Words may be created (**neologism**) or selected by patients using their own internal logic and special symbolism.
   b. **Abnormal concept formation is a perceptual defect** in which patients are unable to exclude irrelevant or competing ideas from their consciousness; their thinking becomes overinclusive. Extraneous items and details that have specific meaning to patients are incorporated into the patients' communication but are difficult for listeners to follow.
   c. **Logic in schizophrenia may follow a primitive pattern.** Illogical reasoning, exclusion of important information from the reasoning process, and frank distortion of logical connections occur in schizophrenic patients. Patients assume the existence of causal connections when others perceive no such connections. Patients may treat symbols as if they were actual objects or may inappropriately substitute them for other logical elements.
   d. **Concreteness may substitute for abstraction.** In general, patients with early-onset schizophrenia may experience greater deterioration of abstraction ability than patients with late-onset disease, as measured by psychological tests. Simultaneous preoccupation with symbols and abstractions, as well as the loss of the ability to process these, are features commonly seen among schizophrenic patients.
      (1) The ability to form abstract ideas may be severely impaired.
      (2) The ability to discern abstractions within ideas may become limited, and concrete interpretations of abstract ideas may become predominant.
      (3) The ability to understand metaphors and similes may be lost.
   e. **Language structural problems** are seen in individuals with schizophrenia, but many of these problems are rare. However, unusual, stilted language is common. Examples include:
      (1) **Neologisms**
      (2) **Verbigeration** (the persistent repetition of words or phrases)
      (3) **Echolalia** (a repetition of the words or phrases of the examiner, which is seen in severely disorganized psychotic states)
      (4) **Mutism** (a functional inhibition of speech and vocalization, which is seen in a variety of nonpsychotic and psychotic illnesses)
      (5) **"Word salad"** (a complete lack of language, which is seen in patients with psychosis and several very specific central nervous system [CNS] lesions)
2. **Poverty of content and speech** is seen in several of the schizophrenic spectrum disorders. Speech may be complex, concrete, or limited in overall productivity, but it generally lacks specific information content.
3. **Thought blocking** is an internal interruption in patients' speech and flow of thought. It may appear that a hallucination may interrupt patients, although they may not be able to identify the interruption.

B **Content of thought** refers to the most characteristic feature of schizophrenia, **delusions,** which are defined as fixed, false beliefs. Delusions cannot be changed by reasoning and are inconsistent with the beliefs of the patients' cultural group. However, they may have a culturally based content (e.g., Americans who believe that they are the targets of influence by the Central Intelligence Agency). In some cases, delusions may be so individualistic that no cultural connections can be made.

Delusions may be relatively circumscribed or may pervade all aspects of patients' life and thinking. In some cases, delusions may appear relatively trivial to patients, but more commonly, they become an organizing force in patients' lives. Delusions may be simple in their organization or highly complex and systematized. Sexual, religious, and philosophical content of delusions are common.

1. **Delusions of persecution** are beliefs that others are trying to harm, spy on, influence, or humiliate patients or interfere with their affairs. Persecutory delusions are frequently pervasive and actively incorporate features of patients' lives.

2. **Delusions of reference** are beliefs that random events in the environment have special meaning and are directed specifically at patients (e.g., talking by strangers, television, or radio about patients; random events such as accidents that have been designed to harm or influence patients). **Ideas of reference** differ from delusions of reference in intensity rather than form.

3. **Delusions of influence** are beliefs that patients' thoughts and actions are controlled by outside forces. In extreme cases, patients feel as if they were robots without thoughts and actions of their own. Patients may believe that body parts, frequently the genitals, are manipulated by unseen forces. Likewise, patients may feel as if their thoughts have been removed and replaced by alien thoughts.

4. **Thought broadcasting** involves thoughts leaving a patient's head and going directly to objects in the environment. Patients may experience this as a physical sensation. For those who have not experienced this phenomenon, thought broadcasting is difficult to understand.

5. **Grandiose delusions** are more common in patients with mania than in those with schizophrenia. However, schizophrenic patients may feel as though they are central figures in the complex delusional systems in the environment. Patients' feelings of having special knowledge, having special relationships with important figures, or posing a threat to conspiracies may all be considered grandiose. These grandiose delusions are differentiated from the expansive and positive grandiose delusions that are typical of mania.

6. **Somatic delusions** in schizophrenic patients typically include feelings that the body has been manipulated or altered by outside forces. These somatic delusions must be differentiated from the somatic delusions of other disorders (e.g., having cancer or a decaying body), which are typical of major depression with melancholic features. Patients with somatic delusions may feel that:
   a. An electronic device has been placed in their body.
   b. Their body is under the control of others.
   c. Portions of their body are not their own.

C **Perceptual disorders** include a variety of distortions of sensory experiences and their interpretation. **Recent data suggest that a fundamental perceptual defect in schizophrenia is the inability to habituate and suppress extraneous environmental stimuli or internal thought processes.** However, it must be emphasized that **no perceptual disturbance is pathognomonic of schizophrenia.** Perceptual distortions may occur in healthy people as well as in patients with mood disorders or organic mental syndromes.

1. **Hallucinations** are sensory experiences that occur without corresponding environmental stimuli.
   a. **Auditory hallucinations** range from unformed buzzing sounds to complex voices holding conversations. The most characteristic auditory hallucinations of schizophrenia include hearing voices speaking about a patient in the third person, hearing voices making derogatory comments about the patient, and hearing one voice telling the patient to commit some action.
      (1) The voices may be muffled or distinct, familiar or unfamiliar, single or multiple, and of either gender. Patients may hear their own voice spoken aloud.
      (2) **Command hallucinations** are a special form of auditory hallucination in which voices tell a patient to commit some action. In some patients, these hallucinations are so persistent that they become difficult to resist. Patients who hear command hallucinations telling them to harm themselves or others must be considered dangerous.
   b. **Visual hallucinations** are also experienced by schizophrenic patients, although they are more common in other disorders, particularly organic mental disorders. These hallucinations may be simple, but they are most characteristic of schizophrenia when they are complex and related to a patient's delusional system (e.g., a visit from aliens).

    c. Other hallucinations may be tactile, gustatory, olfactory (frequently an unpleasant and indescribable odor), or **somatic.** Similar to visual hallucinations, these hallucinatory experiences also occur in individuals with other disorders (e.g., olfactory hallucinations in complex partial seizures). In schizophrenic patients, they are frequently connected to delusional systems.

2. **Illusions** are misperceptions or misidentifications of identifiable environmental events or objects that may occur in any sensory modality. Illusions are common in a variety of disorders and occur in normal individuals as well. In schizophrenic patients, illusions may be variants of a normal experience given a delusional explanation.

    a. "Déjà vu" feelings are those in which unfamiliar situations feel strangely familiar. These illusions also occur as a normal phenomenon and in several forms of epilepsy.

    b. "Jamais vu" feelings are defined as those in which familiar situations feel novel and unfamiliar. These illusions also occur in epilepsy.

    c. Hypersensitivity to light, sound, or smell is common in schizophrenia and other disorders such as migraine headaches.

    d. Distorted perceptions of time also occur in a variety of conditions such as dissociative states and anxiety.

    e. Misperceptions of movement, perspective, and size, which are typical of organic conditions and anxiety, also occur in schizophrenia.

    f. Changes in body perception of one's own body or the body of others also occur.

D **Cognitive dysfunction** contributes to the many day-to-day challenges of living with schizophrenia and are at the root of problems with form and content of thoughts.

1. **Executive functioning is impaired,** demonstrated by:
     a. Difficulty making decisions
     b. Difficulty with abstract concepts
     c. Loss of mental flexibility

2. **Memory and attention are impaired,** with particular difficulty with working memory.

3. **Learning is impaired,** with loss of progress in education and difficulty in job performance.

E **Affect** is defined as the observable manifestations of mood and emotion. Affective findings in patients with schizophrenia may be, in some cases, unreliable because of the parkinsonian effects of the antipsychotic drugs and cultural differences in body language. Affective disturbances in schizophrenia include **blunted affect, flat affect,** and **inappropriate affect.**

F **Sense of self** is the perception of one's individuality, separateness from others, and continuity in space and time. The erosion of the sense of self may lead to the delusions of reference and of influence found in schizophrenia.

1. **In normal individuals,** a solid sense of self is thought to be the basis of good self-esteem and an ability of the individual to weather losses, disappointments, and slights from others.

2. **In schizophrenia,** as well as in other conditions, a disrupted sense of self may manifest as:
     a. Loss of self-esteem
     b. An inability to separate oneself from events in the environment (i.e., feeling that one's thoughts have harmed another person)
     c. Projection of one's own fears or suspicions onto others
     d. Experiencing the self and others as dichotomous opposites (i.e., all good or all bad) with little integration of the opposing features

G **Volitional symptoms** are among the most persistent and intractable features of schizophrenia. Difficulties initiating and maintaining purposeful and goal-directed activity and interest in the environment may account for the difficulties many patients with schizophrenia experience in maintaining stable work and living situations.

1. **Interest** in the environment may be difficult to generate and maintain for schizophrenic patients. This difficulty may be related to ambivalence or to an inability to generate interest internally. It may result from conflicting wishes or desires.

2. **Initiative,** or the ability to begin a goal-directed activity, is often lacking in advanced cases of schizophrenia. Patients may experience difficulty finding housing, financial support, and other needs as a consequence of this symptom. They may also be unable to initiate spontaneous movement without direction from others.

3. **Drive** is the ability to pursue a goal-directed activity after it has been started. Difficulties in maintaining goal-directed behavior appear to be common in, although not unique to, schizophrenia. These difficulties may be a result of the cognitive symptoms experienced by these patients or the inability to sustain thoughts amid the perceptual and cognitive disturbances of schizophrenia.

4. **Ambition** may be preserved in the absence of drive and initiative, as in patients whose grandiose wishes are to be film or music stars, or ambition may be absent. Unrealistic ambitions combined with the patients' delusions may be an organizing principle for complex dysfunctional patterns of behavior.

H **Relationship to the external world** may change. Patients with schizophrenia tend to become increasingly preoccupied with internal events and decreasingly influenced by external events. Preoccupation with delusional and hallucinatory symptoms and difficulty in communicating with others may lead to withdrawal from the world, which is called autism in its extreme form. **Social behavior** may then become impaired. In early and severe cases of schizophrenia, patients may display a loss of the social skills, body language, and empathic abilities that permit successful interaction with others and pursuit of social and vocational functioning. Frequently, normal individuals perceive schizophrenic persons as bizarre, hostile, or socially inept. Impairment of social skills; disturbances of thought, perception, speech, and behavior; or long-term institutionalization may result in schizophrenic patients who are severely socially debilitated and who may live on the fringe of society, often subject to homelessness. In the past, these same individuals may have been long-term institutionalized patients.

I **Motor activity** may change. Some alterations in motor activity and behavior may be associated with the pharmacologic treatment of schizophrenia.

1. **Quantitative changes.** The amount of activity and its "driven" quality ranges from the extremes of agitation in excited catatonic states and acute psychotic exacerbations to the withdrawn and inactive states associated with catatonic stupor and chronic institutionalization. **Akathisia, bradykinesia,** and **tardive dyskinesia** are commonly associated with the effects of antipsychotic medications rather than with schizophrenia.

   a. **Catatonic stupor** is a state of dramatic motor inactivity in which patients may, if untreated, be immobile for weeks or months at a time. Patients may be unable to initiate eating, drinking, or elimination. As patients recover, it is clear that they have been aware of events in the environment. Patients in a catatonic state may require aggressive medical care to avoid dehydration, electrolyte disturbances, and infections. In some cases, catatonic stupor may change abruptly to catatonic excitement. Medical illnesses and affective disorders are the most common causes of catatonia.

   b. **Catatonic excitement,** a hypermetabolic state, is a psychiatric emergency. A patient's activity and speech may be excessive, driven, and purposeless. Patients in this state may be violent. Before pharmacologic treatment and electroconvulsive therapy (ECT) were available, patients in this state frequently died of acute hyperthermia. Organic conditions (e.g., use of phencyclidine) and mania may also cause catatonic excitement.

2. **Qualitative changes.** Psychopharmacologic interventions frequently confuse the clinical picture of movement abnormalities by adding features of parkinsonian movement difficulties and the choreoathetotic movements of tardive dyskinesia. Even without pharmacologic treatment, patients with schizophrenia may exhibit a variety of movement abnormalities (e.g., increased flexor muscle tone, unusual mannerisms, bizarre gestures).

   a. **Catatonic posturing** is demonstrated by patients who assume strange postures and hold them for long periods.

      (1) In **catatonic rigidity,** patients resist being moved from their unusual rigid postures.

      (2) In **waxy flexibility,** patients' limbs may be moved like wax, and they hold the newly assumed position for long periods.

    b. Echopraxia is the behavioral equivalent of echolalia. Patients involuntarily mimic the movements of another person.

    c. Automatic obedience refers to the following of directives in an unquestioning, robot-like manner.

    d. Mannerisms and grimacing refer to patients' artificial and stilted appearance. Inappropriate silliness is evident, particularly in hebephrenic patients and patients with frontal lobe damage, and is frequently accompanied by unusual mannerisms. Particular mannerisms may have special meanings that are connected to delusions or hallucinations. Grimacing movements may be subtle or pronounced but may be mistaken for the orofacial dystonias of tardive dyskinesia.

    e. Stereotyped behaviors (stereotypy) involve the purposeless repetitive movements (or verbalizations) seen in a variety of conditions. These movements may involve the entire body such as rocking or may involve repetition of complex gestures. The movements may have magical significance or may be purposeless to the patient.

    f. Perseveration is involuntary repetition of a task. For example, patients who are asked to copy a series of circles may continue to copy the figures until they run off the page. Patients may repeat an answer to a question until asked to stop. Perseveration is also seen in patients with organic mental syndromes, particularly those with damage to premotor areas.

V COURSE

The course of schizophrenia may be highly variable, ranging from the presence or absence of a prodromal phase, remission or lack of symptoms between episodes, a downward deteriorating course, or full or social recovery. Course and prognosis vary widely depending on a variety of social, economic, and treatment factors as well as the diagnostic criteria used to define the population.

A Onset   The **peak time of onset** of schizophrenia is late adolescence and early adulthood, a time of multiple stresses related to leaving home, choosing a career, and developing relationships. Onset tends to be earlier for men than women, and a smaller peak occurs in the fourth decade, particularly among women.

    1. It has been proposed that separation from parents unmasks psychological deficits that have been present since childhood.

    2. Other studies suggest that these intense stresses are responsible for activating the processes that result in schizophrenia.

    3. A third explanation for the late adolescent time of onset involves the final maturation of the brain in the late teenage years. This final stage of neurodevelopment may leave the brains of persons with schizophrenia more vulnerable to stress.

    4. Patients with **early onset** tend to have more disorganized features and a worse prognosis for recovery and preservation of function than do patients with late onset.

    5. Patients with **late onset** tend to have more paranoid features and a better prognosis and preservation of function than do patients with early onset.

B Precipitating events   Initiating factors are now viewed as stressors that may activate a predisposition to the development of schizophrenia. They can also occur in other psychiatric illnesses such as bipolar disorder.

    1. **Psychosocial stressors.** Cultures experiencing social and economic stress are associated with high rates of schizophrenia. However, it cannot yet be determined which stressors produce schizophrenia in vulnerable individuals.

    2. **Traumatic events.** On a case-by-case basis, specific traumatic events that appear to precipitate schizophrenic symptoms can be isolated. However, it is not clear that either the level of stress or loss for schizophrenic individuals is different than might be experienced by normal individuals.

    3. **Drug and alcohol abuse.** Certain drugs (e.g., amphetamines, cocaine, hallucinogens, phencyclidine, cannabinoids, anticholinergics) and alcohol may precipitate psychotic symptoms. Whether these drugs cause schizophrenia-like syndromes or precipitate the development of

schizophrenia in vulnerable individuals is not clear. Some patients use substances as self-medication to dispel unwanted symptoms. For example, nicotine, which is frequently used by patients with schizophrenia, may alleviate negative symptoms by stimulating dopaminergic neurons in the frontal lobes. Anxiolytic substances may be used to combat side effects of antipsychotics such as akathisia.

C Clinical course

1. **Initial presentation.** The onset of schizophrenia is variable and has prognostic significance.
   a. Schizophrenia may present abruptly with confusion, agitation, affective involvement, hallucinations, and delusions occurring after an identifiable stressor. This clinical picture may develop in a period as short as 1 or 2 days; however, relatively few of these patients develop schizophrenia with the chronic course required for a *DSM-IV-TR* diagnosis. Instead, they meet the criteria for **brief psychotic disorder** or **schizophreniform disorder,** which has a less than 6-month course.
   b. **Trema** (German for "stage fright") is characterized by anxious, irritable, and depressed feelings that may last from a few days to 1 month or longer. These feelings may be a reaction to perceptions that something is going wrong. As this condition progresses, patients may feel as though the environment is odd and ominous. Such a trema may progress to frank psychosis or may resolve as if a discrete episode.
   c. An **insidious prodromal phase** portends a bad prognosis when psychotic features eventually appear. In general, the prognosis is worse if patients experience substantial deterioration in functioning without ever having achieved a high level of psychosocial functioning before the onset of psychotic symptoms. This course may be associated with subsequent high levels of negative symptoms. Symptoms observed in patients with this pattern of onset include:
      (1) Social withdrawal
      (2) Impairment in role functioning (e.g., as a student, parent, spouse)
      (3) Peculiar behavior
      (4) Neglect of grooming and personal hygiene
      (5) Blunted or inappropriate affect
      (6) Vague, digressive, overelaborative, or circumstantial speech, or poverty of speech or content of speech
      (7) Odd beliefs that are inconsistent with the cultural group of which the patient is a member, or magical thinking that influences behavior
      (8) Unusual perceptual experiences such as recurrent illusions, "telepathy," or recurrent déjà vu experiences
      (9) Marked lack of initiative, drive, ambition, interest, or energy
      (10) Diminished ability to correctly perceive social cues, particularly abstract social cues

2. **Acute phase.** Schizophrenia cannot be diagnosed without an acute phase involving worsening psychotic symptoms such as positive symptoms of delusions, hallucinations, catatonia, or agitation, and the possible worsening of negative symptoms.

3. **Stabilization phase.** This period, which may last as long as 6 months or more, involves gradually decreasing severity of symptoms (usually positive symptoms) from the acute phase.

4. **Stable phase.** This phase, which can last months to years, is characterized by little variation in symptom severity. Significant resolution of positive symptoms from the acute phase may occur, with some patients appearing asymptomatic. Negative symptoms may be more evident with attenuation of positive symptoms. Most patients recover some social function but continue to experience some symptoms.

5. **Deterioration from a previous level of functioning** is a key feature of schizophrenia. Role performance in relationships, work, self-care, or school is impaired. Patients often do not return to their previous level of functioning. Residual symptoms may interfere with social functioning. However, some recent studies challenge the assumption that this deterioration is uniform and lifelong.
   a. **Patterns of long-term courses.** Onset may be acute or insidious. The course may involve a single continuous episode of symptoms, be episodic, or evolve from episodic to continuous. The outcome may range from eventual severe impairment to complete recovery. Almost all

combinations of these elements are possible. Up to 30% of schizophrenic patients experience the insidious onset of symptoms, continuous course, and eventual severe impairment.

   b. **Patterns of recovery.** It should be noted that much of the data on the prognosis of schizophrenia is based on observations of patients who have recognized disease of less than 10 years or of patients whose behaviors may represent adaptations to institutionalized life. In addition, the prognosis may depend on socioeconomic factors and the availability of adequate psychosocial interventions. Many of the following factors may be viewed as intermediate-term prognostic factors. Different measures of recovery produce different outcome estimates.

   (1) **Social recovery** is often defined as economic and residential independence with little disruption in social relationships. Social recovery is often more common than complete remission of symptoms because many patients still suffer from negative symptoms. Several studies suggest that over a period of 15 years or longer, more than two-thirds of schizophrenic patients experience either complete, or "social," recovery with adequate treatment.

   (a) Errors in this measurement are possible because it is tied to the status of the economy and to the level of tolerance for social deviance in the culture.

   (b) Rates of social recovery tend to be higher than those for complete recovery.

   (2) **Complete recovery** implies complete remission of psychotic symptoms and a return to previous levels of social and occupational functioning.

   (3) **Hospitalization rates** have been used to measure recovery failures. Although these values are the easiest to determine, they are probably the least accurate measure of the course of schizophrenia. Rates of rehospitalization may depend on a variety of factors, ranging from the available health care resources and service delivery systems to community acceptance of deviant behavior.

D **Prognostic variables**   Early in the course of schizophrenia, a number of variables have been identified that predict a short to intermediate course of schizophrenia. Long-term prognostic factors have not been identified. Positive symptoms (see I A 1) carry much less ominous prognostic implications than do negative symptoms (see I A 2).

   1. **Separation of good from poor prognostic factors.** Patients currently meeting *DSM-IV-TR* diagnostic criteria for schizophrenia tend to exhibit a poorer prognosis in part because the definition excludes the following diagnoses that tend to have better outcomes.

      a. Acute psychotic disorders are now considered to be **schizophreniform disorder** or **brief psychotic disorder** if they do not continue for the 6-month course required for a diagnosis of schizophrenia.

      b. Patients with mood disorders in addition to psychotic symptoms are now diagnosed as having **schizoaffective disorder, major depression with psychotic features,** or **bipolar disorder.**

      c. Many patients previously considered to be schizophrenic are now included in diagnostic categories of **delusional disorder** and **borderline personality disorder.**

   2. **Poor prognostic factors.** Patients with a predominance of negative symptoms, poor cognitive performance on neuropsychological testing, and abnormalities on computed tomography (CT), MRI, and PET scans are reported to have poor outcomes.

E **Quality of life**

   1. **Social network.** Compared with normal individuals, patients with chronic schizophrenia tend to have small social networks. Whereas the social networks of normal individuals may be composed of 20 to 30 individuals, chronic schizophrenic patients may have networks as small as three to five people. The networks of people with chronic mental illnesses also tend to be highly interconnected.

      a. Before the onset of illness, schizophrenic patients have fewer and less satisfactory social relationships than people with affective disorders or normal subjects.

      b. The existence of social connections outside the family is associated with a good prognosis.

      c. In contrast to affective psychosis, family involvement can have positive or negative prognostic significance.

   2. **Impaired educational achievement.** Despite normal or high intelligence, many schizophrenic patients are unable to complete educational plans after the onset of illness.

3. **Impaired work performance.** Employment appears to improve the prognosis of schizophrenic patients. However, these patients may have significant difficulties finding employment, particularly during economic depressions. Schizophrenic patients often have jobs that require less skill than their education and intelligence suggest.

4. **Marital relationships.** Marriage rates for individuals with schizophrenia are lower than rates for the general population. Schizophrenic men tend to be married less frequently than schizophrenic women.

5. **Crime.** Most individuals with schizophrenia are no more violent than average persons, except for a small subset of persons with a history of violent actions when experiencing psychosis. The publicity of some violent crimes committed by persons with schizophrenia can exaggerate the public perception of dangerousness. There is evidence that when services are not provided to schizophrenic persons through the mental health system, they may enter the criminal justice system, usually for minor, nonviolent crimes.

6. **Premature death.** The risk of death in young schizophrenic patients is several times higher than in the general population. As schizophrenic individuals become older, their risk of mortality approaches that of the general population.
   a. Schizophrenic patients risk premature death from suicide, homicide, and medical illnesses (e.g., cardiovascular disease, infectious diseases, cancer).
   b. Another particular risk factor for people with schizophrenia is smoking. Some evidence suggests that smoking briefly "normalizes" some average evoked potential abnormalities associated with schizophrenia, leading to the hypothesis that schizophrenic patients may smoke heavily as a form of self-treatment of symptoms. The neoplasms that are common in patients with schizophrenia are those associated with smoking.

7. **Homelessness.** An estimated 5% to 8% of people with schizophrenia are homeless. Many more live in substandard housing or depend on relatives to maintain their standard of living, including housing.

8. **Psychiatric comorbidity.** Patients with schizophrenia are reported to suffer from other psychiatric symptoms, including anxiety, depression, and obsessive-compulsive symptoms. It is not clear in all cases that these reports represent carefully screened populations (e.g., excluding autistic people from the sample) or that depressive symptoms have been differentiated from deficit symptoms.

VI   DIFFERENTIAL DIAGNOSIS

The diagnosis of schizophrenia is made after a complete clinical and historical evaluation of an individual patient. **Symptoms must be present for at least 6 months** to make the diagnosis of schizophrenia. If the duration is less than 6 months, a variety of other diagnoses are appropriate, including schizophreniform disorder, brief psychotic disorder, psychotic disorder not otherwise specified, and acute psychotic symptoms in borderline personality disorder.

A **Organic mental disorders and syndromes (psychotic symptoms attributable to a medical condition)**

1. An acute medical illness that affects the brain, with psychotic symptoms, is called a **delirium.**

2. Long-term, supposedly irreversible, medical or neurologic syndromes with cognitive and psychiatric features are called **dementias.** Dementias often mimic the negative symptoms of schizophrenia.

3. To differentiate schizophrenia from organic mental syndromes, psychiatrists must rely on a high index of suspicion, an exacting mental status examination, physical and neurologic examinations, and sometimes a neuropsychological examination.
   a. Localized brain illnesses and injuries may produce **focal abnormalities,** resulting primarily from localized damage to the brain that can mimic a variety of cognitive, behavioral, and even linguistic findings found in schizophrenia.
   b. **Nonfocal,** or generalized, **alterations** in brain function can manifest as acute confusion and psychotic symptoms suggestive of schizophrenia. Visual hallucinations are somewhat more common, and auditory hallucinations are less common in organic mental syndromes.

4. **Medical disorders** known to cause psychiatric symptoms should be considered when evaluating patients (Table 2–4).

TABLE 2–4   Medical Disorders That Can Mimic Schizophrenia

Disorders	Comments
Vascular disorders	Vascular disorders must be considered in older patients. Cerebral vasculitis is particularly apt to mimic schizophrenia.
Autoimmune diseases	SLE is notorious for mimicking schizophrenia. Steroids used in treatment of autoimmune disease may cause organic mental syndromes.
Nutritional deficiencies	Overdoses of vitamins are also part of the differential diagnosis.
Metabolic disturbances	
Alcoholism	Delirium tremens and alcoholic hallucinations are frequently mistaken for acute schizophrenia.

Sleep disorders
  Sleep apnea
  Kleine-Levin syndrome
  Narcolepsy
	Patients with narcolepsy are more likely to present with symptoms of depression than schizophrenia.

Hydrocephalus
  Obstructive hydrocephalus
  Normal-pressure hydrocephalus	

Epilepsy
  Complex partial seizures
  Absence seizures	

Degenerative diseases	Degenerative diseases occur more often in older people, who have a low probability of developing schizophrenia.

Congenital disorders
  A subclinical form of PKU
  Smaller twin
  Minimal brain dysfunction
	The development of schizophrenia is associated with the smaller of a pair of twins who has poor motor function and slow development, theoretically as a result of intrauterine insult. Children and adolescents who demonstrate symptoms of minimal brain dysfunction may develop schizophrenia.

Infections
  Bacteria
  Fungi
  Viruses
  Parasites
	Bacterial infection, particularly associated with meningitis, may be the cause of an organic mental syndrome. Although rare, parasitic infection may result in a dramatic organic mental syndrome.

Toxicity
  Drug abuse
  Abuse of gasoline and toluene-based inhalants
  Carbon monoxide
  Lead
  Agricultural and industrial chemicals
  Prescribed medication
    Digitalis
    Anticholinergics
    Antihypertensives
    CNS depressants
    Steroids	

Traumatic insults to the brain
  Acute subdural hematomas
  Chronic subdural hematomas
  Direct trauma
  Postconcussion syndrome
  Left temporal lobe damage
	Left temporal lobe damage is particularly likely to produce schizophrenia-like symptoms.

Endocrine disorders
  Thyroid problems
  Parathyroid problems
  Pituitary adenomas
  Pheochromocytoma	

Neoplasms	In addition to primary and metastatic tumors of the brain, tumors in other parts of the body may cause psychiatric symptoms and cognitive deficits through paraneoplastic effects.

CNS = central nervous system; PKU = phenylketonuria; SLE = systemic lupus erythematosus.

B **Mood disorders.** These conditions are often accompanied by symptoms that are confused with those of other psychotic illnesses, including schizophrenia. For example, depression with severe melancholic features is, in some studies, a more common cause of the catatonic syndrome than schizophrenia. Mood-congruent delusions and hallucinations are a common feature of severe mood disorders.

1. **Manic episodes**
   a. Manic patients who present with irritability, suspicions of persecution, delusions, and hallucinations may be indistinguishable from patients with schizophrenia. At the height of a manic episode, patients may demonstrate bizarre behaviors, incoherence, and other features thought to be pathognomonic of schizophrenia. Careful family histories and longitudinal observations may be required to differentiate among these conditions.
   b. If organic causes for the manic syndrome and personality disorder have been ruled out, a manic episode by definition implies that the patient suffers from **bipolar disorder.** Patients with bipolar disorder usually suffer from both manic and depressive episodes at some time in their lives. However, only mania is present in a few patients.

2. **Major depressive episodes** (including those associated with bipolar disorder). Patients with severe depression may present with paranoid symptoms, social withdrawal, and severely restricted affect, all of which are suggestive of schizophrenia. Patients who develop melancholic features and delusions concerning cancer—a rotting body, guilt, and other mood-congruent delusions—particularly resemble schizophrenic individuals. Likewise, indecisiveness, slowing of thoughts, and lack of spontaneity in speech and behavior may resemble the negative symptoms of schizophrenia. Recent studies suggest that depression, at least in the first episode of psychosis, may be part of the overall illness pattern, which remits along with other acute symptoms and without additional treatment. This implies that separating depressive symptoms from acute psychotic symptoms may be unwarranted.

3. **Postpsychotic depression.** There is some controversy regarding whether postpsychotic depression represents a true depression with the same biologic features as a major depressive episode or if it represents a phase of predominant negative symptoms of schizophrenia. Likewise, oversedation and parkinsonian symptoms may resemble the clinical picture of depression.
   a. During a first psychotic episode, different criteria reveal that up to 75% of patients suffer from depressive symptoms. However, 98% of these symptoms remit with the resolution of psychosis. This suggests that antidepressant treatment should not be initiated except in patients for whom depression persists after the resolution of the psychotic episode.
   b. Since the introduction of the atypical antipsychotics, some patients have had dramatic recoveries from psychosis only to realize that they have lost out on many things. Depression related to life circumstances is best addressed through psychotherapy.

4. **Schizoaffective disorder** (Table 2–5). Patients present with either a manic episode or a major depressive episode with acute psychotic symptoms suggestive of schizophrenia or an episode of psychotic symptoms without mood symptoms (in an individual in whom a mood disorder has been previously diagnosed). Criteria for diagnosing this disorder are:
   a. A family history that is more positive for mood disorder than for schizophrenia
   b. A prognosis intermediate between mood disorders and schizophrenia

---

TABLE 2–5 *DSM-IV-TR* **Diagnostic Criteria for Schizoaffective Disorder**

A. An uninterrupted period of illness during which there is either a major depressive episode or manic episode concurrent with symptoms that meet criterion A for schizophrenia

B. During the same period of illness, there have been delusions or hallucinations for at least 2 weeks in the absence of prominent mood symptoms

C. Symptoms meeting criteria for a mood episode are present for a substantial portion of the total duration of the active and residual periods of the illness

D. Not caused by the direct effects of substance abuse

Specify type:
  Bipolar type: If manic episode or both manic and major depressive episodes
  Depressive type: If major depressive episode only

Reprinted with permission from the Diagnostic and Statistical Manual of Mental Disorders, Fourth Edition, Text Revision, (Copyright 2000). American Psychiatric Association.

TABLE 2–6 *DSM-IV-TR* Diagnostic Criteria for Brief Psychotic Disorder

A. Presence of at least one of the following symptoms:
   1. Delusions
   2. Hallucinations
   3. Disorganized speech (e.g., frequent derailment or incoherence)
   4. Grossly disorganized or catatonic behavior
B. Duration of an episode of the disturbance is at least 1 day and no more than 1 month, with eventual return to premorbid level of functioning. (When the diagnosis must be made without waiting for the expected recovery, it should be qualified as "provisional.")
C. Not better accounted for by a mood disorder (i.e., no full mood syndrome is present) or schizophrenia and not caused by the direct effects of a substance or general medical condition

Specify if:
With marked stressor(s) [brief reactive]: If symptoms occur shortly after and apparently in response to events that, singly or together, would be markedly stressful to almost anyone in similar circumstances in the person's culture
Without marked stressor(s): If psychotic symptoms do not occur shortly after or are not apparently in response to events that, singly or together, would be markedly stressful to almost anyone in similar circumstances in the person's culture
With postpartum onset: If onset within 4 weeks postpartum

Reprinted with permission from the Diagnostic and Statistical Manual of Mental Disorders, Fourth Edition, Text Revision, (Copyright 2000). American Psychiatric Association.

   c. Response to combinations of medications and treatments used for both schizophrenia and mood disorders

C **Other psychoses**

1. **Brief psychotic disorder** (Table 2–6). Similar to schizophreniform disorder, this diagnostic category describes patients who were considered schizophrenic under previous diagnostic criteria but whose good prognosis differentiates them from the patients diagnosed as schizophrenic under current criteria. The illness of a brief psychotic disorder lasts **between 1 day and 1 month.** Clearly, the differential diagnosis for acutely psychotic persons is very large, with a need to rule out medical conditions, substance abuse, and mood disorders.

2. **Schizophreniform disorder** (Table 2–7). This diagnostic category was created to differentiate those who were previously regarded as "good prognosis" schizophrenic patients from "poor prognosis" schizophrenic patients. Patients with symptoms suggestive of schizophrenia for whom no organic cause for psychotic symptoms has been found and who meet the diagnostic criteria for schizophrenia, except that their symptoms have lasted less than 6 months, are appropriately diagnosed as having schizophreniform disorder. A few patients with schizophreniform disorder eventually meet the criteria for schizophrenia. However, the majority of patients with schizophreniform disorder recover without ever having met the diagnostic criteria for schizophrenia.

TABLE 2–7 *DSM-IV-TR* Diagnostic Criteria for Schizophreniform Disorder

A. Meets criteria A, D, and E for schizophrenia
B. An episode of the disorder lasts at least 1 month but less than 6 months

Prognostic features should be specified in the diagnosis:
   With good prognostic features (at least two of the following):
   1. Onset of prominent psychotic symptoms within 4 weeks of the first noticeable change in usual behavior or functioning
   2. Confusion or perplexity at the height of the psychotic episode
   3. Good premorbid social and occupational functioning
   4. Absence of blunted or flat affect
Without good prognostic features:
   Should be specified if good prognostic features are absent

Reprinted with permission from the Diagnostic and Statistical Manual of Mental Disorders, Fourth Edition, Text Revision, (Copyright 2000). American Psychiatric Association.

TABLE 2–8 *DSM-IV-TR* **Diagnostic Criteria for Delusional Disorder**

A. Nonbizarre delusions (i.e., involving situations that could occur in real life such as being followed, poisoned, or infected; having a disease; being loved at a distance) of at least 1 month's duration
B. Has never met criterion A for schizophrenia (for more than a few hours)
C. Apart from the impact of the delusion(s) or its ramifications, functioning is not markedly impaired, and behavior is not odd or bizarre
D. If mood episodes have occurred concurrently with delusions, total duration has been brief relative to the duration of the delusional periods
E. Not caused by the direct effects of a substance (e.g., drugs of abuse, medication) or a general medical condition

Specify type:
Erotomanic type: Delusions that another person, usually of higher status, is in love with the individual
Grandiose type: Delusions of inflated worth, power, knowledge, identity, or special relationship to a deity or famous person
Jealous type: Delusions that one's sexual partner is unfaithful
Persecutory type: Delusions that one (or someone to whom one is close) is being malevolently treated in some way
Somatic type: Delusions that the person has some physical defect or general condition
Mixed type: Delusions characteristic of more than one of the above types but no one theme predominates
Unspecified type

Reprinted with permission from the Diagnostic and Statistical Manual of Mental Disorders, Fourth Edition, Text Revision, (Copyright 2000). American Psychiatric Association.

---

3. **Delusional disorder** (Table 2–8). Without an accurate history and attempts to corroborate the patient's complaints, delusional disorder may be easily mistaken for schizophrenia. Although the delusions may be quite elaborate, they must not be bizarre.

a. If persons have negative symptoms, hallucinations, disorganized speech, or disorganized or catatonic behavior for more than a few hours, the diagnosis of schizophrenia should be made. The delusions may be plausible (e.g., being under surveillance, being poisoned or contaminated, being in love with someone famous, having a serious illness). Patients lack the deterioration of global functioning generally seen in schizophrenia, and many of them are able to maintain employment throughout much of their illness.

b. Because patients are convinced of the validity of their complaints, they may not seek treatment for their condition, which often develops later in life than schizophrenia. Initial physician contact and treatment may occur as part of evaluation for commitment or a forensic evaluation after arrest. Patients with delusional disorder can be highly resistant to treatment with psychotherapy or medications.

4. **Psychotic disorder not otherwise specified.** This diagnosis of exclusion is reserved for patients who have some diagnostic features of schizophrenia but who do not meet all the diagnostic criteria. This diagnosis is appropriate for patients with nonorganic psychotic presentations, which, after exhaustive examination, do not fit another diagnostic criterion for classification of psychotic symptoms.

D **Other disorders** If there is **no episode of acute psychosis,** other diagnoses may be appropriate. Patients who fit the current diagnostic criteria for schizophrenia are unlikely to be confused with other diagnostic groups. However, symptoms suggestive of schizophrenia may be found in a number of conditions, which must be ruled out (see Table 2–4).

1. **Personality disorders.** With the decline of the use of such terms as "process schizophrenia" and "pseudoneurotic schizophrenia," there has been less diagnostic confusion between schizophrenia and personality disorders. However, in the case of several specific personality disorders, features of the clinical presentation may be confused with those of schizophrenia. Personality disorders most likely to be confused with schizophrenia include the following (using *DSM-IV-TR* nomenclature):

a. **Paranoid personality disorder** involves interpreting the actions of others as deliberately demeaning or threatening. Behavior is characterized by questioning the loyalty of others, holding grudges about insults or slights, and lacking trust in others. This disorder can be differentiated from paranoid schizophrenia in that it lacks acute psychotic episodes and extreme deterioration.

    b. **Schizoid personality disorder** is often found among biologic relatives of schizophrenic patients, which suggests that these disorders share some undetermined genetic commonality. The lack of social interests of affected patients results in a restricted lifestyle, which may be confused with the social deterioration of schizophrenia. However, the lack of hallucinations and delusions differentiates these individuals from schizophrenic patients.

    c. **Schizotypal personality disorder** is also frequently found among biologic relatives of schizophrenic individuals. Because of the odd beliefs, magical ideation, and eccentric behavior and appearance of these patients, this disorder may be confused with schizophrenia. However, it can be differentiated from schizophrenia because of the lack of a history of an acute phase (see V C 2).

      (1) Phenomenologic investigations suggest that extreme social anxiety may be the genetic link between schizophrenia and schizotypal relatives.

      (2) Further refinements of this diagnosis and its relationship to genetic factors in schizophrenia may involve differentiation of affective versus nonaffective subtypes of this disorder (which may be more appropriately assigned to borderline personality disorder).

      (3) Some evidence suggests that people who suffer from schizotypal personality disorder may suffer from similar sensory gating problems as do people with schizophrenia.

    d. **Borderline personality disorder** is characterized by suffering from a lifelong pattern of unstable relationships, rapid mood swings, and an unstable self-image. In severe cases, psychotic features may appear in response to stress, but they are rarely of sufficient duration or intensity to make a diagnosis of schizophrenia. The intense reexperiencing of trauma that occurs in some cases of this disorder may be mistaken for psychosis.

    e. **Other personality disorders** exhibit symptoms of sufficient severity that they may sometimes be misdiagnosed as schizophrenia by incautious clinicians.

      (1) **Dependent personality disorder** may be mistaken for exhibiting schizophrenic ambivalence, lack of drive, and fear of being alone.

      (2) **Obsessive-compulsive personality disorder** may demonstrate such restrictions of affective expression that it is mistaken for the flattened affect described in former diagnostic systems for schizophrenia. In addition, ambivalence, circumstantial speech, and other features may give the impression of schizophrenia without a diagnostic evaluation.

  2. **Developmental disabilities.** Asperger syndrome (a high-functioning form of autism), in particular, may be mistaken for schizophrenia if *DSM-IV-TR* criteria are not used. Patients suffering from this disorder are often eccentric, emotionally labile, and anxious, and they demonstrate poor social functioning, repetitive behavior, and fixed habits. Affect may be interpreted as bizarre or flat. Social interactions are severely impaired by a lack of empathy or understanding of other people, and motor performance is clumsy and poorly coordinated. Because these patients do not generally have positive symptoms, they may be most easily mistaken for "simple schizophrenics" by casual diagnosticians.

E **Religious and cultural subgroups** Diagnosticians from one culture may confuse beliefs and behavior patterns associated with another culture with symptoms of schizophrenia. A member of one group or culture who evaluates members of another religious group must not consider the religious beliefs of the other person to be psychotic if the beliefs are held by a group of people of which the patient is a member. Likewise, physicians from another culture must not interpret cultural differences in body language and acceptable affective expression as bizarre. To best avoid this diagnostic confusion, individuals should consult physicians from their own culture or clinicians experienced with that culture.

VII   TREATMENT

Schizophrenia is not currently considered curable, and most patients experience symptoms off and on for the rest of their lives. Therefore, it is important to take a **recovery-oriented approach** that disregards a sole goal of symptom reduction, instead assisting the patient to achieve optimum functioning in a community of his or her choosing with as much autonomy as possible. Significant improvement is more likely for the following schizophrenic patients: those with a late onset of illness, those from developing countries, and those recovering in times of economic prosperity. Perhaps because of a later onset, women tend to have a better prognosis for schizophrenia in many parts of the world.

A Overview

1. Treatment programs for persons with schizophrenia must be individualized and comprehensive, taking into account the biologic, psychological, and social needs of each patient. Attention must also be paid to the continuity of care. The care setting should be as nonrestrictive as possible, and every attempt should be made to reintegrate patients into the community.

2. Modern treatment methods in the United States make it possible for about 90% of schizophrenic patients to recover sufficiently to live outside the hospital most of the time. Some studies suggest that about 75% of individuals who meet the diagnostic criteria for schizophrenia experience substantial or complete recovery 20 to 25 years (or longer) after the onset of illness.

3. Guidelines for the modern treatment of schizophrenia are now available from several sources.
   a. Treatment guidelines published by the American Psychiatric Association in 2004 are part of a series of practice guidelines in psychiatry.
   b. The *Expert Consensus Guidelines,* first published in *The Journal of Clinical Psychiatry* in 1997 and revised in 2008, make specific recommendations on the uses of antipsychotic medications.
   c. The *Texas Medication Algorithm* most recently updated in 2008 by the State of Texas Department of Mental Health and Mental Retardation presents a concise guide to medication choices in the treatment of schizophrenia.
   d. In 1998 the recommendations of the *Schizophrenia: Practice Outcomes Research Team* published in *Schizophrenia Bulletin* presented multidisciplinary treatment guidelines and provided a comprehensive look at treatment of persons with schizophrenia in the community.

B Hospitalization Hospitals were once the primary treatment setting for persons with schizophrenia; at one time, it was not uncommon for affected individuals to spend the rest of their lives in hospitals. Hospitalization now usually focuses on more acute issues, with a minority of patients in long-term hospitalization.

1. **Indications.** Hospitalization is indicated because of specific problems associated with a person's illness rather than because of the appearance of symptoms (Table 2–9).
   a. First episodes of psychosis and unusual presentations of psychotic conditions in patients with more chronic forms of schizophrenia may warrant hospitalization.
   b. Hospitalization is not necessarily indicated for an exacerbation of psychotic symptoms if adequate community alternatives are available.

2. **Goals**
   a. **Protection.** The hospital should be a safe environment where physical needs can be met, stresses can be minimized, and impulses can be controlled.
   b. **Diagnosis.** Twenty-four–hour care allows for extensive observation and evaluation of a patient's problems, strengths, history, support, and response to treatment. In addition, access to

TABLE 2–9 Hospitalization of Patients with Schizophrenia

Problems Requiring Short-term Hospital Care	Problems Requiring Long-term Hospital Care
Risk of suicidal and homicidal ideation	Lack of appropriate community mental health resources
Command hallucinations of a threatening nature, with the clinician's assessment that the patient may act on these hallucinations	Provision of rehabilitative services before discharge to community programs
Extreme fear	Care for a severely debilitated schizophrenic patient
Significant confusion	Treatment of significant comorbidity from medical illnesses, substance abuse, medication complications
	Protection from self-inflicted harm or danger to others

sophisticated diagnostic laboratory and neuroradiologic tests gives physicians the opportunity to differentiate schizophrenia from psychotic disorders resulting from medical conditions.

   c. Therapy. Various kinds of treatments, including antipsychotic medications, vocational and psychosocial rehabilitation, and family education, which are all designed to return the patient to the community, can be started in the hospital. Atypical antipsychotics, cognitive and behavioral treatments, and structured schedules may help decrease negative symptoms. There is no evidence that inpatient psychotherapy without medication is of any benefit.

3. Side effects of hospitalization

   a. Possible loss of self-esteem and social stigmatization as a result of being on a "mental ward"

   b. Possible loss of social supports in the community

   c. Loss of social and living skills required to live in the world outside the hospital (i.e., institutionalism) with prolonged hospitalization

4. Changing role of the hospital. Changing views concerning the importance of hospitalization in the treatment of patients with schizophrenia result from economic pressures and increasing beliefs about the superiority of community treatment over hospitalization.

   a. Current trends. Where adequate community treatment systems exist, it is presumed that community programs will assume many of the treatment functions of the inpatient unit. Present trends include major reductions in length of stay and frequency of hospitalization, with a focus on acute stabilization and discharge as well as an emphasis on diagnostic clarification rather than on psychotherapeutic treatment.

   b. Alternatives to hospitalization. Particularly in the public sector, attempts are being made to provide community-based alternatives to hospitalization. Some of these alternatives involve houses in the community where physicians, nurses, and others provide acute stabilization of psychotic symptoms and rapid reintegration into the community. In other cases, motels and therapeutic foster homes have been used for these purposes.

      (1) In general, these settings are not as well set up to handle violence and to deal with a medical evaluation as hospitals, but they provide less disruption for shorter periods of time.

      (2) These facilities are probably most appropriate for patients whose illnesses are well known, not for first-episode psychotic patients.

5. Therapeutic milieu. The therapeutic environment of the inpatient ward is known as the "therapeutic milieu." Inpatient psychiatric wards frequently use the therapeutic milieu as a major treatment modality for schizophrenic patients. Formal milieu therapy depends on attention to the social structure of the ward and on adequate numbers of well-trained staff. Interactions between staff, patients, and formal social organizations (e.g., the patient's ward government) are tools regularly used in milieu therapy. Trends are away from emphasis on milieu therapy because of decreasing lengths of hospital stay and a change of the focus of the hospital stay to diagnosis, rehabilitation programs, and psychoeducational activities.

   a. Structure. One aspect of the staff's role in the therapeutic milieu is to support the patient's impaired reality testing, impulse control, and modulation of environmental stimulation. The staff works to reduce the patient's anxiety and control injurious behavior. The structure of the ward should contain regular, structured activities; time alone; and help with personal hygiene and self-care. Milieu therapy avoids intense probing and anxiety-provoking psychotherapeutic interventions, which can be overwhelming for psychotic patients.

   b. Flexibility. The milieu should be flexible enough to respond to the changing needs of individuals with regard to length of stay, extent of restrictions, contact with family, group involvement, and activity levels. For example, as a patient's positive symptoms resolve, efforts may be initiated to increase the patient's socialization with other patients, engage the patient in structured recreational and vocational activities, and encourage the patient's participation in the ward government.

   c. Ward community. The other patients, as individuals and as a group, are used as therapeutic agents in the therapeutic milieu. Open, direct communication and individual responsibility are encouraged. The more organized and improved patients can provide hope and act as models for patients in earlier stages of recovery. As a group, patients are encouraged to make decisions about daily activities of the ward and to help change the maladaptive behavior of patients through open feedback.

    d. Side effects. Target-symptom–oriented treatment plans and posthospitalization care plans that involve all staff, including staff from programs outside the hospital, may remedy the side effects of milieu treatment.

       (1) Premature and harsh confrontation from staff and other patients or too much pressure for recovery may exacerbate psychotic symptoms or delay recovery.

       (2) A structured, tolerant atmosphere may promote dependence on the ward, making it difficult to return to the community.

       (3) Excessive demands for participation may cause overstimulation and disorganization.

       (4) Patients who are in more advanced recovery stages may take advantage of those who are not doing so well, unless interactions between patients are monitored carefully.

       (5) Staff may retain patients in the ward milieu longer than is desirable, creating a tendency for patients to return prematurely to the ward without ever developing a relationship with community services. This appears to be a problem with neophyte therapists who become enmeshed with patients and their social networks, believing that only they really understand the patient. This may result in a fragmentation of team efforts and poor communication with outpatient therapists. Good supervision can reduce this risk to the continuity of care.

    e. Organizational continuity. With shorter lengths of stay and an increasing reliance of treatment systems on community-based treatment, hospitals need to be a more highly integrated member of the overall mental health treatment system. Case managers from the community are increasingly involved in ward treatment. Diagnostic and treatment information must be relayed between community and hospital staff, and inpatient treatment objectives must be jointly negotiated between systems. Survival of inpatient, hospital-based treatment programs for patients with schizophrenia may increasingly depend on the ability of the inpatient units to respond to needs of the community mental health system.

C **Group therapy**   Group therapy has long been a mainstay of the treatment of schizophrenic patients in both inpatient and outpatient settings. It is best used in conjunction with other forms of therapy, particularly medications.

   1. Although there is a paucity of well-controlled studies of group therapy in schizophrenia, the studies that do exist support the contention that group therapy focused on communication, alleviation of symptoms, and social skills produces improvements in social integration. Patients in such group therapy also have fewer readmissions to the hospital than do patients who receive only social skills training.

   2. There is little evidence that open-ended, insight-oriented group therapy is effective in the treatment of schizophrenic patients.

D **Individual psychotherapy**   Supportive and adaptive therapeutic techniques that are oriented to helping patients adapt to the details of daily life are far more effective in the management of schizophrenic patients than are insight-oriented techniques that focus on patients' inner experiences. Cognitive and behavioral therapies may reduce deficit symptoms in schizophrenia.

   1. Therapeutic relationship

    a. Supportive psychotherapy is characterized by warm, open relationships that focus on promoting patients' self-esteem and helping them learn about their real strengths and limitations. Effective therapy focuses on practical and concrete issues.

    b. Attempts to establish a **close or intense therapeutic relationship** may exacerbate symptoms in patients who are highly suspicious or who feel overwhelmed by interpersonal relationships.

    c. Nondirective and affectively restricted therapeutic styles may also cause patients to experience anxiety and exacerbations of symptoms. Insight-oriented psychotherapy alone has not proved to be effective in individuals with schizophrenia.

   2. Therapeutic techniques. The principles of psychotherapy of schizophrenic patients are as follows:

    a. Education. One of the main techniques of the therapist is to teach patients about their illness. The therapist should teach techniques of managing stress, understanding symptoms, and knowing the value of compliance with pharmacologic treatments. This approach encourages patients to assume responsibility for their own treatment.

b. **Focusing on problem solving.** The therapist focuses on helping patients solve concrete problems that arise in daily life. The therapist may offer possible solutions to problems presented by patients, including an analysis of possible positive and negative outcomes of each solution. The therapist attempts to develop problem-solving skills for patients in financial, interpersonal, residential, and other areas of patients' daily lives.

c. **Setting reasonable expectations for change.** Therapists who have unreasonable expectations for a "cure" may convey these expectations to patients in a counterproductive manner. Therapists who have generally positive expectations for improving functioning and life satisfaction appear to be correlated with good patient outcomes.

d. **Expressing emotions effectively.** Therapies that encourage expression of emotion for its own sake or for "cathartic" value may trigger exacerbations in some patients. The therapist should encourage a discussion of private feelings and how to deal with these feelings but not encourage full-blown expressions of anger and hostility.

e. **Crisis intervention.** The therapist may be able to intervene in crises in patients' lives to prevent serious escalations. Unlike the passive roles in other forms of therapy, the therapist may need to become active in working with patients' families, landlords, or social agencies to reduce the escalation of crises into psychotic episodes.

f. **Concrete limit setting.** The therapist may need to set concrete limits such as avoiding substance abuse and violence. These discussions frequently include discussions of consequences of harmful behaviors.

g. **Managing dependence.** One of the functions of the therapy of schizophrenic patients is to increase patients' appropriate socialization with other people in the community. In meeting this goal, therapists encourage patients to rely on a large network of people in the community rather than on only the therapist.

h. **Illness self-management.** The therapist and a patient construct "experimental" designs intended to help the patient observe factors that may make both the positive and negative symptoms of illness better or worse. Patients may learn how to initiate activity, reduce social isolation, and control symptoms with medications, as well as many other self-management skills.

i. **Cognitive remediation.** In contrast to rehabilitation, which focuses on relearning concrete social and functional skills, cognitive remediation attempts to reverse neuropsychological performance deficits that are characteristic of schizophrenia. This approach involves the use of behavioral techniques and education to improve outcome, which is assessed by methods such as the Wisconsin Card Sort Test. This approach has produced improvements in patients with brain injury and autism but is new in its application to individuals with schizophrenia.

E Community treatment   The majority of patients with schizophrenia now receive most of their treatment in the community.

1. The cornerstone of modern treatment of schizophrenia is **case management.** For community treatment to work, the sometimes disparate goals of multiple public and private agencies must be managed to provide an individualized treatment plan for a particular patient. Although physicians sometimes play the role of case manager, social workers, nurses, or rehabilitation counselors usually assume this role. Sometimes even patients who are trained to help others negotiate their way through the often complex treatment system may serve as case managers.

a. **Linkage.** The primary role of the case manager is to help patients establish and maintain access to various community resources. This can be a significant challenge because some patients' cognitive difficulties make it impossible for them to successfully apply for and obtain services such as housing, disability benefits, and vocational rehabilitation. Case managers often provide transportation to help patients keep appointments and commitments with various community programs. Case managers also maintain lines of communication to help ensure that the involved agencies efficiently share information.

b. **Treatment planning and monitoring.** Case managers are frequently the clinicians responsible for maintaining the treatment record and ensuring that services are delivered appropriately. In some settings (e.g., high-caseload clinics), this is primarily a paperwork-related task to ensure quality assurance and availability of treatment history. In more effective clinical settings (e.g., low-caseload clinics), the case manager is the clinician who is most involved in the case of a particular patient, maintaining contact on a frequent basis and checking for signs of relapse, noncompliance, and adverse effects.

    c. Intensive case management. This treatment approach can help persons with severe schizophrenia stay in the community. In this type of program, case managers serve only a few clients (e.g., eight to 12 per caseload) and often assess and work with their clients on a daily basis. Some intensive programs provide access to members of the treatment team 24 hours a day, 7 days a week. This enables more effective monitoring of treatment response and can allow for rapid response to crisis, in hopes of reducing the need for expensive hospitalization. Intensive treatment can involve such methods as monitored medication administration.

    d. Advocacy. The case manager may need to seek resources and services for schizophrenic patients. **Case-specific advocacy** is aimed at gaining resources for the individual patient, and **class-specific advocacy** is aimed at gaining services, resources, or access to services for a group of patients.

2. Because returning patients to productive lives in the community has become a priority, **psychosocial rehabilitation** has become a significant part of treatment programs. Goals of these programs are to reduce symptoms, remediate disabilities, and overcome handicaps associated with schizophrenia. In the past, patients who left inpatient institutions had insufficient skills necessary for independent living; they lacked the skills in social interactions required to gain or retain employment and to form social support networks needed for survival. Preliminary data suggest that patients who participate in psychosocial rehabilitation programs suffer relapse at a lower rate than control subjects. These programs focus on the following issues:

    a. Social skills training. Patients require the skills necessary to communicate with both strangers and familiar people involved in their lives. More effective social skills can reduce the socially inappropriate behavior and symptom-based communications that can lead to patients' becoming social outcasts in their own communities.

    b. Living skills acquisition. Patients who have become ill before establishing independence and those who have lived in institutions for much of their lives may be unable to shop for themselves, prepare food, or maintain their own living space.

    c. Housing. Many persons with schizophrenia have difficulty finding and maintaining housing. Modern community mental health programs offer supervised housing during the transition period between hospitalization and residential living while patients try to establish independence.

    d. Managing finances. The management of money, even if it is received monthly, may pose substantial problems for some patients. In extreme cases, patients may spend or lose an entire monthly check in a few days or weeks. To better ensure patients do not go without food, housing, or medications because of mismanaged finances, modern treatment programs may offer financial management assistance. This frequently takes the form of **designated payee** services in which a patient's disability check is received and distributed by a third party or agency.

    e. Managing the illness. Patients are taught to manage medication administration, watch for side effects, and report potentially dangerous developments in the treatment system in an appropriate and assertive manner.

    f. Recreational activities. Patients are taught to pursue recreational and physical activities to reduce stress and promote general health.

F **Self-help programs**

1. Consumer clubhouses. Some persons with schizophrenia receive the majority of their treatment and support from consumer-operated self-help organizations. Programs for mentally ill people such as the internationally known Fountain House are a source of support and self-esteem for persons suffering from major mental illness. Psychosocial rehabilitation, vocational training, housing assistance, and financial management services are offered by some consumer-operated, not-for-profit organizations. Such programs are the chief source of specially trained persons with mental illness, who, in turn, become providers of services to persons with schizophrenia.

2. Illness self-management. The objective of this treatment method is to train patients with persistent schizophrenic symptoms to manage their own illnesses to a greater extent than previously encouraged by the mental health treatment system. Several forms of this training exist, but most encourage the development of skills in several specific areas.

  a. **Symptom control** includes learning to recognize and respond to signs of relapse, differentiating relapse from medication side effects, and working with persistent symptoms.

  b. **Substance avoidance** focuses on avoiding alcohol abuse and the use of street drugs.

  c. **Medication management** requires an understanding of how medications work; how they are taken; and how different side effects should be managed, including when to seek medical help.

  d. **Learning to work with the health care system** involves education about how to communicate with health care providers, navigate the service delivery system, and advocate for oneself.

3. **Advocacy movement.** Advocacy groups have brought about significant changes in the amount of attention paid to the struggles of persons with schizophrenia. The **National Alliance for the Mentally Ill (NAMI)** has brought much attention to the need for more research into effective treatments for severe and persistent mental illnesses. NAMI is also a major voice of parents, siblings, and children who care for persons with illnesses such as schizophrenia. The organization offers valuable educational programs to help dispel the stigma associated with schizophrenia and help families better understand the symptoms of schizophrenia.

G Pharmacologic treatment

1. **First-generation antipsychotics.** Since the 1960s first-generation antipsychotics (e.g., chlorpromazine, perphenazine, and haloperidol) have been the mainstay of the pharmacologic treatment of schizophrenia. All first-generation antipsychotics exert primary effects by blocking dopamine receptors, particularly D-2 receptors.

  a. **Efficacy**

    (1) **Acute treatment.** Therapy with first-generation antipsychotics is frequently successful, with amelioration of symptoms such as hallucinations, delusions, and agitation. First-generation antipsychotics are less effective with chronic or well-organized delusions, and they have little effect on negative symptoms such as apathy, anhedonia, and amotivation.

    (2) **Maintenance treatment.** Dopamine blockers have a proven record in reducing the risk of relapse, particularly when used in conjunction with a comprehensive treatment plan.

      (a) Within 1 month of discharge, 7% of patients with schizophrenia have relapsed, and nearly 50% relapse within 1 year of discharge.

      (b) Two groups of schizophrenic patients may not be effectively treated with maintenance antipsychotics:

        (i) Patients who have had a single acute psychotic episode

        (ii) Very deteriorated chronic schizophrenic patients who may be refractory to treatment

  b. **Choice of agent.** At least nine first-generation antipsychotics are readily available in the United States, and more agents are available in other nations. The choice of the proper agent is more of an art than a science, and as both the physician and patient gain experience, the job becomes easier.

    (1) Route of administration is an important consideration, particularly when the patient's presentation or history suggests the need for acute parental administration or use of longer-acting depot injections.

    (2) Side-effect profile is also important. Matching the potential side effects to the patient's presentation or history may be effective. For example, more sedating drugs may be chosen for more agitated patients, or drugs with more adrenergic blockade may be avoided in older patients or in those with cardiac histories.

  c. **Dosage**

    (1) **Acute psychosis.** The equivalent of 200 to 400 mg chlorpromazine initially given in divided doses is adequate. In most patients, significant effects are reached in 3 to 10 days, but some patients may require 30 or more days to respond. Massive doses of 1,000 to 2,000 mg are sometimes used, but controlled studies indicate that this approach is no more effective than standard dosing. However, a small subset of patients apparently respond only to very high doses.

    (2) **Stabilization phase.** After patients with acute symptoms have begun to respond to treatment, the dosage is frequently titrated toward a maintenance level. This may involve a

titration phase that attempts to balance symptom control and possibly incapacitating side effects (e.g., sedation, orthostatic hypotension).

    (3) Maintenance phase. The goal of the maintenance phase is to keep patients as free from symptoms as possible while avoiding any potentially incapacitating side effects. Physicians may recommend that patients who are prone to violent outbursts or self-destructive behavior tolerate a higher level of side effects to minimize risk of harm. At this point, once-a-day administration is sufficient for almost all patients. In some patients, weekly dosage adjustments may be necessary, depending on the severity of their illness. In other individuals, no dosage adjustments are necessary for months at a time.

    (4) Nonresponse. It is not uncommon to see relapses in patients whose schizophrenia was once under control because they no longer respond to an agent.

        (a) The choice of medication should be reassessed. Several alternative drugs are available. Use of an agent in another chemical class may help, or the addition of augmenting medication may be indicated.

        (b) Incapacitating side effects (e.g., akathisia, severe parkinsonism) may interfere with response to typical antipsychotics. The occurrence of tardive dyskinesia may necessitate the switch to another drug such as an atypical antipsychotic.

        (c) Blood levels should be obtained when possible. The results may indicate if an effective therapeutic blood level has been reached or exceeded. Noncompliance can sometimes also be identified.

        (d) Although waiting weeks to months to ascertain response is not inappropriate, this approach can rarely be implemented in this day of reduced hospital length of stay and community treatment.

  d. Route of administration

    (1) Oral forms. Almost all antipsychotics are available in pill, capsule, or elixir preparations for ease of administration. However, many patients with schizophrenia may have trouble adhering to an orally administered regimen.

    (2) Parenteral forms. Intramuscular and intravenous preparations of most first-generation antipsychotics are available. The parenteral route is necessary for patients who are too agitated or incapacitated to comply with treatment.

    (3) Long-acting injections. Depot formulations of two first-generation and three second-generation antipsychotics (fluphenazine, haloperidol, olanzapine, paliperidone, and risperidone) are available that are generally effective for 2 weeks (fluphenazine and risperidone) and 4 weeks (haloperidol, olanzapine, and paliperidone). Patients who prefer not to have to take medication on a daily basis may seek this route of administration. Physicians should also consider using this route in patients with a history of dangerous behavior and established noncompliance.

  e. Adverse effects

    (1) Extrapyramidal syndromes (EPSs) result from blockade of dopamine receptors in the basal ganglia and occur more commonly with the high-potency antipsychotics.

        (a) Acute dystonic reactions, which are more common in young male patients early in treatment, involve sudden tonic contractions of the muscles of the tongue, neck (**torticollis**), back (**opisthotonos**), mouth, and eyes (**oculogyric crises**). As well as being extremely frightening, such reactions can be dangerous if the patient's airway is compromised. These patients can be effectively treated with benztropine (1 to 2 mg intramuscularly) or diphenhydramine (25–50 mg intramuscularly or intravenously). Prophylaxis is accomplished with regular, orally administered anticholinergic medication.

        (b) Drug-induced parkinsonism is characterized by cogwheel rigidity, bradykinesia, tremor, loss of postural reflexes, mask-like facies, and drooling. It is more common in elderly patients, and although it usually occurs in the first weeks of treatment, it may appear at varying times with varying doses. It can be effectively treated with any of the antiparkinsonian medications (see Appendix) and may also respond to a decrease in the antipsychotic dosage. Antiparkinsonian agents can often be tapered off after 4 to 8 weeks of maintenance treatment for about half of patients taking typical antipsychotics. If these EPSs remain unresponsive, a trial of an atypical antipsychotic is indicated.

(c) **Akathisia** is a syndrome of motor restlessness, which may involve the entire body but is often most obvious in patients' inability to keep their legs and feet still. It can be mistaken for anxiety, agitation, or an increase in psychotic symptomatology. The akathisia may respond to antiparkinsonian agents, but if the patient responds poorly, a decrease in dosage or change to another antipsychotic is indicated. In some cases, akathisia can be successfully treated with propranolol, benzodiazepines, or vitamin E.

(d) **Antipsychotic-induced catatonia,** which occurs more commonly with the high-potency agents, is characterized by withdrawal; mutism; and motor abnormalities, including rigidity, immobility, and waxy flexibility. Although it can be mistaken for a worsening of patients' psychotic symptoms, it is a complication of antipsychotic therapy. It may represent a variant of the neuroleptic malignant syndrome. It should be treated by temporarily discontinuing antipsychotic therapy and, on resolution, changing to a different class of antipsychotic. Amantadine, 100 mg orally three times daily, may also be helpful.

(e) **Tardive dyskinesia** is a late-onset movement disorder that is thought to result from a disturbance in the dopamine–acetylcholine balance in the basal ganglia. Mechanisms theorized to account for this phenomenon include an increase in the numbers or sensitivity of dopamine receptors in certain parts of the brain after chronic blockade with antipsychotics. However, these theories do not fit all the data about the physiology of this condition.

   (i) **Fasciculations of the tongue** may be the earliest symptom, followed by **lingual–facial hyperkinesias,** which are persistent involuntary chewing, smacking, or grimacing movements.

   (ii) **Choreoathetotic movements of the extremities and trunk,** including the respiratory muscles, can be extremely disabling in severe cases. The symptoms are often noticeable when there is a dosage reduction or discontinuation of antipsychotic medication, but they can usually be detected by close examination between antipsychotic doses.

   (iii) The syndrome can usually be reversed if it is detected early and antipsychotics are discontinued.

   (iv) In severe cases, tardive dyskinesia may be irreversible and can progress with continued antipsychotic treatment.

   (v) Symptoms are worsened by anticholinergic medication, which should be discontinued if possible.

   (vi) Increased doses of antipsychotics may cause apparent temporary improvement by increasing the dopamine receptor blockade. However, this ultimately causes further progression of the movement disorder.

   (vii) Patients should be screened every 6 months for early signs and should be maintained on the lowest possible dose to minimize this serious complication of long-term antipsychotic use.

   (viii) Patients withdrawn abruptly from antipsychotics sometimes demonstrate a **withdrawal–emergent dyskinesia** with transient features of tardive dyskinesia that lasts for several days. It is unclear whether this syndrome is an early form of tardive dyskinesia or has another pathophysiologic mechanism.

(2) **Neuroleptic malignant syndrome,** a potentially life-threatening complication of antipsychotic therapy, is characterized by muscular rigidity, fever, autonomic instability, and an altered level of consciousness. Onset of the full-blown syndrome is rapid over 1 to 2 days after a period of gradual progressive rigidity. Treatment involves immediate discontinuation of the antipsychotic medication and support of respiratory, renal, and cardiovascular functioning and possibly treatment with dantrolene or bromocriptine.

(3) **Anticholinergic effects occur with low-potency antipsychotics at a higher rate than with the high-potency antipsychotics.** Anticholinergic effects are often seen as a direct result of treatment with a combination of drugs, including antipsychotics, anticholinergic agents used to treat parkinsonian side effects of the antipsychotics, and the inappropriate use of medications from other classes such as the tricyclic antidepressants. In extreme cases of polypharmacy, combinations (e.g., a low-potency antipsychotic, a tricyclic antidepressant,

and one or more anticholinergic agents) may produce a **life-threatening anticholinergic delirium.** Clinicians must watch for the development of increasing psychotic symptoms with the addition of more or different medications to a patient's treatment plan and should suspect anticholinergic delirium in these circumstances. **Anticholinergic side effects include the following:**

  (a) **At low doses,** effects include blurred vision when changing from close to distant objects, dry mouth, urinary retention in men with enlarged prostate glands, and constipation.

  (b) **Anticholinergic poisoning** occurs at **high doses.** Signs and symptoms include restless agitation; confusion; disorientation; hallucinations; delusions; hot, flushed, dry skin; pupil dilation; tachycardia; decreased bowel sounds; and urinary retention. Central anticholinergic poisoning may occur without obvious physiologic signs, making iatrogenic anticholinergic poisoning a particularly insidious risk of polypharmacy.

  (c) **Anticholinergic abuse.** Because of the ability of anticholinergic agents to alter consciousness, patients sometimes abuse prescriptions for anticholinergic agents. Clinicians should treat parkinsonian symptoms with drugs with low antimuscarinic effects (e.g., amantadine) in at-risk patients.

  (4) **Cardiovascular effects** of antipsychotics most commonly include orthostatic hypotension, particularly in elderly patients, which results from adrenergic blockade. This symptom is most commonly associated with the low-potency antipsychotics. In rare cases, antipsychotics may be associated with serious ventricular arrhythmias with electrocardiographic (ECG) abnormalities (i.e., T-wave changes, prolonged QT intervals) and with cardiac repolarization abnormalities. Risks of all cardiovascular complications are greatest with the low-potency antipsychotics.

  (5) **Hypothalamic effects** may include changes in libido, appetite, and temperature regulation. Hypersecretion of prolactin by the hypothalamus can be induced by dopaminergic blockades. Hyperprolactinemia may result in loss of sexual functioning, amenorrhea, breast enlargement, and galactorrhea.

  (6) **Jaundice** and elevation of liver enzymes may occur with any of the antipsychotics. Physicians should monitor patients for signs of hepatic problems and consider testing of liver enzyme and bilirubin levels when indicated.

  (7) **Agranulocytosis** is a rare and unpredictable reaction to antipsychotics and many other types of medications. Patients should be told to report spontaneous bruises, infections that do not resolve, or cuts that do not heal. Agranulocytosis can usually be reversed when detected early enough but has caused death in patients who are taking antipsychotics.

  (8) **Dermatologic effects** include allergic rashes, which respond to discontinuation of the drug, and photosensitivity, which can be treated with sunscreen.

  (9) **Ophthalmologic effects** include a pigmentary retinopathy associated with thioridazine in doses greater than 800 mg/day. Rarely, lens and corneal pigmentation has been reported with chlorpromazine, thioridazine, and thiothixene after long-term treatment. Blurred vision and worsening of narrow-angle glaucoma secondary to anticholinergic effects are more common.

2. **Second-generation antipsychotics.** The newest drugs for the treatment of schizophrenia are sometimes referred to as atypical antipsychotics. They have begun a new era in the treatment of schizophrenia, helping some patients who were previously thought to be resistant to treatment and decreasing the risk of EPSs and tardive dyskinesia.

  a. **Clozapine.** This agent was the first second-generation antipsychotic marketed as such in the United States.

   (1) **Pharmacology**

     (a) Structurally, clozapine is a dibenzodiazepine.

     (b) The specific mechanism of action of clozapine and all second-generation antipsychotics is not yet fully understood. To a small extent, clozapine blocks D-1 receptors in the mesolimbic and cortical areas of the brain but has little effect on dopamine receptors in the striatum, possibly accounting for some of its unique properties such as significant improvement in negative symptoms while causing few EPSs.

(2) Clinical effects. The effects of clozapine differ significantly from those of earlier antipsychotic agents. In addition to reducing the positive symptoms of schizophrenia, clozapine reduces negative symptoms in some patients. It appears to have a markedly reduced propensity to produce complications such as neuroleptic malignant syndrome, EPS, and tardive dyskinesia. Clozapine also appears to convey particular benefits reducing suicidal or aggressive behaviors in patients with psychosis.

(3) Use. The physician must register with a system of care, which includes a pharmacist and a clinician to perform monitoring functions. Initially, weekly blood tests must be performed, and patients must be located if they fail to report for tests. Clearly informing patients of all the risks is quite complicated.

(4) Dosage and administration. It is recommended that clozapine be initiated at 12.5 mg once or twice a day, very slowly increasing to an average of 300 to 600 mg/day over a 2-week period. In severe cases, doses may be gradually titrated up to 900 mg/day. A fast dissolving form of clozapine is available, but there are no short- or long-acting intramuscular formulations.

(5) Side effects. Significant adverse effects may occur.

    (a) The risk of life-threatening **agranulocytosis** requires intensive monitoring of the patient's complete blood count (CBC) and state of health. Patients may not be started on clozapine if their initial white count is below $3,500/mm^3$. White blood cell count and absolute neutrophil count must be done weekly for the first 6 months and then possibly less frequently if counts have been stable. **Febrile conditions** occur in the first few weeks after initiation of the drug. However, febrile conditions may represent infections secondary to agranulocytosis. Therefore, any fever in a patient taking clozapine must receive an aggressive and expert workup.

    (b) Seizures may occur with clozapine treatment, particularly at higher dosages.

    (c) Cardiovascular adverse events with clozapine have included **myocarditis, heart failure, and respiratory or cardiac arrest,** necessitating the slow titration of dosage.

    (d) Sedation can be excessive, particularly in the early stages of treatment. **Excessive salivation,** especially at night, may be a serious problem for some patients. Unlike sedation, excessive salivation seems to be a more persistent side effect. Although some treatments (e.g., anticholinergic drugs) are available, each treatment carries its own risks.

    (e) Weight gain may occur in more than 50% of patients taking clozapine. Development of **metabolic syndrome** with hyperglycemia and hyperlipidemias must be monitored on a regular basis.

    (f) Other side effects such as nausea and gastrointestinal (GI) disturbances are fairly common. Headache occurs fairly often.

(6) Special issues. Because of potentially lethal agranulocytosis, clozapine is available in the United States under a unique prescribing arrangement. About 30% of treatment-resistant schizophrenic patients may benefit significantly from clozapine, but the many significant side effects still limit the clinical use of the medication to patients who have more severe schizophrenia or who have failed trials of other atypical antipsychotics.

b. Risperidone

  (1) Pharmacology

    (a) Structurally, risperidone is a benzisoxazole.

    (b) The specific mechanism of action of risperidone is best attributed to antagonism of dopamine D-2 receptors and serotonergic 5HT-2 receptors.

  (2) Clinical effects. At lower doses risperidone relieves positive symptoms well, while negative symptoms may also improve but not to the same degree as with clozapine. At high doses **extrapyramidal symptoms** become more likely with risperidone, unlike with clozapine.

  (3) Use. Prescribing risperidone has few unusual precautions other than monitoring for metabolic syndrome, as with all antipsychotics.

  (4) Dosage and administration. Risperidone is usually administered in twice-daily doses, starting at 1 mg twice daily and increasing to 3 mg twice daily over the first few days. Convenient dosage forms (as low as 0.25 mg) have made this drug popular for treating patients requiring only minimal dosages of antipsychotics. A rapidly dissolving sol-tab is available for patients who have difficulty taking tablets. Risperidone was the first second-generation antipsychotic available in a long-acting (2 weeks) depot antipsychotic formulation.

(5) **Side effects.** Unfortunately, at higher dosages, risperidone begins to exert less specific blockade of dopamine receptors and can cause EPSs in some patients.

(a) Because **increased prolactin secretion** is common (as with older dopamine-blocking agents), galactorrhea, gynecomastia, amenorrhea, and sexual performance dysfunction can be expected in some patients.

(b) **QTc prolongation** may occur but is rarely clinically significant.

(c) Weight gain is not common with risperidone use, but patients must be monitored for weight, hyperglycemia, hypertension, and dyslipidemias.

(d) **Other side effects** include insomnia, agitation, dizziness, and constipation.

c. **Paliperidone**

(1) **Pharmacology**

(a) Paliperidone is a human active metabolite of risperidone.

(b) The specific mechanism of action of paliperidone is best attributed to antagonism of dopamine D-2 receptors and serotonergic 5HT-2 receptors.

(2) **Clinical effects.** Paliperidone relieves positive symptoms well, while negative symptoms may also improve.

(3) **Use.** Prescribing paliperidone has few unusual precautions other than monitoring for metabolic syndrome, as with all antipsychotics.

(4) **Dosage and administration.** Paliperidone is usually administered as a 6-mg extended-release tablet in the morning. Some patients may benefit from only 3 mg daily, while some may need 9 or 12 mg daily. Once effectiveness and tolerability are established with oral administration, some patients may benefit from switching to paliperidone palmitate, a long-acting (4-week) depot antipsychotic formulation.

(5) **Side effects.** At higher dosages, paliperidone would be expected to exert less specific blockade of dopamine receptors, causing EPSs in some patients.

(a) Because **increased prolactin secretion** is common (as with older dopamine-blocking agents), galactorrhea, gynecomastia, amenorrhea, and sexual performance dysfunction can be expected in some patients.

(b) **QTc prolongation** may occur but is rarely clinically significant.

(c) Weight gain is not common with paliperidone use, but patients must be monitored for weight, hyperglycemia, hypertension, and hyperlipidemias.

(d) **Other side effects** include insomnia, agitation, dizziness, and constipation.

d. **Olanzapine.** Olanzapine can be very effective for treating negative symptoms, and it is not commonly known to cause EPSs.

(1) **Pharmacology**

(a) Structurally, olanzapine is a thienobenzodiazepine.

(b) The specific mechanism of action of olanzapine is best attributed to antagonism of dopamine D-2 receptors and serotonergic 5HT-2 receptors. Blockade of histamine receptors may be responsible for the sedation known to occur with olanzapine.

(2) **Clinical effects.** The effects of olanzapine more closely approximate clozapine than any other second-generation antipsychotic, with significant relief from both positive and negative symptoms. It has a markedly reduced propensity to produce complications such as neuroleptic malignant syndrome, EPSs, and tardive dyskinesia.

(3) **Use.** Prescribing olanzapine is relatively easy, as there are multiple dosage options and multiple routes of administration.

(4) **Dosage and administration.** Usually olanzapine is administered in once-daily doses, starting at 5 to 10 mg/day and increasing up to 30 mg/day over the first few days. An orally disintegrating tablet is available for patients who have difficulty taking oral medications. Olanzapine is one of only three second-generation antipsychotics currently available in a fast-acting intramuscular injectable formulation. Very recently a long-acting, once-monthly injectable form of depot olanzapine pamoate monohydrate became available in the United States.

(5) Side effects. Unfortunately, at higher doses, weight gain becomes a concern with olanzapine. Up to 50% of olanzapine patients experience weight gain and worrisome rates of hyperglycemia and hyperlipidemias.

    (a) Other side effects include sedation, dry mouth, and constipation.

e. Quetiapine. Quetiapine can be very effective for treating negative symptoms, and some patients report decreased symptoms of anxiety.

    (1) Pharmacology

        (a) Structurally, quetiapine is a dibenzothiazepine derivative.

        (b) The specific mechanism of action is best attributed to antagonism of dopamine D-2 receptors and serotonergic 5HT-2 receptors. Very rapid dissociation from the D-2 receptor may account for the striking lack of EPSs with quetiapine.

    (2) Clinical effects. Lower doses of quetiapine are used for their tranquilizing effect. Higher doses are needed to achieve relief from severe symptoms of schizophrenia. Patients report more relief from anxiety than with any other second-generation antipsychotic.

    (3) Use. Prescribing quetiapine has no unusual precautions other than monitoring for metabolic syndrome, as with all antipsychotics.

    (4) Dosage and administration. Quetiapine is usually administered in twice-daily doses, starting at 100 to 200 mg/day and increasing up to 800 mg/day over the first week. An extended-release formula allows for more rapid titration.

    (5) Side effects. Sedation is the most commonly reported side effect of quetiapine.

        (a) Weight gain is known to occur with quetiapine, and patients must be monitored for metabolic syndrome.

f. Ziprasidone. Ziprasidone can be very effective for treating both positive and negative symptoms, and some patients report improvement in depressed moods.

    (1) Pharmacology

        (a) Structurally, ziprasidone is a benzothiazolylpiperazine.

        (b) The specific mechanism of action is attributed to blockade of both dopamine and serotonin receptors. Ziprasidone uniquely provides partial agonist activity at the 5HT-1a receptor and reuptake inhibition of serotonin and norepinephrine, possibly creating an antidepressant effect.

    (2) Clinical effects. The effects of ziprasidone do not differ significantly from those of other second-generation antipsychotic agents.

    (3) Use. Prescribing ziprasidone has no unusual precautions other than monitoring for metabolic syndrome, as with all antipsychotics. However, ziprasidone should not be administered to patients with a family history of prolonged QT syndrome or recent cardiac problems that can increase the QT interval.

    (4) Dosage and administration. Ziprasidone is usually administered in once-daily doses, starting at 40 to 80 mg daily and increasing up to 200 mg/day over the first week. Ziprasidone is one of only three atypical antipsychotics currently available in an intramuscular injectable formulation.

    (5) Side effects. Agitation is the most commonly reported side effect of ziprasidone, with some patients developing akathisia.

        (a) QTc prolongation is known to occur with ziprasidone, requiring electrocardiographic clearance in patients with cardiac histories.

        (b) Weight gain is not common with ziprasidone, but patients must still be monitored for weight, hyperglycemia, hypertension, and hyperlipidemias.

        (c) Other side effects include dizziness, GI effects, sedation, and lightheadedness.

g. Aripiprazole. Aripiprazole can be very effective for treating negative symptoms.

    (1) Pharmacology

        (a) Structurally, aripiprazole is a quinolone derivative.

        (b) The specific mechanism of action of aripiprazole is best attributed to antagonism of dopamine D-2 receptors and serotonergic 5HT-2 receptors. However, aripiprazole actually can function as a partial agonist to dopamine D-2 receptors, resulting in minimal risk of EPSs and hyperprolactinemia.

    (2) Clinical effects. Although blockade of some dopamine and serotonin receptors occurs, partial agonist activities at D-3 and 5HT-1a make aripiprazole unique among the second-generation antipsychotics and a unique option for patients who have adverse effects or limited response to other agents.

(3) **Use.** Prescribing aripiprazole is relatively easy, as there is a narrow range of dosage options and it has the fewest side effects of any other antipsychotic.

(4) **Dosage and administration.** Aripiprazole is usually administered in once-daily doses, starting at 10 to 15 mg/day and increasing up to 30 mg/day over the first few weeks. There is both a rapidly dissolving tablet form and a quick-acting intramuscular injectable form.

(5) **Side effects.** Agitation, anxiety, and insomnia are reported side effects of aripiprazole, and some patients find these side effects difficult to tolerate.

(a) Patients rarely gain weight while taking aripiprazole, but weight, hyperglycemia, and hyperlipidemia must be monitored with all atypical antipsychotics.

(b) **Other side effects** include GI effects and lightheadedness.

h. **Iloperidone** is one of the newest second-generation antipsychotics, just becoming widely available in 2010.

(1) **Pharmacology**

(a) Structurally, iloperidone is a piperidinyl-benzisoxazole derivative.

(b) The specific mechanism of action of iloperidone is best attributed to antagonism of dopamine D-2 receptors and serotonergic 5HT-2 receptors. α-1 Receptor blockade may also contribute to the effectiveness of iloperidone.

(2) **Clinical effects.** Iloperidone reduces both positive and negative symptoms in some patients. There is some risk of hypotension from α-1 receptor blockade.

(3) **Use.** Prescribing iloperidone may be complicated initially and a slow titration schedule should be used to avoid hypotension.

(4) **Dosage and administration.** It is recommended that iloperidone be initiated at 1 mg twice daily, slowly adding 1 mg bid daily over a 1-week period to get to a target dose of 12 mg bid.

(5) **Side effects.** Sedation and dizziness were the most commonly reported side effects of iloperidone, with some patients developing syncope.

(a) **QTc prolongation** is known to occur with iloperidone, requiring electrocardiographic clearance in patients with cardiac histories.

(b) Because **increased prolactin secretion** is common (as with older dopamine-blocking agents), galactorrhea, gynecomastia, amenorrhea, and sexual performance dysfunction can be expected in some patients.

(c) Weight gain has been noted with iloperidone, and patients must be monitored for weight, hyperglycemia, hypertension, and hyperlipidemias.

(d) **Other side effects** include dry mouth, GI effects, and tachycardia.

i. **Asenapine** is one of the newest second-generation antipsychotics, just becoming widely available in 2010.

(1) **Pharmacology**

(a) Structurally, asenapine is a dibenzo-oxepino pyrrole.

(b) The specific mechanism of action of asenapine is best attributed to antagonism of dopamine D-2 receptors and serotonergic 5HT-2 receptors.

(2) **Clinical effects.** Asenapine reduces both positive and negative symptoms in some patients.

(3) **Use.** Prescribing asenapine is relatively uncomplicated, as there is a rather limited dosage range.

(4) **Dosage and administration.** It is recommended that asenapine be initiated at 5 mg twice daily. A few patients may benefit from increasing to 10 mg bid. Asenapine is only available in the United States in a sublingual tablet form.

(5) **Side effects.** Somnolence and akathisia were the more commonly reported side effects of asenapine.

3. **Other pharmacologic agents.** Although antipsychotics are the drugs of choice in the treatment of schizophrenia, it is sometimes necessary to turn to other classes if patients are nonresponsive or intolerant of side effects of antipsychotics. Augmentation strategies for nonresponse are covered in some of the schizophrenia treatment algorithms.

a. **Anticonvulsants and lithium.** The addition of a mood stabilizer is recommended for the treatment of patients who have not achieved a satisfactory response to trials of antipsychotics alone.

(1) **Valproate** can be effective. This agent can be added to clozapine to treat clozapine-induced seizures without substantially increasing the risk of agranulocytosis.

(2) **Carbamazepine** can also be effective but should never be used with clozapine.

(3) Newer anticonvulsants such as **gabapentin, topiramate,** and **lamotrigine** may also be useful in adjunctive treatment.

(4) In patients with significant affective symptoms, including signs of mood swings, **lithium** has also been found to be an effective adjunctive agent.

b. **Antidepressants.** Patients with a history of schizophrenia may develop full diagnostic criteria of depression. All classes of antidepressants are worth trying for patients with signs of **significant schizophrenia and depression.**

Some of the **newer antidepressants,** such as the selective serotonin reuptake inhibitors (SSRIs), may be useful in patients in whom **panic attacks** or **obsessive-compulsive disorder (OCD)–like syndromes** occur. According to some reports, atypical antipsychotics may precipitate OCD symptoms.

c. **Anxiolytics and sedatives.** Agitation in schizophrenia can be severe and life threatening.

(1) **Benzodiazepines** are frequently used in the short-term treatment of agitation in schizophrenia. These agents, particularly lorazepam, are also the drugs of choice in adjunctive management of catatonic schizophrenia. However, although patients with both akathisia and tardive dyskinesia may respond to benzodiazepines, long-term use of these drugs can be problematic; as many as 50% of all patients with schizophrenia have had substance abuse problems. Benzodiazepines should be avoided when clozapine is used, and they should never be used when the clozapine dose is being titrated initially.

(2) **Barbiturates** are no longer commonly used in the therapy of schizophrenia, but they are sometimes used as a treatment of last resort in agitated psychotic patients who do not respond to high doses of antipsychotics and benzodiazepines.

d. **β-Blockers.** These agents are effective in the treatment of akathisia, and they may be effective against some medication-induced tremors. Propranolol is frequently used for this purpose, and longer-acting, less lipophylic agents may be more convenient in long-term treatment. In addition, propranolol has shown promise in treating some cases of severe psychosis and cases of severe aggression. Pindolol, which actually has some serotonergic activity, may have other uses in psychiatry (e.g., as an adjunct treatment with antidepressants).

H **Electroconvulsive therapy (ECT)** Until modern medications for use in schizophrenia treatment were developed, ECT was the only effective treatment option available. ECT still plays an important role in the therapy of treatment-resistant schizophrenia. Current treatment algorithms indicate that ECT should be considered after three or four drug trials. ECT is likely most effective in patients with affective symptoms and in catatonia.

1. **Indications**

a. When life-threatening circumstances such as severe catatonia or extreme suicidal ideation are present

b. When massive doses of antipsychotics become disabling and patients can be maintained on standard doses of antipsychotics after ECT

c. When patients are clearly refractory to standard treatments and augmentations

2. **Difficulties.** The negative public perception of ECT and risks of anesthesia make this a difficult course when treating schizophrenia outside of academic centers. It can be very difficult to establish informed consent to use ECT in patients with schizophrenia.

Study Questions

Directions: *Each of the numbered items or incomplete statements in this section is followed by answers or by completions of the statement. Select the ONE lettered answer or completion that is BEST in each case.*

1. A 34-year-old woman complains that she is gaining weight since she started taking chlorpromazine for chronic undifferentiated schizophrenia. A complete review of systems and history shows evidence of breast enlargement and lactation. However, a serum pregnancy test is negative. Which of the following antipsychotics would be a good choice for a treatment change?

- [A] Fluphenazine   T
- [B] Haloperidol   T
- [C] Paliperidone   A
- [D] Perphenazine   T
- [E] Aripiprazole   A

2. A 32-year-old woman is brought to the emergency department by her family. They report that she has been acting strangely for the past 2 weeks since coming home abruptly from a job assignment out of state. In addition, they mention her rapid speech. The woman states that she has been hearing voices and seeing small creatures out of the corner of her eye. She presents with an agitated and restless manner. Which of the following is the next appropriate treatment step?

r/o med condition

- [A] Interview the family to complete a genogram.
- [B] Start a second-generation depot antipsychotic.
- [C] Perform a complete physical examination and consider laboratory tests.
- [D] Send the patient to the nearest state hospital for treatment.
- [E] Order psychological testing.

3. A 40-year-old man presents to a mental health center complaining that his neighbors have been spying on him. He reports a complicated delusion: the Federal Reserve Bank is conspiring to take away his home. He denies any hallucinations or mood changes, and he has been able to work as a truck mechanic without loss of function. Which of the following diagnoses is most appropriate?

- [A] Schizophreniform disorder
- [B] Major depression with psychotic features
- [C] Schizoaffective disorder
- [D] Delusional disorder
- [E] Schizophrenia

4. A 29-year-old man who lives in a group home and takes perphenazine on a daily basis develops a high fever and muscle rigidity. The man undergoes examination and testing at the local emergency department, where a creatine phosphokinase value comes back as 10,000. Which of the following therapeutic steps should be taken next?

NMS

- [A] Send the patient home on an atypical antipsychotic.
- [B] Send the patient home with instructions to take acetaminophen every 4 hours.
- [C] Admit the patient to a state hospital.
- [D] Admit the patient to an intensive care unit.
- [E] Send the patient home on benztropine (2 mg tid).

5. The patient described in Question 4 has been hospitalized but plans to return to the community. The treating psychiatrist recommends which of the following changes in the medication regimen?

- [A] Changing to fluphenazine decanoate
- [B] Decrease dose of perphenazine
- [C] Adding lithium
- [D] Adding trihexyphenidyl
- [E] Changing to clozapine   A to atypical

6. A disheveled 27-year-old man presents with bizarre movements, agitated behavior, and rapid and unintelligible speech. The patient has had signs of psychosis for much of the past few months, and the family reports that the patient twice spent a month in state psychiatric hospitals. Which of the following schizophrenic subtypes can most appropriately be applied to this patient?

- A Chronic undifferentiated
- B Catatonic
- C Residual
- D Paranoid

7. A 45-year-old woman with no psychiatric history presents with disheveled appearance, almost mute speech, and thought blocking of several months' duration. She also fears that her internal organs have been stolen by a transplant surgeon to be used in a military robot. Which of the following diagnoses is most appropriate?

- A Schizoaffective disorder
- B Borderline personality disorder
- C Delusional disorder
- D Schizophrenia
- E Bipolar disorder

8. A 24-year-old man is discharged from the psychiatric ward with a diagnosis of paranoid schizophrenia. Four weeks after discharge, he tells his psychiatrist that he stopped taking his medications 2 days ago. Which of the following interventions is most appropriate?

- A Discharge the patient from the clinic.
- B Hospitalize the patient in a psychiatric ward.
- C Refer for psychotherapy.
- D Switch to a depot antipsychotic.
- E Inquire about side effects from the medication.

9. The patient described in Question 8 reports that although he receives Social Security Disability Income (SSDI), he has not been able to afford all of his medication. Which of the following interventions is most appropriate?

- A Rehospitalize the patient in a psychiatric ward.
- B Switch to a less expensive antipsychotic.
- C Inquire into how he has budgeted his money.
- B Refer the patient for psychotherapy.
- E Discharge the patient from the clinic.

10. The patient described in Question 8 reports that he has been giving much of his money away to panhandlers. Which of the following interventions is most appropriate?

- A Inquire into how he can get a larger disability check.
- B Rehospitalize the patient in the psychiatric ward.
- C Refer the patient for case management.
- D Refer the patient for psychosurgery.
- E Discharge the patient from the clinic.

Directions: *The response options for items 11–14 are the same. Select one answer for each question in the set. Match the clinical picture with the type of drug that could change the situation.*

- A Anticholinergics
- B Depot haloperidol
- C Barbiturates
- D Benzodiazepines
- E Aripiprazole

11. A patient who is sometimes agitated has been tried on several different first- and second-generation antipsychotics with little success. D → calm his ass down

12. A patient who responded to perphenazine develops a pill-rolling tremor and shuffling gait.

A

13. A patient has a positive response to antipsychotic medication in the hospital but becomes noncompliant shortly after five discharges in 1 year.

B

14. A patient has hallucinations that respond to haloperidol but severe negative symptoms prevent successful discharge from the state hospital.

E

Directions: *The response options for items 15–18 are the same. Select one answer for each question in the set. Match the following diagnostic criteria with the most likely diagnosis.*

[A] Brief psychotic disorder
[B] Delusional disorder
[C] Schizophreniform disorder
[D] Schizophrenia
[E] Schizoaffective disorder

15. A patient presents with hallucinations and bizarre delusions lasting 6 weeks.

C

16. A patient presents with periods of mood disturbance with psychosis and periods of psychosis without mood disturbance over the past 3 years.

E

17. A patient presents with a second lifetime episode of hallucinations and bizarre delusions that again lasts only a few days.

A

18. A patient who otherwise appears normal presents with a 5-month belief that a prominent racecar driver has fallen madly in love with him; he believes she demonstrates her love by painting the patient's age as the number on her car.

B

Answers and Explanations

1. The answer is E [*VII G 2 g*]. Aripiprazole does not cause hyperprolactinemia, which can occur with fluphenazine, haloperidol, paliperidone, and perphenazine.

2. The answer is C [*VI A 3*]. Acute medical causes of psychotic symptoms must be ruled out through a complete physical examination and any indicated medical tests.

3. The answer is D [*VI C 3 a, b*]. Delusional disorder often occurs later in life and lacks the global functional deterioration seen in individuals with schizophrenia and schizophreniform disorder. Diagnosis of schizoaffective disorder or psychotic depression requires substantial mood changes.

4. The answer is D [*VII G 1 e (2)*]. Neuroleptic malignant syndrome is potentially life threatening and requires admission to an intensive care unit for support of respiratory, renal, and cardiovascular functioning.

5. The answer is E [*VII G 2 a*]. Switching to an atypical antipsychotic would reduce the risk of another episode. Clozapine would be the best choice of antipsychotic. Lithium is not indicated by this history. Trihexyphenidyl will not help neuroleptic malignant syndrome.

6. The answer is B [*IV I 1 a, b*]. Catatonia is distinguished by either a dramatic increase or dramatic decrease in motor activity. Chronic undifferentiated, paranoid, and residual subtypes do not involve significant changes in movements.

7. The answer is D [*V A*]. In women, the onset of schizophrenia can occur much later than in men. Individuals with bipolar disorder or schizoaffective disorder would normally have had prior episodes. This patient has deteriorated too much to have delusional disorder and has been psychotic too long to have psychosis in a personality disorder.

8. The answer is E [*VII G 1 b (2), c (4) (b)*]. Side effects are a common cause of nonadherence to treatment. Consideration of side effects and their importance should be the first step in evaluation of nonadherence. Nonadherence to treatment is a common clinical challenge and must be managed in a way that keeps the patient in treatment.

9. The answer is C [*VII E 2 d, e*]. Nonadherence to a medication regimen for financial reasons may have a complex cause and must be thoroughly investigated. This patient does not meet current admission criteria for rehospitalization. Do not automatically switch to a cheaper medication because free drug programs or other psychosocial interventions may keep this patient on the best regimen. Psychotherapy can help but cannot replace medication in most cases.

10. The answer is C [*VII E 1, 2 d*]. Financial management poses a substantial problem for many patients but can be improved through case management and/or psychosocial rehabilitation.

11. The answer is D [*VII G 3 c (1)*]. The agitation of akathisia can be treated with benzodiazepines. Anticholinergics rarely work to reduce akathisia. Barbiturates are used only in extremely rare cases of prolonged agitation. Depot antipsychotics could prolong the time at risk for akathisia. Aripiprazole may cause agitation and akathisia.

12. The answer is A [*VII G 1 e (1) (a)*]. Anticholinergics are indicated for treating extrapyramidal syndromes (EPSs) that occur as a result of antipsychotic use. The pill-rolling tremor and shuffling gait of EPSs often respond to anticholinergics. Use of an atypical antipsychotic is not always the best choice when a patient already responds to a typical antipsychotic. Benzodiazepines and barbiturates are not the primary choice for treating EPSs. Aripiprazole would be a second choice if EPSs did not respond to treatment.

13. The answer is B [*VII G 1 d (3)*]. Depot antipsychotics are a proven way to better ensure compliance in such a "heavy-dose" patient. Compliance cannot be assured with the other options.

14. The answer is E [*VII G 2*]. Any second-generation antipsychotic would be the best treatment for negative symptoms. Negative symptoms are the primary indication for use of the more expensive second-generation antipsychotics. There is no reason to expect a response to anticholinergics, benzodiazepines, barbiturates, or depot haloperidol.

15. The answer is C [*VI C 2*]. Schizophreniform disorder involves psychotic symptoms lasting longer than 2 weeks but less than 6 months.

16. The answer is E [*VI B 4*]. Schizoaffective disorder involves both periods of mood disturbance with psychosis and periods of psychosis without mood disturbance.

17. The answer is A [*VI C 1*]. Brief psychotic disorder involves periods of psychosis lasting less than 1 month. This disorder can recur later in life.

18. The answer is B [*VI C 3*]. Delusional disorder lacks the global functional deterioration seen in schizophrenia and schizophreniform disorder. In the erotomanic type of delusional disorder, patients believe someone (usually of a higher status) has fallen in love with them. Brief psychotic disorder involves periods of psychosis lasting less than 1 month.

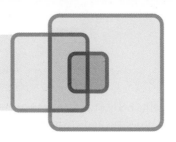

chapter 3

Mood Disorders

MEERA NARASIMHAN

I INTRODUCTION

The prominent feature of mood disorders is a **disturbance of mood** along the happy–sad axis. The *Diagnostic and Statistical Manual of Mental Disorders,* 4th edition, text revision (*DSM-IV-TR*), classifies mood disorders to include **major depressive disorder, bipolar I disorder, bipolar II disorder, dysthymic disorder, cyclothymic disorder, mood disorder caused by a general medical condition, and substance-induced mood disorder.**

The etiology and classification of mood disorders have been researched since the middle of the nineteenth century. As in other areas of psychiatry and medicine, prevailing theories have viewed mood disorders both as a biologically based illness and as a psychologically based illness.

A Nineteenth century In the **mid- to late nineteenth century,** a number of clinicians began to see the possibility of differentiating forms of "insanity."

1. **Emil Kraepelin** noted that some psychotic patients endorsed a cyclical pattern and prominent mood symptoms (manic depression), while others had a more chronic pattern that also featured cognitive impairment (i.e., **dementia praecox,** now called **schizophrenia**).

2. At the turn of the twentieth century, neuropathologists found abnormal brains in patients with Alzheimer disease and neurosyphilis. Many assumed that brain disease was also the cause of schizophrenia and depression.

B Twentieth century In the twentieth century, particularly in the United States, psychoanalytic theorists believed that many mood disorders stemmed from the psychological response to loss. Experts often differentiated between **endogenous** (caused by biologic factors) and **exogenous** (caused by loss or other environmental stresses) depression.

1. The **first half of the century** laid greater emphasis on psychological factors and limited research efforts on the neurochemical and neuroanatomic aspects of mood disorders.

2. In the **1950s,** the serendipitous observation that two drugs affect depression stimulated appreciation of the biologic underpinnings of mood disorders.
   a. **Iproniazid,** which was being studied as a treatment for tuberculosis, elevated the mood of (often depressed) patients. Knowledge that this drug acted as a **monoamine oxidase (MAO) inhibitor** led to speculation that low levels of monoamines (e.g., norepinephrine [NE], serotonin [5-HT], dopamine) might play a role in the etiology of depression.
   b. **Reserpine,** an antihypertensive drug that **depletes monoamines** presynaptically, caused depression in some patients.

C Twenty-first century As advances in understanding the neurobiologic underpinnings of mood disorders continue, experts currently believe that the interaction of biologic (neurochemical, neuroanatomic, and genetics) and psychosocial factors determines which individuals have a predilection to develop mood disorders. The exogenous–endogenous dichotomy is no longer seen as a critical distinction because patients with and without obvious environmental causes of depression can have similar prognoses and treatment responses.

Over the years there has been a growing body of evidence to suggest that mood disorders result from a complex interplay between biologic processes and environmental factors suggestive of a multifactorial etiology.

A Genetic factors Both major depressive and bipolar disorders run in families, which does not necessarily indicate genetic transmission. However, a variety of research techniques have shown the etiology of mood disorders to be at least partly genetic.

1. **Family studies**
   a. **Major depressive disorder.** Approximately 50% of individuals with major depressive disorder have a first-degree relative with a mood disorder, which is more often depression than bipolar disorder. Whereas concordance for identical twins is approximately 50%, siblings (including fraternal twins) have an approximate 15% risk. When one twin of a concordant pair has major depression, the other twin usually has depression rather than bipolar illness.
   b. **Bipolar disorder.** Approximately 90% of people with bipolar illness have a first-degree relative with a mood disorder, either bipolar or depressive. Estimates of concordance range between 33% and 90% for monozygotic twins and between 5% and 25% for other siblings. If the twin of a bipolar patient becomes ill, the twin will usually have a bipolar disorder.

2. **Adoption studies** in both major depression and bipolar disorder have supported a genetic etiology.

3. **Linkage studies.** Genetic epidemiologic studies have shown that genetic factors play an important role in the pathophysiology of mood disorders; therefore, molecular genetics studies using either the linkage approach or the candidate gene approach and association studies have been performed extensively .
   a. Linkage studies have shown some candidate locations that have been reproduced in two or more studies, such as 1q21-42, 4p16, 10q21-26, 11p15, 12q11-32, 18p11, 18q21-22, 22q11-13, Xp11, and Xq24-28.
   b. Studies have suggested that bipolar disorder is inherited in some families in an **X-linked pattern.**
   c. **Other linkage sites may be on chromosomes 4, 11** (the site of the gene for tyrosine hydroxylase), **18, and 21.** As of yet, no single chromosomal site seems to play a dominant role in the development of bipolar disorder, but several genes may interact to confer risk.
   d. A majority of the association studies have until now focused on the neurotransmitter system as a candidate molecule, including serotonin transporters, serotonin receptors, dopamine receptors, tyrosine hydroxylase, monoamine oxidase A (MAO-A), catechol-O-methyltransferase (COMT), and tryptophan hydroxylase.

4. **Expanding triplet repeats.** This factor (i.e., repeating nucleotide bases), seen in the genetic basis of Huntington disease, may account for the finding that bipolar illness has an earlier onset and more severe symptomatology in subsequent generations of some families.

5. **Pharmacogenetic studies** also have been carried out in this field to identify candidate genes that may help predict treatment response and move the field toward personalized medicine.

B Neurochemical factors A number of neurotransmitters, including the monoamines **NE, dopamine, and 5-HT,** have been implicated, and there has been emerging evidence of the role of **γ-aminobutyric acid (GABA) and neuropeptides** in mood disorders.

1. **NE** is associated with mood disorders, based on a variety of findings.
   a. Many effective antidepressant medications (e.g., desipramine, nortriptyline) block **NE** reuptake immediately and **downregulate β-receptors** after several weeks. Because the latter effect correlates with the onset of action, it has been speculated that **adrenergic function may be abnormal in depression.**
   b. Measurements of NE or its metabolites in cerebrospinal fluid (CSF), plasma, and urine are variable. Metabolites of NE are generally diminished in depression.
   c. Increased NE activity has been speculated to be involved in mania.

2. **5-HT** has been of more interest since the primarily serotonergic antidepressants were introduced.
   a. The **selective serotonin reuptake inhibitors (SSRIs)** such as fluoxetine have proved to be effective antidepressants.
   b. Some studies have found 5-HT and 5-hydroxyindoleacetic acid (5-HIAA, a serotonin metabolite) in low levels in depressed patients; 5-HT depletion (e.g., by a tryptophan-depleted diet) can worsen depression.
3. **Dopamine** is also linked to depression, but the link is not as strong as with NE and 5-HT.
   a. Bupropion is an effective antidepressant that is dopaminergic without directly affecting 5-HT or NE transmission.
   b. Parkinson disease, which involves dopaminergic dysfunction, often leads to depressive symptoms.
   c. Dopaminergic agents such as the stimulants methylphenidate and modafinil can be effective antidepressants in some patients.
4. **Other neurotransmitters,** including GABA and neuropeptides, have also been implicated in mood disorders.

C Other biologic factors

1. **Neuroendocrine regulation** appears to be related to mood disorders.
   a. The hypothalamic–pituitary–adrenal (HPA) axis may be disrupted in depression, as the dexamethasone suppression test (DST) demonstrates. Normally, administration of dexamethasone (a synthetic corticosteroid) suppresses the HPA axis, and serum cortisol levels decrease. However, depressed patients have been found to exhibit **nonsuppression** (cortisol remains elevated). The DST is not sufficiently selective or specific to be used in routine clinical care, but it points to endocrine involvement.
   b. **Hypothyroidism** may mimic depression, and **hyperthyroidism** may mimic mania. In addition, a subset of depressed patients release a low amount of thyroid-stimulating hormone (TSH) after being given thyrotropin-releasing hormone (TRH).
2. **Sleep and circadian rhythm**
   a. Sleep disturbances are among the most common symptoms in patients with mood disorders, and patients with mood disorders exhibit higher rates of sleep disturbances than the general population. Insomnia and hypersomnia are associated with an increased risk for the development or recurrence of mood disorders and increased severity of psychiatric symptoms.
   b. **Polysomnography** reveals that depressed patients have **shortened rapid eye movement (REM) latency** (i.e., the time from falling asleep to the first REM period is about 60 minutes rather than 90 minutes). Other abnormalities of sleep architecture are also found in mood disorders.
   c. **Sleep deprivation** is an effective treatment for depression, although depression returns after the next night's sleep.
3. **Kindling** is a phenomenon observed when repeated, subthreshold stimulation of the brain eventually results in seizure activity. It has been postulated that bipolar illness follows a similar paradigm. The temporal pattern may be suggestive: some patients have a first episode of illness in response to stress (e.g., a loss), with subsequent episodes following lower-grade stress, and spontaneous episodes eventually occurring.

D Psychological and social factors

1. **Stress** commonly precedes the first episode of both major depression and mania (e.g., job loss, loss of a loved one, divorce). It has been speculated that such stress can precipitate brain changes, which make an individual more vulnerable to future mood episodes.
2. **Loss of a parent** before the age of 11 years has been linked to depression in adulthood.
3. Some psychodynamic theorists have proposed that depression represents **anger turned inward;** that is, a person becomes angry at a loved one (often one who was lost), but because such anger is intrapsychically unacceptable, the patient experiences depression and self-hatred.

4. Animal studies have led to the model of depression as **learned helplessness.** An animal exposed to inescapable shock will, over time, fail to escape the shock even when given the opportunity. Antidepressant medications reverse this behavior.

5. Depressed individuals often express inaccurate, negative cognitions including negative view of self, their future, and the world (e.g., "I've never done anything right"). **Cognitive therapy** is aimed at changing these distortions and improving depressive symptoms in many individuals.

III DIAGNOSIS/DIFFERENTIAL DIAGNOSIS

(A) **Identification of mood episodes** Diagnosis of a mood disorder requires the identification of discreet mood episodes, which by themselves are not actual diagnoses but serve as building blocks to help the clinician in making the diagnosis of a mood disorder. The *DSM-IV-TR* defines **four types of mood episodes:** major depressive episode, manic episode, mixed episode, and hypomanic episode. The criteria for each type require that the mood symptoms lead to serious distress or dysfunction and that they are not caused by the effects of drugs, alcohol, or a medical condition.

1. **Major depressive episode (MDE).** The criteria for MDE are shown in Table 3–1. Symptoms must represent a change from baseline and must persist for at least 2 weeks to be characteristic of MDE. Five or more of the following must be present:
   a. Patients must exhibit **either depressed mood or a notable decrease in interest or pleasure.** Another name for the inability to experience pleasure is **anhedonia.** Loss of interest commonly extends to **loss of libido.**
   b. Patients typically exhibit **neurovegetative symptoms** of depression such as changes in sleep. Sleep impairment may involve initial insomnia (trouble falling asleep), middle insomnia (awakening during the night), or terminal insomnia (early morning awakening).

TABLE 3–1 *DSM-IV-TR* **Diagnostic Criteria for a Major Depressive Episode**

A. At least five of the following symptoms have been present during the same 2-week period and represent a change from previous functioning; at least one of the symptoms is either (1) depressed mood or (2) loss of interest or pleasure.
  1. Depressed mood most of the day, nearly every day, as indicated by either subjective report (e.g., feels sad or empty) or observation made by others (e.g., appears tearful); in children and adolescents, irritable mood suffices
  2. Markedly diminished interest or pleasure in all, or almost all, activities most of the day, nearly every day (as indicated either by subjective account or observation made by others)
  3. Significant weight loss or weight gain when not dieting (e.g., >5% of body weight in 1 month) or decrease or increase in appetite nearly every day; in children, consider failure to make expected weight gains
  4. Insomnia or hypersomnia nearly every day
  5. Psychomotor agitation or retardation nearly every day (observable by others, not merely subjective feelings of restlessness or being slowed down)
  6. Fatigue or loss of energy nearly every day
  7. Feelings of worthlessness or excessive or inappropriate guilt (which may be delusional) nearly every day (not merely self-reproach or guilt about being sick)
  8. Diminished ability to think or concentrate, or indecisiveness, nearly every day (either by subjective account or as observed by others)
  9. Recurrent thoughts of death (not just fear of dying); recurrent suicidal ideation without a specific plan; or a suicide attempt or a specific plan for committing suicide
B. The symptoms cause clinically significant distress or impairment in social, occupational, or other important areas of functioning.
C. The symptoms are not caused by the direct effects of a substance (e.g., drugs of abuse, medication) or a general medical condition (e.g., hypothyroidism).
D. The symptoms are not better accounted for by bereavement (after the loss of a loved one, the symptoms persist for longer than 2 months or are characterized by marked functional impairment, morbid preoccupation with worthlessness, suicidal ideation, psychotic symptoms, or psychomotor retardation).

Reprinted with permission from the Diagnostic and Statistical Manual of Mental Disorders, Fourth Edition, Text Revision, (Copyright 2000). American Psychiatric Association.

     c. Significant weight loss or weight gain when not dieting (a change of ≥5% of the body weight in a month) often occurs, along with an increase or a decrease in appetite.

          Whereas sleep and appetite usually decrease in MDE, patients with **atypical depression** report excessive and increased appetite with weight gain.

     d. **Fatigue** and **impaired concentration** are common.

     e. **Psychomotor activity** may be increased (agitation, including pacing and hand wringing) or decreased (retardation, including soft speech, lack of eye contact, and immobility).

     f. Feelings of **worthlessness** and **guilt** are often present. The guilt may be **delusional** (i.e., a fixed, false belief such as thinking that one has committed a great crime or caused a natural disaster).

     g. **Thoughts of death** or **suicidal ideation** are also common. Suicidal ideation can range from passive ideas (e.g., wishing one would develop cancer) to active plans.

2. **Manic episode.** This features a distinct period of elevated or irritable mood that lasts at least 1 week. *DSM-IV-TR* criteria are given in Table 3–2. Features of mania include the following:

     a. **Grandiosity** involves an elevated opinion of one's features and accomplishments. Manic patients may feel extraordinarily attractive, engage in name dropping, exaggerate educational and career achievements, and feel superior to other people. **Grandiose delusions** may also be seen. For example, a patient may believe that he has achieved world peace or owns a billion-dollar company.

     b. During a manic episode, **most patients need little sleep.** Whereas depressed individuals complain about their short nights, patients with mania feel well rested after only 2 or 3 hours of sleep.

     c. **Pressured speech,** as observed by clinicians, may reflect **flight of ideas** or **racing thoughts.**

     d. Manic patients are **easily distracted/inattentive** and become interested in various environmental stimuli. This can lead to difficulty in engaging patient during the interview. During mental status testing, vigilance tests such as the continuous performance task (CPT) show evidence of this dysfunction.

     e. An **increase in goal-directed activities** as well as participation in **potentially dangerous activities** such as gambling, sexual promiscuity, or reckless driving often occurs.

3. **Mixed episode.** This describes a period during which patients satisfy criteria for **both manic episode and MDE over a 1-week period.** Such patients might exhibit pressured speech, irritability, and the need for little sleep, while feeling worthless and suicidal.

TABLE 3–2 DSM-IV-TR Diagnostic Criteria for a Manic Episode

A. A distinct period of abnormally and persistently elevated, expansive, or irritable mood lasts at least 1 week (or any duration if hospitalization is necessary).

B. During the period of mood disturbance, at least three of the following symptoms have persisted (four if the mood is only irritable) and have been present to a significant degree:

  1. Inflated self-esteem or grandiosity

  2. Decreased need for sleep (e.g., feels rested after only 3 hours of sleep)

  3. More talkative than usual or pressure to keep talking

  4. Flight of ideas or subjective experience that thoughts are racing

  5. Distractibility (i.e., attention too easily drawn to unimportant or irrelevant external stimuli)

  6. Increase in goal-directed activity (e.g., socially, at work or school, or sexually) or psychomotor agitation

  7. Excessive involvement in pleasurable activities that have a high potential for painful consequences (e.g., the person engages in unrestrained buying sprees, sexual indiscretions, or foolish business investments)

C. The mood disturbance is sufficiently severe to cause marked impairment in the occupational functioning or in usual social activities or relationships with others or to necessitate hospitalization to prevent harm to self or others or psychotic features are present.

D. The symptoms are not caused by the direct effects of a substance (e.g., drugs of abuse, medication) or a general medical condition (e.g., hyperthyroidism).

Note: Manic episodes that are clearly precipitated by somatic antidepressant treatment (e.g., medication, electroconvulsive therapy, light therapy) should not count toward a diagnosis of bipolar I disorder.

Reprinted with permission from the Diagnostic and Statistical Manual of Mental Disorders, Fourth Edition, Text Revision, (Copyright 2000). American Psychiatric Association.

TABLE 3–3 Differentiation of Mood Disorders

Diagnosis	Major Depressive Episode	Milder Depression	Manic or Mixed Episode	Hypomania
Major depressive disorder	+	±	−	−
Dysthymic disorder	−*	+	−	−
Bipolar I disorder	±	±	+	±
Bipolar II disorder	+	±	−	+
Cyclothymia	−	+	−†	+

+ = This syndrome must be present to make the diagnosis; − = this syndrome must be absent to make the diagnosis; ± = this syndrome may be present or absent.
*A major depressive episode must not occur during the first 2 years of the illness.
†A manic episode must not occur during the first 2 years of the illness.

4. **Hypomanic episode.** This is similar in many ways to a manic episode but is less severe. Differences in the criteria include the following:
   a. The episode need only last 4 days.
   b. The episode must not include psychotic features (e.g., delusions) and is not severe enough to cause severe social or occupational impairment.

B **Diagnosis of mood disorders**   Differentiation of the mood disorders listed below depends on the presence or absence of the mood episodes discussed in III A 1–4. Table 3–3 may help clarify the various diagnoses.

1. **Major depressive disorder**
   a. **Diagnostic criteria.** The diagnosis requires the presence of one or more MDE and the absence of any manic, hypomanic, or mixed episodes.
   b. **Associated clinical features or specifiers**
      (1) **Psychotic features.** These conditions, which are seen in some patients, are most often **mood congruent** (i.e., the content of the delusion or hallucination reflects depression). A mood-congruent delusion might be the belief that one has committed terrible crimes or sins. A mood-congruent hallucination might be a voice that tells one to die or says that one is a loser.
      (2) **Melancholic features.** A more severe subtype of major depression, melancholia features more profound anhedonia and neurovegetative symptoms. Early morning awakening, anorexia, and significant weight loss are common (see III C 3).
      (3) **Catatonic features** are characterized by motoric immobility, excessive motor activity, echolalia, echopraxia, and abnormal posturing.
      (4) **Atypical features** are characterized by mood reactivity, weight gain, heaviness in the limbs, and interpersonal rejection sensitivity.
      (5) **Postpartum onset** is characterized by an episode that occurs within 4 weeks postpartum.
      (6) **Mortality and morbidity.** In addition to the risk of suicide, affected patients have a higher risk of illness or death from medical causes. While 50% of patients do go on to attempt suicide, only 10% to 15% are successful.
      (7) **Psychiatric comorbidity.** Patients are at risk for several other psychiatric conditions (e.g., alcohol or other substance abuse, anxiety disorders).
   c. **Epidemiology**
      (1) **Risk and prevalence.** The lifetime prevalence of developing major depressive disorder is about 17% overall; the prevalence in women is roughly twice the prevalence in men. The risk is similar in different countries and across races. The rate of completed suicide is 10% to 15%.
      (2) **Age of onset.** The age of onset can range from childhood to old age; the mean age of onset is about 40 years old.
      (3) **Recurrence.** Approximately 50% of people who have one episode of major depression will have one or more additional episodes. After two episodes, the recurrence rate is about 70%, and after three episodes, it is about 90%.

d. **Differential diagnosis.** The symptoms of major depressive disorder can overlap with symptoms of many other illnesses.

(1) **Other psychiatric disorders.** Conditions with symptoms that are similar to major depressive disorder include dysthymic disorder, adjustment disorder with depressed mood, schizoaffective disorder, dementia, anxiety disorders, and personality disorders.

(2) **Substance-induced mood disorders.** Causes may include intoxication with depressogenic substances (e.g., alcohol, opiates, barbiturates); withdrawal from stimulants (e.g., cocaine, amphetamines); treatment with medications such as steroids, some antihypertensives (i.e., reserpine, propranolol), and cimetidine; and hepatitis C treatment (interferon).

(3) **Mood disorders caused by a general medical condition.** Depression has been associated with a number of medical illnesses, including hypothyroidism, stroke, anemia, pancreatic cancer, epilepsy, Parkinson disease, sleep apnea, and tuberculosis.

(4) **Normal bereavement.** Many symptoms of a major depressive episode may be features of normal bereavement. In such cases, a diagnosis of major depressive disorder is not usually made unless the MDE criteria are still met 2 months after the loss. Some symptoms such as hallucinations unrelated to the loss and prolonged functional impairment are atypical of normal bereavement and more suggestive of major depression. One must recognize that the symptoms and duration of "normal" bereavement vary among cultures. The *DSM-IV-TR* has classified bereavement as a "V" code.

2. **Dysthymic disorder**

a. **Diagnostic criteria**

(1) Patients present with a **depressed mood for most of the day** (at least 2 years in duration for adults and 1 year for children and adolescents) that has **not** been **severe enough to meet the criteria for MDE.** Instead of the five symptoms required of MDE, patients must have two of the following: increase or decrease in appetite or sleep, low energy, low self-esteem, poor concentration or decision-making ability, and hopelessness.

(2) If patients experience an MDE after 2 years of having a dysthymic disorder, more than one diagnosis is made (dysthymic disorder and major depressive disorder).

(3) In addition, patients must never have met criteria for manic episode, mixed episode, or hypomanic episode.

b. **Associated clinical features.** Dysthymic disorder is associated with social impairment, health problems, alcohol and other drug abuse, and major depressive disorder. Coexistence of dysthymic disorder and major depression is sometimes referred to as **double depression.**

c. **Epidemiology.** The lifetime risk of dysthymic disorder is about 5% overall; the prevalence rate in women is about twice that in men. Patients who develop dysthymic disorder before age 21 years are more likely to develop major depressive disorder later.

d. **Differential diagnosis.** The possible diagnoses are similar to those of major depressive disorder (see III B 1 d).

3. **Bipolar I disorder.** Bipolar is a misnomer for this illness because a single manic episode is a prerequisite for the diagnosis (i.e., one only needs one "pole"). However, most patients experience both manic and depressive symptoms, and the first episode may be manic, hypomanic, depressed, or mixed.

a. **Diagnostic criteria.** Patients have experienced **at least one manic or mixed episode** unless the symptoms were caused by a substance (including antidepressants) or a general medical condition. MDEs may or may not have ever been present.

b. **Associated clinical features**

(1) **Psychotic features.** Delusions, hallucinations, and disorganization can be seen during manic episodes, with severity similar in degree to that in schizophrenia. These are most often **mood congruent.** A mood-congruent delusion in mania might be the belief that one is a famous singer or an actor or has the ability to predict the future. A mood-congruent hallucination might involve hearing the voice of God.

(2) Morbidity and mortality. Attempted and completed suicide are both common, with rates of completed suicide as high as 25%. Comorbid medical problems can worsen the prognosis given elevated rates of noncompliance stemming from grandiosity or impaired judgment. Reckless behavior can increase the risk of sexually transmitted diseases and accidents.

(3) Psychiatric comorbidity. Alcohol and other forms of drug abuse frequently complicate manic episodes and can carry into other phases of this disorder. Other comorbid disorders include eating disorders, anxiety disorders, and attention deficit hyperactivity disorder (ADHD).

c. Epidemiology. The lifetime risk of bipolar I disorder is about 1%, and it is similar in men and women and across racial groups. The mean age of onset is 30 years. More than 90% of people who have a manic episode will have additional episodes of mania or major depression.

d. Differential diagnosis

(1) Other psychiatric disorders. Similar symptoms are seen in bipolar II disorder and cyclothymic disorder. When psychotic symptoms exist, it can be difficult to differentiate bipolar I disorder from schizophrenia or schizoaffective disorder. However, if a patient has ever had delusions or hallucinations for at least 2 weeks in the absence of mania or major depression, then a psychotic disorder (rather than a mood disorder with psychotic features) must be diagnosed. Narcissistic personality disorder also has some overlapping features.

(2) Substance-induced mood disorder. Intoxication with stimulants such as cocaine or amphetamine can mimic mania. Antidepressant drugs can occasionally cause patients to "switch" from depression to mania in individuals with a predisposition for bipolarity. Other prescription medications (e.g., corticosteroids, dopamine agonists, anticholinergics, cimetidine) can also precipitate manic symptoms.

(3) Mood disorder caused by a general medical condition. Manic symptoms can be seen with infectious diseases, AIDS, endocrinopathies (e.g., Cushing disease, hyperthyroidism), lupus, and a variety of neurologic disorders (e.g., epilepsy, multiple sclerosis [MS], Wilson disease).

4. Bipolar II disorder. This disorder was officially recognized for the first time in the *DSM-IV.*

a. Diagnostic criteria. Patients have had **at least one MDE and one hypomanic episode** in the absence of any manic or mixed episodes.

b. Associated features. Suicide is a risk, particularly during depressive episodes. As with major depression and bipolar I disorder, comorbidity with substance abuse or anxiety disorders is common.

c. Epidemiology. The lifetime risk is approximately 0.5% and is higher in women than in men. There do not appear to be racial differences.

d. Differential diagnosis. The possible diagnoses are similar to those of bipolar I disorder (see III B 3 d).

5. Cyclothymic disorder. This disorder is characterized as dysthymic disorder with intermittent hypomanic periods. It is a chronic illness similar to dysthymic disorder.

a. Diagnostic criteria. A patient who, over at least 2 years (1 year in children and adolescents), experiences repeated episodes of hypomania and depression (not severe enough to meet criteria for major depressive disorder) is diagnosed with cyclothymic disorder. During the first 2 years, a patient may not have an MDE, manic episode, or mixed episode. If such episodes occur after 2 years, more than one diagnosis may be made (e.g., cyclothymic disorder and bipolar I disorder).

b. Associated features. Substance abuse and social and occupational dysfunction are common.

c. Epidemiology. The lifetime risk of cyclothymic disorder is about 1%; it is slightly higher in women than in men. The age of onset is usually in the teens or early adulthood, and the course tends to be chronic. Up to 50% of people with cyclothymic disorder may ultimately go on to develop bipolar disorder.

d. Differential diagnosis. Possible diagnoses are similar to those for bipolar I disorder. In addition, the features of cyclothymic disorder must be differentiated from the mood swings seen in borderline personality disorder.

6. Mood disorder caused by a general medical condition and **substance-induced mood disorder.** These conditions are two other mood disorder diagnoses in the *DSM-IV-TR*. As noted previously, other mood disorder diagnoses (e.g., major depressive disorder) are not made if medical illness or drug use appears to be the cause of the symptoms. Clinical examples include the following:

  a. A 70-year-old man recently suffered a myocardial infarction and now has the symptoms of an MDE. The appropriate diagnosis is mood disorder caused by a cardiovascular disease, with a major depressive-like episode.

  b. A 25-year-old woman who presents to an emergency department with manic behavior reports having used cocaine in the past 24 hours. In the emergency room 36 hours later she reports feeling very depressed and suicidal. The diagnosis is cocaine-induced mood disorder.

C Mood disorder specifiers The *DSM-IV-TR* provides a number of specifiers that better describe a current or most recent mood episode.

  1. Severity or remission status (with or without psychosis). Mood episodes can be described in two ways: as mild, moderate, or severe and as partial or full remission. When symptoms are severe, the **presence or absence of psychotic features** should be noted. When psychotic features are present, they should be described as mood congruent or mood incongruent.

  2. Catatonic features. This specifier is used when a mood episode features two of the following: immobility; excess purposeless activity; negativism or mutism; posturing, mannerisms, or stereotypic behaviors; and echolalia or echopraxia.

  3. Melancholia. This more severe presentation of depression is more common in inpatients and those with psychotic features. This specifier describes patients who exhibit (during the worst of the episode) a **loss of almost all pleasure** and three of the following:

   a. A distinct quality to the sad mood (e.g., it does not resemble normal grief or sadness)
   b. Symptoms that are worse in the morning
   c. Early morning awakening
   d. Marked psychomotor changes
   e. Marked anorexia or weight loss
   f. Excessive guilt

  4. Atypical features of depression. Symptoms that are opposite to what is commonly observed, particularly increased weight or sleep, occur. Affected patients exhibit mood brightening in the face of positive events and can also report heaviness in their limbs and chronic rejection sensitivity.

  5. Other specifiers. Postpartum onset (onset within 4 weeks postpartum; a nonpsychotic depression may occur in 10% to 20% of women. Note: Postpartum psychosis occurs in about one per 1,000 births), **seasonal pattern** (two seasonally linked MDEs in the past year, with full remission also occurring seasonally), and **rapid cycling** (four or more mood episodes in the past 12 months, with remission or a polarity switch between episodes) may occur.

IV TREATMENT

A Overall treatment planning Despite some variation in symptoms and severity, some general guidelines are appropriate in most cases.

  1. Treatment setting
   a. Type of clinician. Most patients with mood disorders are treated by clinicians other than mental health professionals.
    (1) Primary care physicians provide much of the care for disorders that respond well to medication. However, this can present several problems, including:
      (a) Inadequate diagnosis or missed diagnosis
      (b) Limited time for supportive therapy (which improves compliance by monitoring for a lack of efficacy, intolerability, and treatment response)
    (2) Psychiatrists are able to provide both medication and psychotherapy.
    (3) Psychologists, psychiatric social workers, and other mental health professionals often provide assessment and psychotherapy.
   b. Location of treatment. Patients with mood disorders are most often treated in **outpatient settings,** although dangerous or disorganized patients and those who have failed outpatient treatment may require **hospitalization.** Patients receive daytime support, supervision, and therapy at a **psychiatric day hospital,** an intermediate setting in which patients return home at night.

2. **Diagnostic evaluation.** The various mood disorders are treated quite differently. Therefore, it is important to establish, for instance, if a patient with a current MDE has a history of mania. Comorbid psychiatric and medical problems must also be identified or ruled out. Such an evaluation can be performed in either an inpatient or outpatient setting.

3. **Assessment of safety.** Mood disorders carry a risk of suicide. All clinicians who deal with these patients must be familiar with assessment of suicidal risk so that appropriate steps can be taken (e.g., **voluntary or involuntary hospitalization**) when needed to ensure patients' safety. In addition, bipolar patients may engage in behavior that, although not suicidal, is dangerous to themselves or others. Evidence of such behavior (e.g., reckless driving, accidents, and injuries) requires similar steps to protect the patient.

B Treatment of major depressive disorder

1. **Hospitalization.** While most patients with major depression can safely be treated as outpatients, a subset of patients require hospitalization, which can serve several functions.
   a. **Safety** for a suicidal or severely psychotic patient can often be best ensured in a hospital.
   b. **Treatment** can, at times, be more rapidly instituted in the hospital setting.
      (1) Medication doses can be advanced more rapidly in a setting where side effects can be rapidly identified and alleviated.
      (2) Electroconvulsive therapy (ECT), at times an outpatient procedure, is more commonly performed on inpatients.
      (3) **Novel treatments** include repetitive transcranial magnetic stimulation (rTMS) and vagus nerve stimulation (VNS).
   c. **Support** in the form of individual and group therapies, as well as general staff availability, is intensive in a hospital setting.

2. **Outpatient treatment.** Various levels and modalities of outpatient treatment are available.
   a. A **combination of psychotherapy and medication** is optimum for some patients with major depression, particularly those who have chronic conditions, have psychiatric comorbidity, or are refractory to pharmacotherapy alone. One clinician (e.g., a psychiatrist) or different clinicians (a multidisciplinary team approach; e.g., an internist and a social worker) may provide this treatment.
   b. Several **models of psychotherapy** for depression have been used.
      (1) **Psychodynamic** (psychoanalytically oriented) **psychotherapy** is commonly used with depressed patients, although it is also the least well studied.
      (2) The two modalities of psychotherapy that have the best available evidence are **cognitive therapy** (focuses on cognitive distortions) and **interpersonal therapy** (focuses on patients' interpersonal problems) and have been found in controlled studies to be effective treatments for depression.
   c. Because **support** appears to be an important variable both in treatment and safety, a number of supportive measures (in addition to individual therapy) are often used.
      (1) **Family or friends** are often involved in some phase of treatment.
      (2) **Day hospitalization** may be used instead of or as a transition from inpatient hospitalization.
      (3) **Supportive living arrangements** (group homes) may be recommended for patients with more refractory symptoms, more limited social supports, or comorbid factors.

3. **Somatic therapies.** All of the somatic therapies listed have proved similarly effective in treating patients with MDEs. Response to all of the antidepressant medications takes time, with full response usually seen within 4 to 6 weeks. When choosing a treatment for an individual patient, the clinician must consider prior treatment response in the patient or a family member, potential adherence issues, comorbid psychiatric or medical problems, and factors that might make side effects of a particular drug more problematic. Recently the Food and Drug Administration included a suicide warning for all antidepressants, warranting a careful assessment and follow-up for individuals started on these treatments.
   a. **Tricyclic antidepressants (TCAs)** had been the standard drug treatment over the past several decades, and they are still used for some patients. TCAs are hepatically metabolized, are renally excreted, and have a narrow therapeutic index requiring drug level monitoring. Relatively long half-lives allow once-daily dosing. Cardiotoxicity shared by these drugs leads to the lethality of overdose.

(1) **Tertiary tricyclics** (e.g., imipramine, amitriptyline) are the oldest members of this class. A side-effect profile includes prominent antihistaminergic effects that can result in sedative effects and anticholinergic effects that can result in dry mouth and constipation, which limits their use.

(2) **Secondary tricyclics** (e.g., nortriptyline, desipramine) tend to be less anticholinergic, less sedating, and less likely to cause orthostatic hypotension.

b. **MAO inhibitors,** discovered in the 1950s, have not been popular because of the **hypertensive crisis** that these drugs may precipitate when they interact with sympathomimetic agents (including a diet high in tyramine, which is found in ripe cheese, for example). Other side effects include orthostatic hypotension, weight gain, and insomnia. A new class of **reversible inhibitors of monoamine oxidase A,** which may be as effective as the standard MAO inhibitors but much safer, is being clinically tested and is not yet available in the United States. In the past few years a selegiline transdermal patch received approval for depression. It is currently the only skin patch that is approved to treat depression. While most monoamine oxidase inhibitors work equally on both MAO-A and MAO-B enzymes, the selegiline transdermal patch works more on MAO-B than on MAO-A and does not require dietary restrictions in doses below 12 mg/day.

c. **SSRIs,** which were introduced in the 1980s, have the advantages of once-daily dosing and a wide therapeutic index. **Fluoxetine, sertraline, paroxetine, fluvoxamine, citalopram,** and **escitalopram** are currently available. Limitations include side effects (e.g., nausea, insomnia, anxiety, sexual dysfunction) and drug interactions:

(1) SSRIs affect the hepatic P450 system, but each drug inhibits the isoforms (such as 2D6 or 2C19) to different degrees. To avoid a particular drug interaction, clinicians may choose one SSRI over another.

(2) Combination with other serotonergic drugs can precipitate a potentially lethal **serotonin syndrome** featuring restlessness, confusion, diaphoresis, and myoclonus.

d. **Triazolopyridines** include **trazodone** and **nefazodone.** Both of these agents have a short half-life (necessitating multiple daily dosing) and a wide therapeutic index. Whereas trazodone is very sedating, nefazodone is not; neither drug has prominent anticholinergic effects. Male patients taking trazodone run a risk of developing **priapism.** Nefazodone has been associated with liver failure and is contraindicated in those with liver disease.

e. **Bupropion,** an aminoketone, blocks the reuptake of dopamine rather than 5-HT or NE. Although it is rarely lethal in overdose, it has a narrow therapeutic index and has the potential to result in **seizures** in higher doses. Side effects include restlessness, sweating, tremors, and constipation. The incidence of sexual side effects is low. Bupropion is contraindicated in patients with comorbid eating disorders. It does come in a sustained-release and an extended-release preparation.

f. **Venlafaxine,** which has been called a selective 5-HT–NE reuptake inhibitor, has a wide therapeutic index. An extended-release formulation allows once-daily dosing. Side effects are dose dependent and resemble those associated with SSRIs and an increase in diastolic blood pressure. **Duloxetine** is a serotonin norepinephrine reuptake inhibitor (SNRI). Common side effects include nausea, dry mouth, sleepiness, constipation, decreased appetite, and increased sweating.

also used for diabetic neuropathic pain!

g. **Mirtazapine,** an antagonist of α_2 (i.e., adrenergic, inhibitory) autoreceptors, acts presynaptically but by a different mechanism. It also blocks some postsynaptic serotonergic and histaminergic receptors. Mirtazapine results in increased noradrenergic and serotonergic activity, has fewer sexual side effects, is very sedating, and is anxiolytic.

h. **ECT,** when performed with present-day equipment and anesthetic procedures, is a safe and effective treatment for major depressive disorder. Transcranial magnetic stimulation and vagal nerve stimulation have been approved for major depression and treatment-resistant depression, respectively, for routine clinical practice. Studies on deep brain stimulation and magnetic seizure therapy are under way.

(1) The use of ECT remains limited because of bias remaining from the years when it was a much cruder procedure. Use of ECT is often reserved for patients with psychotic depression and those who have failed or are unable to tolerate trials of antidepressant medications.

(2) Common **complications** are confusion immediately after the procedure and memory loss, which usually resolves within 6 months. There is no evidence that ECT causes permanent brain damage.

C **Treatment of bipolar I and bipolar II disorders**

1. **Hospitalization.** As is the case with major depressive disorder, a subset of patients with bipolar disorder require hospitalization, usually because of the risks of suicide during the depressed phase or out-of-control behavior during the manic phase.
   a. **Containment of manic behavior** can prevent potentially disastrous consequences for affected patients, including financial loss, arrest, and destroyed relationships.
   b. **Initial or reinstituted treatment** with antipsychotic medication and mood stabilizers can be accomplished rapidly in the hospital.
   c. **Compliance** is often an issue in the treatment of patients with bipolar disorder, so intensive psychoeducation and the involvement of family and friends are important goals of hospitalization.

2. **Outpatient treatment**
   a. **A combination of psychotherapy and medication** is important.
      (1) **Compliance** is a formidable challenge in clinical practice, particularly because many patients with bipolar disorder prefer hypomania or mania to euthymia. When manic symptoms begin, they believe that they know better than their physicians. A strong **therapeutic alliance** and frequent visits aid compliance and enable early intervention if signs of mania begin. **Family-focused therapy** (psychosocial program involving available family), **cognitive therapy,** and **psychoeducation** have been shown to decrease the number of relapses.
      (2) During a depressed phase, psychotherapeutic approaches as noted for major depression are appropriate.
   b. Approximately one-third of patients with bipolar disorder develop a degree of **chronic functional impairment.** These patients may benefit from programs such as **day hospitals, vocational rehabilitation,** or **supportive living arrangements.**

3. **Somatic therapies.** Several drugs have been found to possess **mood-stabilizing** properties (i.e., they are effective in treating both mania and depression) in bipolar patients. **ECT** is also effective for both phases of the illness.
   a. **Lithium,** traditionally the first-line treatment for bipolar disorder, has been found effective as an acute treatment for mania and depression and as a prophylactic agent.
      (1) During **acute mania,** approximately 80% of patients respond to lithium, although such response may take 1 to 2 weeks. Antipsychotic drugs are often coadministered during this initial period to control behavior and psychosis.
      (2) During **acute bipolar depression,** approximately 80% of patients also respond to lithium, although it may take 6 to 8 weeks to see the full effect.
      (3) Lithium is effective at preventing future episodes of depression and mania, with **relapse rates** reduced by approximately 50% compared with placebo.
      (4) **Side effects** of lithium include tremor, sedation, nausea, polyuria, polydipsia, memory problems, and weight gain. Hypothyroidism occurs in some patients.
      (5) Lithium is **renally excreted** (it is treated by the kidney like sodium), so impaired renal function can lead to toxicity.
      (6) Lithium has a **narrow therapeutic index,** and high serum levels can lead to seizures, confusion, coma, and cardiac dysrhythmia. In the case of severe overdose, dialysis is effective. The danger of lithium toxicity requires extra care for patients taking nonsteroidal anti-inflammatory agents (except sulindac and acetylsalicylic acid [ASA]) and thiazide diuretics because these drugs reduce lithium clearance.
   b. **Valproate** has been found in many studies to be as effective as lithium in treating bipolar illness.
      (1) In patients with **acute mania,** some evidence suggests that whereas valproate may be a more effective treatment than lithium for mixed episodes, lithium may be more effective for traditional manic episodes.

    (2) The role of valproate in **bipolar depression** is less clear.

    (3) As a **prophylactic agent,** valproate appears to have a role, particularly in the case of **rapidly cycling patients.**

    (4) Side effects include dose-related symptoms (e.g., nausea, tremor, sedation, hair loss, weight gain) and rare, idiosyncratic responses, including hepatic failure, pancreatitis, and agranulocytosis.

    (5) Valproate is **hepatically metabolized,** so patients who take it are vulnerable to pharmacokinetic drug interactions.

    (6) Valproate has a **wide therapeutic index,** although it can be fatal in overdose.

  c. Carbamazepine

    (1) Carbamazepine appears to be effective in patients with **acute mania** and **bipolar depression.**

    (2) When used for **prophylaxis,** it appears to reduce the frequency and severity of manic and depressive episodes.

    (3) Common, dose-related **side effects** include blurred vision, ataxia, nausea, fatigue, hyponatremia, and asymptomatic leukopenia. Rare, idiosyncratic effects include agranulocytosis, liver failure, Stevens-Johnson syndrome, and pancreatitis.

    (4) Carbamazepine is **hepatically metabolized** and induces its own metabolism (so dosage adjustment may be needed over time). Pharmacokinetic drug interactions are seen with other hepatically metabolized drugs.

    (5) Carbamazepine is **toxic at high doses** (serum levels must be monitored) and can be lethal in overdose.

  d. Second-generation antipsychotics

    (1) Olanzapine, risperidone, ziprasidone, aripiprazole, and **quetiapine** have all been shown in clinical trials to be effective as monotherapy for acute treatment of mania. Evidence suggests that quetiapine and the combination of olanzapine and fluoxetine are effective for the treatment of acute depressive episodes in patients with bipolar disorder. Quetiapine monotherapy and olanzapine and fluoxetine combination are approved for the treatment of bipolar depression.

    (2) Each of these drugs has also been shown to be effective as adjunctive therapy.

    (3) In varying degrees, these medications are associated with an increased risk of developing **diabetes mellitus** and **dyslipidemia.** Weight, blood pressure, glucose, and lipids should be monitored in patients taking these medications.

  e. Lamotrigine

    (1) Lamotrigine has been shown to be clinically effective as a maintenance treatment for bipolar disorder.

    (2) Except for a rash, lamotrigine has minimal side effects compared with placebo.

    (3) Lamotrigine seems to prevent depressive episodes better than manic episodes.

  f. Several other drug classes also have a role in the treatment of bipolar disorder.

    (1) Benzodiazepines, particularly **clonazepam,** may be used to treat mania. Sedation and a full night's sleep can markedly improve symptoms in some patients.

    (2) Anticonvulsants including oxcarbazepine, topiramate, gabapentin, and tiagabine as monotherapy or in combination with other mood stabilizers have been shown to be somewhat effective in treating manic symptoms.

    (3) Antidepressants are frequently used in the depressed phase of bipolar illness, either alone or in combination with an agent such as lithium. However, this practice is not well studied. Clinicians must be cautious because most antidepressant agents have been reported to precipitate mania in some patients.

D Treatment of dysthymia and cyclothymia Evidence-based therapy for these disorders is less well established than that for treatment of mania and depression.

  1. Dysthymia. Traditionally, dysthymia was treated with psychotherapy. The condition was believed to be poorly responsive to antidepressant medication.

    a. It now appears that this disorder may respond to drug treatment with **SSRIs, SNRIs,** and **MAO inhibitors.**

    b. Cognitive therapy and **behavioral therapy** are the two kinds of psychotherapy with the best evidence-based treatment data.

2. **Cyclothymia.** Therapy may involve mood-stabilizing drugs. Antidepressants frequently precipitate manic symptoms. Supportive psychotherapy is also important.

BIBLIOGRAPHY

American Psychiatric Association: *Guideline Watch: Practice Guideline for the Treatment of Patients with Bipolar Disorder,* 2nd ed. Washington, DC, American Psychiatric Association, 2005.

American Psychiatric Association: *Guideline Watch: Practice Guideline for the Treatment of Patients with Major Depressive Disorder,* 2nd ed. Washington, DC, American Psychiatric Association, 2005.

Study Questions

Directions: *Each of the numbered items in this section is followed by possible answers. Select the ONE lettered answer that is BEST in each case.*

QUESTIONS 1–2

A 50-year-old female secretary presents to her internist with a 2-month history of worsening depression, insomnia, weight loss, poor concentration, paranoia, fatigue, and suicidal ideation. She believes that she caused the death of her boyfriend, who was killed in a car accident.

1. At this time, which of the following diagnoses is most likely an explanation for her symptoms?
- [A] Dysthymic disorder
- [B] Bipolar I disorder
- [C] Major depressive disorder with psychotic features
- [D] Schizophrenia
- [E] Somatization disorder

2. The patient's belief about her boyfriend would best be described as which of the following?
- [A] A mood-congruent delusion
- [B] A mood-incongruent delusion
- [C] A melancholic symptom
- [D] Thought broadcasting
- [E] Thought insertion

Directions: *Each set of matching questions in this section consists of a list of five to nine lettered options followed by several items. For each numbered item, select the ONE lettered option that is most closely associated with it. Each lettered option may be selected once, more than once, or not at all.*

QUESTIONS 3–5

Match each clinical feature with the associated drug.
- [A] Carbamazepine
- [B] Lamotrigine
- [C] Lithium
- [D] Olanzapine
- [E] Valproate

3. This drug is effective for maintenance treatment of bipolar disorder. Side effects may include a rash.

B

4. The toxicity of this drug can result in coarse tremors, slurring of speech, delirium, and death.

C

5. This agent may be particularly effective in bipolar patients who exhibit rapidly cycling illness and is metabolized hepatically.

E

QUESTIONS 6–8

For each of the following patients, select the most likely diagnosis.
- [A] Adjustment disorder with depressed mood
- [B] Bipolar I disorder
- [C] Bipolar II disorder

[D] Cyclothymic disorder
[E] Dysthymic disorder
[F] Major depressive disorder
[G] Mood disorder caused by a general medical condition
[H] Normal bereavement
[I] Substance-induced mood disorder

6. A 45-year-old woman reports an almost 1-year history of poor sleep, low energy, and a general feeling of hopelessness. She suffered a myocardial infarction 5 weeks ago and since has no interest in life, stopped going to work because she could not concentrate, and felt so run down that she could hardly get out of bed. She began to feel suicidal. She denies any significant use of any drugs other than her cardiac medications.

G

7. A 25-year-old man was recently admitted to the surgical unit with multiple fractures and internal injuries he received in a motorcycle accident. He suffered no apparent head trauma. While he was in college, he twice experienced episodes that each lasted for a week or two in which he felt "on top of the world," needed little sleep, went out every night with friends, and ordered expensive electronic equipment that he later had to return. He did not seek or receive treatment for these episodes. He does report drinking 5 beers a day. His laboratory values are within normal limits except for a blood alcohol of .7.

Bipolar II ?   *C*

8. A 60-year-old woman with no psychiatric history has been feeling sad, anxious, and lonely since her husband died suddenly about 3 weeks ago. She feels depressed, has difficulty falling asleep almost every night, and has lost 5 pounds. Although she has continued to work, she has become isolated from her friends and believes that she will never recover from the loss. She denies suicidal ideation and hallucinations. She is physically healthy and denies alcohol or drug use.

H

QUESTIONS 9–11

Choose the most appropriate treatment for each of the following psychiatric outpatients.

[A] Bupropion
[B] Cognitive therapy
[C] Day hospitalization
[D] Mirtazapine *(Remeron)*
[E] Lithium
[F] Nortriptyline
[G] Amitriptyline
[H] Valproate

9. A 30-year-old woman with major depressive disorder says that she has difficulty sleeping most of the nights in a week, and she wants something to help her sleep. She was treated using medication for her first episode of depression at age 17, but she does not recall the name of the drug. At that time, she was briefly hospitalized because of an overdose attempt with her antidepressant.

D

10. A 27-year-old man has recently been diagnosed with major depressive disorder. He is able to work. Despite having a previously successful social life, he has become very isolated socially. He views himself negatively and is very pessimistic. Because he has a mother and a sister with depression who have troubling side effects on their antidepressant medications, the man is very reluctant to take antidepressant drugs.

B

11. A 55-year-old man was recently discharged from a brief inpatient stay for mania. He has had frequent hospitalizations for agitation, grandiosity, and psychosis, which always responded well to lithium. However, it appears that he takes his medication erratically, and his poor treatment adherence contributes to the relapses. He was recently also diagnosed with hypertension, and his internist plans to start him on hydrochlorothiazide. More recently symptoms of psychosis, being followed, and spending a lot of time reading the bible and talking in tongues have been his presenting symptoms.

H

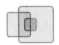

Answers and Explanations

1–2. **The answers are 1-C, 2-A** [*III A 1, B 1 b (1)*]. This woman meets all the criteria for major depressive disorder. Dysthymia alone could not account for her current symptoms, which are consistent with a major depressive episode (MDE). MDE can be a feature of several mood disorders, including major depressive disorder, bipolar I and bipolar II disorders, somatization disorder, and substance-induced mood disorder. To differentiate these, one would need a history of any prior mood episodes, concurrent medical problems, and drug and alcohol use. She also reports paranoia, suggesting psychotic features.

Believing that thoughts can cause someone to die is delusional. Because the patient's symptoms are those of an MDE and the delusion has a depressing content (causing someone to die), the belief would be described as a mood-congruent delusion. Thought insertion is the belief that thoughts have been placed into the patient's head, and thought broadcasting is the belief that others can hear the patient's thoughts. Neither is related to this case. Delusions can occur in melancholic patients, but they are not a specific symptom of melancholia.

3–5. **The answers are 3-B** [*IV C 3 e*], **4-C** [*IV C 3 a*], and **5-E** [*IV C 3 b*]. Although both lithium and lamotrigine have been shown to be effective for maintenance treatment of patients with bipolar disorder, lamotrigine can cause a rash as a side effect.

Lithium, usually considered a first-line treatment for bipolar disorder, has side effects that include tremor, sedation, nausea, polyuria, polydipsia, memory problems, weight gain, and hypothyroidism. Toxic effects of this medication can result in coarse tremors, slurring of speech, delirium, and coma and may require hemodialysis .

Valproate is a mood stabilizer that appears to be particularly effective in patients who have a pattern of rapid cycling illness (i.e., at least four episodes of mood disorder within a 12-month period). It is metabolized hepatically.

6–8. **The answers are 6-G** [*III B 6*], **7-C** [*III B 4*], and **8-H** [*III B 1 d (4)*]. The 45-year-old woman developed a major depressive episode (MDE) secondary to having suffered a heart attack. She has all the symptoms of an MDE but with an onset after the myocardial infarction. Also, the cardiac medications she has started need to be further explored. Medication like propranolol in higher doses can be depressogenic.

The man in the hospital appears to have a history of bipolar II disorder, with two hypomanic episodes. He is recovering from medical problems (fractures and internal injuries), but there is no evidence of a medical condition known to cause mood symptoms physiologically. In addition, although he recently experienced a severe psychosocial stressor (his accident), a diagnosis of adjustment disorder would not be appropriate because his symptoms meet criteria for another Axis I disorder (in this case, bipolar II disorder).

The recently widowed woman has many features of an MDE, but this condition is consistent with normal bereavement. Her symptoms are not in excess of what one would expect to see after the loss of a husband, so a diagnosis of an adjustment disorder or major depressive disorder is not appropriate. Features that might lead to the diagnosis of major depressive disorder in a grieving individual include prominent psychotic features, serious or prolonged functional impairment, suicidal ideation, or the presence of an MDE for more than several months. Cultural factors regarding the severity and time course of normal bereavement should be considered.

9–11. **The answers are 9-D** [*IV B 3 g*], **10-B** [*IV B 2 b*], and **11-H** [*IV C 3 b*]. Of the listed antidepressants, the 30-year-old woman with multiple depressive disorder and prominent insomnia would best be treated with mirtazapine, which is a sedating antidepressant with a wide therapeutic index. Amitriptyline, although sedating, could be lethal if she overdosed on her medication again. Fluoxetine and bupropion can both cause restlessness and may worsen her insomnia. Fluoxetine has a wide therapeutic index, but bupropion can cause seizures in cases of overdose.

The 27-year-old man with major depressive disorder who is reluctant to take medication may do well with cognitive therapy. His negative view of himself is the sort of cognitive distortion seen in depressed patients and one that can respond to work with a cognitive therapist. If the man does later agree to take medication, bupropion might be a good choice because in view of his family history, this man is at risk for developing bipolar illness. Bupropion is less likely than many other antidepressants to precipitate mania. There is no indication that this man requires the level of support and supervision provided by a psychiatric day hospital, although if his condition deteriorated, this might be an option.

Of the choices given, valproate, with its wider therapeutic index and known efficacy in patients with bipolar disorder, would be the best option for an individual with bipolar disorder. Although he is known to respond well to lithium, the addition of hydrochlorothiazide, a thiazide diuretic, to lithium could be dangerous in light of his difficulty with medication compliance. Thiazide diuretics decrease lithium clearance, resulting in higher serum levels. In compliant patients, the lithium dosage could be adjusted accordingly and maintained at a safe level. However, in this patient, there would be a risk of the lithium level fluctuating downward (becoming ineffective) and upward (becoming toxic). Valproate may also be indicated because this patient might meet criteria for rapid cycling, as the clinical vignette suggests. Given his history of psychosis, olanzapine or any of the atypical antipsychotics may be viable treatment options. Day hospitalization, although not effective alone in preventing relapses, might also provide support and improve compliance.

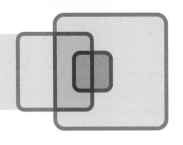

chapter 4

Anxiety Disorders

JEFFREY D. RAYNOR

I OVERVIEW

Anxiety is abnormal fear out of proportion to any external stimulus. Significant anxiety is experienced by 10% to 15% of general medical outpatients and 10% of inpatients. Of the physically healthy population, 25% of individuals are anxious at some point in their lives. Approximately 7.5% of these people have a diagnosable anxiety disorder in any given month. Anxiety either may be a physiologic response to a perception of internal or external danger or may be spontaneous.

A **Signs and symptoms of anxiety** Patients may describe a subjective feeling of anxiety, or they may report physical or other psychological complaints.

1. **Psychological symptoms**
   a. Apprehension, worry
   b. Anticipation of misfortune
   c. Sense of doom or panic
   d. Hypervigilance
   e. Irritability
   f. Fatigue
   g. Insomnia
   h. Derealization (the world seems strange or unreal)
   i. Depersonalization (feeling unreal or changed)
   j. Difficulty concentrating

2. **Somatic (physical) symptoms**
   a. Headache
   b. Dizziness
   c. Lightheadedness
   d. Palpitations, chest pain
   e. Nausea, diarrhea
   f. Frequent urination
   g. Lump in the throat
   h. Motor tension
   i. Restlessness
   j. Shortness of breath
   k. Paresthesias
   l. Dry mouth

3. **Physical signs**
   a. Diaphoresis
   b. Cool, clammy skin
   c. Tachycardia, arrhythmias
   d. Flushing, pallor
   e. Hyperreflexia
   f. Tremor
   g. Easy startling
   h. Fidgeting

B **Panic anxiety versus generalized anxiety**

1. **Panic anxiety** arises spontaneously and does not have particular content associated with it.
   a. Panic anxiety may evolve gradually from spontaneous subclinical (limited symptom) anxiety attacks to full-blown panic attacks.
   b. The direct psychological effects of these attacks may include unrealistic fears of occult disease and anticipatory anxiety about panic attacks.
   c. Behavioral manifestations of panic anxiety may include avoidance of only situations in which panic attacks might occur or generalized avoidance (agoraphobia).
   d. Efforts to control anxiety with drugs or alcohol, depression, and social isolation often result from chronic panic anxiety.

2. **Generalized anxiety** involves excessive worry about actual circumstances, events, or conflicts.
   a. Panic anxiety and generalized anxiety often accompany each other. Whereas subpanic anxiety may mimic generalized anxiety, anticipatory anxiety is a type of generalized anxiety.
   b. Whereas panic anxiety does not involve fear of any specific circumstance, generalized anxiety involves worry about specific circumstances.
   c. Symptoms of generalized anxiety fluctuate more than those of panic anxiety.

C **Diagnostic categories of anxiety**   Information about symptoms and diagnostic criteria is taken from the *Diagnostic and Statistical Manual of Mental Disorders,* 4th edition, text revision (*DSM-IV-TR*). In addition to the specific symptoms listed with each category, all *DSM-IV-TR* criteria for anxiety disorders include significant distress or interference with normal functioning or routines caused by the symptoms.

1. **Panic disorder**
   a. **Symptoms.** Panic disorder (Table 4–1) consists of recurrent panic attacks (Table 4–2) characterized by sudden apprehension or fear and usually accompanied by autonomic arousal. Panic disorder seems to be associated with abnormal responsiveness to carbon dioxide, resulting in overreaction to a sense of suffocation. The disorder may be accompanied by agoraphobia.
   b. **Treatment.** Antidepressants (selective serotonin reuptake inhibitors [SSRIs], serotonin norepinephrine reuptake inhibitors [SNRIs], tricyclic antidepressants [TCAs]), benzodiazepines, and cognitive behavioral therapy have all demonstrated efficacy.

2. **Agoraphobia**
   a. **Symptoms.** Anxiety about being in situations from which escape might be difficult or embarrassing or for which help may not be available in the event of panic or other forms of discomfort or distress is characteristic of agoraphobia. Common agoraphobic situations include being away from home, sitting in the middle of a row of seats in a theater, being on a bridge or in an elevator, or traveling in a car or airplane. Such situations are either avoided or are endured only by having a companion nearby. Otherwise, remaining in the situation causes marked distress or panic.
   b. **Association with panic disorder.** If agoraphobia complicates panic disorder, the diagnosis is **panic disorder with agoraphobia.** If agoraphobia occurs in the absence of panic disorder, the diagnosis is **agoraphobia without a history of panic disorder.**

TABLE 4–1   *DSM-IV-TR* Diagnostic Criteria for Panic Disorder (With or Without Agoraphobia)

A. Both (1) and (2)
  1. Recurrent unexpected panic attacks
  2. At least one attack followed by 1 month (or more) of one (or more) of:
     a. Persistent concern about additional attacks
     b. Worry about the implications of the attack or its consequences (e.g., losing control, having a heart attack, "going crazy")
     c. A significant change in behavior related to the attacks
B. Presence or absence of agoraphobia
C. Not due to direct effect of a substance or general medical condition
D. Not better accounted for by another mental disorder

Reprinted with permission from the Diagnostic and Statistical Manual of Mental Disorders, Fourth Edition, Text Revision, (Copyright 2000). American Psychiatric Association.

TABLE 4–2 *DSM-IV-TR* **Diagnostic Criteria for Panic Attack**

A discrete period of intense fear or discomfort, in which four (or more) of the following symptoms developed abruptly and reached a peak within 10 minutes:
1. Palpitations, pounding heart, or accelerated heart rate
2. Sweating
3. Trembling or shaking
4. Sensations of shortness of breath or smothering
5. Feeling of choking
6. Chest pain or discomfort
7. Nausea or abdominal distress
8. Feeling dizzy, unsteady, lightheaded, or faint
9. Derealization (feelings of unreality) or depersonalization (being detached from oneself)
10. Fear of losing control or going crazy
11. Fear of dying
12. Paresthesias (numbness or tingling sensations)
13. Chills or hot flushes

Reprinted with permission from the Diagnostic and Statistical Manual of Mental Disorders, Fourth Edition, Text Revision, (Copyright 2000). American Psychiatric Association.

3. **Generalized anxiety disorder**
   a. **Symptoms.** Generalized anxiety disorder is characterized by excessive worries about a variety of stressors (Table 4–3). The level of anxiety is typically out of proportion to the severity of the stressor.
   b. **Treatment.** SSRIs, SNRIs, buspirone, benzodiazepines, and sometimes β-adrenergic blockers and cognitive behavioral therapy have proven to be efficacious. Relaxation training, hypnosis, biofeedback, supportive therapy, and other forms of psychotherapy may also be helpful.

4. **Obsessive-compulsive disorder (OCD)**
   a. **Symptoms.** OCD is characterized by recurrent obsessions and compulsions that are significantly distressing or time consuming (Table 4–4).
   b. **Treatment**
      (1) **Pharmacologic therapy.** SSRIs such as fluoxetine, paroxetine, sertraline, fluvoxamine, and the serotonergic TCA clomipramine have demonstrated efficacy. Higher doses of SSRIs are sometimes required.
      (2) **Psychotherapy.** Cognitive behavioral therapies involving exposure and response prevention (ERP) have proven to be effective. There is some evidence supporting augmentation with ERP after partial response or nonresponse to SSRIs. When coupled with relapse prevention

TABLE 4–3 *DSM-IV-TR* **Diagnostic Criteria for Generalized Anxiety Disorder**

A. Excessive anxiety and worry (apprehensive expectation), occurring more days than not for at least 6 months, about a number of events or activities.
B. It is difficult to control the worry.
C. The anxiety and worry are associated with three (or more) of the following six symptoms (with at least some symptoms present for more days than not for the past 6 months).
   Note: Only one item is required in children.
   1. Restlessness or feeling keyed up or on edge
   2. Being easily fatigued
   3. Difficulty concentrating or mind going blank
   4. Irritability
   5. Muscle tension
   6. Sleep disturbance (difficulty falling or staying asleep, or restless unsatisfying sleep)
D. The focus of the anxiety and worry is not confined to features of an Axis I disorder.
E. Cause clinically significant distress or impairment in functioning.
F. Not due to the direct physiologic effects of a substance or a general medical condition and does not occur exclusively during a mood disorder, a psychotic disorder, or a pervasive developmental disorder.

Reprinted with permission from the Diagnostic and Statistical Manual of Mental Disorders, Fourth Edition, Text Revision, (Copyright 2000). American Psychiatric Association.

TABLE 4–4 *DSM-IV-TR* Diagnostic Criteria for Obsessive-Compulsive Disorder

A. Either obsessions or compulsions:
Obsessions as defined by (1), (2), (3), and (4):
  1. Recurrent and persistent thoughts, impulses, or images experienced as intrusive and inappropriate and causing marked anxiety or distress
  2. Not simply excessive worries about real-life problems
  3. The person attempts to ignore or suppress such thoughts, impulses, or images, or to neutralize them with some other thought or action.
  4. The person recognizes them as product of his or her own mind (not imposed from without as in thought insertion).
Compulsions as defined by (1) and (2):
  1. Repetitive behaviors or mental acts that the person feels driven to perform in response to an obsession, or according to rules that must be applied rigidly
  2. Aimed at preventing or reducing distress or preventing some dreaded event or situation; however, they either are not connected in a realistic way with what they are designed to neutralize or prevent or are clearly excessive.
B. The person has recognized the obsessions or compulsions are excessive or unreasonable. Note: This does not apply to children.
C. Obsessions or compulsions cause marked distress, are time consuming (>1 hour/day), or significantly interfere with functioning.
D. Obsessions or compulsions are not restricted to another Axis I disorder.
E. Not due to direct effects of a substance or general medical condition.

Reprinted with permission from the Diagnostic and Statistical Manual of Mental Disorders, Fourth Edition, Text Revision, (Copyright 2000). American Psychiatric Association.

---

techniques, therapy can produce more lasting benefits than medication alone. Other cognitive therapies and specialized techniques such as "stop thinking" can also be helpful.

    (3) Other treatment modalities. Ablative neurosurgery is occasionally used for severe and very treatment-refractory OCD. Deep brain stimulation now offers a reversible alternative to surgery.

5. **Specific phobias**
  a. Symptoms. These phobias involve excessive or irrational fear in response to the presence or anticipation of a specific object or situation (e.g., height, spiders, blood). Although the anxiety is recognized as inappropriate, the phobic stimulus is avoided or endured only with intense distress. Specific phobias often reflect universal reactions to stimuli that many people may find uncomfortable but evoke intense anxiety in a particular patient.
  b. Subtypes
    (1) Animal type. Fear of animals or insects usually begins in childhood.
    (2) Natural environmental type. This type involves fear of storms, height, and other events in the environment and also usually begins in childhood.
    (3) Blood–injection–injury type. This is a fear of seeing blood or injury or receiving an injection. It is often familial and is associated with fainting (vasovagal syncope).
    (4) Situational type. This type involves fear of specific situations such as elevators, bridges, and enclosed places but without panic disorder or other agoraphobic symptoms. However, situational phobia is similar to panic disorder with agoraphobia in its age of onset, familial aggregation, and gender ratios.
    (5) Other type. This category includes irrational fears of other stimuli, such as illness, or fears of falling if not near a wall or other means of physical support (**space phobia**).
  c. Treatment. Specific phobias are usually treated with behavioral therapies.
6. **Social phobia**
  a. Symptoms. A marked and persistent fear of humiliating oneself in social or performance situations that involve social scrutiny may be characteristic. Panic attacks may occur in social situations.
  b. Treatment. Social phobia is typically treated with SSRIs, SNRIs, cognitive behavioral therapy, and occasionally β-adrenergic blocking agents.

TABLE 4–5 *DSM-IV-TR* **Diagnostic Criteria for Posttraumatic Stress Disorder**

A. The person has been exposed to a traumatic event in which both of the following were present:
   1. The person experienced, witnessed, or was confronted with actual or threatened death or serious injury, or a threat to the physical integrity of self or others.
   2. The person's response involved intense fear, helplessness, or horror. **Note:** In children, this may be expressed instead by disorganized or agitated behavior.
B. The traumatic event is persistently reexperienced in one (or more) of the following ways:
   1. Recurrent and intrusive distressing recollections of the event
   2. Recurrent distressing dreams of the event
   3. Acting or feeling as if the traumatic event were recurring
   4. Intense psychological distress at exposure to internal or external cues that symbolize or resemble an aspect of the traumatic event
   5. Physiologic reactivity on exposure to internal or external cues that symbolize or resemble an aspect of the traumatic event.
C. Persistent avoidance of stimuli associated with the trauma and numbing of general responsiveness, as indicated by three (or more) of the following:
   1. Efforts to avoid thoughts, feelings, or conversations associated with the trauma
   2. Efforts to avoid activities, places, or people that arouse recollections of the trauma
   3. Inability to recall an important aspect of the trauma
   4. Markedly diminished interest or participation in significant activities
   5. Feeling of detachment or estrangement from others
   6. Restricted range of affect (e.g., unable to have loving feelings)
   7. Sense of a foreshortened future (e.g., does not expect to have a career, marriage, children, or a normal life span).
D. Persistent symptoms of increased arousal, as indicated by two (or more) of the following:
   1. Difficulty falling or staying asleep
   2. Irritability or outbursts of anger
   3. Difficulty concentrating
   4. Hypervigilance
   5. Exaggerated startle response.
E. Duration of the disturbance (symptoms in Criteria B, C, and D) is more than 1 month.
F. The disturbance causes clinically significant distress or impairment in social, occupational, or other important areas of functioning.

Reprinted with permission from the Diagnostic and Statistical Manual of Mental Disorders, Fourth Edition, Text Revision, (Copyright 2000). American Psychiatric Association.

7. **Posttraumatic stress disorder (PTSD)**
   a. **Symptoms.** This syndrome of distress, reexperiencing, avoidance, and arousal develops after exposure to traumatic events (Table 4–5).
   b. **Treatment.** Cognitive therapy may be helpful in restructuring thoughts about the traumatic event. Some patients may benefit from therapeutic reexposure to traumatic events (through writings, guided imaging, etc.). Eye movement desensitization and reprocessing (EMDR) has proven helpful in many patients with PTSD. EMDR involves processing distressing memories while engaged in guided eye movement. Discussing recently experienced traumas (sometimes called "debriefing") is not generally helpful, but psychological first aid measures can be effective in decreasing distress in the immediate aftermath of a traumatic event. SSRIs have demonstrated efficacy in non–combat-related PTSD, but less so for combat-related PTSD. SNRIs, mirtazapine, prazosin, atypical antipsychotics, and anticonvulsants have demonstrated efficacy.
8. **Acute stress disorder (ASD).** A traumatic event, which is defined exactly as in PTSD, produces anxiety or arousal, avoidance, reexperiencing, and acute or delayed dissociative symptoms such as detachment or absence of emotional responsiveness, decreased awareness of surroundings, derealization, depersonalization, or dissociative amnesia. Three or more of these symptoms (including emotional numbing) must be present to make the diagnosis. Acute stress disorder begins within 1 month of the event and lasts 2 days to 4 weeks. The diagnosis is changed to PTSD after acute stress disorder has been present for 1 month. Recent research suggests that because the presence of dissociation soon after a trauma does not identify a distinct subgroup of traumatized individuals, acute stress disorder may be just a variant or, at most, a precursor of PTSD.

9. **Anxiety disorder caused by a general medical condition.** This diagnosis refers to anxiety caused by medical and surgical disorders.

10. **Substance-induced anxiety disorder.** This diagnosis is made when a psychoactive substance is responsible for anxiety symptoms.

II PSYCHOLOGICAL COMPONENTS OF ANXIETY

A significant number of patients display anxiety symptoms that do not meet criteria for any specific *DSM-IV-TR* diagnosis but still cause significant distress or disability.

A **Situational anxiety**   Severe stress may temporarily overwhelm any person's ability to cope.

1. **Symptoms.** A relatively minor situation may feel overwhelming because it recalls other situations in which the individual was unable to cope or that aroused unresolved conflict. The intensity and nature of anxiety that evolves from a stressful situation can vary greatly based on the resiliency of the patient. Whereas a relatively well-adjusted patient may experience mild, transient symptoms, a marginally compensated patient may have persistent, severe anxiety when faced with the same stressor.

2. **Treatment.** Patients should be encouraged to talk about what the stress means to them. Feelings of helplessness can be decreased by helping the patient to put the situation into words. The use of relaxation techniques and related therapies may also be effective.

B **Anxiety about death**   Even nonfatal illnesses may remind individuals of their mortality.

1. **Symptoms.** Persistent fear of death, even in terminally ill patients, often symbolizes concern about loss of control, pain, isolation, helplessness, and the prospect of losing important relationships.

2. **Treatment.** Reassurance that patients will not be left alone and in pain often decreases the apparent fear of death.

C **Anxiety about mutilation, loss of prowess, or loss of attractiveness** is especially common in medically ill patients who feel that love, approval, and self-esteem depend on their strength or beauty.

1. **Symptoms.** Illness or injury may threaten the patient's appearance or prowess, resulting in anxiety. Such patients may attempt self-reassurance by demonstrating attractiveness or strength in inappropriate or even dangerous ways (e.g., a 25-year-old athlete hospitalized with a severe cardiac condition is found doing push-ups in his room despite warnings about overexertion).

2. **Treatment.** Patients should be reassured that they still possess valued traits. Involving the patient's family should be considered.

D **Anxiety about loss of self-esteem**   Patients whose self-esteem is fragile are especially vulnerable to experiencing illness as an imperfection, weakness, or failure, which can lead to attempts to bolster a sense of self-worth by boasting about importance and superiority.

1. **Symptoms.** Patients may adopt a self-important air, insisting on being treated only by the most senior or well-known physicians and treating others as worthless inferiors. Attempts to convince these patients that they are not as important as they think they are only increase their insecurity, which is covered up with greater protestations of their own importance and, by comparison, the unimportance of others.

2. **Treatment.** Patients should be approached with appropriate deference and should be reassured that they are still important. Reasonable requests for special consideration (e.g., a telephone for a patient in the intensive care unit) during an acute illness should be granted.

E **Separation anxiety**   Regressed adults (i.e., those who function psychologically more as children than as adults) may become frightened when they are separated from important caregivers. This state commonly is encountered in physically ill patients, psychotic patients, and those with Cluster B or C personality disorders.

1. **Symptoms.** Separation distress may be expressed directly as anxiety or indirectly as complaints of pain or, when left alone, by calls for assistance with trivial matters.

2. Treatment. Family and close friends should be encouraged to be with the patient as much as possible. The nursing staff should be encouraged to visit the patient frequently for brief periods before the patient asks for help to avoid teaching the patient that the only way not to be left alone is to complain. The patient's room should be close to the nurse's station to facilitate frequent, brief visits. A roommate should be provided.

(F) Stranger anxiety

1. Symptoms. Patients who suffer from separation anxiety may also react adversely to unfamiliar people, including new physicians, nurses, and visitors. In hospitalized adults, this can lead to distress at shift changes or in other situations in which there are new caregivers.

2. Treatment. As much continuity in personnel as possible should be provided (e.g., the same nurse should be assigned to the patient every day). Having staff from the previous shift introduce new nurses may ease the transition between shifts. Unfamiliar visitors should be limited. Changes in roommates should be minimized. A careful mental status examination is necessary to be certain that patients are not reacting adversely to changes in the environment because of developing delirium.

(G) Anxiety about loss of control

1. Symptoms. Illness and hospitalization may be threatening to people who have a strong need to feel in complete control of their life and environment, especially when others must make decisions for them. Patients may attempt to gain a sense of control by refusing to comply with the physician's advice, becoming excessively demanding, making the physician feel helpless, or otherwise asserting control over those who are in a caregiving role or who are healthy.

2. Treatment. Patients should be allowed as much control as possible over their treatment. For example, the patient's opinion about therapeutic decisions should be solicited, and the patient should be consulted about which treatment schedules seem most reasonable to the patient.

(H) Anxiety about dependency Patients who fear loss of control also commonly have anxiety about being dependent on others, which is usually a necessary component of any serious illness. Fear of dependency is common in people whose normal dependency needs were not met in childhood (e.g., because of parental illness or unavailability).

1. Symptoms. Extremely strong dependency wishes, which have remained unchanged since childhood, threaten to break through when patients encounter a mild illness that could place them in a dependent position. Because patients are afraid that they will not be able to control their dependency needs, they reject attempts of others to be helpful and become hostile toward potential caregivers. Affected individuals may also assert their independence by being noncompliant, failing to keep appointments, or ignoring signs of increasing illness.

2. Treatment. When possible, patients should be reassured that the illness and the dependency required by it are temporary. They should be helped to maintain as much independent function as possible.

(I) Anxiety about intimacy

1. Symptoms. Patients with concerns about dependency may also be afraid of becoming too close emotionally to caregivers or loved ones. To protect themselves, they maintain a greater-than-normal emotional distance. They experience distress in response to expressions of friendliness or intimacy and may attempt to ward off (e.g., through hostility) people who are nice or express concern.

2. Treatment. Intimacy should not be forced. The patient's sense of formality (e.g., by always using the patient's last name) should be respected.

(J) Anxiety about being punished

1. Symptoms. Patients with an underlying sense of guilt about real or imagined transgressions may have a conscious or unconscious expectation of punishment. They may attempt to relieve guilt or avoid worry about when they will be punished by means of self-inflicted punishment (e.g., through an unhappy marriage, repeated accidents, not recovering from an illness, and other self-destructive behaviors).

2. Treatment. The suffering of these patients should be acknowledged, and attempts should be made to uncover the source of their guilt. Psychotherapy may help patients to identify the source of their guilt.

K **Signal anxiety**

1. **Symptoms.** When awareness of a previously unconscious, unresolved psychological conflict is stimulated by some external occurrence (e.g., the patient had mixed feelings about a parent, and the patient's age is the same as that of the parent at the time of death), anxiety may signal the emergence of the conflict. This anxiety may call forth **psychological defenses (ego defenses),** which are unconscious mechanisms that avoid anxiety by keeping the conflict out of the patient's awareness.

   a. **Repression** (forgetting) is an unconscious process by which memories, thoughts, and feelings are excluded from awareness.

   b. **Rationalization** is the act of explaining away psychologically meaningful data (e.g., "I'm anxious only because of a low blood sugar").

   c. **Reaction formation** is feeling the opposite of one's true emotion in order not to be aware of it (e.g., experiencing excessive affection toward someone who actually elicits hostility).

   d. **Isolation of affect** is experiencing the content of a thought without its associated emotions.

   e. **Denial** is remaining unaware of some aspect of reality (e.g., feeling that one does not have to be afraid of the consequences of an illness because one is not really sick).

   f. **Projection** is attributing one's own motives to someone else.

   g. **Projective identification** is incompletely projecting an intense emotional state, usually anger, onto another individual while inducing the emotion in the object of the projection through provoking behavior. Patients then experience the original emotion, but they feel that the only reason they have the emotion or thought is that they are attempting to protect themselves from the other individual's affect.

2. **Treatment.** When it is possible and practical, an attempt to resolve the underlying conflict should be undertaken. When patients cannot tolerate awareness of their motives, they should be helped to develop less disabling defenses against them (e.g., isolation of the affect rather than denial of it, or denial of anxiety rather than denial of the situation that causes it). Behavioral and adjunctive measures (e.g., relaxation training), which are useful for control of situational anxiety, may help lessen signal anxiety.

III DIFFERENTIAL DIAGNOSIS

A **General medical disorders** Before investigating psychological causes of anxiety, it is important to exclude the possibility of physical disorders in which anxiety may be a presenting complaint even before other signs of disease become evident.

1. **Cardiovascular disorders**
   a. Arteriosclerotic heart disease
   b. Paroxysmal tachycardia
   c. Mitral valve prolapse
   d. Hyperdynamic β-adrenergic circulatory state

2. **Pulmonary disorders**
   a. Pulmonary embolism
   b. Hypoxemia
   c. Asthma
   d. Chronic obstructive lung disease

3. **Disorders of the endocrine system and metabolism**
   a. Hypoglycemia
   b. Hyperthyroidism or hypothyroidism
   c. Hypocalcemia
   d. Cushing syndrome
   e. Porphyria

4. **Tumors**
   a. Insulinoma
   b. Carcinoid tumor
   c. Pheochromocytoma

5. **Neurologic disorders**
    a. Multiple sclerosis (MS)
    b. Temporal lobe epilepsy
    c. Delirium and dementia
    d. Ménière disease

6. **Infections**
    a. Tuberculosis
    b. Brucellosis

B Substance-related disorders

1. Abstinence syndromes (e.g., withdrawal from central nervous system [CNS] depressants such as alcohol, tranquilizers, sleeping pills)

2. Intoxication with sympathomimetics

3. Akathisia

4. Caffeinism

5. Chinese restaurant syndrome, resulting from the ingestion of monosodium glutamate (MSG)

6. Nicotine

C Anxiety that mimics general medical illness Anxiety may also mimic physical disease. For example, patients with hyperventilation syndrome complain of shortness of breath, weakness, paresthesias, headache, and carpopedal spasm. These patients are often unaware of feeling anxious about anything except being short of breath. Symptoms abate when the patient is calmed and the respiratory rate decreases. Treatment consists of instructing the patient to breathe into a paper bag, which is held over the nose and mouth. Carbon dioxide accumulates and reverses the respiratory alkalosis caused by hyperventilation.

D Other psychiatric conditions

1. **Depression.** Approximately 70% of depressed patients also feel anxious, and 20% to 30% of apparent cases of anxiety are caused by an underlying depression. Approximately 40% to 90% of patients with panic disorder become depressed, and 20% to 50% of depressed patients have panic attacks. A depressive diagnosis is changed to an anxiety disorder, and vice versa, in about 25% of patients initially diagnosed with a depressive or anxiety disorder. Depressed patients with blood relatives who are anxious are more likely to experience anxiety plus depression than those with a family history of depression only.

2. **Psychosis.** As control of mental processes is lost, patients who experience psychotic disorganization often display considerable anxiety, which may initially obscure the underlying severe disturbance of thinking, affect, or behavior.

3. **Mania.** Bursts of overstimulation, excess energy, and racing thoughts may be experienced as panic attacks, especially in younger patients.

4. **Delirium and dementia.** Anxiety is the most common emotion experienced by patients with acute organic mental syndromes (delirium) who are frightened by a sudden disruption of cognitive abilities, as well as by patients with dementia, whose mental syndromes are made worse by an intercurrent illness or by a sudden change in the environment (e.g., a change in the roommate of a hospitalized demented patient).

5. **Adjustment disorder with anxiety.** Within 3 months of exposure to an obvious stress, patients experience anxiety or impairment in excess of that which would normally be expected. Anxiety and other symptoms appear soon after the onset of an event that most people would consider upsetting but not life threatening, unlike with PTSD, and the symptoms are expected to resolve within 6 months of the stress abating or the patient achieving a new level of functioning.

6. **Factitious disorder.** Rarely, individuals consciously simulate a mental disorder, including anxiety disorders, for the sole purpose of becoming a patient. The patient often relates an improbable history and has been hospitalized numerous times, often under different names.

7. **Malingering** refers to the conscious simulation of a condition for some obvious gain (e.g., obtaining benzodiazepines). Malingering is more common in patients with a history of lying, drug abuse, and antisocial behavior.

IV   TREATMENT

A **Psychotherapy**   This mode of treatment involves group or individual sessions with a trained therapist who may utilize a variety of methods to decrease symptoms of anxiety. Psychotherapy is effective for individuals alone or in combination with medication.

1. **Supportive therapy.** This type of psychotherapy is useful for acutely ill patients, patients under severe stress, and patients with limited emotional and psychosocial resources (e.g., because of social isolation or other psychiatric illness).
   a. **Support of defenses.** The principal therapeutic approach involves encouraging defenses that are as adaptive as possible. For example:
      (1) A 62-year-old man with severe coronary artery disease experiences anxiety about having a myocardial infarction. Bouts of anxiety have caused frequent episodes of angina and increased risk of a cardiac event. He uses denial to control his anxiety, but this leads to chronic noncompliance with his cardiac medications. In supportive therapy, the goal would be to decrease his use of denial and encourage other ways to control anxiety (distraction, discussing feelings with others, etc.).
      (2) A 35-year-old woman with chronic schizophrenia struggles with paranoia and disturbing hallucinations, despite compliance with medication. Supportive therapy would attempt to decrease her distress by helping with more modifiable problems such as improving hygiene and increasing social interactions.
      (3) People who are anxious because they feel out of control may gain a sense of mastery through intellectualization.
   b. **Reality testing.** With patients who tend to distort reality and misinterpret events, the physician may offer alternative explanations. Tactfully pointing out lapses in reality testing helps patients assess the situation more objectively.
   c. **Advice.** Help with problem solving is appropriate, especially when patients attempt to avoid anxiety through destructive or self-destructive behavior. For example, a patient might be advised to stop attempting to relieve anxiety by arguing with a spouse and to go for a walk instead.
   d. **Adaptive behavior.** Such patient behavior should be reinforced (encouraged). Therapists may encourage such behavior through modeling in their interactions with the patient.

2. **Psychodynamic psychotherapy.** Motivated patients with the capability to understand themselves may gain control of their symptoms by uncovering the psychological meaning of the anxiety and resolving unconscious conflicts. Conflicts related to early childhood experiences (particularly with parental figures) are often repeated in the patient–therapist relationship through a process called transference. Before applying psychodynamic psychotherapy, it is important to assess a patient's ability to be aware of emotions without acting on or being overwhelmed by them. Components of expressive psychotherapy include:
   a. **Clarification** of the patient's statements in order to make them more comprehensible
   b. **Confrontation** of aspects of reality or the patient's emotions that the patient is ignoring (e.g., "You say that you are not anxious, but you look very nervous")
   c. **Interpretation** of unconscious thoughts and feelings to bring them into the patient's awareness (e.g., "Do you think that you are anxious around your boss because he is so much like your father?")

3. **Cognitive behavioral therapy.** These treatment methods are effective for phobias, panic anxiety, generalized anxiety, PTSD, acute stress disorder, and OCD.
   a. **Systematic desensitization includes:**
      (1) The therapist teaches patients deep muscle relaxation.
      (2) Patients visualize a scene involving thoughts that are the opposite of anxious thinking such as feeling safe, relaxed, and in control.
      (3) Next patients imagine anxiety-provoking situations.

(4) As soon as anxiety begins to emerge, the scene that induces relaxation is evoked until the anxiety ceases.

(5) Anxiety-provoking and comforting scenes are repeatedly paired until the thought of the former no longer causes anxiety.

(6) Beginning with the situation that provokes the least anxiety, patients gradually move up a hierarchy of situations to the ones that are most feared. Hypnosis may be used to facilitate the process.

(7) When patients can visualize the most anxiety-provoking scene while still feeling relaxed, less anxiety is experienced in the corresponding real-life situation.

b. **Graduated in vivo exposure** places phobic patients (who are usually accompanied by a family member, friend, or physician for reassurance) in situations that evoke anxiety. Systematic desensitization may be necessary first if the patient becomes overwhelmingly anxious in the phobic situation. Relaxation techniques and hypnosis are used to change the association between phobic situations and anxiety to an association of those situations with relaxation and control.

c. **Panic control therapy** involves redefining symptoms of a panic attack such as dizziness or shortness of breath as harmless physiologic responses to anxiety rather than signs of a catastrophic illness. This kind of cognitive restructuring is facilitated by actual induction of panic symptoms (e.g., by spinning the patient around in a chair to produce dizziness). Patients are also taught to substitute relaxation for the anxiety that otherwise develops in response to physiologic triggers of a panic attack.

d. **Exposure and response prevention** are the cornerstones of the behavioral treatment of OCD. Patients are exposed to a stimulus that evokes rituals (e.g., touching a toilet seat) and are then helped to refrain from engaging in a compulsive behavior (e.g., hand washing) for increasing lengths of time while using adjunctive techniques to control the resulting anxiety. Response prevention for mental compulsions or obsessions is less effective in the absence of physical compulsions because the latter are easier for other people to restrain.

e. **"Stop thinking"** is a mental variant of response prevention in which patients repeat an obsessive thought until it seems overwhelming and then terminate the thought while saying "stop" out loud.

f. **Adjunctive behavioral techniques** may be useful for patients who suffer from any type of anxiety.

(1) **Relaxation techniques.** These can include muscle relaxation, guided imagery, controlled breathing, or any other activity that contributes to decreased tension.

(2) **Hypnosis.** This altered state of consciousness permits heightened concentration and attention. Hypnosis helps patients concentrate on calming thoughts that are incompatible with anxiety. Patients who have excessive fear of loss of control or who have organic brain disease often cannot be hypnotized.

(3) **Biofeedback.** This technique is useful for patients who prefer a self-administered relaxation technique. The level of muscular tension, usually in the forearm or frontalis muscles, is "fed back" through a visual or auditory stimulus to help patients learn to decrease motor tension and anxiety. It also has been used to treat headaches and mild essential hypertension.

B **Psychopharmacology** Medications can be helpful in the treatment of anxiety disorders, particularly when coupled with appropriate psychotherapy. Some medications provide immediate relief of symptoms (e.g., benzodiazepines), while others have a more gradual effect (e.g., antidepressants). Treatment relying entirely on medication rarely results in long-term recovery.

1. **Selective serotonin reuptake inhibitors**
   a. **Uses.** SSRIs are at least as effective as tricyclic antidepressants in the treatment of a variety of anxiety disorders. A more favorable side-effect and safety profile has made them the first-line pharmacologic treatment for anxiety disorders.

   (1) **Panic disorder.** Fluoxetine, paroxetine, and sertraline are supported by randomized controlled trials and have a Food and Drug Administration (FDA) indication. Citalopram and fluvoxamine also have evidence supporting their efficacy.

   (2) **PTSD.** Sertraline and paroxetine have an FDA indication, although all the SSRIs may be effective. SSRIs are less effective for combat-related PTSD.

    (3) **OCD.** Fluvoxamine, fluoxetine, paroxetine, and sertraline are FDA indicated for the treatment of OCD and are well supported in the literature. Citalopram and escitalopram have also demonstrated positive results.

    (4) **Social phobia.** Sertraline, paroxetine, and fluvoxamine are FDA indicated, although all SSRIs likely have beneficial effects.

    (5) **Generalized anxiety disorder.** Paroxetine and escitalopram are FDA indicated, although all SSRIs likely have beneficial effects.

  b. Administration. Dosing required can vary significantly between patients. The goal should be to determine the lowest effective dose. Patients with severe anxiety or those with panic disorder may benefit from very low doses initially to avoid worsening anxiety. High doses (e.g., 80 mg/day of fluoxetine) are often needed to treat OCD.

  c. Side effects. SSRIs are safer in overdose and better tolerated than TCAs and monoamine oxidase inhibitors (MAOIs).

    (1) Common side effects include gastrointestinal symptoms, irritability, weight gain, insomnia, drowsiness, and sexual dysfunction.

    (2) There may be an increased risk of upper gastrointestinal bleeding in predisposed patients.

    (3) Accelerated bone loss in elderly patients has also been reported.

    (4) The FDA has issued warnings that patients under the age of 25 may experience an increase in suicidal thoughts or behaviors when taking antidepressants. This risk must be weighed against the risk of suicide associated with the illness being treated. The warning also reinforces the importance of monitoring patients closely when starting antidepressants.

    (5) Abrupt discontinuation may lead to a syndrome characterized by dizziness, poor coordination, nausea, headache, and irritability. This is usually temporary and is non–life threatening.

2. Serotonin-norepinephrine reuptake inhibitors

  a. Uses. Venlafaxine has demonstrated efficacy and is FDA approved for panic disorder, generalized anxiety disorder, and social phobia. Duloxetine is FDA indicated for generalized anxiety disorder, although conditions responsive to venlafaxine would likely be responsive to duloxetine as well. SNRIs may also be effective in the treatment of PTSD. There are limited data to support the use of SNRIs in OCD.

  b. Side effects. The side-effect profile is similar to that of the SSRIs, although increases in blood pressure may occur with higher doses of SNRIs. Discontinuation syndrome similar to that seen with SSRIs is not uncommon.

3. Tricyclic antidepressants

  a. Uses. TCAs are effective in both generalized and panic anxiety. Imipramine, clomipramine, nortriptyline, and desipramine have demonstrated efficacy for panic disorder. Clomipramine is a well-proven treatment for OCD, either as monotherapy or as an augmentation to another form of treatment.

  b. Side effects. The most common side effects are anticholinergic effects (dry mouth, constipation, difficulty urinating, increased heart rate, and blurry vision), increased sweating, sleep disturbance, orthostatic hypotension, fatigue, cognitive disturbance, weight gain, and sexual dysfunction. Even a small overdose of a TCA can lead to fatal cardiac toxicity. Given this risk, TCAs are used less frequently than the safer SSRIs and SNRIs.

4. Monoamine oxidase inhibitors

  a. Uses. MAOIs have been used for panic disorder, social phobia, and other anxiety disorders. There are few trials to support the use of MAOIs in anxiety disorders. MAOIs are rarely used due to their less favorable side-effect profile compared to SSRIs and SNRIs.

  b. Side effects and interactions. MAOIs can be sedating or stimulating. These agents can produce hypertensive crises when administered with foods that are high in tyramine content (e.g., aged cheese) and with sympathomimetic substances. Fatal serotonin syndrome, which involves myoclonus, fever, headaches, nausea, seizures, and cardiotoxicity, may occur when MAOIs are combined with SSRIs, dextromethorphan, and other serotoninergic compounds.

5. Buspirone

  a. Uses. Buspirone has partial agonist effects at the serotonin 5-HT$_{1A}$ receptor. Its primary use is generalized anxiety disorder. Unlike benzodiazepines, buspirone does not have a rapid onset of action.

b. **Administration.** Buspirone must be given in divided doses (total: 10–60 mg/day) for 1 month before it is effective.

c. **Side effects.** Buspirone is generally well tolerated. It has few clinically important interactions other than serotonin syndrome when combined with MAOIs. Because higher doses cause dysphoria, patients do not escalate the dose (as may occur with benzodiazepines).

6. **Benzodiazepines** are effective antianxiety drugs. These agents are most useful for acute situational anxiety, anticipatory anxiety associated with panic attacks, generalized anxiety disorder, and panic disorder.

   a. **Uses**

     (1) **Panic anxiety.** The most widely used benzodiazepines for treating panic disorder are the triazolobenzodiazepine **alprazolam** and the anticonvulsant **clonazepam.**

       (a) Alprazolam has high potency (i.e., a small dose produces a large clinical effect), high lipid solubility, a short elimination half-life, and no active metabolites. Clonazepam has high potency, low lipid solubility, a long elimination half-life, and several active metabolites. As a result, alprazolam has a rapid onset and offset of action and requires frequent dosing, and clonazepam can be given less frequently but becomes more sedating with time as the parent drug and its metabolites accumulate.

       (b) Improvement should begin to be apparent within 1 month of treatment with a dosage of 2 to 10 mg/day of alprazolam or 1 to 5 mg/day of clonazepam. If improvement has not begun within 4 to 6 weeks, another medication, such as an antidepressant, should be considered.

       (c) Equivalently high doses of other benzodiazepines (e.g., 20–100 mg of diazepam) appear to be equally effective for panic disorder but are difficult to tolerate and require taking too many pills.

     (2) **Generalized and situational anxiety.** Benzodiazepines are effective for generalized and situational anxiety. They differ mainly in their elimination half-lives, potency, and lipid solubility. These properties vary for different preparations. For example, midazolam has a very short half-life, high potency, and high lipid solubility; diazepam has a long half-life, intermediate potency, and high lipid solubility; and chlordiazepoxide has a long half-life, low potency, and low lipid solubility.

       (a) **Long-acting benzodiazepines** include diazepam, chlordiazepoxide, clorazepate, and clonazepam. Long-acting preparations can be given less frequently during the day, although they are usually administered at least twice daily to minimize oversedating peaks in blood level. Discontinuation syndromes appear more gradually, last longer, and are often more attenuated than after discontinuation of shorter-acting benzodiazepines.

       (b) **Short-acting benzodiazepines** include midazolam, lorazepam, oxazepam, and alprazolam. Short-acting drugs must be given more frequently (as often as every 2 to 3 hours for some patients taking alprazolam). Discontinuation syndromes are more severe and abrupt than with longer-acting benzodiazepines, but these syndromes last a shorter period of time. Alprazolam is also available in an extended-release form, which allows for less frequent dosing.

       (c) Clorazepate is a **diazepam prodrug** that has no action of its own but is metabolized to diazepam after ingestion.

     (3) **Insomnia**

       (a) Benzodiazepines such as flurazepam, temazepam, triazolam, and estazolam are used to treat acute insomnia associated with stress, jet lag, or a change in sleep phase. Any benzodiazepine can be used to treat insomnia.

       (b) Zolpidem, a nonbenzodiazepine hypnotic, is selective for a subtype of the benzodiazepine receptor (type 1 receptor), which results in fewer side effects and withdrawal syndromes. Zaleplon and eszopiclone are also nonbenzodiazepine medications that act on the benzodiazepine type 1 receptor with a side-effect profile similar to that of zolpidem.

   b. **Administration.** Benzodiazepines are most effective when used to treat time-limited anxiety that occurs in response to clear-cut stress and when treatment lasts less than 8 weeks. However, some chronically anxious patients may need long-term therapy. Because generalized anxiety disorder follows a relapsing course, repeated treatment episodes are often necessary.

c. **Addiction.** Benzodiazepine addiction is rare in medical patients. However, individuals with a history of alcohol or drug abuse are at high risk for abusing benzodiazepines. The most frequently abused benzodiazepines are diazepam, alprazolam, and lorazepam. Early requests for refills, use of deception to obtain medication, and "doctor shopping" are indications that a patient may be misusing benzodiazepines.

d. **Abstinence syndromes.** Withdrawal symptoms may appear up to 10 days after abrupt discontinuation of moderate doses of benzodiazepines that have been taken for more than 1 month. Signs and symptoms of withdrawal include anxiety, insomnia, irritability, and, at times, psychosis, delirium, and seizures. Some patients may experience prolonged, attenuated withdrawal symptoms lasting up to 1 year. Withdrawal is more abrupt and severe and seizures are more likely to occur after discontinuation of short-acting benzodiazepines.

e. **Common side effects.** Sedation, memory problems, and impaired psychomotor performance may occur. Tolerance develops to the sedative effects of benzodiazepines but not to the anxiolytic effects or impaired performance. Alcohol and benzodiazepines have additive effects that impair driving. Benzodiazepines may cause or aggravate depression. Because of drug accumulation, use of longer-acting benzodiazepines is a common cause of falls in the elderly.

7. **Antihistamines** (e.g., hydroxyzine, diphenhydramine) are frequently used as antianxiety drugs and hypnotics for elderly patients and for those in whom addiction may be a problem. However, these agents are not as predictably effective as other antianxiety drugs, and their anticholinergic and sedating side effects can aggravate memory loss and loss of coordination.

8. **Antipsychotic drugs**

a. **Uses.** No antipsychotic is specifically indicated for the treatment of anxiety. Second-generation antipsychotics may be useful for augmentation of SSRIs or SNRIs in PTSD patients who have shown a partial response. Antipsychotics may also be helpful as an augmenting agent in the treatment of OCD.

b. **Side effects.** The risk of long-term side effects, especially tardive dyskinesia, likely outweighs the potential benefit of antipsychotic medications in most patients with anxiety disorders. Atypical antipsychotic drugs (e.g., risperidone, olanzapine, quetiapine, clozapine) have a lower risk of tardive dyskinesia but carry a greater risk of metabolic effects (diabetes, dyslipidemia, obesity).

8. **Antihypertensives** such as β-blocking agents (e.g., propranolol) can relieve symptoms for patients whose anxiety is accompanied by signs of adrenergic stimulation (e.g., sweating, tremor) and for patients with performance anxiety. These agents are not as predictably effective as the benzodiazepines or the antidepressants in relieving generalized anxiety. β-Blockers may be useful in relieving stage fright. The α-blocker prazosin has demonstrated efficacy in controlling nightmares related to PTSD.

BIBLIOGRAPHY

American Psychiatric Association: *Diagnostic and Statistical Manual of Mental Disorders,* 4th ed., text revision. Washington, DC, American Psychiatric Association, 2000.

American Psychiatric Association: *Practice Guideline for Treatment of Patients with Panic Disorder,* 2nd ed. Washington, DC, American Psychiatric Association, 2009.

American Psychiatric Association: *Practice Guideline for the Treatment of Patients with Acute Stress Disorder and Posttraumatic Stress Disorder.* Washington, DC, American Psychiatric Association, 2004.

American Psychiatric Association: *Guideline Watch: Practice Guideline for the Treatment of Patients with Acute Stress Disorder and Posttraumatic Stress Disorder.* Washington, DC, American Psychiatric Association, 2009.

American Psychiatric Association: *Practice Guideline for the Treatment of Patients with Obsessive-Compulsive Disorder.* Washington, DC, American Psychiatric Association, 2007.

Study Questions

Directions: *Each of the numbered items or incomplete statements in this section is followed by answers or by completions of the statement. Several items may pertain to one clinical vignette. Select the ONE lettered answer or completion that is BEST in each case.*

QUESTIONS 1–2

A 35-year-old woman presents to your primary care practice saying that she believes she may have suffered a stroke. She describes episodes lasting 5 to 10 minutes in which she sweats profusely, becomes dizzy, and has difficulty swallowing. She says she is terrified by these episodes, which seem to occur whenever she leaves her apartment at rush hour. She asked to be on the night shift at her job, but she has recently stopped working altogether out of fear that she would have a stroke while driving.

1. Provided you find no other cause for her symptoms, which of the following would be the most likely psychiatric diagnosis?

- A Obsessive-compulsive disorder
- B Panic disorder with agoraphobia
- C Panic disorder without agoraphobia
- D Generalized anxiety disorder
- E Schizophrenia

2. Which of the following medications would be most appropriate as a first-line treatment for this patient?

- A Sertraline SSRI
- B Fluphenazine Typical (1st gen antipsychotic)
- C Gabapentin
- D Phenobarbital – barbiturate
- E Lamotrigine

anticonvulsant [C, D, E grouped]

QUESTIONS 3–4

A 20-year-old female patient is receiving inpatient treatment for community-acquired pneumonia. She has a history of borderline personality disorder and multiple admissions to the hospital's psychiatric unit. She rings her call bell every few minutes requesting assistance from her nurse. She insists that the nurse come to her room before she will reveal what she needs. The requests to see her nurse become more frequent after her family leaves or as the change of shifts approaches.

3. Which of the following is the patient most likely experiencing?

- A Anxiety related to psychosis
- B Anxiety about being punished
- C Panic attacks
- D Separation anxiety ~ Cluster B
- E Anxiety about dependency

4. Which of the following would be an appropriate approach to this patient?

- A Firmly refuse her requests as they are inappropriate and excessive.
- B Give the patient quetiapine.
- C Transfer the patient to the psychiatry unit.
- D Discourage family from visiting.
- E Instruct the nurses to make frequent, brief visits to the patient.

5. A 65-year-old man says he has nightmares about seeing his friend killed in combat during his military service many years ago. He is easily startled by loud noises. He is diagnosed with posttraumatic stress disorder. How would his illness differ from an adjustment disorder?

- [A] It only occurs in veterans.
- [B] It is characterized by impairment of social functioning.
- [C] It persists long after the stress has abated.
- [D] It is characterized by preoccupation with the stress.
- [E] It can be accompanied by depression.

6. You are beginning psychodynamic therapy with a patient suffering from generalized anxiety disorder. This type of therapy would include:

- [A] Systemic desensitization   CBT
- [B] Exposure and response prevention   CBT
- [C] Interpretation of unconscious thoughts and feelings -- Psychodynamic
- [D] Giving advice   supportive
- [E] Biofeedback   CBT

7. You are treating a patient with paroxetine for generalized anxiety disorder, but his symptoms are only partially controlled. You would like to start a long-acting benzodiazepine to augment the effect of the selective serotonin reuptake inhibitor (SSRI). Which of the following would you choose?

- [A] Alprazolam short
- [B] Mirtazapine - antidepressant
- [C] Midazolam short
- [D] Lorazepam short
- [E] Clonazepam long   *(Klonopin)*

Directions: *Each of the numbered items or incomplete statements in this section is negatively phrased, as indicated by a capitalized word such as NOT, LEAST, or EXCEPT. Select the ONE lettered answer or completion that is BEST in each case.*

8. All of the following are true regarding side effects of selective serotonin reuptake inhibitors (SSRIs) EXCEPT:

- [A] Abrupt discontinuation may result in a potentially fatal withdrawal syndrome.
- [B] Gastrointestinal side effects are common.
- [C] Risk of accelerated bone loss may increase in elderly patients.
- [D] Sexual dysfunction is a common side effect.
- [E] Patients should be monitored for the emergence of suicidal thoughts.

9. All of the following are physical conditions that may present with anxiety symptoms EXCEPT:

- [A] Mitral valve prolapse
- [B] Hyperthyroidism
- [C] Pulmonary embolism
- [D] Hypoglycemia
- [E] Gout

Answers and Explanations

1. The answer is B [*I C 1*]. The patient presents with intense fears and symptoms of autonomic arousal. This is most consistent with a panic attack. She is also reporting anxiety about having these episodes as well as behavioral avoidance of situations where she might be unable to escape in the event of an attack (e.g., in rush-hour traffic). Her avoidance symptoms indicate the presence of agoraphobia.

2. The answer is A [*I C 1 b, IV B 1*]. Sertraline is a selective serotonin reuptake inhibitor (SSRI), which is a first-line treatment for panic disorder. None of the other listed medications are appropriate first-line treatments for anxiety disorders. Fluphenazine is a first-generation antipsychotic, gabapentin and lamotrigine are anticonvulsants, and phenobarbital is a barbiturate.

3. The answer is D [*II E*]. The patient's frequent attempts to have the nurse come to her room indicate the presence of separation anxiety. Patients with Cluster B personality are more likely to experience this type of anxiety. There is no indication of psychosis or of clearly defined panic attacks. There are also no indications that the patient has fears of punishment.

4. The answer is E [*II E 2*]. Frequent visits to the patient's room will reassure her that making trivial requests is not required to obtain the emotional support she needs. Refusal to provide support or limiting her visitors would likely worsen her anxiety. Neither antipsychotic medication (e.g., quetiapine) nor inpatient psychiatric care would be helpful in controlling the patient's anxiety.

5. The answer is C [*I C 7 a, III D 5*]. All of the listed statements could be true of an adjustment disorder, except that the symptoms persist after the stressor has resolved. An adjustment disorder, by definition, includes symptoms that resolve in the absence of the stressor. PTSD symptoms can persist for many years after a stressful situation has passed.

6. The answer is C [*IV A 2*]. Interpretation of unconscious thoughts or feelings is a technique used in psychodynamic therapy. The other techniques listed are part of either cognitive behavioral (A, B, and E) or supportive (D) therapy.

7. The answer is E [*IV B 6 a (2)*]. Clonazepam is a long-acting benzodiazepine. Alprazolam, lorazepam, and midazolam are all short-acting benzodiazepines. Mirtazapine is an antidepressant.

8. The answer is A [*IV B 1 c*]. There is a withdrawal syndrome associated with selective serotonin reuptake inhibitors (SSRIs) and serotonin norepinephrine reuptake inhibitors (SNRIs), but it is not fatal. All of the other listed items are side effects relevant to SSRIs.

9. The answer is E [*III A*]. Gout does not typically present with anxiety. The other listed items are all physical conditions that can present with a primary complaint of anxiety.

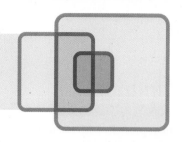

chapter **5**

Cognitive and Mental Disorders Due to General Medical Conditions

KIMBERLY RUDD · ROBERT BREEN

I · INTRODUCTION

In the *Diagnostic and Statistical Manual of Mental Disorders,* 4th edition, text revision (*DSM-IV-TR*), psychopathology that is caused by general medical conditions or by substances (e.g., abused drugs, medications, and toxins) is classified in three distinct groups. This classification replaced such terms as "organic mental disorders" that erroneously implied that other (primary) mental disorders are nonorganic.

A **Delirium, dementia, amnestic, and other cognitive disorders** are characterized by cognitive disturbances. They are caused by general medical conditions or are substance induced.

B **Mental disorders due to general medical conditions,** excluding cognitive disorders, are specific mental disorders due to general medical conditions. Examples include mood disorder due to a general medical condition, psychosis due to a general medical condition, sleep disorder due to a general medical condition, and sexual disorder due to a general medical condition. The description for each of these disorders is found in the *DSM-IV-TR* chapter that describes the primary psychiatric disorders with similar syndromes. For example, the description of mood disorder due to a general medical condition is found in the *DSM-IV-TR* chapter that concerns mood disorders.

1. **Diagnosis.** A mental disturbance is due to a general medical condition when evidence suggests that the disturbance results from the direct physiologic effect of the medical condition.

2. **Etiology.** The proposed general medical etiology should be known to cause the particular mental disturbance, and a temporal relationship should exist between the course of the general medical condition and the mental disturbance.

3. **Differentiation.** The disturbance should not be better explained by a primary mental disorder or one that is substance induced.

C **Substance-induced mental disorders** Specific substance-induced mental disorders are described in the *DSM-IV-TR* with other disorders that have similar presenting syndromes. For example, cocaine-induced psychotic disorder is described in the *DSM-IV-TR* chapter concerning schizophrenia and related psychotic disorders.

1. **Diagnosis.** A mental disturbance is substance induced if evidence suggests that the disturbance developed in association with substance use.

2. **Etiology.** The proposed substance should be known to cause the particular mental disturbance.

3. **Differentiation.** The disturbance should not be better explained by a primary mental disorder or one that is due to a general medical condition.

II COGNITIVE DISORDERS

Cognitive disorders are characterized by the syndromes of delirium, dementia, and amnesia. All are caused by general medical conditions, substances, or a combination of these factors. Disturbances of cognition involve symptoms such as confusion, memory impairment, speech and language difficulties, and impairment of the ability to plan or engage in complex tasks.

A **Delirium (Table 5–1)**

1. **Diagnostic features**
   a. **Disturbance of consciousness.** Individuals have reduced clarity of awareness of the environment. Their ability to focus, sustain, or shift attention is impaired. Affected individuals may appear confused, perplexed, or alarmed. They may have difficulty in responding to reassurance or in following directions.
   b. **Impaired cognition.** Individuals with delirium often have a marked disturbance of recent memory and may be unable to give a meaningful history. They may be disoriented to time and place. Speech may be rambling, incoherent, or sparse. Patients may have trouble finding words or identifying objects or people. Perceptual disturbances may include illusions and hallucinations. Often, actual perceptions are misinterpreted, and ordinary noises or objects are perceived as dangerous or disturbing. Hallucinations are often visual, but other senses can also be involved. Persecutory delusions based on sensory misperceptions are common.
   c. **Short and fluctuating course.** Delirium develops over a course of hours or days and fluctuates in severity. Individuals may have relatively lucid intervals of minutes or hours. Often, delirium worsens at night or during isolation.
   d. **Caused by a general medical condition or by a substance.** A comprehensive medical assessment should be undertaken to establish the relationship of the delirium to a general medical condition or to a substance. The disturbance should not be better explained by a primary mental disorder such as a manic episode occurring during the course of bipolar disorder. A

TABLE 5–1 DSM-*IV-TR* Classifications for Cognitive Disorders

Delirium
Delirium due to a general medical condition
Substance intoxication delirium
Substance withdrawal delirium
Delirium due to multiple etiologies
Delirium not otherwise specified

Dementia
Dementia of the Alzheimer type
Vascular dementia
Dementia due to HIV disease
Dementia due to head trauma
Dementia due to Parkinson disease
Dementia due to Huntington disease
Dementia due to Pick disease
Dementia due to Creutzfeldt-Jakob disease
Dementia due to other general medical conditions
Substance-induced persisting dementia
Dementia due to multiple etiologies
Dementia not otherwise specified

Amnesia
Amnestic disorder due to a general medical condition
Substance-induced persisting amnestic disorder
Amnestic disorder not otherwise specified
Cognitive disorder not otherwise specified

general medical condition is more likely to be responsible for a delirium if its onset or exacerbation corresponds in time period to the course of the delirium and if it has previously been reported to cause delirium. Similarly, it is more likely that a substance is responsible for a delirium if history or laboratory results indicate that use of or withdrawal from the substance corresponds in time period to the delirium and if the substance is known to cause delirium.

    e. **Not explained by delirium.** When delirium is superimposed on a preexisting dementia, it is considered an associated feature of the dementia, not a separate diagnosis, and is coded as the specific type of dementia **with delirium.**

2. **Associated features and diagnoses**
    a. **Disturbance in the sleep–wake cycle.** Individuals with delirium are often somnolent during the daytime or awake and agitated at night. They may have difficulty falling asleep and marked confusion on arousal.
    b. **Disturbance in psychomotor behavior.** Psychomotor behavior may be disorganized, with purposeless movements, psychomotor agitation, or decreased psychomotor activity.
    c. **Emotional disturbances.** Individuals with delirium are often emotionally labile. They may be extremely agitated and frightened or withdrawn and apathetic. Periods of irritability, belligerence, or euphoria can occur. Symptoms of delirium can cause affected individuals to strike out, struggle, or attempt to flee, sometimes resulting in patient injuries.
    d. **Abnormal electroencephalogram (EEG) findings.** EEG abnormalities are common in patients with delirium, usually showing either generalized slowing or fast wave activity. But delirium may occur without EEG changes.
    e. **Evidence of general medical conditions or substance use**
        (1) Individuals with delirium often have signs and symptoms of the underlying general medical condition. Metabolic disturbances and hypoxia due to perfusion or ventilation abnormalities are especially common.
        (2) Individuals with substance-induced delirium may have toxic levels of the responsible substance and other physical problems associated with the substance. Substance withdrawal delirium may occur while patients still test positive for significant amounts of a substance to which they have become tolerant. In many cases, delirium results from multiple concurrent etiologies.

3. **Epidemiology.** Older adults are most susceptible to delirium. Studies indicate that up to 30% to 40% of older patients have delirium at some point during hospitalization. Delirium also may occur in 30% to 40% of hospitalized patients with AIDS. According to the *DSM-IV-TR,* an independent risk factor is male gender.

4. **Etiology.** Delirium most often results from a variety of general medical conditions and from substances that interfere with brain function. Disturbance of the balance between cholinergic and dopaminergic neurotransmission is common in dementia. Some research findings suggest that the reticular activating system may be specifically affected in individuals with delirium.
    a. **General medical conditions** most often associated with delirium include systemic infections, metabolic disturbances, hepatic and renal diseases, seizures, and head trauma.
    b. **Substance-induced delirium** is associated with either intoxication or withdrawal from drugs. Elderly and severely ill individuals are at highest risk of developing substance-induced delirium.

5. **Differential diagnosis.** Delirium must be distinguished from psychosis. The diagnosis of substance-induced delirium should not be made unless the symptoms exceed those that would be expected during typical intoxication or withdrawal.

6. **Treatment.** Delirium is treated by **diagnosis and correction of the underlying physiologic problems.** Environmental measures can reduce overstimulation and aid in orientation but avoid sensory deprivation. Reassurance of the patient and family is important. Antipsychotic medications may aid in control of agitation. Judicious use of benzodiazepines is critical in sedative withdrawal delirium. Appropriate control of pain should be maintained. Restraints may be necessary but may also increase the risk of patient injury.

B **Dementia (Table 5–1)**

1. The essential feature of dementia is progressive deterioration of memory and cognition that is due to general medical conditions or is substance induced. In dementia, cognitive deficits should be apparent even with clarity of consciousness. A disturbance of both memory and at least one of the following aspects of cognition is necessary for a diagnosis of dementia.

   a. **Memory impairment,** the hallmark of dementia, often develops insidiously as the condition progresses. Early on, individuals may appear more absentminded and distracted, misplacing personal objects and becoming disoriented in unfamiliar surroundings. As dementia progresses, recent memories are difficult to recall, learning deficits become more prominent, and individuals may become lost in what were familiar surroundings. Older memories are the most resistant to loss, but individuals with progressive dementia eventually forget even their own names. In addition to social and occupational compromise, memory impairment can lead to physical dangers such as fires from untended cooking, traffic accidents due to inattention, or exposure from wandering away while in a disoriented state.

   b. **Possible cognitive deficits of dementia**
      (1) **Aphasia** is an **impairment or loss of language function.** Affected individuals may have difficulty constructing sentences, finding words, naming objects, maintaining fluency, or comprehending instructions. Speech may become halting or characterized by circumlocution as aphasic individuals become frustrated and attempt to substitute more general words such as "it," "that," or "thing," rather than the correct noun. Communication deteriorates over time, sometimes resulting in mutism.
      (2) **Apraxia** is an **inability to execute previously learned complex motor behaviors** such as bathing, dressing, driving, or drawing. The difficulty is not due to impaired sensory or motor function.
      (3) **Agnosia** is a **failure to recognize or identify previously known objects.** This problem is not due to impaired sensory function. Affected individuals may be unable to recognize common objects or utensils and may not recognize familiar persons.
      (4) **Disturbance in executive function** refers to **impaired ability to think abstractly and plan, initiate, sequence, monitor, and stop complex behavior.** Individuals with dementia may have difficulty conceptualizing or solving problems such as creating a report, making a grocery list, or adjusting the thermostat in a house.

   c. **Insidious and progressive course.** Dementia usually develops over a course of months or years and progresses in severity. Traumatic or infectious dementias may develop more rapidly. Individuals may have brief periods of improvement only to lose some cognitive skills forever as the illness runs its course.

   d. **Caused by a general medical condition or by a substance.** A comprehensive medical assessment should be undertaken to determine the type of dementia and possible treatment. The disturbance should not be better explained by a primary mental disorder such as schizophrenia or a developmental disorder. Some of the medical conditions responsible for dementia are reversible. When a substance is responsible for dementia, abstinence may interrupt progression, but reversibility is limited. Some clinicians distinguish between cortical and subcortical dementias.
      (1) **Cortical dementia** is characterized by the early appearance of aphasia, difficulties with calculation, and memory loss. Disturbances of speech and psychomotor behavior are less predominant.
      (2) **Subcortical dementia** is characterized by the early appearance of problems with executive functioning and recall, dysarthria, motor skill impairment, and personality changes. These symptoms occur in the absence of significant aphasia.

   e. **Not explained by dementia.** When delirium is superimposed on a preexisting dementia, it is considered an associated feature of the dementia, not a separate diagnosis, and is coded as the specific type of dementia **with delirium.**

2. **Associated features and diagnoses**
   a. **Disturbance in the sleep–wake cycle.** Individuals with dementia lose orientation to time and may develop a dysfunctional sleep–wake cycle with agitation at night.

b. Disturbance in psychomotor behavior. Psychomotor behavior may be disorganized, with restlessness, agitation, or decreased psychomotor activity. Specific psychomotor changes are seen in different types of dementia.

c. Emotional disturbances. Individuals with dementia may become emotionally disinhibited and labile. They may have outbursts of anger, anxiety, or despair. Depressive symptoms are common and may exacerbate cognitive deficits.

d. Personality disturbances. Individuals with even relatively mild dementia may undergo marked changes in personality, becoming disinhibited, socially inappropriate, or moody. Irritability and argumentativeness may increase. Expansiveness and euphoria are sometimes present.

e. Psychotic symptoms. Misperceptions are common because some individuals mistake old memories for current events. Delusions of a persecutory nature may be present. Hallucinations can also occur.

f. Neuroimaging. Abnormal findings on computed tomography (CT) and magnetic resonance imaging (MRI) are common and reflect the pathophysiology of the underlying general medical condition. Neurodegenerative diseases often cause generalized or focal cerebral atrophy, with enlarged cerebral ventricles and deepened cortical sulci. Vascular disease, neoplasms, and traumatic injuries may cause focal lesions. Functional MRI (fMRI), positron emission tomography (PET), or single-photon emission computed tomography (SPECT) may reveal evidence of focal hypometabolic activity before structural changes are visible.

g. Evidence of general medical conditions or substance use. Individuals may demonstrate diagnostic signs of the dementia subtype. Neurodegenerative diseases are frequently associated with motor and sensory deficits. Cerebrovascular lesions may be associated with focal motor and sensory deficits and with evidence of systemic vascular disease. Other dementing generalized medical conditions have characteristic physical findings such as evidence of infection, endocrine disturbance, or head trauma. Laboratory findings may reveal evidence of vitamin deficiencies, organ dysfunctions, and tumors. Substance-induced persisting dementia may be associated with physical signs of prolonged substance abuse such as alcohol-related liver disease.

3. Epidemiology. The prevalence of dementia increases with age; it affects 5% of the population older than age 65 years and 50% of the population older than age 85 years.

4. Familial pattern. Some types of neurodegenerative dementias are heritable, such as dementia of the Alzheimer type and Huntington dementia.

5. Etiology. Many medical conditions that involve diffuse or focal cerebral damage can cause dementia. **Neurodegenerative diseases** account for more than 75% of dementias. **Cerebrovascular disease** is the other major cause of dementia. **Traumatic** causes of dementia will become more common as more people survive serious accidents with head injuries. **Infectious** causes of dementia had been on the decline until HIV disease began to spread. **Metabolic, nutritional, endocrine, and substance-induced persisting dementias** also occur.

6. Differential diagnosis. Dementia must be distinguished from other psychiatric conditions. Cognitive functioning often deteriorates in patients with schizophrenia, but when delusions develop in the course of a dementia, the diagnosis is **dementia with delusions.** Delirium may occur superimposed on dementia and should be diagnosed as **dementia with delirium.** Major depressive disorder may occur with cognitive dysfunction equal to dementia, but this should be reversible with effective treatment for depression. When depressive symptoms develop during the course of a dementia, the diagnosis is **dementia with depressed mood.**

7. Treatment of dementia depends on proper diagnosis of the cause.

a. Behavioral interventions involve providing a low-demand environment. Familiar surroundings are reassuring for individuals with memory and cognitive impairment. Predictable routines and orientation with clocks and calendars may keep the day structured. The physical environment should be managed to reduce the risk of injury from falls, and appropriate lighting should correspond with times for activity and rest. Wandering can also be controlled with environmental management, and identification bracelets may aid in recovery of an individual who wanders away.

    b. Family counseling about managing the risks associated with dementia is important. Caring for a person with dementia is challenging, and **respite** is important for caregivers.

    c. Somatic treatments are under development for neurodegenerative dementias. Vascular dementia can be prevented with early control of cerebrovascular disease. Surgery may reverse progressive dementia from an intracranial process. Infectious, metabolic, nutritional, endocrine, and substance-induced persisting dementias may also be reversible.

    d. Agitation occurs in at least half of all cases of dementia. When behavioral measures fail to ameliorate agitation, antidepressants, mood stabilizers, and antipsychotic medications have all been used to manage agitation. The use of substances such as alcohol, anxiolytics, hypnotics, and opioid analgesics often further impairs cognition and should be avoided.

C **Amnestic disorders (Table 5–1)**

  1. Diagnostic features. Memory impairment, which does not occur solely during the course of delirium or dementia, is the essential characteristic.

    a. Memory impairment. As with delirium and dementia, the memory impairment is manifested by difficulty in learning new information and, less often, by an inability to recall previously learned information. Immediate memory is usually relatively intact, but recent memory is severely affected. Individuals may not be able to recount recent events and may be disoriented. Long-term memory is usually preserved.

    b. The memory impairment **does not occur exclusively during the course of delirium or dementia.** In amnestic disorders, other aspects of cognition are relatively intact. Clarity of awareness is preserved.

  2. Associated features and diagnoses

    a. Confusion. Individuals are often confused and disoriented as a result of recent memory impairment, and they may appear to be suffering from delirium.

    b. Confabulation. Individuals with memory impairment may imagine events to account for periods of time that they are unable to recall. They may adamantly defend their ideas.

    c. Emotional changes. Other subtle emotional changes often occur. Individuals sometimes appear inappropriately unconcerned and amotivated. Emotional lability is sometimes present.

  3. Epidemiology. Amnestic disorders are more common in populations with a higher prevalence of alcohol abuse and head trauma. Young adult men and individuals with antisocial personality disorder are at greater risk.

  4. Course. The **onset** of amnesia may be rapid when it results from trauma or acute biochemical injury (e.g., anoxia). More insidious onset is seen with neurodegenerative conditions and with chronic exposure to toxic substances. The **clinical course** depends on the underlying cause, and the symptoms may be transient or chronic.

  5. Etiology. Bilateral damage (transient or chronic) to diencephalic and mediotemporal structures (e.g., mamillary bodies, fornix, hippocampus) may produce memory dysfunction in the absence of other cognitive symptoms. Such damage can be caused by thiamine deficiency associated with alcohol dependence, head trauma, cerebrovascular disease, hypoxia, severe hypoglycemia, local infection (herpes encephalitis), ablative surgical procedures, and seizures. Acute and chronic use of alcohol, anxiolytics, sedatives, and hypnotics can produce amnesia.

  6. Differential diagnosis

    a. Delirium and dementia are both characterized by prominent memory disturbances but are accompanied by other cognitive deficits.

    b. Dissociative disorders also involve disturbances of memory but are often associated with emotional stress and unusual patterns of memory impairment.

    c. Substance intoxication and withdrawal often cause memory impairment, which does not persist.

    d. Age-related cognitive decline is associated with a decreased acuity of memory but not to a degree that causes significant functional impairment.

  7. Treatment. As with delirium and dementia, **stabilization or correction of the underlying general medical condition is the definitive treatment.** Further physical or biochemical cerebral insults should be avoided. Familiar surroundings as well as reassurance and support are helpful as gradual reorientation occurs.

D **Cognitive disorder not otherwise specified**   A variety of cerebral insults can lead to patterns of cognitive deficits, which are not better explained by delirium, dementia, or amnesia.

1. **Mild neurocognitive impairment.** Early in the course of neurodegenerative illness or after mild cerebral damage from various causes, symptoms of cognitive impairment are sometimes evident in the absence of dementia. In addition, subtle changes in personality are often present in individuals with such conditions.

2. **Postconcussional disorder.** Chronic physical discomfort and disturbances in cognition sometimes occur after significant closed-head trauma with transient loss of consciousness and amnesia. In such cases, sleep disturbances, headaches, and dizziness are often present. Automobile accidents are a common cause of concussion injury.

III   MENTAL DISORDERS DUE TO GENERAL MEDICAL CONDITIONS

A **Catatonic disorder due to a general medical condition**

1. **Diagnostic features.** Catatonia is a syndrome characterized by **abnormalities of psychomotor activity,** which include any of the following:
   a. **Motoric immobility** (e.g., catatonic rigidity, waxy flexibility)
   b. **Excessive motor activity** (e.g., catatonic excitement)
   c. Extreme **negativism or mutism** (e.g., passive resistance to instructions, failure to speak)
   d. **Peculiarities of voluntary movement** (e.g., purposeless repeated movements, bizarre posturing)
   e. **Echolalia** (e.g., immediate purposeless repetition of words)
   f. **Echopraxia** (e.g., purposeless imitation of movements)

2. **Etiology.** General medical conditions that cause catatonia include both generalized and focal cerebral insults and systemic illnesses. It is not known whether specific central nervous system (CNS) structures must be affected to produce catatonia.
   a. Neurologic conditions that can produce catatonia include **neoplasms, head trauma, cerebrovascular disease,** and **encephalitis.**
   b. Other general medical conditions associated with catatonia include **hypercalcemia, hepatic encephalopathy, homocystinuria, thiamine deficiency,** and **diabetic ketoacidosis.**

3. **Differential diagnosis.** Individuals with catatonia often appear bizarre and disturbed; this combination makes comprehensive medical assessment particularly difficult. The onset and course of catatonia depend entirely on the underlying general medical condition. Conditions that should be ruled out include the following:
   a. **Delirium** may occur, but when catatonic behavior occurs exclusively during the course of delirium, it is not diagnosed separately.
   b. **Movement disorders,** especially dystonias, can mimic catatonia.
   c. **Schizophrenia, catatonic type,** may be present with catatonia but is accompanied by other signs of schizophrenia. This syndrome is not due to a general medical condition.
   d. **Mood disorders** may occur with catatonia but are accompanied by a mood disturbance such as depression or mania.

4. **Treatment.** Stabilization or correction of the underlying general medical condition is the definitive treatment. Antipsychotic medications or restraints are sometimes indicated to prevent patient injury from disorganized behavior.

B **Personality change due to a general medical condition**   The alteration of personality may include emotional lability, poor impulse control, aggressive or angry outbursts, apathy, or suspiciousness. *DSM-IV-TR* subtypes of personality change due to a general medical condition are designated as labile, disinhibited, aggressive, apathetic, paranoid, other, combined, and unspecified types.

1. **Diagnostic features.** Affected individuals may become reclusive, querulous, or combative.

2. **Etiology.** The **pattern of personality changes** depends in part on the locus of the responsible lesion. Frontal lobe damage is characterized by disinhibition, shallow emotions, and occasionally

euphoria (so-called "**frontal lobe syndrome**"). Many of the same general medical conditions that cause dementia can cause personality change when the lesion is relatively less severe or the clinical course is in its early stages. Head trauma is a major cause of personality change that does not progress to dementia.

3. **Differential diagnosis**
   a. Personality change due to a general medical condition must be distinguished from other mental disorders due to general medical conditions and from those due to substance use or abuse. Dementia and other cognitive disorders are characterized by memory impairment or other cognitive problems.
   b. Other mental disorders, whether they are primary or due to a general medical condition, can secondarily result in personality change such as those that result from depressed mood, delusional beliefs, or immersion in a substance-abusing subculture.

4. **Treatment.** Stabilization or correction of the underlying general medical condition is the definitive treatment for personality disorder due to a general medical condition. Unfortunately, full recovery after traumatic damage does not always occur. Social and occupational rehabilitation plays an important role in treatment, as do counseling and support for patients' families. Medications targeted to the specific symptoms may help, such as mood stabilizers for affective instability.

IV GENERAL MEDICAL CONDITIONS THAT CAUSE MENTAL DISTURBANCES

A) Overview

1. **Examination of patients with mental disturbances.** The general availability of sensitive and specific diagnostic examinations makes it reasonable to screen for general medical conditions in almost all patients who have cognitive or behavioral changes.

2. **Pathophysiology.** General medical conditions and substances can adversely affect cerebral functioning through a number of mechanisms. Effects may be reversible or irreversible, depending on the nature of the lesion.
   a. **Disruption of metabolic homeostasis.** Levels of electrolytes, pH, hydration, and osmolarity can be altered by many metabolic and endocrine disorders and neoplasms.
   b. **Disruption of molecular synthesis.** Synthesis of neurotransmitters, neuroreceptors, cellular structures, and supporting elements can be disrupted by neurodegenerative diseases, endocrine diseases, and nutritional deficiencies.
   c. **Deficiency of substrates.** Oxygen or metabolic substrates for oxidative metabolism may be deficient in patients with pulmonary disease, cerebrovascular disease, nutritional disease, and metabolic diseases.
   d. **Electrophysiologic disruption.** Synaptic transmission can be altered biochemically or by seizures.
   e. **Tissue damage.** Brain tissue can be damaged or destroyed by trauma, infection, or neoplasms.

B) Neurodegenerative diseases can be differentiated between those illnesses that can impact at any age and those that are seen in geriatric populations.

1. **Huntington disease.** This progressive neurodegenerative disease involves **loss of γ-aminobutyric acid (GABA)-ergic neurons of the basal ganglia.** It is manifested by choreoathetosis and dementia.
   a. **Histopathology.** A loss of GABAergic neurons occurs in the striatum. Other neurons may also be involved.
   b. **Gross morphology.** Functional neuroimaging reveals caudate hypometabolism at an early stage. **Atrophy of the caudate nucleus**, with resultant ventricular enlargement, is common.
   c. **Epidemiology.** The prevalence is about one in 100,000. Fifty percent of offspring of patients with Huntington disease develop the illness.
   d. **Etiology.** Huntington disease is caused by a **defect in an autosomal dominant gene (*D4S10*) located on chromosome 4** that consists of unstable expanded cytosine–adenosine–guanine (CAG) repeats. The precise mechanism by which this defect produces the disease is unknown, but it may involve Huntington protein, an abnormal gene product.

   e. Symptoms and course

     (1) The **onset** of clinically evident disease usually occurs at approximately age 40 years, but the variation is wide. Death usually occurs approximately 15 years after onset.

     (2) **Early symptoms** include personality changes and subtle movement disturbances.

     (3) **Later symptoms** include choreoathetosis and dementia. The dementia is characterized by subcortical features, with cognitive slowing and disturbances of executive function. Behavioral disorganization, severe mood instability, and psychotic features are fairly common.

   f. Differential diagnosis. Other causes of dementia should be considered. Schizophrenia (especially with catatonic symptoms), schizoaffective disorders, mood disorders with psychotic and catatonic symptoms, and other psychotic disorders can resemble Huntington disease. Other causes of choreoathetosis, including tardive dyskinesia from antipsychotic medications, are also in the differential diagnosis.

   g. Treatment. There is no proven somatic treatment to reverse or prevent degeneration in Huntington disease. Antipsychotic medications can ameliorate both choreoathetosis and psychotic symptoms. Antidepressant and mood-stabilizing medications may also provide symptomatic treatment. Family counseling, including genetic counseling, is essential. (See Chapter 13 for further neurodegenerative disorders.)

C **Infectious diseases**

  1. Mechanisms. Infectious agents can cause mental disorders in a variety of ways:

   a. Physical destruction of brain tissue

   b. Inflammation of brain tissue, meninges, or cerebral vasculature

   c. Mass effects from infectious lesions

   d. Toxins

   e. Systemic metabolic alterations such as fever, renal failure, hepatic failure, or electrolyte disturbance

  2. Viral encephalitis. This disorder can lead to delirium, sometimes accompanied by headache, fever, and photophobia. Focal CNS herpes virus lesions, usually in the frontal or temporal lobes, can produce anosmia, personality changes, bizarre behavior with possible gustatory and olfactory hallucinations, and complex partial seizures. Rabies encephalitis rapidly produces delirium, with hydrophobia present in half the population. Subacute sclerosing panencephalitis (SSPE) can occur after measles infection in children and progresses from delirium with myoclonus, ataxia, and seizures to chronic dementia.

  3. Chronic viral infections. These disorders can produce progressive destruction of CNS tissue resulting in dementia.

   a. Dementia due to HIV disease. HIV directly **destroys brain parenchyma,** and the course of the dementia is progressive. It becomes clinically apparent in at least 30% of individuals with AIDS. Diffuse multifocal destruction of brain structures occurs, and cognitive impairment may be accompanied by signs of delirium. Motor findings include gait disturbance, hypertonia and hyperreflexia, pathologic reflexes (e.g., frontal release signs), and oculomotor deficits. The differential diagnosis for dementia due to HIV disease includes other HIV-associated general medical conditions that cause dementia, including CNS tumors and opportunistic CNS infections. Mood disturbances in individuals with HIV infection may mimic cognitive impairment.

   b. Dementia due to Creutzfeldt-Jakob disease. This **rare spongiform encephalopathy** is believed to be caused by a slow virus (prion). Affected individuals present with dementia, myoclonus, and EEG abnormalities (e.g., sharp, triphasic, synchronous discharges and, later, periodic discharges). Over a course of several months, symptoms progress from vague malaise and personality changes to dementia. Other findings include visual and gait disturbances, choreoathetosis or other abnormal movements, and myoclonus. Atypical presentations and slower courses have been described in some patients. So-called "new variant" Creutzfeldt-Jakob disease may be related to bovine spongiform encephalopathy. **Kuru,** a slow virus found in New Guinea, causes dementia and motor disturbances.

   c. Progressive multifocal leukoencephalopathy (PML). This demyelinating condition, which is usually caused by papovavirus JC (JCV) infection, occurs predominantly in immunocompromised hosts. Over several months, increasing multiple motor deficits and cognitive deficits lead to death. HIV infection has increased the incidence of PML.

4. **Neurosyphilis** (general paresis). This parenchymal form of CNS tertiary syphilis typically occurs 5 to 30 years after incompletely treated primary syphilis. Personality changes are usually noted before the onset of dementia. Prominent psychotic symptoms are sometimes present. Physical findings include papilledema, optic atrophy, Argyll Robertson pupils (i.e., constriction reaction to near objects [accommodation reflexes present] but not to light [pupillary reflexes absent]), gait disturbances, and spasticity.

5. **Acute bacterial meningitis.** This disease usually has a rapid onset. Affected individuals present with systemic signs of infection (e.g., high fever) that are accompanied by headache, stiff neck, and delirium. In most cases, the causal bacteria are *Streptococcus pneumoniae, Neisseria meningitides,* and *Listeria monocytogenes.*

6. **Chronic meningitis.** This form of meningitis is characterized by a more gradual onset of cognitive impairment, progressing in some cases to delirium. The **most common infections are tuberculosis and cryptococcal and coccidioidal mycoses. Syphilitic meningitis** is a form of tertiary syphilis that usually occurs 1 to 3 years after incompletely treated primary syphilis, and patients present with delirium. **Chronic basilar meningitis** is accompanied by pupillary abnormalities, ptosis, hearing impairment, and facial paralysis. **Chronic hemispheric meningitis** is accompanied by marked cognitive impairments and seizures.

7. **Mass lesions.** Depending on their location, lesions resulting from granulomatous infections or abscesses can cause a variety of cognitive disturbances. **Infections that most commonly produce mass lesions include tuberculosis, parasitic disease (cysticercosis, schistosomiasis), and mycoses.**

D **Myelin diseases**   Several diseases involve myelin, the white matter that sheaths neuronal axons, and are associated with motor and sensory disturbances. Depending on the nature of the disorder and sites affected, cognitive symptoms, personality changes, and mood disturbances can occur.

1. **Acute disseminated encephalomyelitis.** This demyelinating illness of abrupt onset presents with delirium followed by sensory and motor deficits, seizures, and coma. The mortality rate is 50%, and marked residual neurologic and cognitive impairments are present. It sometimes occurs after viral illnesses or vaccinations and may have an immune origin. MRI is diagnostic.

2. **Multiple sclerosis (MS).** A multifocal demyelinating disease of unclear viral or immune origin, MS has a waxing and waning clinical course. Episodes of focal disturbances occur and remit, sometimes with increasing residual motor and sensory deficits. It has an overall prevalence of about 50 in 100,000 and is slightly more common in women, with a peak incidence between age 20 and 40 years. **It is more common in temperate climates**.
   a. **Sensory symptoms** include transient visual impairment (initial presentation in 40% of patients) and impaired vibratory and position sense.
   b. **Transient motor symptoms** include nystagmus, dysarthria, tremor, ataxia, bladder dysfunction, and focal motor weakness.
   c. **Personality changes** depend on the loci of lesions but may include emotional lability, shallow emotions, depression, suspiciousness, apathy, and impulsiveness.
   d. **Cognitive symptoms** occur, and persisting dementia occasionally develops late in the course of the illness. The transient and patchy distribution of lesions often leads to somatic preoccupation in affected individuals, suggesting a somatoform disorder.

3. **Other diseases of myelin.** A number of other leukodystrophies caused by genetic lesions of myelin metabolism cause progressive neurologic impairment and dementia in children and adults. These diseases include metachromatic leukodystrophy (cerebroside sulfatase deficiency), globoid cell (Krabbe) leukodystrophy (galactocerebrosidase deficiency), **amyotrophic lateral sclerosis** (ALS), and adrenoleukodystrophy.

E **Epilepsy**   This disorder is characterized by recurrent seizures and is associated with a variety of mental disturbances that occur both intra- and interictally.

1. **Definition.** Seizures, also referred to as convulsions or ictal episodes, are characterized by transient bursts of abnormal CNS electrical activity that cause disturbances of movement, autonomic activity, and consciousness. Seizure manifestations depend on the location of the seizure focus and the electrophysiologic state of the CNS.

2. **Pathophysiology.** Seizures result from disturbances of the electrophysiologic activity of brain cells, leading to paroxysmal discharges, which spread to large groups of neurons and produce characteristic EEG findings.

3. **Types of seizures**
   a. **Generalized seizures** involve the entire brain.
      (1) **Tonic–clonic (grand mal) seizures** are manifested by loss of consciousness and postural control, followed by generalized muscular rigidity (tonic phase). This is followed by rhythmic contractions (clonic phase) of the upper and lower extremities. Incontinence may occur. EEG tracings show a wide range of abnormalities.
      (2) **Absence (petit mal) seizures** are characterized by brief disruptions of consciousness during which affected individuals may seem inattentive or unresponsive. There may be subtle motor findings such as loss of muscle tone, chewing, or lip-smacking movements. EEG tracings show characteristic bilaterally synchronous 3-Hz spikes and slow wave activity. Absence epilepsy is more common in children.
      (3) **Atonic seizures** (drop attacks) are characterized by brief losses of consciousness and postural tone. Episodes can resemble the cataplexy symptom of narcolepsy.
      (4) **Myoclonic seizures** involve muscle contractions without loss of consciousness. They are seen in individuals with a variety of neurodegenerative diseases.
   b. **Partial seizures** involve specific brain foci.
      (1) **Simple partial seizures** are manifested by motor, sensory, or autonomic disturbances, depending on the location of the seizure focus.
      (2) **Complex partial seizures** cause disturbances of consciousness, including decreased awareness and alterations of cognition, emotion, and sensory experience. Recurrent complex partial seizure is the most common form of adult epilepsy, sometimes called psychomotor epilepsy or temporal lobe epilepsy. During seizure episodes, affected individuals may have dream-like sensations and may exhibit poorly organized behavior that can appear inappropriate, bizarre, or violent. Complex partial seizures may resemble symptoms seen with dissociative fugue and depersonalization disorder. Interictal personality changes may occur.

4. **Etiology.** Focal brain lesions resulting from trauma, infections, and neoplasms may cause seizures. Metabolic disturbances, neurodegenerative diseases, and various substances may also precipitate seizures. Autism and mental retardation are associated with a higher incidence of seizures.

5. **Symptoms**
   a. **Preictal symptoms** are often referred to as an **aura** and can include motor, sensory, emotional, and cognitive experiences. Motor twitching, olfactory hallucinations (e.g., burning rubber), autonomic sensations (e.g., a feeling of epigastric discomfort), peculiar emotion states or reveries, and intrusive thoughts or memories have been described as components of auras.
   b. **Postictal mental symptoms** due to generalized seizures and complex partial seizures are characteristic of resolving delirium. The duration of confusion varies from minutes to hours. Amnesia is usually complete for intraictal events during generalized seizures. Varying degrees of amnesia for events occur during complex partial seizures. After tonic–clonic seizures, focal motor paralysis may be present for minutes, hours, or days (**Todd paralysis**).
   c. **Interictal symptoms** are absent in many patients with epilepsy. Some affected individuals, especially those with complex partial seizure disorders, may develop a variety of personality changes or cognitive deficits. Psychotic symptoms may also occur. Some of these symptoms may be caused by subclinical seizure episodes. With long-standing and poorly controlled seizure disorders, cognitive deficits become more common.

6. **Other psychopathology associated with epilepsy.** Individuals with epilepsy have a higher incidence of mental disorders.
   a. Some mental disorders such as mental retardation and autism may stem from the same cause as the comorbid seizure disorder.
   b. In cognitive disorders and other mental disorders due to general medical conditions, seizures may be the physiologic cause of the comorbid mental disturbance.
   c. Individuals with epilepsy may develop mood, anxiety, or somatoform disorders as a result of the psychological stress associated with the illness. The incidence of suicide is relatively high in individuals with epilepsy.

7. **Differential diagnosis**

a. Seizure-like episodes can occur in **conversion disorder** and **factitious disorder,** but there is rarely incontinence or physical harm (e.g., tongue biting) from tonic–clonic motor activity. Patients with factitious seizures are more likely to suffer from actual seizures as well.

b. **Dissociative disorders** can be manifested by alterations of consciousness and cognition that are suggestive of complex partial seizures. It is sometimes difficult to distinguish between these conditions. Repeated EEGs or 24-hour EEG recordings may be required. Nasopharyngeal EEG leads are sometimes used.

8. **Treatment.** Definitive treatment requires amelioration of the underlying cause through management of systemic illness or surgical removal of seizure foci in the brain. Control of epilepsy can often be attained with anticonvulsant medications. However, these medications themselves may cause cognitive impairment and mental disturbances.

F **Neoplasms** Neoplastic disease can cause mental disturbances through a variety of physiologic mechanisms, including intracranial mass effects, destruction of brain tissue, seizures, metabolic alterations, production of neuropeptides and toxins, and autoimmune reactions.

1. The **type of mental disturbance produced** by neoplasia depends on the nature of the neoplasm, the location of the tumor, the size of the tumor, and the rate of tumor growth.

2. **Rapidly growing intracranial neoplasms** in any location can produce **delirium** accompanied by other signs of increased intracranial pressure, including headache, papilledema, and vomiting. Slowly growing intracranial neoplasms can produce more insidious changes in cognition and personality.

3. The **location of intracranial neoplasms** influences the nature of the mental disturbances and physical findings.

a. **Frontal lobe tumors** may be associated with personality changes, including disinhibition, emotional lability, and apathy.

b. **Parietal lobe tumors** may be associated with sensory deficits, agnosia, and visual neglect.

c. **Temporal lobe tumors** may be associated with complex motor, perceptual, and behavioral symptoms that resemble complex partial seizures.

d. **Occipital lobe tumors** may be associated with visual hallucinations.

e. **Brain stem tumors** may lead to an alert yet immobile and mute state (akinetic mutism or vigilant coma).

4. **Neuropeptide- and hormone-secreting tumors** in any location can produce mental changes through direct effects on CNS activity or by alteration of systemic metabolism.

5. **Paraneoplastic syndromes** are distant effects of neoplasms mediated by tumor-induced autoimmune reactions, tumor-produced neurotoxic substances, and perhaps other mechanisms. Paraneoplastic syndromes can produce mental disturbances. Small-cell lung carcinoma can produce encephalitis and delirium. When limited to limbic structures (limbic encephalitis), the condition can produce memory impairment and personality changes.

6. **Adjustment disorders** arising from the psychosocial effects of neoplastic disease must be considered in the differential diagnosis of mental disorders due to neoplasms.

G **Head trauma** Injury to the head that leads to traumatic brain injury can produce subtle or profound cognitive symptoms and personality changes that may be transient or chronic. Head trauma can cause **brain injury** by direct destruction of brain tissue, by shearing of neuronal axons, by increased intracranial pressure, and by resultant vascular hemorrhage. The symptoms and course of resultant mental disturbances depend on the nature, location, and extent of damage.

1. **Diagnostic features.** When brain injury is caused by head trauma we currently diagnose this as cognitive disorder not otherwise specified in the DSM-IV-TR. However, **postconcussional disorder** is described in research criteria as a disturbance of at least 3 months' duration that sometimes occurs after significant head trauma/cerebral concussion with difficulty in concentration or memory. It is characterized by cognitive, somatic, and behavioral symptoms that include headaches, fatigue, sleep disturbances, dizziness/vertigo, irritability/aggression, anxiety/depression/affective instability, apathy, and personality changes.

2. **Associated symptoms** can be classified as cognitive and behavioral.
   a. Cognitive symptoms can include impaired attention with distractibility, impaired processing speed, difficulty with memory and problem solving, amotivation, and language disabilities.
   b. Behavioral symptoms can include increased impulsivity and aggression, affective lability, sleep disturbances, anxiety, and personality changes. These symptoms can be worsened with alcohol and/or substance use.

3. **Epidemiology.** Head trauma most commonly occurs in individuals between 15 and 25 years of age and is more common in males than females. An estimated 2 million incidents involving head trauma occur annually.

4. **Course.** Six to 12 months after injury, the symptoms remaining from the trauma are more likely to be permanent.

5. **Etiology.** Injury factors can be divided into rotational and skull fractures with acute head trauma, hematomas, contusions, and diffuse axonal injury.
   a. **Acute head trauma** may result in immediate delirium or delirium that occurs after recovery of consciousness. The delirium is of variable duration, from a few seconds to days or weeks. The duration may reflect the extent of overall damage. Recovery is often gradual over several weeks and frequently involves amnesia for events surrounding the trauma.
   b. **Subdural hematomas** arising from head injury (occurring in 10% of individuals with serious head injury) may manifest as headache, cognitive or personality changes, and focal neurologic deficits reflecting the location of the lesion. **Individuals with alcoholism are predisposed to the development of posttraumatic subdural hematomas.**
   c. **Focal contusions** develop during the actual head trauma, when the brain and skull are mismatched in their actions during rapid deceleration and acceleration.
   d. **Diffuse axonal injury** consists of progressive injury during which the axon is stretched, leading to increased permeability, axonal swelling, and subsequent detachment.

6. **Differential diagnosis. Personality change** sometimes results from head trauma, even in the absence of obvious cognitive changes. **Chronic amnestic disorder** can result from damage to diencephalic and mediotemporal lobe structures (e.g., mamillary bodies, hippocampus, fornix). **Dementia due to head trauma** is usually nonprogressive. This condition may persist indefinitely or may gradually ameliorate over many months or years. It is often accompanied by emotional lability and impulsivity. A history of head trauma is a risk factor for the development of dementias caused by neurodegenerative disorders. In **children,** head trauma may lead to either loss of developmental competencies or a slowing of mental development. When either occurs, diagnoses of both mental retardation and dementia may be appropriate.

7. **Treatment.** Social factors including abuse, neglect, and environmental issues should be ruled out. Use of benzodiazepines and anticholinergic and antidopaminergic agents should be minimized because they can lead to impaired cognition and increased sedation and impede neuronal recovery. Patients may be more sensitive to side effects, so they should be started on lower doses than usual and titrated slowly. Selective serotonin reuptake inhibitors (SSRIs) can be used for depression, and anticonvulsants can be used for mood stabilization.

H **Nutritional deficiencies**   Mental disturbances resulting from nutritional deficiencies are characterized by development of cognitive deficits and personality changes with occasional psychotic symptoms. Without treatment, such disorders may progress to dementia.

1. **Etiology.** Several nutritional substances are essential for the structural integrity of the CNS. Deficiencies can be caused by inadequate intake, impaired absorption, and abnormal metabolism. Deficiency diseases are more common in areas of severe food shortage and in individuals with limited or unusual diets or alcoholism. Often, multiple deficiencies and general malnutrition are present in a single individual.

2. **Thiamine (vitamin B$_1$)** is required as a coenzyme for oxidative decarboxylation and for neural conduction.
   a. **Beriberi** results from thiamine deficiency caused by malnutrition. Individuals can present with high-output cardiac failure (**wet beriberi**), peripheral neuropathy with bilateral distal

impairment of motor and sensory skills and reflexes (**dry beriberi**), and CNS damage with motor and cognitive impairments (**cerebral beriberi**).

b. **Wernicke encephalopathy** and **Korsakoff psychosis** describe forms of cerebral beriberi most commonly found in alcohol-dependent individuals.

(1) **Wernicke encephalopathy** is characterized by the rapid onset of ataxia, oculomotor abnormalities (ophthalmoplegia and nystagmus), and delirium. Histopathologic changes occur in the mamillary bodies and walls of the third ventricle. Symptoms usually quickly resolve if thiamine is administered early.

(2) Repeated or incompletely treated encephalopathy may result in alcohol-induced persisting amnestic disorder (**Korsakoff psychosis**), which is not responsive to treatment with thiamine. **Associated symptoms include confabulation, personality changes, and motor deficits.** Dementia may supervene.

3. **Nicotinic acid (niacin)** deficiency (**pellagra**) usually results from a dietary deficiency of tryptophan as a consequence of alcohol dependence, from some vegetarian diets, or from starvation. Symptoms include dermatitis, diarrhea, peripheral neuropathies, cognitive deficits, and personality changes that progress to delirium. Irreversible dementia can result if the deficiency is not treated.

4. **Pyridoxine (vitamin B$_6$)** deficiency leads to dermatitis, neuropathies, and cognitive changes. It is usually found only in association with use of medications (e.g., isoniazid) that act as pyridoxine antagonists.

5. **Cobalamin (vitamin B$_{12}$)** deficiency usually occurs when gastric mucosal cells fail to produce intrinsic factor necessary for ileal absorption of vitamin B$_{12}$. Symptoms include megaloblastic anemia (**pernicious anemia**), paresthesias and other sensory and motor peripheral neuropathies, gait disturbance, and cognitive disturbances. Delirium may occur. If treatment is inadequate, irreversible dementia may supervene.

I **Metabolic disorders**   These conditions can cause mental disturbances through systemic metabolic alterations or by direct toxic effects on the CNS.

1. **Genetic metabolic diseases of childhood** (i.e., disorders of lipid, carbohydrate, and protein metabolism) can produce progressive mental retardation and other neurologic conditions in childhood. Some childhood disorders can be ameliorated by dietary control.

2. **Wilson disease (hepatolenticular degeneration)** is an autosomal recessive genetic illness characterized by abnormal copper metabolism that results in copper deposition. As a result, copper deposition occurs, with damage to the liver, renal tubules, and brain structures (e.g., corpus callosum, putamen). Personality changes may become apparent in early adulthood and progress to dementia if untreated. Gait disturbances, incoordination, and chorea also develop. Treatment often includes a copper-restricted diet and administration of chelating agents (e.g., D-penicillamine, zinc).

3. **Acute intermittent porphyria (AIP),** an autosomal dominant genetic disorder, is characterized by abnormal heme biosynthesis and excessive accumulation of porphyrins. AIP leads to episodes of abdominal pain, motor neuropathies, and mental disturbances that range from personality changes to psychotic symptoms and delirium. This disease is more common in women and is often first apparent in young adulthood. Episodes are sometimes precipitated by use of barbiturates, estrogens, and sulfonamides. Treatment is symptomatic, involving analgesic and antipsychotic medications. Two other porphyrias, hereditary coproporphyria and variegated porphyria, have similar psychiatric symptoms.

4. **Hepatic encephalopathy** results from acute or chronic liver failure. Patients present with delirium accompanied by a characteristic flapping tremor (asterixis). Other symptoms include jaundice, hyperventilation, and EEG abnormalities. Treatment requires a nitrogen-restricted diet.

5. **Uremic encephalopathy** results from acute or chronic renal failure. Patients present with delirium accompanied by diffuse polyneuropathy, twitching, and hiccups. Untreated uremic encephalopathy may result in irreversible dementia. Treatment involves renal dialysis, which can also produce delirium.

6. **Disorders of glucose metabolism**

a. **Hypoglycemic encephalopathy** results from the presence of excessive endogenous or exogenous insulin or the unavailability of glucose. Such episodes are most common after nighttime fasting, after vigorous exercise, or several hours after a heavy meal. Early symptoms include hunger, sweating, tremulousness, and anxiety. When untreated by administration of sugar, symptoms progress to delirium, coma, and seizures. Repeated severe hypoglycemic episodes can result in irreversible cognitive deficits.

    b. **Diabetic ketoacidosis** results from inadequately treated diabetes mellitus and presents with weakness, polyuria, polydipsia, nausea, vomiting, headache, and fatigue. Delirium may supervene. Dementia may result from repeated episodes.

7. **Fluid and electrolyte disturbances** cause mental disturbances that range from personality change to delirium.

8. **Hypoxia** can result from pulmonary, cardiovascular, and hematologic diseases and from toxins (e.g., carbon monoxide). Acute cognitive changes and delirium can occur. Chronic amnestic disorder or dementia is a possible sequela.

J **Endocrine disorders**   These conditions often cause changes in personality, mood, and cognitive function.

1. **Pituitary disorders.** Pituitary tumors may impair cognitive function by causing pressure to hypothalamic and temporal lobe structures. Compression of the optic chiasm can cause bitemporal hemianopia. Endocrine disturbances reflect the area of the pituitary that is affected. Postpartum infarction and hemorrhage into the pituitary result in **Sheehan syndrome,** which is characterized by thyroid and adrenal failure with associated mental disturbances.

2. **Hypothalamic disorders.** Tumors of the hypothalamus may cause appetite and sleep disturbances accompanied by personality changes. Resultant metabolic disturbances from dysregulation of antidiuretic hormone can result in delirium from fluid and electrolyte disturbances.

3. **Thyroid disorders.** Disorders of thyroid metabolism can be caused by genetic lesions; neoplasms of the thyroid gland, pituitary gland, or hypothalamus; autoimmune diseases of the thyroid gland; surgical or radiochemical ablation of the thyroid gland; exogenous thyroxin; and iodine deficiencies.

    a. **Hyperthyroid disorders.** Presenting symptoms include weakness and fatigue, insomnia, weight loss, tremulousness, palpitations, and sweating. Exophthalmos and eyelid lag sometimes occur. Anxiety and restlessness are early mental symptoms, and cognitive impairment and personality changes may emerge. In severe cases, manic and psychotic symptoms can develop. Cognitive deficits in the absence of anxiety can occur in elderly individuals. Treatment results in resolution of the associated mental disturbances.

    b. **Hypothyroid disorders.** Individuals with hypothyroidism (**myxedema**) present with fatigue, somnolence, weakness, dry skin, brittle hair, cold intolerance, and hoarse speech. Depression and irritability are common. Cognitive slowing may progress to dementia. Occasionally, persecutory delusions and hallucinosis develop. Without timely treatment (i.e., exogenous thyroxin, iodine), residual dementia occurs. Untreated hypothyroidism in children results in mental retardation.

4. **Parathyroid disorders.** Disorders of parathyroid metabolism can be caused by genetic lesions, neoplasms of the parathyroid gland and other tissues, and surgical or radiochemical ablation of the parathyroid gland. In addition to parathyroid pathology, abnormal calcium metabolism can also result from diseases with bone lesions such as Paget disease, multiple myeloma, and metastatic disease.

    a. **Hyperparathyroidism** with resultant hypercalcemia can cause muscular weakness, anxiety, and personality changes. Delirium, seizures, and death can occur in parathyroid storm.

    b. **Hypoparathyroidism** with resultant hypocalcemia leads to neuromuscular signs and symptoms, including increased excitability, transient paresthesias, cramping, twitching, tetany, and seizures. Delirium may occur even in the absence of tetany.

5. **Abnormalities of adrenal cortical functioning.** These disorders can be caused by adrenal and pituitary neoplasms, excessive use of exogenous corticosteroids, or sudden cessation of corticosteroid use.

    a. **Adrenocortical hyperactivity (Cushing syndrome)** or excessive levels of exogenous corticosteroids produce a variety of mental disturbances. Restlessness, sleep disturbances, and mood symptoms are common. Mood changes can include agitated depression or manic symptoms. Psychotic symptoms are sometimes seen, and suicide can occur. Treatment of the underlying pathology or gradual tapering of exogenous corticosteroids causes resolution of associated mental disturbances.

    b. Chronic adrenal insufficiency (Addison disease) produces apathy, fatigability, irritability, and depression. Occasionally, psychotic symptoms or delirium occurs. Treatment with corticosteroids eliminates the mental disturbances.

6. Pheochromocytoma. This catecholamine-secreting neoplasm of the adrenal medulla can produce panic attacks, hypertension, excessive perspiration, palpitations, tremulousness, lightheadedness, headaches, and pallor.

K Autoimmune disorders   These conditions can produce cognitive deficits and personality changes resulting from direct damage to brain tissue, damage to cerebral vasculature, and metabolic disturbances due to damage to other organ systems. Treatment of autoimmune disorders with steroids and other immunosuppressants can also produce mental disturbances.

1. Systemic lupus erythematosus (SLE). Characteristic damage to multiple organ systems results from deposition of antinuclear antibody–antigen complexes in renal glomeruli and systemic vascular beds. Arthralgias, cutaneous rashes, adenopathy, pericarditis, pleurisy, and renal failure are common manifestations. Mental disturbances, the initial presentation, eventually occur in at least 50% of SLE patients. Mental symptoms commonly involve personality changes. Mood symptoms and psychotic symptoms are sometimes present, and occasionally, delirium and dementia occur. Treatment with corticosteroids often produces mental disturbances, including psychosis and mood symptoms. SLE is much more common in women.

2. Vasculitides. Individuals with other autoimmune vasculitides may present with psychiatric symptoms when cerebral vasculature is involved. Such vasculitides may be associated with infection, transplant rejection, or other systemic autoimmune disease. Isolated vasculitis of the CNS sometimes occurs without identified associated illness, and affected individuals present with headache, focal neurologic deficits, and altered mental status.

Study Questions

Directions: *Each of the numbered items or incomplete statements in this section is followed by answers or by completions of the statement. Select the ONE lettered answer or completion that is BEST in each case.*

1. On examination in the emergency department, a 32-year-old man has an unsteady gait, mild bilateral oculoparesis, and spider angiomas. He is confused and agitated. Which of the following agents is the best immediate pharmacologic treatment?

- [A] Anticoagulants
- [B] Acetylcholinesterase (AChE) inhibitors
- [C] Pentobarbital
- [D] Salicylates
- [E] Thiamine

2. A 46-year-old woman has been found unconscious in her garage. Her car was running, and all the doors to the garage were closed. On examination, the woman is confused. Which of the following is the most likely cause of her confusion?

- [A] Dissociative fugue
- [B] Gasoline inhalation
- [C] Hypoglycemia
- [D] Hypoxia
- [E] Lead poisoning

3. A 58-year-old man has gradually become more apathetic and moody. At times, he is confused and forgetful. His gait is unsteady, his deep tendon reflexes are diminished, and he complains of tingling in his legs. Which of the following disorders is the most likely diagnosis?

- [A] Cerebellar neoplasm
- [B] Cobalamin (vitamin B_{12}) deficiency
- [C] Hyperthyroidism
- [D] Manganese intoxication
- [E] Multiple sclerosis (MS)

4. A 26-year-old woman presents with a history of episodic anxiety, emotional lability, confusion, and abdominal pain. She takes birth control pills but uses no other substances. Which of the following disorders is the most likely diagnosis?

- [A] Absence (petit mal) seizures
- [B] Acute intermittent porphyria (AIP) → *can be ppt by estrogens/ barbiturates*
- [C] Exposure to organophosphates
- [D] Premenstrual syndrome
- [E] Wilson disease (hepatolenticular degeneration)

5. A 29-year-old man presents with a history of three distinct episodes of emotional lability. Five years ago, when the first episode occurred, he experienced a right visual field deficit that resolved after 3 months. Two years ago, during another episode, he experienced transient mild ataxia. He now has a 2-month history of chronic fatigue, nonrestorative sleep, anxiety attacks, and irritability. Which of the following disorders is the most likely diagnosis?

- [A] Cobalamin (vitamin B_{12}) deficiency
- [B] Herpes encephalitis *seizures/Bizarre behavior*
- [C] Multiple sclerosis (MS)
- [D] Neurosyphilis *Psychosis*
- [E] Systemic lupus erythematosus (SLE) *mood disturbance*

6. A 39-year-old man with Down syndrome has exhibited increasing forgetfulness and angry outbursts over the past several months. He has become neglectful of personal hygiene and has trouble finding items in his room. Which of the following conditions is the most likely cause of these problems?

- (A) Alzheimer disease
- (B) Cerebrovascular disease
- (C) Intracranial neoplasm
- (D) HIV
- (E) Thiamine deficiency

7. A 23-year-old woman with no history of alcohol abuse reports that she has been troubled by morning episodes of tremulousness, anxiety, tachycardia, and sweating. Which one of the following test results is most likely to be abnormal?

- (A) Serum ammonia measurement
- (B) Serum glucose measurement
- (C) Serum sodium measurement
- (D) Thyroid function test
- (E) Toxicologic screen

8. A 28-year-old woman presents with complaints of irritability and moodiness. She gives a history of brief episodes of auditory hallucinosis and suspiciousness. Her speech is slightly slurred. Which one of the following conditions is the most likely diagnosis?

- (A) Folate deficiency
- (B) Hyperparathyroidism
- (C) Pick disease
- (D) Sydenham chorea
- (E) Wilson disease

Answers and Explanations

1. The answer is E [*IV H 2 b*]. This case is most suggestive of Wernicke encephalopathy, which is a delirium characterized by gait disturbance, oculomotor abnormalities, and cognitive impairment. This delirium is caused by acute thiamine deficiency, usually resulting from alcohol abuse. Treatment involves rapid administration of thiamine. Pentobarbital is likely to worsen the symptoms. Salicylates, anticoagulants, and acetylcholinesterase (AChE) inhibitors would have no effect.

2. The answer is D [*IV I 8*]. The particular circumstances strongly suggest that the woman has been exposed to levels of carbon monoxide sufficient to interfere with the oxygen-carrying capacity of her hemoglobin. Thus, cerebral anoxia and delirium have resulted. Although the other choices can cause cognitive disturbances, they are less likely causes in this case.

3. The answer is B [*IV H 5*]. The evidence of gradual cognitive, motor, and sensory impairments is most suggestive of cobalamin deficiency. Megaloblastic anemia is likely to be present. Although multiple sclerosis (MS) might also cause such impairments, the course would most likely wax and wane. A patient with a neoplasm is more likely to present with seizures. Hyperthyroidism causes increased reflexes and palpations.

4. The answer is B [*IV I 3*]. The woman's history is characterized by episodes of cognitive impairment, personality changes, mood disturbance, and abdominal pain. The episodes started when she began using estrogen. This pattern is most suggestive of acute intermittent porphyria (AIP), a disorder of heme synthesis that includes wine-colored urine. AIP is most common in women; often, it is first evident in the third decade of life and can be precipitated by use of estrogens and barbiturates.

5. The answer is C [*IV D 2*]. The man has experienced relapsing and remitting symptoms involving a variety of central nervous system (CNS) sites, a course that is characteristic of multiple sclerosis (MS). The visual deficit is suggestive of optic nerve involvement, which is often an early symptom of this illness and is uncommon in any of the other choices. The peak incidence of diagnosis of MS is approximately age 30 years. Cobalamin deficiency causes megaloblastic anemia. Herpes encephalitis produces bizarre behavior and seizures. Psychosis is prominent in patients with neurosyphilis. Mood disturbance is seen in individuals with systemic lupus erythematosus.

6. The answer is A [*II B*]. The symptoms are very suggestive of dementia, with impairment in memory and other cognitive processes. Alzheimer disease causes 55% of cases of dementia. It is usually seen in older individuals, but individuals with Down syndrome are very likely to develop this disease by age 40 years.

7. The answer is B [*IV I 6*]. The patient describes an episodic disturbance that occurs in the morning. This episode is most suggestive of hypoglycemia, which most often occurs after nighttime fasting or after vigorous exercise. Symptoms are strongly reminiscent of anxiety attacks. Hyperthyroidism might also manifest as anxiety and tremulousness, but it would not be limited to the morning. Ammonia levels are associated with liver disease secondary to alcohol abuse. Sodium is likely to be normal without gastrointestinal disturbance. Thyroid symptoms would occur at other times. Toxicology screen is less productive, unless ingestion occurred within a few hours.

8. The answer is E [*IV I 2*]. Wilson disease (hepatolenticular degeneration) usually becomes symptomatic in the second or third decade of life. The initial signs often include personality and mood changes. Transient episodes of psychosis may occur. The disease process involves the putamen and the corpus callosum, resulting in movement or muscular signs such as the dysarthria manifested here. Hyperparathyroidism is associated with anxiety and personality change, and folate deficiency is associated with birth defects. Pick disease causes dementia. Sydenham chorea is noted for movements.

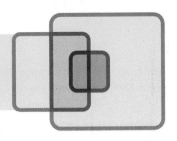

chapter **6**

Substance-Related Disorders

ANGELA D. HARPER

I   **INTRODUCTION**

The *Diagnostic and Statistical Manual of Mental Disorders*, 4th edition, text revision (*DSM-IV-TR*), recognizes two broad categories of disorders related to the use of psychoactive substances. Substance use disorders are syndromes of pathologic use of a substance, and substance-induced disorders are disturbances of thinking, emotion, or behavior caused by intoxication with or withdrawal from a psychoactive substance.

A **Substance use disorders** are subdivided into two categories: substance dependence and substance abuse.

  1. **Substance dependence** is a pathologic pattern of substance use that results in impairment or distress. Substance dependence is diagnosed when three or more of the following consequences of substance use occur together at any time in the same year:
     a. **Tolerance,** which is defined as:
        (1) A requirement for increased amounts of the substance to achieve the same effect
        (2) Decreased effect with continued use of the same amount of the substance
     b. **Withdrawal,** which is defined as:
        (1) Typical withdrawal syndrome for the substance (see I B 2)
        (2) The substance or a related compound is taken to relieve or avoid withdrawal symptoms
     c. Use of the substance in greater amounts or for a longer time than was originally intended
     d. Unsuccessful attempts or wishes to cut down on or control substance use
     e. Significant amounts of time spent in activities necessary to obtain or use the substance or recover from its effects
     f. Giving up important social, occupational, or recreational activities because of substance use
     g. Continued use of the substance despite knowledge that it is causing or aggravating physical or mental problems

  2. **Physiologic dependence** is defined in the *DSM-IV-TR* as the presence of either tolerance or withdrawal (see I A 1 a, b).

  3. **Substance abuse,** according to the *DSM-IV-TR,* is a maladaptive pattern of abuse with fewer and different consequences than substance dependence. Substance abuse is diagnosed if one of the following four problems has occurred over a 12-month period and if the patient does not meet criteria for substance dependence:
     a. Failure to fulfill major role obligations
     b. Recurrent use of a substance in situations in which it is hazardous (e.g., while driving)
     c. Recurrent legal problems resulting from substance use
     d. Continued use of a substance despite social or interpersonal problems caused by the substance (e.g., arguments with a spouse about substance use, getting into fights when drunk)

B **Substance-induced disorders** include a diverse group of physical and mental syndromes caused by psychoactive substances or their withdrawal:

  1. **Substance intoxication** is a reversible, substance-specific syndrome (see II).

  2. **Substance withdrawal** is a substance-specific syndrome that appears when a substance is withdrawn (see III).

3. **Substance-induced delirium** is an acute disturbance of cognition and awareness caused by taking a psychoactive substance. Of the substances in the *DSM-IV-TR* considered to be psychoactive, only nicotine is not thought to cause delirium.

4. **Substance-withdrawal delirium** is caused by withdrawal of alcohol, sedative-hypnotics, anxiolytics, and related substances.

5. **Substance-induced persisting dementia,** which is caused by intoxication with or withdrawal from substances (e.g., alcohol, inhalants, sedatives), is characterized by memory impairment plus one or more of four signs of cognitive dysfunction. These signs include **aphasia, apraxia, agnosia,** and **disrupted executive function.** Signs of dementia persist after intoxication or withdrawal has cleared.

6. **Substance-induced, persisting amnestic disorder** consists of impairment of recall of previously learned material or of the ability to learn new information. It is associated with the use of alcohol, sedative-hypnotics, anxiolytics, and related substances. The memory disorder persists after intoxication or withdrawal has resolved.

7. **Substance-induced psychotic disorder** is characterized by prominent hallucinations or delusions caused by substances such as alcohol, amphetamines, cannabis, cocaine, hallucinogens, inhalants, opioids, phencyclidine, and sedatives. According to the *DSM-IV-TR*, this diagnosis cannot be based on hallucinations if the patient realizes that the hallucinations are caused by the substance, although the significance of this distinction is not established scientifically. If transient psychotic symptoms are associated only with delirium caused by substance intoxication or withdrawal, the diagnosis is substance-induced delirium or substance-induced withdrawal delirium.

8. **Substance-induced mood disorder** is depressed or manic mood that either is clearly caused by substances such as alcohol, amphetamines, cocaine, hallucinogens, inhalants, opioids, phencyclidine, sedatives, and anxiolytics or develops within 1 month of using these substances.

9. **Substance-induced anxiety disorder** (see Chapter 4) consists of generalized anxiety, panic attacks, obsessions, or compulsions that either are clearly caused by a substance or develop within 1 month of substance use or withdrawal.

10. **Substance-induced sexual dysfunction** either develops within 1 month of substance intoxication or is clearly caused by substances such as alcohol, amphetamines, cocaine, opioids, and a number of medications (e.g., reserpine, serotonin reuptake inhibitors, monoamine oxidase [MAO] inhibitors).

11. **Substance-induced sleep disorder** either is obviously caused by a psychoactive substance or appears within 1 month of substance use or withdrawal. Typical offending agents include alcohol, amphetamines, caffeine, cocaine, opioids, sedatives, hypnotics, and anxiolytics.

12. **Hallucinogen-persisting perception disorder (flashbacks)** is the reexperiencing of perceptual symptoms that were caused by intoxication with a hallucinogen but occur after the drug is no longer being taken. Because hallucinogens act on the serotonin 5HT-2 receptor, medications that increase synaptic serotonin availability (e.g., selective serotonin reuptake inhibitors [SSRIs]) may overstimulate receptors previously sensitized by hallucinogens to produce flashbacks years after substance discontinuation.

C **Addiction** is a term used by some clinicians to refer to overwhelming involvement with seeking and using drugs or alcohol and a high tendency toward relapse after substance withdrawal. It is, therefore, a quantitative description of the degree to which drug use pervades an individual's life. Addiction may be described as a form of substance dependence, as defined in I A.

1. It is possible for an individual to develop tolerance and undergo withdrawal without being addicted; that is, the individual's life is not organized around finding and using the drug. This is common in patients who become physically dependent on narcotics, tranquilizers, or sedatives during treatment of prolonged illness or insomnia but who do not experience intrusion of drug use into many aspects of their lives.

2. It may be possible to be addicted in the sense that drug-seeking behavior is paramount in an individual's life without being physically dependent.

D **Substances subject to dependence and abuse** The *DSM-IV-TR* categorizes substance-related disorders according to which of 13 types of substances is used. All of these substances are believed to be associated with dependence and abuse, except caffeine (which in the *DSM-IV-TR* is said to produce neither syndrome but recently has been shown to produce physical dependence) and nicotine (which causes dependence only). Any of these substances may produce the other syndromes listed in I B. The specific substance categories include:

1. Alcohol
2. Amphetamines
3. Caffeine
4. Cannabis
5. Cocaine
6. Hallucinogens
7. Inhalants
8. Nicotine
9. Opioids
10. Phencyclidine
11. Sedatives, hypnotics, and anxiolytics
12. Polysubstance
13. Other (e.g., digitalis, amyl nitrite)

II INTOXICATION SYNDROMES

Because the manifestations and treatment of intoxication with different drugs can vary drastically and may require different treatments, it is crucial to be able to differentiate between common intoxication syndromes.

A **Alcohol** often is combined with other substances. The odor on the patient's breath that is characteristically associated with alcohol intoxication is caused by impurities in the preparation and is unreliable in diagnosing intoxication. In addition, head injuries and metabolic encephalopathies (e.g., ketoacidosis) often are mistaken for alcohol intoxication. Blood and urine screens may help to make the diagnosis. The central nervous system (CNS) concentration of alcohol parallels the concentration in the blood.

1. **Alcohol intoxication** is diagnosed in the *DSM-IV-TR* when the following signs appear in association with drinking:
   a. Slurred speech
   b. Loss of coordination
   c. Unsteady gait
   d. Nystagmus
   e. Impaired attention or memory
   f. Stupor or coma

2. **Mild intoxication** is characterized by disorganization of cognitive and motor processes. The first functions to be disrupted are those that depend on training and previous experience. As intoxication becomes more noticeable, the following changes occur:
   a. **Overconfidence.** If performance is initially impaired by psychological inhibitions, an individual may transiently function better after ingestion of small amounts of alcohol. However, although the intoxicated individual tends to feel more efficient, all aspects of physical and mental performance are impaired by alcohol.
   b. **Mood swings, emotional outbursts,** and **euphoria** may occur.
   c. **Initial enhancement of spinal reflexes** may develop as they are released from higher inhibiting circuits, followed by progressive general anesthesia of CNS functions.
   d. **An increased pain threshold** may be evident, but other sensory modalities are unaffected.
   e. **Nausea, vomiting, restlessness,** and **hyperactivity** may be present.

 3. **Severe intoxication** is characterized by:
   a. Stupor or coma
   b. Hypothermia
   c. Slow, noisy respiration
   d. Tachycardia
   e. Dilated pupils (may be normal in some intoxicated individuals)
   f. Increased intracranial pressure
   g. Death (rare in the absence of ingestion of additional substances, trauma, infection, or unconsciousness lasting longer than 12 hours)

 4. **Treatment** depends on whether or not the patient is conscious.
   a. **Conscious patients** need little treatment beyond waiting for the alcohol to be metabolized.
      (1) Stimulants and caffeine do not hasten sobriety.
      (2) Restraint for severe agitation is safer than administration of tranquilizers or sedatives, which may potentiate the CNS depressant effects of alcohol.
      (3) In low doses, antipsychotic drugs (e.g., ziprasidone or haloperidol given intravenously or risperidone or olanzapine given orally) may decrease hyperactivity without increasing sedation.
   b. **Stuporous or unconscious patients** should be kept warm with legs elevated. It also may be necessary to:
      (1) Prevent aspiration, especially if gastric lavage is performed.
      (2) Treat increased intracranial pressure with mannitol or by other measures (e.g., corticosteroids) in addition to the normal management of overdoses of CNS depressants.
      (3) Remove alcohol by hemodialysis in extreme situations.

B Sedatives, hypnotics, and anxiolytics

 1. **Specific substances**
   a. Benzodiazepine tranquilizers (e.g., diazepam, oxazepam, chlordiazepoxide, lorazepam, clorazepate, alprazolam, clonazepam)
   b. Benzodiazepine hypnotics or sleeping pills (e.g., flurazepam, temazepam, triazolam, estazolam)
   c. Barbiturates (e.g., phenobarbital, amobarbital, pentobarbital, secobarbital)
   d. Drugs related to barbiturates: ethchlorvynol, glutethimide, propanediols (e.g., meprobamate), methyprylon, paraldehyde, and others
   e. Chloral compounds (e.g., chloral hydrate)

 2. **Mild to moderate intoxication** with benzodiazepines, barbiturates, and related compounds causes:
   a. Euphoria
   b. Hypalgesia (increased pain threshold)
   c. Increased seizure threshold
   d. Sedation
   e. Paradoxical excitement in:
      (1) Susceptible individuals
      (2) Elderly persons
      (3) Children
      (4) People with preexisting neurologic impairment
   f. Nystagmus, dysarthria, ataxia, impaired attention and memory
   g. Psychomotor impairment
   h. Postural hypotension

 3. **Severe intoxication** usually is caused by purposeful overdoses in suicide attempts and accidental overdoses by addicts. A few patients, especially those with preexisting brain disease, may take too much medication because of drug automatism (the patient forgets that the drug has already been taken and continues to take more pills, usually in an effort to get to sleep). Severe intoxication can cause:
   a. Stupor and coma
   b. Respiratory depression
   c. Depressed reflexes

    d. Hypotension

    e. Decreased cardiac output

    f. Hypoxemia

    g. Bullous skin lesions and necrosis of sweat glands

    h. Hypothermia

    i. Coma

    j. Death

        (1) Death from barbiturate intoxication usually is caused by pneumonia or renal failure.

        (2) Short-acting preparations (e.g., amobarbital) are more lethal at lower doses than are long-acting compounds (e.g., phenobarbital).

        (3) Death from an overdose of benzodiazepines alone is rare. However, combinations of benzodiazepines and other CNS depressants, especially combinations with alcohol, can be fatal.

4. Treatment of CNS depressant intoxication involves emesis if the ingestion has occurred within 30 minutes of initiation of treatment and the gag reflex is intact. Gastric lavage should be performed for less recent ingestions of substances that have not been fully absorbed. A cathartic agent should be given to decrease intestinal absorption of the drug. For severe poisoning, the following steps are taken:

    a. Protection of the airway

    b. Oxygen administration

    c. Ventilation when necessary

    d. Prevention of further loss of body heat

    e. Correction of hypovolemia and maintenance of blood pressure with dopamine

    f. Forced diuresis with maximal alkalinization of the urine

    g. Hemodialysis

C **CNS stimulants**

1. Specific substances

    a. Amphetamines and related compounds include the prescription drugs dextroamphetamine, methylphenidate, and pemoline sodium and the illicit drugs methamphetamine (speed), cocaine, and smokable cocaine (crack). Medical indications for amphetamines include:

        (1) Attention deficit disorder

        (2) Depression in elderly patients

        (3) Depression in medically ill patients who cannot tolerate antidepressants

        (4) Augmentation of antidepressants in patients with treatment-resistant depression

        (5) Narcolepsy

    b. Cocaine is used to treat nosebleeds and is sometimes used as a local anesthetic in the ears, nose, and throat

    c. Phenmetrazine

    d. Phenylpropanolamine

    e. Antiobesity drugs. Long-term treatment of obesity with stimulants is almost always unsuccessful because of tolerance

2. Mild to moderate intoxication produces:

    a. Elevated mood

    b. Increased energy and alertness

    c. Increased ability to perform repetitive tasks when the individual is tired or bored

    d. Decreased appetite

    e. Talkativeness

    f. Anxiety and irritability

    g. Insomnia

    h. Hypertension or hypotension

    i. Increased or decreased heart rate

    j. Hyperthermia

    k. Nausea or vomiting

    l. Loss of appetite and weight

3. **Severe intoxication** may produce agitation, anger, and psychosis. Although tolerance develops to many of the effects of stimulants, there is no tolerance to the tendency to develop psychotic symptoms, which may be indistinguishable from those of functional paranoid psychoses. **Signs and symptoms** include:

   a. Visual, auditory, and tactile hallucinations
   b. Delusions, especially of being infested with parasites
   c. Paranoia and loose associations in a clear sensorium
   d. Mania
   e. Fighting
   f. Hypervigilance
   g. Dilated pupils
   h. Elevated blood pressure and pulse (may be normal in some chronic abusers)
   i. Arrhythmias
   j. Seizures
   k. Exhaustion
   l. Coma
   m. Intracranial hemorrhage
   n. Multiple cerebral infarcts

4. **Treatment**
   a. Hypertension and hyperthermia can be treated with **phentolamine.**
   b. Psychotic symptoms can be treated with **haloperidol,** which antagonizes the dopaminergic properties of stimulants.

D **Hallucinogens and phencyclidine**

1. **Specific substances**
   a. Lysergic acid diethylamide (LSD)
   b. Psilocybin
   c. Mescaline
   d. 2,5-Dimethoxy-4-methylamphetamine (STP)
   e. Phencyclidine (PCP)

2. **Intoxication** depends on the substance.
   a. Most hallucinogen intoxications produce:
      (1) Dilated pupils
      (2) Increased heart rate and blood pressure
      (3) Fever
      (4) Paranoia in a clear sensorium
      (5) Illusions
      (6) Hallucinations
      (7) Depersonalization
      (8) Anxiety
      (9) Distortion of time sense
      (10) Inappropriate affect
   b. **PCP intoxication** also can cause:
      (1) Violent behavior
      (2) Hyperactivity
      (3) Hyperacusis
      (4) Mutism
      (5) Echolalia
      (6) Analgesia
      (7) Nystagmus
      (8) Ataxia
      (9) Muscular rigidity
      (10) Focal neurologic signs
      (11) Seizures

(12) Coma

(13) Intracranial hemorrhage

3. **Treatment** of intoxication and "bad trips" depends on the substance.

   a. The psychological effects of most hallucinogens are usually decreased by reassurance in a quiet setting. Oral administration of diazepam is sometimes a useful adjunct.

   b. Patients intoxicated with PCP may react violently to any environmental stimulation, including attempts at reassurance. They should generally be left alone in a quiet area. If they become violent, they may be sedated with intravenously administered haloperidol or diazepam. Seizures should be treated with intravenous administration of diazepam.

E **Cannabis** Specific substances include marijuana, hashish, and Δ-tetrahydrocannabinol (TCH).

1. **Intoxication by marijuana and related substances** rarely produces hallucinations. More common effects include:

   a. Euphoria

   b. Anxiety

   c. Increased appetite

   d. Increased suggestibility

   e. Distortion of time and space

   f. Red conjunctivae

   g. No change in pupils

   h. Dry mouth

   i. Tachycardia

2. **Treatment.** The psychological effects of the cannabis group of drugs, similar to those of most hallucinogens, are generally eased by reassurance in a quiet setting. Oral administration of diazepam is sometimes useful.

F **Opioids** Many street preparations are adulterated with quinine, procaine, lidocaine, lactose, or mannitol and are contaminated with bacteria, viruses, or fungi.

1. **Specific substances**

   a. Morphine

   b. Heroin

   c. Hydromorphone

   d. Oxymorphone

   e. Levorphanol

   f. Codeine

   g. Hydrocodone

   h. Oxycodone

   i. Methadone

   j. Meperidine

   k. Alphaprodine

   l. Propoxyphene

   m. Pentazocine, which has both narcotic antagonist and agonist properties

2. **Mild to moderate intoxication** may produce:

   a. Analgesia without loss of consciousness

   b. Drowsiness and mental clouding

   c. Nausea and vomiting

   d. Apathy and lethargy

   e. Euphoria

   f. Itching

   g. Constricted pupils

   h. Constipation

   i. Flushed, warm skin caused by cutaneous vasodilation

   j. Dysarthria

   k. Impaired attention and memory

   l. Illusions

3. **Severe intoxication** is associated with:
   a. Miosis
   b. Respiratory depression, which may recur up to 24 hours after apparent recovery from an overdose with most narcotics and up to 72 hours after apparent recovery from a methadone overdose
   c. Hypotension or shock
   d. Depressed reflexes
   e. Coma
   f. Pulmonary edema
   g. Seizures (with propoxyphene or meperidine)

4. **Treatment**
   a. Severe intoxication is treated primarily by **supportive care.**
   b. **Naloxone,** a narcotic antagonist, can:
      (1) Reverse coma and apnea (The effects of concomitantly self-administered drugs [e.g., barbiturates] are not altered, and detoxification from these drugs also should be undertaken.)
      (2) Precipitate a severe abstinence syndrome in narcotic-dependent patients
      (3) Cause vomiting

G **Inhalants** Sniffing ("huffing") inhalants is becoming an increasingly severe problem among children and adolescents. Because brain damage may occur with repeated use, and no antidote or specific treatment of intoxication exists, it is important to identify the problem and institute remedial therapy.

1. **Specific substances**
   a. Gasoline
   b. Glue
   c. Paint thinner
   d. Solvents
   e. Spray paints

2. **Intoxication** may cause:
   a. Dizziness
   b. Euphoria
   c. Altered states of consciousness
   d. Confusion
   e. Nystagmus
   f. Ataxia
   g. Dysarthria
   h. Lethargy
   i. Depressed reflexes
   j. Psychomotor retardation
   k. Tremor
   l. Muscular weakness
   m. Blurred vision
   n. Delirium

3. Chronic use may result in dementia.

4. There is no specific treatment for inhalant dependence and abuse other than prevention of further access to the substance.

H **Anticholinergic drugs** A number of psychiatric medications have anticholinergic side effects. Some anticholinergic substances grow wild, and some are included in various herbal medications.

1. **Specific substances**
   a. Most over-the-counter cold and sleeping preparations
   b. Atropine
   c. Belladonna
   d. Henbane

    e. Scopolamine

    f. Antiparkinsonian drugs (e.g., trihexyphenidyl, benztropine)

    g. Tricyclic and tetracyclic antidepressants and paroxetine

    h. Low-potency neuroleptics (e.g., thioridazine)

    i. Jimson weed

    j. Mandrake

    k. Propantheline

2. **Intoxication** with anticholinergic substances is coded as "other intoxication" in the *DSM-IV-TR* and may produce:

    a. Confusion

    b. Memory loss

    c. Delirium

    d. Hallucinations

    e. Amnesia

    f. Body image distortions

    g. Drowsiness

    h. Psychosis

    i. Tachycardia

    j. Decreased peristalsis

    k. Fever

    l. Warm, dry skin

    m. Fixed, dilated pupils

    n. Coma

3. **Treatment** is primarily directed toward protecting the patient and waiting for the drug to be metabolized. Intravenous administration of physostigmine can temporarily reverse coma or severe hyperpyrexia but should be used cautiously. Relief is transient because of the short half-life of the drug; gastrointestinal and cardiac side effects may be significant. Persistent signs of intoxication can be treated with longer-acting cholinesterase inhibitors such as donepezil (Aricept).

I. **Club drugs** are the newest category of drugs that hit the scene in nightclubs and "raves" or all-night dance parties during the 1990s. These so-called "designer drugs" are most popular in young adults.

1. **Specific substance**

    a. GHB (GABA-hydroxybutyrate)

    b. MDMA (3,4–methylenedioxymethamphetamine) or Ecstasy or "X"

    c. Ketamine or "Special K"

2. **Intoxication**

    a. Euphoria and disorientation

    b. Relaxation and emotional warmth

    c. Increased sexuality

    d. Amnesia

    e. Disinhibition

    f. Hypertension and hyperthermia

    g. Dehydration and tachycardia

    h. Jaw clenching and bruxism

    i. Liver or renal failure in extreme cases

3. **Treatment** is similar to that of other stimulants. Supportive care such as adequate rehydration is crucial. Occasionally, the use of alprazolam for extreme agitation is needed.

III   SUBSTANCE WITHDRAWAL

Substance withdrawal produces substance-specific, physiologically determined syndromes that appear after abrupt withdrawal or decrease in dosage of the drug. Withdrawal from some compounds produces mild syndromes. Withdrawal from others produces phenomena that are uncomfortable but not dangerous. Life-threatening abstinence syndromes result from abrupt discontinuation of a few substances. Blood levels are often zero in abstinence syndromes.

A Alcohol abstinence syndromes

1. Alcohol withdrawal ("the shakes") usually appears within a few hours of stopping or decreasing alcohol consumption. Generally, this lasts for 3 to 4 days; occasionally, it may last as long as 1 week.

   a. **Signs and symptoms** include:
      (1) Tachycardia
      (2) Tremulousness
      (3) Diaphoresis
      (4) Nausea
      (5) Orthostatic hypotension
      (6) Malaise or weakness
      (7) Anxiety
      (8) Irritability

   b. **Treatment**
      (1) The standard practice has been to administer a mid- to long-acting benzodiazepine, such as diazepam or chlordiazepoxide, in a tapering dose over 4 to 5 days.
      (2) Thiamine can be given parenterally at 100 mg/day for 3 days if one is extremely concerned about the patient's nutritional status, but this is usually not necessary.

2. **Major motor seizures ("rum fits")**
   a. **Symptoms.** Major motor seizures occur during the first 48 hours of alcohol withdrawal in a small percentage of patients.
   b. **Treatment** is via intravenous administration of diazepam. Phenytoin is not administered unless the patient has epilepsy.

3. **Alcohol withdrawal delirium (delirium tremens)** begins on the second or third day (rarely later than 1 week) after withdrawal or decrease of alcohol intake. It occurs in fewer than 5% of alcohol-dependent patients, usually after they have been drinking heavily for at least 5 to 15 years. If seizures also occur, they always precede the development of delirium. If a patient decompensates to the point of delirium tremens, the mortality rate is approximately 10%.

   a. **Symptoms** of delirium tremens include:
      (1) Delirium
      (2) Autonomic hyperactivity (e.g., increased pulse rate, increased blood pressure, and sweating)
      (3) Agitation
      (4) Vivid hallucinations
      (5) Gross tremulousness

   b. **Treatment**
      (1) Hydration
      (2) Vital signs every hour
      (3) A benzodiazepine (e.g., diazepam) administered in divided doses. The maximum dosage depends on the amount that it takes to keep the patient calm, comfortable, and seizure free.
      (4) An antipsychotic drug such as haloperidol or risperidone in severe cases of agitation or psychosis
      (5) Consider parenteral administration of thiamine if necessary.
      (6) Consider the addition of valproic acid as a seizure prophylaxis, as augmentation to the benzodiazepine, and to assist in keeping the patient calm and comfortable if the patient is not responding well to the benzodiazepine alone.

4. **Alcohol hallucinosis** (alcohol-induced psychotic disorder with hallucinations in the *DSM-IV-TR*) is a rare condition that develops within 48 hours of cessation of drinking or at the end of a long binge with gradual decreases in blood alcohol levels.

   a. **The principal symptom** is vivid auditory hallucinations without gross confusion. Usually, the patient hears threatening or derogatory voices that discuss the patient in the third person or speak directly to the patient. Command hallucinations are absent. Symptoms usually last a few hours or days, but in approximately 10% of patients, they may persist for weeks or months. Occasionally, the syndrome may become chronic, in which case it may be indistinguishable from schizophrenia.

    b. Treatment. Antipsychotic drugs may relieve hallucinations in patients who do not improve spontaneously. Although they are not well studied for alcohol hallucinations, the atypical antipsychotic drugs (e.g., risperidone, ziprasidone) are good initial choices because they are better tolerated than neuroleptics such as haloperidol.

B **Withdrawal from sedatives, hypnotics, and anxiolytics** produces syndromes that vary in time of onset, duration, and severity. Withdrawal syndromes are likely to occur after chronic use of 400 to 600 mg/day of pentobarbital, 3,200 to 6,400 mg/day of meprobamate, and 40 to 60 mg/day of diazepam or their equivalents. Milder withdrawal syndromes may develop in individuals taking lower doses for longer periods of time. It is difficult to predict whether an individual will develop a withdrawal syndrome and how severe it may be.

  1. Symptoms usually begin within 12 to 24 hours, peak at 4 to 7 days, and last about 1 week after withdrawal from short-acting compounds such as pentobarbital and alprazolam. Withdrawal from long-acting compounds such as diazepam or phenobarbital begins later (4–10 days after drug discontinuation) and reaches its peak more slowly (around the seventh day). Signs and symptoms include:

    a. Anxiety and agitation

    b. Orthostatic hypotension

    c. Weakness and tremulousness

    d. Hyperreflexia and clonic blink reflex

    e. Fever

    f. Diaphoresis

    g. Delirium

    h. Seizures

    i. Cardiovascular collapse

  2. Treatment. Withdrawal from CNS depressants can be life threatening, so treatment is mandatory when the syndrome is diagnosed. Although some patients with uncomplicated withdrawal may be managed as outpatients, hospitalization is required for the management of more severe and complicated withdrawal to ensure compliance with the treatment protocol and adequate coverage if the condition worsens. Treatment is not as effective if it is initiated after the appearance of delirium.

    a. Because all CNS depressants produce cross-tolerance, a known compound (pentobarbital or phenobarbital) is substituted for the offending substance to suppress the abstinence syndrome and is then gradually withdrawn. The amount of phenobarbital or pentobarbital that the patient is likely to tolerate—and that therefore will suppress withdrawal—can be calculated by observing the results of administering 200 mg of pentobarbital or 60 to 100 mg of phenobarbital when the patient no longer appears to be intoxicated (usually within 12 to 16 hours after discontinuation of the offending substance).

      (1) If the patient becomes severely intoxicated or falls asleep with the test dose, tolerance does not exist, and the patient does not need further treatment.

      (2) If the patient develops moderate symptoms after the test dose (e.g., dysarthria, nystagmus, ataxia without sleepiness), moderate tolerance exists, suggesting that the patient requires 200 to 300 mg/day of pentobarbital or 60 to 90 mg/day of phenobarbital.

      (3) Absence of symptoms or nystagmus without other signs of intoxication in response to the test dose indicates significant tolerance. The patient should then be administered a total daily (divided) dose of 600 to 1,000 mg of pentobarbital or 180 to 300 mg of phenobarbital every 6 hours to suppress withdrawal.

      (4) Tolerance also may be assessed by giving successive 60- to 100-mg doses of phenobarbital every 1 to 4 hours until the patient is intoxicated. The amount necessary to produce definite signs of intoxication (to a maximum of 500 mg/day) is then administered in divided doses every 6 hours to suppress the abstinence syndrome.

    b. As soon as the patient is stabilized, the dose of pentobarbital is decreased by 10% every 1 to 2 days. Phenobarbital, which is longer acting, may be withdrawn more rapidly. Reappearance of abstinence phenomena indicates that the dose needs to be reduced more gradually. Unexpected intoxication during the phenobarbital protocol indicates accumulation of the barbiturate and a need for faster dosage reduction.

    c. Because cross-tolerance exists between barbiturates and alcohol, phenobarbital or pentobarbital can also be used to suppress alcohol abstinence syndromes, as well as withdrawal from more than one CNS depressant.

    d. Benzodiazepines can also be used to suppress withdrawal from any cross-reacting CNS depressant. With the exception of alcohol withdrawal, standardized protocols using benzodiazepines have not been established, however.

C **Stimulant withdrawal**   There is no observable physiologic disruption with stimulant withdrawal; psychological and behavioral manifestations may be severe, however.

    1. Symptoms
        a. Increased sleep
        b. Nightmares caused by rapid eye movement (REM) rebound
        c. Fatigue
        d. Lassitude
        e. Increased appetite
        f. Depression ("cocaine blues")
        g. Suicide attempts
        h. Craving for the drug

    2. Treatment
        a. Antidepressants (e.g., bupropion, venlafaxine, desipramine) are helpful for withdrawal depression.
        b. Hospitalization may be necessary if the patient is suicidal.

D **Cessation of hallucinogens** does not produce a significant abstinence syndrome.

    1. Symptoms. Flashbacks (brief reexperiences of the hallucinogenic state) may be precipitated by marijuana, antihistamines, and SSRIs.

    2. Treatment. Reassurance that symptoms will subside and administration of a benzodiazepine are usually sufficient therapy.

E **Opioid withdrawal** is not life threatening; however, it may be extremely uncomfortable.

    1. Symptoms usually appear 8 to 10 hours after cessation of morphine. The onset is slower when long-acting drugs, such as methadone, have been withdrawn. Symptoms peak at 48 to 72 hours and disappear in 7 to 10 days. Disturbances include:
        a. Lacrimation and rhinorrhea
        b. Sweating
        c. Restlessness and sleepiness
        d. Gooseflesh
        e. Dilated pupils
        f. Irritability
        g. Violent yawning
        h. Insomnia
        i. Coryza
        j. Craving for the drug

    2. Treatment
        a. Buprenorphine was introduced in the late 1990s. Administered intramuscularly up to four times a day with a daily taper, it is highly effective for acute opiate withdrawal. Buprenorphine is a partial agonist/antagonist to the mu receptor. If given too soon after the patient's last use of opiates, acute and painful withdrawal will occur because of buprenorphine's antagonistic properties. The patient must show clear evidence of opiate withdrawal before receiving the first dose. A sublingual form of buprenorphine that is absorbed in the mucosal lining of the oral membranes may also be used. It is given in divided doses of 2 to 6 mg up to four times a day and tapered until detox is complete.
        b. The effects of narcotic withdrawal are lessened by **methadone** substitution. When the patient demonstrates objective signs of withdrawal, a sufficient dose of methadone to suppress

abstinence, or a maximum dose of 20 to 50 mg/day (never more than 100 mg), is administered. The dose of methadone is then decreased by 10% to 20% at each reduction, every few days. Although any licensed physician may prescribe methadone for pain, the use of methadone to detoxify a narcotic addict (as well as methadone maintenance to prevent relapse of addiction) violates federal law in any setting other than a federally approved site for the treatment of narcotic addiction.

c. **Clonidine** administered at 0.1 to 0.3 mg three times per day for 2 weeks may help to suppress withdrawal symptoms, although it can cause hypotension. Clonidine should be tapered rather than abruptly discontinued because rapid withdrawal causes rebound hypertension.

F **Anticholinergic drug withdrawal** occasionally produces influenza-like syndromes, depression, mania, or seizures. Discontinuation of clinically significant doses taken for more than 1 month should, therefore, be gradual. Treatment is with atropine or reintroduction of the offending agent with more gradual discontinuation.

G **Nicotine withdrawal** has been found to be a significant impediment to smoking cessation.

1. **Symptoms** include malaise, irritability, anxiety, and craving for tobacco.

2. **Treatment** includes over-the-counter nicotine patches containing gradually decreasing doses of nicotine. This is most effective when it is combined with a behavioral program. Clonidine administered as described in III E 2 c or by means of a patch may be a useful adjunct. Nicotine lozenges and inhalers are also available. Bupropion, a norepinephrine/dopamine antagonist, and varenicline, a nicotinic receptor partial agonist, are prescription smoking cessation aids. The Food and Drug Administration (FDA) has required both medications to carry a black box warning due to side effects including depression and suicidal ideation.

H **Caffeine withdrawal** produces insomnia, depression, and headaches. Gradual reduction of intake may prevent withdrawal symptoms.

IV PRINCIPLES OF TREATMENT OF SUBSTANCE-RELATED DISORDERS

Certain approaches are useful for treatment of abuse and dependence with all substances.

A **Detoxification** It is impossible to address the causes of substance abuse and dependence while the patient continues to use the substance. The first goal of treatment, therefore, is to withdraw the substance.

B **Insistence on abstinence** A few individuals may be able to use addicting substances in moderation after successful treatment of dependence or abuse, but it is impossible to identify them. Complete abstinence is safest.

C **Avoidance of other substances associated with dependence or abuse** Frequently, people who have been dependent on alcohol or another substance ask to be treated with benzodiazepines or related compounds for anxiety or insomnia. Acceding to this request is dangerous for several reasons:

1. It introduces another substance that can be associated with dependence.

2. Taking a pill for rapid relief of dysphoria reinforces the association between taking the drug and feeling better, thereby increasing the tendency to go back to the drug of choice for the same result.

3. There is no evidence that tranquilizers decrease the use of alcohol as a self-treatment for anxiety, and some reports suggest that using benzodiazepines increases the risk of relapse of alcoholism.

4. Controversy surrounds the use of stimulants such as methylphenidate and dextroamphetamine to treat attention deficit hyperactivity disorder (ADHD) in individuals who are presumed to have used cocaine and other illicit stimulants as self-treatments for ADHD. It is usually safer to use treatments for ADHD with a lower risk of dependence and abuse (e.g., bupropion, venlafaxine, desipramine).

D **Involvement of the family** Family members may encourage use of the substance in the patient, especially if there is family strife that everyone is able to ignore because all attention is focused on the identified patient. For example, a family may ignore or overlook sexual abuse of one child by focusing attention on another child's problem with drugs or alcohol. A spouse may also be drug dependent. The family can be important allies in insisting that the patient deal with the problem. Similarly, it is very difficult to prevent use of a substance by a patient whose spouse continues to use that substance or is not willing to reduce its availability in the home. Encouragement of families to enlist the help of **Al-Anon** is often helpful when treating a patient with addiction issues.

E **Unscheduled toxicology screens** Despite technical problems that may reduce reliability, periodic urine screens often are essential in identifying relapse and noncompliance.

F **Self-help groups** Peer support groups provide credibility and encouragement from individuals who have had similar problems and who are adept at dealing with common resistances to treatment. Twelve-step programs have been developed for most substances.

G **Sanctioned treatment** When a patient is forced to remain in therapy by a legal sanction (e.g., threatened loss of driver's license or professional license for relapse), the outcome is better than when the patient is free to withdraw from therapy at any time.

H **Contingency contracting** Contingency contracting provides a powerful negative contingency for leaving treatment or relapsing and a positive contingency for remaining drug free. In the most widely used form of contingency contracting, the patient agrees in advance that the therapist will notify an employer or licensing body if relapse occurs. The patient may leave a letter with the therapist outlining the problem, which is to be mailed if a urine screen result is positive or the patient does not keep an appointment. Some patients deposit a sum of money with the therapist; a certain amount is then paid back to the patient for each week of abstinence. When the contingency for relapse is a report to the appropriate medical licensing authority, the relapse rate of substance-dependent physicians is less than 25%.

I **Change of peer group** For many patients, especially adolescents, substance use is encouraged by peers. Such individuals must be helped to find a different peer group in which substance use is not a prerequisite to social support.

V ALCOHOLISM

Alcoholism affects approximately 12% of the population at some point during their lifetimes. Alcohol abuse or dependence usually develops during the first 5 years of regular use of alcohol.

A **Three patterns of chronic alcohol abuse** have been described:
1. Regular daily excessive drinking
2. Regular heavy drinking on weekends only
3. Long periods of sobriety interspersed with binges that last days, weeks, or months

B **Familial influences** seem to play a role in the development of alcoholism. Individuals are at an increased risk of being alcoholic if they have:
1. A family history of alcoholism, especially if the individual is the son of an alcoholic father
2. A family history of teetotalism (i.e., avoidance of alcohol under any circumstance)
3. An alcoholic spouse

C **Diagnostic clues** to alcoholism include:
1. Inability to decrease or discontinue drinking
2. Binges lasting at least 2 days
3. Occasional consumption of a fifth of spirits or the equivalent in wine or beer in a single day
4. Blackouts (transient amnesia for events that occur while the patient is intoxicated)
5. Continued drinking despite a physical illness that is exacerbated or caused by drinking

6. Drinking nonbeverage alcohol (e.g., shaving lotion)

7. Drinking in the morning

8. Withdrawal syndromes

9. Apparent sobriety in the presence of an elevated alcohol level in the blood, indicating tolerance to the sedative effects of alcohol

10. Arrest for driving under the influence (DUI)

11. Frequent trips to the emergency room for falls or other "accidents"

12. Absenteeism from work

D **Physical, psychiatric, and social complications**

1. **Physical complications,** which may be caused by associated nutritional deficiencies or by a direct toxic effect of alcohol, are not uncommon in patients who drink more than 3 to 6 oz of whiskey a day or the equivalent. More familiar syndromes include:

   a. Cerebral atrophy

   b. Wernicke encephalopathy

   c. Korsakoff psychosis

   d. Nicotinic acid deficiency encephalopathy

   e. Polyneuropathy

   f. Cardiomyopathy

   g. Hypertension

   h. Skeletal muscle damage of uncertain clinical significance

   i. Gastritis

   j. Peptic ulcer

   k. Constipation

   l. Pancreatitis

   m. Cirrhosis

   n. Impotence

   o. Various anemias

   p. Teratogenicity

      (1) **Fetal alcohol syndrome,** characterized by mental retardation, microcephaly, slowed growth, and facial abnormalities, may be a risk even if moderate amounts of alcohol are consumed during pregnancy.

      (2) Because safe quantities have not been established, complete abstinence from alcohol during pregnancy is recommended. If a patient does drink, she should be advised to do so on a full stomach to minimize rapid increases in blood alcohol levels. Folate supplementation may have the potential to ameliorate the risk of fetal malformations, but it has not been shown to make it possible to drink safely during pregnancy.

   q. **Accidents**

      (1) Almost half of all traffic fatalities involve alcohol.

      (2) Drunk drivers who are killed in motor vehicle accidents are four to 12 times more likely than drivers who are not killed to have had a previous arrest for driving under the influence, indicating that drinking and driving is a recurrent problem. Many people continue to drink and drive after their licenses are revoked.

2. **Psychiatric complications.** The major psychiatric complication of alcoholism is **suicide.** More than 80% of individuals who kill themselves are depressed, alcoholic, or both. Alcohol is a frequent component of many suicides, even in patients who are not alcoholic.

   a. Seventy-five percent of alcoholics have no other primary psychiatric diagnoses, although depression is a common complication of the direct effects of alcohol on the brain and the consequences of drinking on the patient's life.

   b. Alcoholism may be an attempt at self-treatment of another psychiatric disorder, such as depression, anxiety, mania, psychosis, or posttraumatic stress disorder. This possibility should be considered when psychiatric symptoms clearly preceded heavy drinking. However, the history often is unreliable, and only a trial period of abstinence reliably distinguishes between primary alcoholism and alcohol abuse that is secondary to another condition. If psychological distress resolves after a period of abstinence, alcoholism is likely to have been a cause rather than a result of the psychiatric disorder.

   c. Alcoholism is a common comorbid condition with mood disorders, anxiety disorders, and personality disorders. In such situations, both conditions must be treated.

3. **Social complications** occur with the use of all psychoactive substances. The on-the-job accident rate is increased three to four times in workers who use psychoactive substances. Alcohol and other drugs cause sexual, marital, and legal problems.

E **Specific treatment approaches** result in approximately one-third of patients remaining sober, one-third enjoying a period of sobriety followed by relapse, and one-third continuing to drink. Useful interventions include the following:

1. **Confrontation of denial.** The major obstacles to therapeutic success are the patient's denial of the severity of the problem and his or her wish to continue drinking. Repeated statements that the patient is not in control of the drinking and repeated confrontation with the complications of the alcoholism may be necessary before the patient agrees to treatment.

2. **Insistence on abstinence.** Because it is not possible to identify in advance the very few patients who may be able to succeed with controlled drinking, total abstinence is the only realistic goal.

3. **Assessment of motivation.** The patient who is willing to consider abstaining completely for 1 month has at least some motivation to give up alcohol completely. If the patient insists on some continued alcohol intake (usually while assuring the doctor that it will be easy to keep from drinking excessively), treatment is less likely to be successful. Further therapeutic efforts may be unsuccessful until the patient is willing to give up alcohol completely for at least a brief period of time.

4. **Disulfiram.** Many alcoholics' efforts at abstinence are supported by disulfiram, which causes severe nausea and vomiting when it interacts with alcohol. Even if the patient does not need the drug, willingness to take it is a favorable prognostic sign. The only contraindications to the use of disulfiram are organic brain syndromes, severely impaired liver function, or other conditions that might interfere significantly with compliance. The usual dose is 250 to 500 mg/day. Vitamin C and antihistamines may abort the alcohol–disulfiram reaction. Disulfiram may, in rare instances, increase liver enzymes; therefore, yearly monitoring of liver functioning is recommended. Patients must be warned about not using metronidazole, alcohol-containing mouthwash, and certain cough syrups because these substances will produce the disulfiram reaction.

5. **Naltrexone** is approved for reduction of craving for alcohol, although its effectiveness has been limited.

6. **Acamprosate** is approved and designed to reduce the craving for alcohol while still allowing the patient to consume alcohol and not get sick. It works on GABA and glutamate neurotransmission. The patient must abstain from alcohol for 5 days before taking the medication for it to be effective.

7. **Involvement of the family.** The patient's family can be an important source of support, or the family may openly or covertly encourage the patient to go on drinking.
   a. A family "intervention," in which all family members confront the patient's drinking, helps the patient to deal with denial.
   b. Refusal by the spouse to remain with the patient unless he or she stops drinking may be the only force strong enough to convince the patient to agree to a trial of abstinence. Such threats should be mobilized only when they are a true expression of the spouse's feelings, or they will not be credible.
   c. Contingency contracting that involves remaining in the hospital may be very effective.
   d. Employers and other important individuals in the patient's life should also be involved in treatment whenever possible.

8. **Alcoholics Anonymous (AA).** AA is a highly useful treatment group and has actually been found to be the most effective treatment model in maintaining sobriety in multiple studies. Other peer counseling programs also provide peer support and encouragement for patients to stop drinking.

9. **Behavior therapy.** Punishing drinking (e.g., with disulfiram) and rewarding sobriety (e.g., by paying the patient for abstinence through contingency contracting) are useful for patients who consider their drinking a bad habit. Expressive psychotherapy is appropriate for patients who believe that their drinking is motivated by unresolved emotional conflicts.

10. **Ongoing emotional support by the primary physician.** Primary care physicians provide an important source of encouragement for patients to confront the problem and to maintain sobriety. The physician should accept periodic relapses in a nonjudgmental manner. If the patient refuses specific therapy for alcoholism, the physician should continue to be available to the drinking patient in case a psychosocial crisis precipitates the patient's wishing to become involved in treatment.

VI   OPIOIDS

Opioid dependence and abuse is a major public health problem. The incidence of heroin use increased during the 1960s, and use of this drug is now a problem in smaller communities in the United States as well as in large cities. After a period of decreased use, narcotic use is undergoing a resurgence in middle-class groups.

A **The epidemiology** of narcotic use, particularly heroin, deserves consideration. Between 2% and 3% of adults age 18 to 25 years have tried heroin at some time in their lives. Abuse of narcotics usually occurs in the context of abuse of other drugs. Using "soft" drugs such as marijuana seems to break down a psychological barrier to using "hard" drugs. Approximately 50% of individuals who abuse narcotics become physically dependent. Most addicts tend to become abstinent over time. Often they finally discontinue drug dependence approximately 9 years after its onset.

1. **Patterns of narcotic abuse vary widely.** Some addicts, particularly those who are maintained on methadone, lead productive lives and enjoy good health. For others, the need to obtain illicit drugs and money to buy them leads to prostitution and other crimes. However, to a significant extent, personality and behavior before drug use predict behavior while using opioids. Many narcotic abusers lead an antisocial lifestyle that persists until the drug is withdrawn. These individuals differ from those with antisocial personality disorder who are also narcotic abusers in that the antisocial behavior in persons with the personality disorder antedated substance abuse. Because of physical complications of abuse and a lifestyle associated with violence, the death rate is two to 20 times higher (10 in 1,000) in opioid addicts than it is in the general population. Patterns of narcotic use and dependence are as follows:

   a. **Acquired during medical treatment.** A small but definite percentage of narcotic users become dependent in the course of medical treatment. This can often provide a gateway into obtaining greater quantities off the streets when their physicians finally cut off their supply or may lead them into harder drugs, such as heroin.

   b. **Recreational use.** More commonly, narcotic abuse develops when an adolescent or young adult who is engaged in experimental or recreational drug use progresses to use of more dangerous substances. Although between 60% and 90% of adolescents experiment to some extent with drugs (experimentation with drugs has been reported in children as young as age 5 years), the number who go on to opioid dependence is not great. Progression to dependence on CNS stimulants and depressants is more common.

   c. **Methadone maintenance.** A significant number of individuals who have become dependent on opioids receive methadone from organized treatment programs.

   d. **Health care personnel.** The incidence of narcotic addiction is higher in physicians, nurses, and other health care personnel than in any other group of individuals with comparable education and socioeconomic class. Most physician–addicts initially use a narcotic to relieve depression, fatigue, or a physical ailment rather than for pleasure. The pattern and consequences of the addiction are no different than they are for other addicts, except that health care personnel are more likely to make drugs available to themselves through prescriptions written for real and imaginary patients. Health care professionals are often caught diverting narcotics from the floor medication dispensers, from partially used vials of medication, or even from patients.

2. **Epidemic transmission.** Heroin abuse tends to be transmitted in an epidemic fashion among individuals who know each other. These epidemics begin slowly, peak rapidly, and then decline quickly. They tend to abate completely after 5 to 6 years.

    a. **Susceptibility** to heroin addiction varies in different populations. Young African American men are at highest risk, and women seem to be at lower risk.

    b. **Dependence** is initiated in a susceptible individual by someone known to the individual who is already addicted. The risk of such initiators exposing their acquaintances to heroin use continues for about 1 year. Drug "pushers" actually cause few new cases of dependence, although they obviously are a major source of the drug.

    c. **Heroin abuse** tends to spread until all susceptible individuals within a given group have been exposed. New addicts then tend to expose their friends in other circles, who produce a third generation of abusers.

3. **Drug cultures.** When cultural norms support heroin use and relatively pure preparations are available, a large percentage of users become dependent.

    a. More than 40% of the U.S. Army–enlisted men stationed in Vietnam reported trying narcotics at least once, and approximately 50% of those who tried it became physically dependent at some time during their stay in Vietnam. However, very few individuals who became dependent on narcotics in Vietnam continued drug use when they returned to the United States. This suggests that removal of peer group support for drug abuse, removal of the easy availability of drugs, and, possibly, removal of major environmental stresses ended the reasons for drug abuse.

    b. Most individuals in the United States who become dependent on narcotics have a psychological predisposition to abuse and tend to remain in peer groups that encourage substance use. Relapse is likely when they return to an environment in which drugs are available and friends and colleagues condone abuse.

4. **Psychiatric illness.** Approximately 50% to 87% of people with opioid dependence suffer from another psychiatric illness, especially depression, anxiety states, and borderline and antisocial personality disorders. Individuals from disorganized social backgrounds are also more susceptible to narcotic dependence. A combination of a susceptible psychosocial constellation, availability of narcotics, an environment that encourages abuse, and friends or colleagues who already are users may be necessary for the development of addiction.

B **Medical complications** of narcotic abuse may result from contaminants of illicit preparations and the patient's lifestyle.

1. **Sexually transmitted diseases** are common in female drug abusers as a result of engaging in prostitution to obtain the narcotic.

2. **Fatal overdose** caused by fluctuations in the purity of available compounds is common.

3. **Anaphylactic reactions** may be caused by the intravenous injection of impurities.

4. **Hypersensitivity reactions** to impurities may also cause the formation of granulomata and neurologic, musculoskeletal, and cutaneous lesions.

5. **Infections** commonly caused by contaminated products and shared needles include hepatitis, endocarditis, septicemia, tetanus, and formation of pulmonary, cerebral, and subcutaneous abscesses. Up to two-thirds of individuals in narcotic treatment centers test positive for HIV.

6. **Suicide and death** at the hands of associates are more common in narcotic abusers than in the general population.

C **Treatment** of opioid dependence requires a multidisciplinary approach.

1. **Methadone maintenance** for the treatment of addiction can only be carried out by a federally approved program.

    a. If the patient has strong psychosocial supports available and is highly motivated to discontinue drug use, the patient can be withdrawn from opioids immediately using methadone (see III E 2 b).

    b. If supports are weak or motivation to undergo withdrawal is uncertain, a period of methadone maintenance is instituted while motivation, social supports, and the relationship with the treatment team are strengthened. The usual dosage of methadone in this setting is 40 to 150 mg/day. The role of methadone is to take away craving and prevent a "high" from self-administered opiates because of the blockage of the mu receptor by the methadone. Patients must come to the clinic 6 out of 7 days a week for the first 90 days. If their urine is clean, they "phase up" to the next level, which allows them less restrictions every 3 months.

(1) The patient must have clear-cut signs of addiction (e.g., intoxication, needle tracks, and medical or psychosocial consequences of abuse) to qualify for methadone maintenance.

(2) Periodic unscheduled urine and blood screens are performed to assess compliance with the program. Persistent noncompliance (i.e., continued self-administration of narcotics, cocaine, benzodiazepines) results in dismissal.

(3) Very gradual withdrawal from methadone is attempted when the patient seems ready. Most addicts note some abstinence symptoms when the dosage is reduced below 20 mg/day, and reduction in dosage by as little as 1 mg/week below this level may be necessary for the detoxification of long-term methadone users.

2. **L-α-Acetylmethadol (LAAM),** also known as methadyl acetate, a long-acting preparation, suppresses narcotic withdrawal for 72 hours. When it is used instead of methadone for maintenance, less frequent administration of the drug is necessary. However, more patients drop out of LAAM maintenance than methadone maintenance.

3. **Naltrexone,** a long-acting narcotic antagonist, has been used in a manner analogous to disulfiram to precipitate withdrawal when narcotics are used.

4. A combination medication of **buprenorphine and naloxone** can be prescribed on an outpatient basis by physicians who have completed a training course on the use of this medication. Naloxone was added so that if anyone tried to inject the drug, the addict would experience the antagonist effect of the drug. The combination is given in pill form and instead of being used for detoxification, it is used for opiate replacement and maintenance. Patients usually take 8 to 24 mg/day in divided doses. Similar to methadone, it reduces craving and prevents a high if opiates are used while taking it. Benefits of this combination over methadone are that a 30-day prescription can be given instead of going to a methadone clinic every day. Patients must be very motivated and reliable for this treatment to work. Each doctor with the required certification may provide treatment for 30 patients in his or her practice. Once a physician has held the prescription licensure for a year, he or she may apply for an "exemption" to treat up to 100 patients thereafter.

5. **Therapeutic communities** play an important role in the treatment of narcotic addiction. Confrontation by fellow addicts of lying and rationalization of drug use has more credibility to an addict than therapies that are administered by professionals. Most of the time, this occurs during 12-step meetings.

6. **Residential treatment.** If outpatient therapy is unsuccessful, residential treatment is necessary to remove the patient from easy access to the drug and from associates who encourage continued narcotic use. Group confrontation and support are used extensively in these settings. Compliance with treatment is higher when it is mandated by the courts than when it is voluntary and the patient is free to withdraw at any time.

7. **Licensure restrictions.** Physicians and nurses who abuse narcotics are increasingly being identified by state licensing bodies and professional societies. Treatment programs have been very successful when the problem is identified early and when continued licensure for medical practice is made contingent on documentation of ongoing abstinence (i.e., contingency contracting).

8. **Prevention of addiction in a medical setting.** Health care providers should not permit fears of addiction from interfering with the administration of appropriate doses of narcotics to patients in pain. The following guidelines apply to the administration of opioids to patients at risk of dependence:

a. Adequate doses of narcotics should be administered to patients with bona fide acute pain syndromes. As a result of tolerance, addicts generally require higher doses than other patients.

b. Narcotics should be administered on a set schedule rather than as needed. This approach prevents patients from becoming preoccupied with pain and its relief and provides a constant blood level that results in lower individual doses being necessary.

c. An addict should not be detoxified during an acute physical illness.

d. Prescriptions should not be written for outpatients with suspicious complaints or those with a high abuse potential, as indicated by:
   (1) Losing prescriptions or running out of medication early
   (2) Requests for a specific drug
   (3) History of abuse of alcohol or other drugs
   (4) Physician shopping
   (5) Claims that a physician who originally wrote a prescription is unavailable
   (6) Threats when narcotics are not prescribed
   (7) Dishonesty with the physician
   (8) When a narcotic is not the standard of care for that particular complaint (e.g., migraine headaches, fibromyalgia, general back pain)

VII TRANQUILIZERS AND SLEEPING PILLS

Abuse of and dependence on tranquilizers and sleeping pills are created or encouraged in everyday medical practice more often than opioid dependence and abuse.

(A) Manifestations of dependence and abuse Barbiturates and related compounds are particularly prone to pathologic use. Whereas benzodiazepines with short half-lives are more prone to dosage escalation to reduce interdose withdrawal, highly lipid-soluble benzodiazepines produce a more rapid effect that may be experienced as a high. Diazepam, which is very lipid soluble; lorazepam, which has a short half-life; and alprazolam, which has both properties, are the most commonly abused benzodiazepines. Dependence may first be suspected only when an abstinence syndrome that responds to phenobarbital or pentobarbital appears in a patient who is admitted to the hospital and is denied access to the abused substance.

1. Because they suppress REM sleep, barbiturates and related sedatives (e.g., secobarbital, glutethimide, ethchlorvynol) subject the patient who uses them to a **rebound of REM sleep,** usually in the form of **nightmares,** when the drug is discontinued. Although it seems to the patient that he or she cannot sleep without the drug, continued drug use serves only to prevent withdrawal and suppress REM rebound, and escalating doses often are needed to accomplish this result.

2. When barbiturates and related compounds are used as tranquilizers, drug withdrawal tends to be mistaken for a return of anxiety, which leads to an increase in dosage to suppress the symptoms. Fear of withdrawal symptoms then leads to continued drug use and an inability to function without the drug, as well as other manifestations of dependence.

3. Symptoms of benzodiazepine withdrawal may persist for months after drug discontinuation, leading to prolonged use of the benzodiazepine to suppress withdrawal.

(B) Identification and management of abuse Misuse of sedatives and tranquilizers can be minimized if the physician does not prescribe barbiturates for insomnia and anxiety or benzodiazepines for patients with a history of substance dependence. Identification and management of problems with CNS depressants involve the following steps:

1. A **detailed history** of amounts and kinds of all prescription and nonprescription drugs that have ever been taken should be obtained. Often, the patient continues to take drugs that were prescribed by a physician that he or she is no longer seeing.

2. **Prescriptions** for a patient who has terminated treatment should be **discontinued.**

3. **Toxicology screening** in patients who abuse any drug should be performed to identify mixed abuse. Drugs are not present in the blood of a patient who is experiencing a withdrawal syndrome.

4. **Regular appointments** should be scheduled for patients who have been taking barbiturates for years and who are reluctant to discontinue them. Assurance of an ongoing relationship with a physician the patient trusts may make the patient more willing to consider tapering drug intake. Insistence on discontinuation of barbiturates and related medications is mandatory for patients who escalate the dose, have withdrawal symptoms, or experience psychomotor impairment.

5. **Hospitalization** should be considered for detoxification of patients with severe or mixed dependence. This permits adequate treatment of what may be life-threatening withdrawal and ensures compliance with the withdrawal protocol.

VIII COCAINE

Cocaine abuse and dependence have become extremely serious public health problems. One-fourth of young adults have used cocaine, and adverse consequences are common.

A Routes of administration   Cocaine may be self-administered by three routes.

1. **Nasal** administration is associated with the onset, over a period of about 20 minutes, of euphoria that lasts approximately 1 hour.

2. **Intravenous** administration produces immediate euphoria.

3. **Crack,** an easily synthesized compound that is not inactivated by high temperature, is **smoked,** producing immediate euphoria.

B Addictive potential   Contrary to the popular wisdom of a few years ago, cocaine is highly addictive. The advent of crack and the flooding of the market with cheap cocaine have made cocaine a drug of abuse at all socioeconomic levels.

1. Animals will choose self-administration of cocaine over food and water until they die.

2. Some patients report feeling addicted from the very first dose of cocaine.

3. Crack is the cheapest and most addictive form of cocaine.

4. Cocaine often is used in conjunction with other substances, especially alcohol and tranquilizers.

C Psychomotor impairment   In one report, more than 50% of a group of drivers who were stopped by the police for reckless driving and who were not intoxicated with alcohol were intoxicated with cocaine, marijuana, or both.

D Psychiatric disorders   Cocaine use may be a means of self-treatment for certain psychiatric disorders, especially depression and attention deficit disorder. Some individuals who suffer from bipolar disorder abuse cocaine to achieve a sense of control over excitement and mood swings that occur spontaneously without the drug. In any of these situations, cocaine is so inherently rewarding that attempts to treat the comorbid condition without treating cocaine abuse are invariably unsuccessful. In addition, as a potent kindling stimulus, cocaine exacerbates mood instability in bipolar disorder.

E Treatment   The same approaches that have been applied to abuse of opioids and alcohol have been found helpful in the treatment of cocaine abuse and dependence.

1. **Bupropion and possibly venlafaxine** are thought to potentially reduce craving because of their action on dopamine.

2. **Amantadine** decreases cocaine craving in the first few weeks after withdrawal. It may also be useful in long-term treatment.

3. **Cognitive therapy** has been found to have a delayed onset of action in promoting abstinence from cocaine. The benefits of medications tend to dissipate after the medication is discontinued.

4. **Topiramate and disulfiram** are being considered as potential treatments for cocaine craving.

IX CANNABIS

Cannabis abuse and dependence is often not considered an important problem. However, in addition to producing medical and psychological complications, marijuana has been shown in adolescents to serve as a "gateway drug." That is, use of marijuana reduces the threshold for using more dangerous substances, with progression from use of alcohol and marijuana to use of hallucinogens, stimulants, and narcotics.

A Manifestations of dependence and abuse   Chronic marijuana use results in an amotivational syndrome that may persist after drug discontinuation. Intellectual function may also be impaired. Although marijuana traditionally has not been thought to cause physical dependence, recent reports indicate that people who use this substance regularly experience craving for the drug and prolonged dysphoria with drug withdrawal that is reduced by restarting the drug.

B **Treatment**

1. No medication is specifically useful in the treatment of marijuana use, although 5HT-3 antagonists may turn out to reduce the craving and "highs" that reinforce marijuana use.

2. As with any substance, reducing access to the drug, learning other means of coping with stress, changing peer groups, toxicology screens, and involving the family are essential components of any treatment plan.

Study Questions

Directions: *Each of the numbered items or incomplete statements in this section is followed by answers or by completions of the statement. Select the ONE lettered answer or completion that is BEST in each case.*

1. Joe is a 27-year-old male who requires more alcohol and cocaine to get the same high. He is hanging out with a rough crowd and engaging in riskier behavior to obtain drugs. He has tried to quit but can't seem to stop. He thinks he may have even had a seizure on one occasion. He has stolen from his parents to get high. He has been getting in trouble with the law and shows little remorse. All of the following features of Joe's addiction meet the criteria for substance dependence EXCEPT:

- [A] Overwhelming involvement in seeking and using a drug
- [B] Physical dependence
- [C] Attempts to quit
- [D] Antisocial behavior
- [E] Tolerance and withdrawal

2. A patient presents to the emergency room after overdosing on phenobarbital. Which of the following symptoms is indicative of barbiturate intoxication?

- [A] Agitation
- [B] Confusion
- [C] Disorientation
- [D] Nystagmus
- [E] Postural hypotension

can be sx of withdrawal or intoxication

3. A patient presents to the emergency room with a blood alcohol level of 10 mg/100 ml, but there is no clinical evidence of intoxication. It is a reasonable assumption that the patient:

- [A] Is tolerant to opioids → *no cross - tolerance (benzos?)*
- [B] Is dependent on alcohol
- [C] Has pancreatitis
- [D] Is impotent
- [E] Has cerebral atrophy

4. A patient with depressed reflexes, decreased respirations, pinpoint pupils, hypotension, and lethargy is carried into a walk-in clinic by a friend. What is the most likely cause of the emergency?

- [A] Alcohol intoxication
- [B] Cocaine intoxication
- [C] Opiate intoxication
- [D] Marijuana intoxication
- [E] Benzodiazepine intoxication

5. A law school student suddenly starts acting quite bizarre while studying for a major exam in the library. His friends have become concerned that he could be "buying" amphetamine salts to get through school. All of the following would be expected if he were having a stimulant-induced psychosis EXCEPT:

- [A] Clear sensorium
- [B] Depression → *happens in withdrawal*
- [C] Loose associations
- [D] Paranoia
- [E] Tactile hallucinations

6. You are working in an outpatient drug and alcohol rehabilitation clinic. You are counseling a long-term marijuana user who believes that marijuana is a "safe drug." He should be concerned about possible long-term negative consequences of his use, which include all of the following EXCEPT:

[A] Physical dependence can develop.

[B] Its use increases the likelihood of narcotic use.

[C] Overdose causes seizures.

[D] Chronic use causes an amotivational state.

[E] It causes tachycardia.

7. A patient is in the hospital for heroin detoxification. He just received his first injection of buprenorphine. Thirty minutes later, he begins vomiting, sweating, and cramping. What happened?

[A] He is allergic to buprenorphine.

[B] He does not really use heroin.

[C] He lied about when he last used.

[D] He has the stomach flu.

[E] The nurse gave him disulfiram instead of buprenorphine.

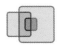 # Answers and Explanations

1. The answer is D [*I A*]. While personality disorders are often common in alcohol and drug dependency problems, their presence is not necessary in order to confirm a diagnosis. Physical dependence, tolerance, withdrawal, and increasing time spent acquiring substances are all seen with alcohol and drug dependency problems.

2. The answer is D [*II B 1 c, 2 e; III B 1*]. Both intoxication and withdrawal from barbiturates may cause confusion, delirium, anxiety, agitation, and postural hypotension. If caused by withdrawal, these signs improve with administration of a barbiturate. Nystagmus, which is a sign of intoxication but not of withdrawal, may appear.

3. The answer is B [*V C 9*]. Absence of intoxication in the presence of a high blood alcohol level indicates that the patient is tolerant to the central nervous system depressant effects of alcohol, which is a major criterion for alcohol dependence. Pancreatitis, impotence, and cerebral atrophy are complications of alcoholism that should be investigated, but these are not diagnosed by a blood alcohol level. Because opioids and alcohol are not cross-tolerant, tolerance to alcohol does not provide any information about tolerance to opioids.

4. The answer is C [*II F 2 g*]. Similar to alcohol, barbiturates, and benzodiazepines, narcotics can produce depression of consciousness, reflexes, blood pressure, and respiration. Narcotics cause constricted rather than dilated pupils. Opioid intoxication can be diagnosed with intravenous naloxone.

5. The answer is B [*II C 3*]. Stimulant psychosis often is associated with paranoia and loose associations in a clear sensorium, which may make it indistinguishable from schizophrenia. Tactile hallucinations and delusions of infestation with parasites also may occur. Depression is usually associated with stimulant withdrawal, not stimulant intoxication.

6. The answer is C [*II E 1, IX A*]. Contrary to popular wisdom, physical dependence on marijuana may occur, and withdrawal symptoms may appear with discontinuation. Marijuana has been found to be a "gateway drug" that lowers the threshold for use of "harder" drugs. Marijuana use can produce tachycardia and an amotivational state. Overdose can cause distortions in time sense and injected conjunctivae, but not seizures.

7. The answer is C [*III E 2 a*]. The patient is going into acute opiate withdrawal 30 minutes after receiving his first buprenorphine injection. He most likely told the nursing staff and physician that he had used his last dose of heroin several hours earlier from the time of his admission than he actually did. He probably feared going into withdrawal and did not wait long enough for withdrawal signs to appear before getting his first dose of buprenorphine. As a result, buprenorphine's antagonistic properties knocked off the remaining heroin still attached to the mu receptors and put the patient into acute opiate withdrawal. *powerful M binding*

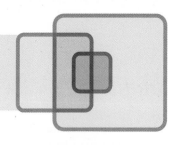

chapter **7**

Personality Disorders

ROBERT BREEN • JOSHUA THORNHILL

I | INTRODUCTION

Individuals have a repertoire of coping devices or defenses that allows them to maintain an equilibrium between their internal drives and the world around them. This repertoire is **personality—the set of characteristics that defines the behavior, thoughts, and emotions of individuals.** The characteristics become ingrained and dictate people's lifestyles.

A **Personality traits**   In general, personality traits are viewed as the result of cultural and societal influences as well as the child-rearing practices of the individual family. Studies in child development suggest that genetically determined temperamental factors may also be involved in personality development. Certain genetic characteristics may make the occurrence of a specific behavioral response more likely, thus leading to a specific personality style. When this stable pattern of response leads to problems, a personality disorder may exist. **A personality disorder is present when personality traits are inflexible and maladaptive and deviate from the expectations of the individual's culture, causing either significant impairment in social or occupational functioning or subjective distress.** Manifestations of a personality disorder are usually recognized by adolescence and continue into adulthood. However, symptoms may become less obvious in later years.

B **Expression of symptoms**   Personality disorders are among the most common emotional disorders seen in psychiatric practice, particularly in the outpatient clinic. The patient's perception of the problem and the expression of symptoms, however, are different from those demonstrated in other psychiatric illnesses, making treatment difficult. Patients with personality disorders may complain of mood disturbances, particularly depression or anxiety. They may exhibit:

1. **Ego-syntonic symptoms,** in which patients do not recognize that anything is wrong with them that needs to be changed. They view existing disturbances as being the result of the world's being out of step with them.

2. **Ego-dystonic symptoms,** in which patients may be experiencing internally distressing symptoms that are self-induced but are still unable to alter their behavior

C **Clinical picture**   Symptoms of personality disorders generally affect other individuals and involve work, play, and all relationships.

1. **Individuals have trouble in their work settings.** They have often had many jobs and work below their capacities.

2. **Social relationships are disrupted or absent.** Individuals with personality disorders can be irritating and infuriating to those involved with them, and the reactions of these involved individuals are often more pronounced than the disorder itself.

3. **Patients may seek help as a result of a concurrent medical or surgical problem or because of a primary emotional distress.** In any case, these patients may elicit strong negative reactions in the physicians and other health care personnel who take care of them.

4. **In general, patients with personality disorders tolerate stress poorly** and seek help to alleviate the outside stress rather than to change their character. If stress is great, as it can be in those who are physically ill, patients may regress.

D Biology

1. **Genetics.** Twin and adoption studies show strong genetic components to **personality traits.** Less is known about **personality disorder.**

2. **Familial associations.** There is an increased risk of both Axis I and Axis II disorders in families of persons with personality disorders.

E Diagnosis

1. **Comorbid Axis I disorders are common.** The majority of persons with personality disorder also have one or more Axis I disorders. It is sometimes difficult to diagnose a specific personality disorder when a patient has a mix of traits. However, the ***Diagnostic and Statistical Manual of Mental Disorders,* 4th edition, text revision (*DSM-IV-TR*), allows for the diagnosis of more than one personality disorder if a patient meets the diagnostic criteria for several disorders.** Diagnosis of a personality disorder should be made carefully in individuals who are reacting to a major environmental or social stress; for example, some young men develop maladaptive coping mechanisms in the military that they do not otherwise use.

2. **Axis I disorders make the assessment of personality disorder more difficult.** For example, a diagnosis of personality disorder should not be made in a person with schizophrenia unless the personality disorder *clearly* preceded the onset of schizophrenia.

3. Diagnosis of a personality disorder is only made after dysfunction can be determined in **at least two of the following four areas:**
   a. Cognition (perceiving or interpreting oneself, others, or events)
   b. Affect (range, intensity, lability, or appropriateness of emotional response)
   c. Interpersonal functioning
   d. Impulse control

II CLUSTERS OF PERSONALITY DISORDERS

Ten specific personality disorders are described in the *DSM-IV-TR*. Because of the similarities in symptoms or traits, they are grouped into three clusters:

A Cluster A   The **odd or eccentric group** includes the **paranoid, schizoid, and schizotypal personality disorders.**

1. Affected individuals use the **defense mechanisms of projection and fantasy** and may have a tendency toward psychotic thinking.
   a. **Projection** involves attributing to another person the thoughts or feelings of one's own that are unacceptable (e.g., prejudice, excessive fault finding, paranoia).
   b. **Fantasy** is the creation of an imaginary life with which the patient deals with loneliness. A fantasy can be quite elaborate and extensive.
   c. **Paranoia** is a feeling of being persecuted or treated unfairly by others. Paranoid patients may feel that others are talking about or making fun of them.

2. Biologically, patients with Cluster A personality disorders may have a **vulnerability to cognitive disorganization when stressed.**

3. **Schizotypal patients** have been found to have some of the same biologic markers seen in schizophrenic individuals, including low levels of monoamine oxidase (MAO) activity in platelets and disorders of smooth pursuit eye movements.
   a. It has been speculated that not everyone who has a genetic vulnerability to schizophrenia becomes psychotic, but some of these individuals may be diagnosed as having a schizotypal personality disorder.
   b. In families with a history of schizophrenia, the number of relatives with schizotypal personality disorder is also increased.

B **Cluster B** The **dramatic, emotional, and erratic group** includes **histrionic, narcissistic, antisocial, and borderline personality disorders.**

1. Affected individuals tend to use certain **defense mechanisms such as dissociation, denial, splitting, and acting out.**
   a. **Dissociation** involves the "forgetting" of unpleasant feelings and associations. It is the unconscious splitting off of some mental processes and behavior from the normal or conscious awareness of the individual. When extreme, this can lead to multiple or disorganized personalities.
   b. **Denial** is closely associated with dissociation. In denial, patients refuse to acknowledge a thought, feeling, or wish but are unaware of doing so.
   c. **Splitting,** often seen in patients with borderline personalities, occurs when these individuals view other persons as "all good" or "all bad." Affected patients cannot experience an ambivalent relationship and cannot even be ambivalent in regard to their own self-image.
   d. **Acting out** involves the actual motor expression of a thought or feeling that is intolerable to a patient; this can involve both aggressive and sexual behavior. Patients with these types of personality disorders may be biologically vulnerable to stress (i.e., a tendency to low cortical arousal causes them to easily overstimulate) and a wide variation of autonomic and motor activities. Thus, a psychobiologic pattern may develop, which increases the potential for acting out that is not associated with any particular anxiety.

2. **Mood disorders** are common and may be the chief complaint.

3. **Somatization disorder** is associated with histrionic personality disorder.

C **Cluster C** The **anxious and fearful group** includes **avoidant, dependent, and obsessive-compulsive** personalities.

1. Affected individuals use **defense mechanisms of isolation, passive aggression, and hypochondriasis.**
   a. **Isolation** occurs when an unacceptable feeling, act, or idea is separated from the associated emotion. Patients are orderly and controlled and can speak of events in their lives without feeling.
   b. **Passive aggression** occurs when resistance is indirect and often turned against the self. Thus, failing examinations, clownish conduct, and procrastinating are aspects of passive-aggressive behavior.
   c. **Hypochondriasis** is often present in patients with personality disorders, particularly in dependent, passive-aggressive patients. Biologically, these patients may have a tendency toward higher levels of cortical arousal and an increase in motor inhibition. Thus, stressful stimuli may lead to high anxiety or affective arousal.

2. Twin studies have demonstrated some **genetic factors** in the development of Cluster C personality disorders. For example, obsessive-compulsive traits are more common in monozygotic twins than in dizygotic twins. **Patients with obsessive-compulsive disorder (OCD) are not at increased risk for obsessive-compulsive personality disorder and vice versa.**

III **SPECIFIC CLUSTER A PERSONALITY DISORDERS**

These disorders—schizoid, paranoid, and schizotypal personality disorders—do not occur exclusively during the course of schizophrenia, a mood disorder with psychotic features, another psychotic disorder, or a pervasive developmental disorder. If criteria are met before the onset of schizophrenia, a premorbid condition exists (e.g., schizoid personality disorder [premorbid]).

A Schizoid personality disorder

1. **Definition.** This disorder is characterized by a pervasive pattern of detachment from social relationships and a restricted range of expression of emotions in interpersonal settings that begins by early adulthood.

2. **Symptoms.** Schizoid personality disorder is present in a variety of contexts, as indicated by **at least four** of the following:
   a. **No desire or enjoyment of close relationships,** including being part of a family
   b. **Choice of solitary activities** (almost always)

      c. Little, if any, **interest in having sexual experiences** with another person

      d. Enjoyment of few, if any, **activities**

      e. Lack of close friends or confidants other than first-degree relatives

      f. Apparent indifference to the praise or criticism of others

      g. Emotional coldness, detachment, or flattened affect

3. **Prevalence.** Because **patients** with schizoid personality disorder **rarely seek treatment,** the **prevalence** of this condition is unknown.

4. **Medical–surgical setting.** Illness brings these patients into close contact with caregivers, which is often seen as a threat to their equilibrium. Patients may intensify their aloofness and are likely to leave the hospital against medical advice if they are intruded on too much. Physicians should respect the patient's distance, should expect the development of trust to take a long time, and should not demand emotional reactions from the patient.

5. **Treatment.** Individuals with schizoid, paranoid, and schizotypal personality disorders do not usually seek treatment. If treatment is sought, physicians should be respectful but scrupulously honest in dealing with patients.

      a. Individual psychotherapy is usually the preferred approach.

      b. Group therapy can be more successful if patients can tolerate it.

B **Paranoid personality disorder**

1. **Definition.** Paranoid personality disorder consists of a pervasive distrust or suspiciousness of others such that their motives are interpreted as malevolent.

2. **Symptoms.** Paranoid personality disorder is indicated by **at least four** of the following:

      a. Suspicion, without sufficient basis, of exploitation or deceitfulness on the part of others

      b. Preoccupation with unjustified doubts about the loyalty or trustworthiness of friends or associates

      c. Reluctance to confide in others because of unwarranted fear that the information will be used maliciously against oneself

      d. Reading hidden, demeaning, or threatening meanings into benign remarks or events

      e. Persistently bearing grudges (i.e., unforgiving of insult, injuries, or slights)

      f. Perception of attacks on character or reputation that are not apparent to others; **quick, angry reactions** or counterattacking

      g. Recurrent suspicions, without justification, regarding the fidelity of a spouse or sexual partner

3. **Prevalence.** The prevalence of paranoid personality disorder is believed to be 0.5% to 2.5% of the general population.

4. **Medical–surgical setting**

      a. Patients. Illness tends to exacerbate the personality style of paranoid patients. Affected individuals tend to become more guarded, suspicious, and quarrelsome. In addition, they are frequently overly sensitive to slights and project their concerns onto others. They complain more often.

      b. Physicians. Clinicians should not expect to be trusted and should not impose closeness on these patients but should remain professional and even a little aloof. Although physicians should be courteous and honest and should respect the defenses of paranoid patients, they should be straightforward about all necessary diagnostic tests and procedures, laboratory results, and treatment regimens.

5. **Treatment.** Individuals with paranoid personality disorders, like those with schizoid personalities, rarely seek treatment. If treatment is sought, physicians should be respectful but scrupulously honest. For example, if a patient finds something amiss (e.g., lateness for an appointment), the therapist should admit fault and apologize immediately. The goal of treatment is to help patients understand that not all problems are caused by others.

      a. Individual therapy is usually the preferred approach.

      b. Occasionally, patients can tolerate **group therapy,** but great care must be taken in the selection of patients.

      c. Therapists need to avoid getting too close to patients too quickly. Some patients may become agitated and threatened, which causes a hostile defensiveness. **Limits** then must be set.

   d. Antipsychotic medications can be used in small doses for short periods of time to manage agitation. However, physicians should explain the side effects.

C Schizotypal personality disorder

   1. **Definition.** The central features of this disorder are pervasive patterns of "strange" or "odd" behavior, appearance, or thinking. These peculiarities are not so severe that they can be termed schizophrenic, and there is no history of psychotic episodes.

   2. **Symptoms.** A pervasive pattern of social and interpersonal deficits marked by acute discomfort with, and reduced capacity for, close relationships is indicative. Cognitive or perceptual distortions and eccentricities of behavior also occur. Schizotypal personality disorder is indicated by the presence of **at least five** of the following:
      a. Ideas of reference (excluding delusions of reference)
      b. Odd beliefs or magical thinking that influence behavior and are inconsistent with subcultural norms (e.g., belief in superstitions, clairvoyance, telepathy, or "sixth sense"; in children and adolescents, bizarre fantasies or preoccupations)
      c. Unusual perceptual experiences, including bodily illusions
      d. Odd thinking and speech (e.g., vague, circumstantial, metaphorical, overelaborate, or stereotyped)
      e. Suspiciousness or paranoid ideation
      f. Inappropriate or constricted affect
      g. Behavior or appearance that is odd, eccentric, or peculiar
      h. Lack of close friends or confidants other than first-degree relatives
      i. Excessive social anxiety that does not diminish with familiarity and tends to be associated with paranoid fears rather than negative judgments about oneself

   3. **Prevalence.** Several studies indicate that 3% of the population has this disorder.

   4. **Medical–surgical setting.** The problems posed by treating patients with schizotypal personality disorder and a medical or surgical illness are similar to those encountered with schizoid patients. Schizotypal individuals tend to put off caregivers. Illness threatens their isolation.

   5. **Treatment.** If treatment is sought, physicians should be honest in dealing with patients. The odd behavior of these patients can cause uneasiness in physicians, who must avoid all ridicule. Physicians should not expect to develop a warm relationship with patients and should respect the patients' need for psychological distance.
      a. Group therapy is associated with a greater chance of success than individual psychotherapy.
      b. However, only certain patients can tolerate group therapy.

IV   SPECIFIC CLUSTER B PERSONALITY DISORDERS

A Antisocial personality disorder

   1. **Definition.** Individuals have a **history of continuous and chronic antisocial behavior in which the rights of others are violated.**
      a. The **essential defect** is one of character structure in which affected individuals are seemingly **unable to control their impulses** and postpone immediate gratification.
      b. Affected individuals **lack sensitivity** to the feelings of others. They are egocentric, selfish, and excessively demanding; in addition, they are usually free of anxiety, remorse, and guilt.
      c. Violation of the law and customs of the local community is characteristic. The terms "sociopath" and "psychopath" have been applied to individuals with particularly deviant antisocial personalities.
      d. Personality disorders are considered lifelong conditions, and the signs of conduct disorder must be present in adolescence. The criteria for conduct disorder (i.e., a childhood pattern of antisocial and oppositional behavior) should be met.
      e. Persons who use illegal substances satisfy many of the criteria of antisocial personality disorder as a result of their pursuit of these substances. However, the diagnosis of antisocial personality disorder is not appropriate if the diagnostic criteria are all drug related and the patient shows some remorse about victimizing others.

2. **Symptoms.** Factors indicative of antisocial personality disorder include:
   a. Current age of **18 years or older**
   b. Evidence of a **conduct disorder** (e.g., a childhood pattern of antisocial and oppositional behavior) with onset before age 15 years
   c. A pervasive **pattern of disregard for and violation of the rights of others** occurring since age 15 years, as indicated by at least three of the following:
      (1) **Failure to conform to social norms** with respect to lawful behaviors, as indicated by repeatedly performing acts that are grounds for arrest
      (2) **Deceitfulness,** as indicated by repeated lying, use of aliases, or conning others for personal profit or pleasure
      (3) **Impulsivity or failure to plan ahead**
      (4) **Irritability and aggressiveness,** as indicated by repeated physical fights or assaults
      (5) **Reckless disregard for the safety** of oneself or others
      (6) **Consistent irresponsibility,** as indicated by repeated failure to sustain consistent work behavior or honor financial obligations
      (7) **Lack of remorse,** as indicated by being indifferent to or rationalizing having hurt, mistreated, or stolen from another person
   d. Antisocial behavior that does not occur exclusively during the course of schizophrenia or a manic episode

3. **Prevalence.** In the United States, it is estimated that 3% of men have the disorder.

4. **Etiology.** The etiology of antisocial personality disorder is unclear.
   a. There is often **a family history** of antisocial personality disorder in both men and women. Both **environmental and genetic factors** play a role. A sociopathic father is predictive of an antisocial personality regardless of whether the child is reared in the presence of the father. Family problems with alcoholism also increase the risk of antisocial behavior.
   b. Some antisocial behavior is precipitated by **brain damage secondary to closed-head trauma or encephalitis.** In these cases, the proper diagnosis is **personality change caused by a general medical condition.** The causative factors are generally believed to be biologic.
   c. Other studies indicate that **inconsistent and impulsive parenting** can be more damaging than the loss of a parent.

5. **Medical–surgical setting.** The emergency department is a common site of interaction between physicians and patients with antisocial personality disorder. Impulsivity may lead to fights, suicide attempts, or other injuries. Substance abuse is a common complication.
   a. Patients may be superficially charming when under stress and not cause any particular problems initially. However, they tend to be manipulative if given a chance and resist following the rules of the hospital.
   b. Young patients have particular difficulty with the authority of physicians and tend to be noncompliant with treatment. In the hospital setting, they are generally disruptive, and when threatened, they are likely to leave the hospital against medical advice.

6. **Treatment**
   a. Setting **firm behavioral limits** is crucial. In general, **inpatient settings** are the only places where behavior can be controlled. Outpatient treatment is rarely satisfactory because patients avoid treatment as soon as they experience any unpleasant effects.
   b. **Group therapy** is more helpful than individual therapy because the patient sees it as less authoritative. Inpatient groups can confront antisocial behavior because a group of antisocial personalities is made up of experts at recognizing this behavior. Group treatment may involve therapeutic communities as well.
   c. **Medication to control aggression** may be useful in patients with brain dysfunction. β-Blockers, selective serotonin reuptake inhibitors (SSRIs), and bupropion have been used.
   d. Treatment of comorbid substance abuse is often necessary.

B Borderline personality disorder
   1. **Definition**
      a. **Origin of term.** The term "borderline" originated with the concept that this disorder was on the border between neurosis and psychosis.

   b. Important features. Essential features are **instability of self-image, interpersonal relationships, and mood.** An identity disturbance is usually present and is manifested by an uncertainty about sexual orientation, goals, types of friends, and self-image.

2. **Symptoms.** A pervasive pattern of instability of interpersonal relationships, self-image, affects, and control over impulses beginning by early adulthood is characteristic. Borderline personality disorder, which may be present in a variety of contexts, is indicated by **at least five** of the following:
   a. Frantic efforts to avoid real or imagined abandonment
   b. Unstable and intense interpersonal relationships characterized by alternating between extremes of idealization and devaluation
   c. Identity disturbance, that is, persistent and markedly disturbed, distorted, or unstable self-image or sense of self
   d. Impulsivity in at least two areas that are potentially self-damaging (e.g., spending, sex, substance abuse, reckless driving, binge eating)
   e. Recurrent suicidal behavior, gestures, or threats, or **self-mutilating behavior**
   f. Affective instability caused by a **marked reactivity of mood** (e.g., intense episodic dysphoria, irritability, or anxiety usually lasting a few hours and only rarely more than a few days)
   g. Chronic feelings of emptiness
   h. Inappropriate, intense anger or **lack of control of anger** (e.g., frequent displays of temper, constant anger, recurrent physical fights)
   i. Transient, stress-related paranoid ideation or severe dissociative symptoms

3. **Prevalence.** This disorder may be present in 2% of the population. The diagnosis is made predominantly (about 75%) in women. Of the individuals with this diagnosis, 90% also have one other psychiatric diagnosis, and 40% have two other diagnoses.

4. **Etiology.** Almost all theories related to the cause of the borderline personality have postulated problems in early development. **Severe abuse in childhood** (verbal, physical, and sexual) is a common finding. **Neurocognitive deficits** and **decreased serotonin** levels are also found.

5. **Medical–surgical setting.** When individuals with a borderline personality become ill, they exhibit an increase in stress and the potential for an exacerbation of symptoms related to the personality disorder.
   a. The illness can signify a threat to any emotional homeostasis that has developed.
   b. Splitting is used as a defense to divide others. The hospital staff may unconsciously take sides and, with the patient, view situations or people as "all good" or "all bad." This split often occurs between physicians and nurses. The intensity of the feelings provoked by patients may make medical treatment difficult.

6. **Treatment**
   a. Psychological therapy. This type of treatment may involve three approaches.
      (1) The **psychodynamic approach** aims to understand the underlying psychopathology. In general, standard long-term psychotherapy is difficult because patients tend to regress, and the reactions of therapists are intense.
      (2) **Treatment oriented toward supportive reality** is confrontational rather than interpretational. Therapists help patients recognize the feelings that are being provoked and their connection with behavior. Therapists set limits and provide structure. This approach is more appropriate in the general hospital setting.
      (3) **Dialectic behavioral therapy,** a form of cognitive therapy, has been developed to help individuals with borderline personality disorder gain better control of unstable emotions and impulsive actions. This form of therapy focuses on helping patients achieve some behavioral stability before beginning the sometimes volatile work of therapy for trauma and abuse.
   b. Pharmacologic treatment. This type of therapy is clinically important, and modest improvement in patient mood and behavior can be obtained with pharmacotherapy.
      (1) Modern **antidepressants** such as SSRIs have helped some patients control impulsivity and self-injury while improving their mood. The older MAO inhibitors (e.g., tranylcypromine) have been effective in improving mood but not in causing behavioral changes.
      (2) **Anticonvulsants** such as carbamazepine and valproate have helped decrease behavioral dyscontrol and stabilize mood.

(3) Both typical and atypical **antipsychotic medications,** when given in low doses, have been shown to be effective in decreasing behavioral dyscontrol and reducing occasional psychotic symptoms.

(4) Benzodiazepines are usually contraindicated for most patients because they may cause disinhibition, and drug abuse problems are common.

C **Narcissistic personality disorder**

1. **Definition.** Individuals have a grandiose sense of their own importance but are also extremely sensitive to criticism. They have little ability to empathize with others, and they are more concerned about appearance than substance.

2. **Symptoms.** Narcissistic patients have a pervasive pattern of grandiosity (in fantasy or behavior), need for admiration, and lack of empathy that begins in early adulthood and is present in a variety of contexts. Narcissistic personality disorder is indicated by **at least five** of the following:

   a. A grandiose sense of self-importance (e.g., **exaggeration of achievements and talents,** expectation for recognition as superior without commensurate achievements)
   b. Preoccupation with fantasies of unlimited success, power, brilliance, beauty, or ideal love
   c. Belief in being "special" and unique and can only be understood by, or should associate with, other special or high-status people (or institutions)
   d. Requirement for excessive admiration
   e. A **sense of entitlement** (i.e., unreasonable expectations of especially favorable treatment or automatic compliance with their views)
   f. Behavior that is **interpersonally exploitative** (i.e., take advantage of others as a means to achieve their own ends)
   g. Lack of empathy (i.e., unwilling to recognize or identify with the feelings and needs of others)
   h. Jealousy or belief that others are envious
   i. Arrogance; demonstration of haughty behavior or attitude

3. **Associated features**
   a. Depression or a depressed mood is common.
   b. Painful preoccupation with appearance occurs.
   c. Features of other Cluster B disorders are often present.

4. **Prevalence.** The prevalence of narcissistic personality disorder is believed to be about 1% of the general population.

5. **Medical–surgical setting**
   a. Patient reactions. Individuals react to illness as a threat to their sense of grandiosity and self-perfection. Intensification of characteristic behavior and either overidealization or devaluation of physicians is usually apparent. Patients expect special treatment.
   b. Physician or caregiver reactions. Patients tend to provoke negative reactions in caregivers. Feelings of both anger and boredom can be expected. Narcissistic personality traits are sometimes encountered in physicians, complicating work with difficult patients.

6. **Treatment**
   a. Individual psychotherapy, with an attempt at understanding the pain suffered by patients, is the treatment of choice.
   (1) The therapist must deal with transitions from being overidealized to being devalued.
   (2) These transitions can be stormy, and they occur when the therapist has misunderstood the patient or has not been perfectly empathic. It is important that the physician not be defensive about mistakes.
   b. Group therapy in combination with individual therapy can be useful in helping patients obtain feedback about the effects they have on others.

D **Histrionic personality disorder**

1. **Definition.** Affected individuals are flamboyant, seek attention, and demonstrate an excessive emotionality. Their emotions are shallow and shift rapidly. Typically, they are attractive and seductive and, like narcissistic persons, overly concerned with their appearance.

2. **Symptoms.** A pervasive pattern of excessive emotionality and attention seeking that begins by early adulthood and is present in a variety of contexts is characteristic. Histrionic personality disorder is indicated by **at least five** of the following:

a. Feeling of discomfort in situations in which the individual is not the **center of attention**

b. Interaction with others that is often characterized as **inappropriately sexually seductive** or **provocative**

c. **Insincere affect** (i.e., display of rapidly shifting and shallow expression of emotions)

d. Consistent **use of physical appearance to draw attention** to oneself

e. **Speech that is excessively impressionistic** and lacking in detail

f. **Self-dramatization,** with a theatrical and exaggerated expression of emotion

g. **Suggestibility** (i.e., easily influenced by others or circumstances)

h. **Exaggeration of importance** of relationships and acquaintances

3. **Associated features.** As with all of the Cluster B disorders, mood and somatization disorders, especially depression, are common.

4. **Prevalence.** The prevalence of histrionic personality disorder is estimated to be about 2% to 3% of the general population. The condition is diagnosed in women much more often than in men. Men who exhibit similar behavior patterns are often diagnosed as narcissistic.

5. **Medical–surgical setting**

a. Physicians may find patients charming and fascinating, especially when they are of the opposite sex.

b. Patients often think of illness as a threat to their physical attractiveness. They may view illness as a punishment for their thoughts or feelings, and men may see it as a threat of mutilation.

c. Male patients may behave in an inappropriate sexual manner with female nurses and physicians; the sexual behavior may be a cover for deeper concerns about dependency. These patients learn that they can be taken care of by being sexually attractive, and this behavior is accentuated under the stress of illness. Physicians should approach patients as professionals and remind them that the roles are set. At the same time, it is important to remain noncritical.

6. **Treatment**

a. **Psychotherapy,** either individual or group, is generally the treatment of choice. In general, therapists help patients become aware of the real feelings underneath the histrionic behavior.

b. **Antidepressant medications,** especially MAO inhibitors and SSRIs, have been useful in treating mood disorders associated with this personality type.

V   SPECIFIC CLUSTER C PERSONALITY DISORDERS

A Avoidant personality disorder

1. **Definition.** Although individuals with avoidant personality disorder are timid and shy, they do wish to have friends, unlike schizoid patients. Because they are so uncomfortable and afraid of rejection or criticism, they avoid social contact. In addition, they are self-critical and have low self-esteem. If affected individuals are given strong guarantees of uncritical acceptance, however, they will make friends and participate in social gatherings.

2. **Symptoms.** A pervasive pattern of social inhibition, feelings of inadequacy, and hypersensitivity to negative evaluation that began by early adulthood is indicative. Avoidant personality disorder, which is present in a variety of contexts, is indicated by at least four of the following:

a. **Avoidance of occupational activities that involve significant interpersonal contact** because of fears of criticism, disapproval, or rejection

b. **Unwillingness to become involved with people** unless certain of being liked

c. **Restraint in intimate relationships** because of the fear of being shamed or ridiculed

d. **Preoccupation with worry about being criticized or rejected** in social situations

e. **Inhibition in new interpersonal situations** because of feelings of inadequacy

f. **Belief that they are socially inept, personally unappealing, or inferior** to others

g. **Unusual reluctance to take personal risks** or engage in any new activities because they may prove embarrassing

3. **Associated features.** Social phobias and agoraphobia may be present, but they are also separate disorders that need to be ruled out.

4. **Prevalence.** The prevalence of avoidant personality disorder is believed to be about 0.5% to 1% of the general population.

5. **Medical–surgical setting.** Unlike schizoid patients, avoidant patients may do well in the hospital, where they are undemanding and generally cooperative. Illness can allow them to be taken care of and establish relationships with the staff. However, avoidant patients are sensitive to criticism and may misinterpret equivocal statements as being derogatory or ridiculing and withdraw emotionally.

6. **Treatment**
   a. **Psychotherapy,** either individual or group, can be useful. Patients respond to genuine caring and support.
   b. **Assertiveness training** may provide new social skills.

B **Dependent personality disorder**

1. **Definition.** These passive individuals allow others to direct their lives because they are unable to do so themselves. Other people such as spouses or parents make all the major life decisions, including where to live and what type of employment to obtain.
   a. The **needs of dependent individuals are placed secondary to those of the people on whom they depend** to avoid any possibility of having to be self-reliant. Dependent persons lack self-confidence and see themselves as helpless or stupid.
   b. Some authorities believe that the presence of this disorder depends to a large extent on **cultural roles** (i.e., some groups of people are "expected" to assume dependent roles on the basis of certain criteria such as gender or ethnic background).

2. **Symptoms.** A pervasive and excessive need to be taken care of, which leads to submissiveness, clinging behavior, and fear of separation, is characteristic. This behavior begins by early adulthood and is present in a variety of contexts, as indicated by **at least five** of the following:
   a. **Inability to make everyday decisions** without an excessive amount of advice and reassurance from others
   b. **Need for others to assume responsibility** for most major areas of their life
   c. **Difficulty expressing disagreement** with others because of fear of loss of support or approval (realistic fears of retribution should not be included here)
   d. **Difficulty initiating projects** or doing things on their own (as a result of a lack of self-confidence in judgment or abilities rather than a lack of motivation or energy)
   e. **Go to excessive lengths to obtain nurturance and support** from others, to the point of volunteering to do things that are unpleasant
   f. **Feelings of discomfort or helplessness when alone** because of exaggerated fears of being unable to care for oneself
   g. **Urgent seeking of another relationship** as a source of care and support when a close relationship ends
   h. **Unrealistic preoccupation with fears** of being left to take care of oneself

3. **Associated features.** Children who have had a chronic physical illness or who have had separation anxiety may be at risk for this disorder in adulthood. Depression is common.

4. **Prevalence.** The prevalence is unknown, but passive-dependent traits are common.

5. **Medical–surgical setting**
   a. Being sick usually means being taken care of, and one might expect that dependent individuals would be good patients. However, **illness may provoke intolerable feelings of fear of abandonment and helplessness in these patients.** There is a pull to regress to an earlier state of dependency, which may frighten patients because of its intensity. Feelings of dependency increase. Generally, dependent individuals become demanding and complaining when they are sick.
   b. **Physicians need to set limits.** It is important for physicians, nurses, and other staff to meet with these patients to plan what kind of care is going to be given. For instance, it should be clear to patients how often the nurse will come by to check on them. If this is not done early, the negative reactions that these patients provoke can lead to punitive behavior on the part of the caregivers.

6. **Treatment**
   a. **Psychotherapy** can be very useful in the treatment of dependent patients. The focus is on the current behavior and its consequences. Therapists should be careful when there is a challenge to a pathologic but dependent relationship. Patients may leave therapy rather than give up such a relationship.
   b. Behavioral therapies, including **assertiveness training,** can be helpful.

C **Obsessive-compulsive personality disorder**

1. **Definition.** Affected individuals are perfectionistic, inflexible, and unable to express warm, tender feelings. They are preoccupied with trivial details and rules and do not appreciate changes in routine. **Obsessive-compulsive disorder (OCD)** is an Axis I anxiety disorder that involves irresistible obsessions and compulsions and should be distinguished from obsessive-compulsive personality disorder.

2. **Symptoms.** Individuals with obsessive-compulsive personality disorder display a pervasive pattern of preoccupation with orderliness, perfectionism, and environmental and interpersonal control, at the expense of flexibility, openness, and efficiency. This behavior begins by early adulthood and is present in a variety of contexts, as indicated by at least four of the following:
   a. **Preoccupation with details, rules, lists, order, organization, or schedules** to the extent that the major point of the activity is lost
   b. **Perfectionism that interferes with task completion** (e.g., inability to complete a project because one's own overly strict standards are not met)
   c. **Excessive devotion to work and productivity** to the exclusion of leisure activities and friendships (not accounted for by obvious economic necessity)
   d. **Overconscientiousness, scrupulousness, and inflexibility about matters of morality, ethics, or values** (not accounted for by cultural or religious identification)
   e. **Inability to discard worn-out or worthless objects** even when they have no sentimental value
   f. **Reluctance to delegate tasks or to work with others** unless they submit to exactly their way of doing things
   g. Adoption of a **miserly spending style toward both oneself and others** (money is viewed as something to be hoarded for future catastrophes)
   h. **Rigidity and stubbornness**

3. **Associated features.** People with this disorder have few friends. They are difficult to live with and tend to drive people away. They may do very well in jobs that require detail and precision with little personal interaction. Hypochondriasis may develop later in life.

4. **Prevalence.** This disorder is more common in men and is believed to occur in about 1% of the general population.

5. **Medical–surgical setting**
   a. Illness may be **perceived by compulsive individuals as a threat to their control** over impulses. Generally, stress increases compulsive behavior with an intensification of self-restraint and obstinacy.
      (1) Patients become more inflexible than before, which may lead to complaints about the sloppiness of the hospital and imprecision of the care being given.
      (2) When these patients are critical of failure to meet their standards, physicians should avoid defensive, authoritarian rebuttal. There is a fear of losing control of a situation on the part of these patients, and this may lead to a struggle for control with their physicians.
   b. **Control should be shared with patients in as many ways as possible.** Patients should be allowed to participate actively in the decisions and details of their actual medical care. This may include charting medication times, carefully calculating caloric intake, and monitoring fluid intake and output.

6. **Treatment.** In general, individuals with compulsive personalities recognize that they have problems, unlike those with the other personality disorders. These patients know that they suffer from their inability to be flexible, and they realize that they do not permit themselves to have good feelings.

  a. **Individual psychotherapy** can be helpful, but treatment is difficult because these patients use the defense of isolation of affect. **Group therapy may be more useful.**
  b. Therapy should **focus on current feelings and situations,** and excessive time should not be spent on examining the psychological etiology of the condition. Struggles for control should be avoided. Depression, when present, should be treated.

VI PERSONALITY DISORDERS NOT OTHERWISE SPECIFIED (NOS)

Patients may not always present with all the criteria for a specific personality disorder but still have clinically significant distress or impairment. In other situations, patients may present with symptoms of more than one personality disorder in a cluster. The NOS designation would then be appropriate if criteria were not met for any one disorder. This category also can be used when clinicians decide that a specific personality disorder not included in the *DSM-IV-TR* is appropriate, for example, **passive-aggressive personality disorder** or **depressive personality disorder.**

BIBLIOGRAPHY

American Psychiatric Association: *Diagnostic and Statistical Manual of Mental Disorders,* 4th ed., text revision. Washington, DC, American Psychiatric Association, 2000.

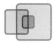

Study Questions

Directions: *Each of the numbered items in this section is followed by possible answers. Select the ONE numbered answer that is BEST in each case.*

QUESTIONS 1–3

A 28-year-old law student is admitted to the hospital for gallbladder problems. He is stubborn and rigid and expects staff to adhere to his exact ways of doing things. He refuses to stop working on school papers. He reports that his girlfriend has threatened to leave him unless he changes his inflexible ways and throws out some of a large collection of useless junk.

1. Which personality disorder diagnosis appears most appropriate?
   - [A] Antisocial
   - [B] Avoidant
   - [C] Histrionic
   - [D] Obsessive-compulsive
   - [E] Schizotypal

2. You expect the patient may act out in which of the following fashions when under stress in the hospital?
   - [A] Strange behavior may put off caregivers
   - [B] Sees hospitalization as a threat to his control
   - [C] Can be charming but in a manipulative fashion; resists rules
   - [D] Uses splitting, possibly dividing the staff, who might take sides
   - [E] Likely to be cooperative and do well with the attention

3. You might recommend which of the following interventions to the staff regarding the patient?
   - [A] Set firm limits; consider an antidepressant.
   - [B] Set firm limits on patient and staff roles; remain noncritical.
   - [C] Odd behavior may make staff uneasy, but avoid ridicule.
   - [D] Similar patients generally do well, but avoid criticism.
   - [E] Share control with the patient in as many ways as possible.

QUESTIONS 4–7

You are called to the emergency room (ER) to see a 24-year-old woman who is waiting for stitches for a wrist laceration. She has been seen in the ER seven times previously for self-inflicted wrist lacerations. She reports rapid mood swings, impulsivity, a chronic feeling of emptiness, and periods in which she feels paranoid when under stress.

4. Which personality disorder diagnosis appears most appropriate?
   - [A] Antisocial
   - [B] Borderline
   - [C] Obsessive-compulsive
   - [D] Paranoid
   - [E] Schizoid

5. You expect that this patient may act out in which fashion when under stress in the hospital?
   - [A] Strange behavior may put off caregivers
   - [B] Can be charming but in a manipulative fashion
   - [C] Likely to be charming and fascinating; sense of attractiveness may be threatened by illness

D Uses splitting, possibly dividing the staff, who might take sides
E Likely to be cooperative and do well with the attention

6. For this patient, you might recommend which of the following interventions to the staff?
   A Be straightforward, explain everything, and expect distrust.
   B Odd behavior may make staff uneasy, but avoid ridicule.
   C Set firm limits and consider an antidepressant.
   D Similar patients generally do well, but avoid criticism.
   E Share control with the patient in as many ways as possible.

7. Which of the following medications has been useful in decreasing self-injury in patients with a similar diagnosis?
   A Alprazolam *abuse potential*
   B Diazepam
   C Diphenhydramine
   D Fluoxetine *stimulants CI*
   E Methylphenidate

QUESTIONS 8–9

A 35-year-old man presents requesting psychotherapy for problems with reacting angrily to his coworkers. The patient reports persistent fear that he will lose his job "due to a system that has it out for me." He reports distrust of others and a "look out for number one" philosophy.

8. Which personality disorder diagnosis appears most appropriate?
   A Antisocial
   B Avoidant
   C Narcissistic
   D Obsessive-compulsive
   E Paranoid

9. You might recommend which form of treatment for this patient? *Psychotherapy > Pharmacotherapy*
   A Start a monoamine oxidase (MAO) inhibitor antidepressant to reduce impulsivity.
   B Refer him straight to group therapy.
   C Start an antipsychotic and plan to explain treatment for side effects only if they occur.
   D Cautiously begin individual psychotherapy.
   E Tell the patient there is no hope for treatment and you will not take his money.

QUESTIONS 10–12

A 35-year-old single man is admitted to the hospital for deep vein thrombosis. He has been inappropriately provocative and seductive toward the female staff. Dramatic and suggestive, he appears obsessed with his attractiveness. He exaggerates his familiarity with some staff members and displays shallow, shifting emotions.

10. Which personality disorder diagnosis appears most appropriate?
    A Antisocial
    B Avoidant
    C Histrionic
    D Obsessive-compulsive
    E Paranoid

11. You expect this patient may act out in which fashion when under stress in the hospital?

[A] Aloof; may want to leave against medical advice
[B] Will likely be charming and fascinating; his sense of attractiveness may be threatened by illness
[C] Very guarded, suspicious, and quarrelsome
[D] Will use splitting, possibly dividing the staff, who might take sides
[E] Will see hospitalization as a threat to his control

12. For this patient, you might recommend which of the following interventions to the staff?

[A] Be straightforward, explain everything, and expect distrust.
[B] Set firm limits and consider an antidepressant.
[C] Similar patients generally do well, but avoid criticism.
[D] Share control with the patient in as many ways as possible.
[E] Set firm limits on patient and staff roles; remain noncritical.

QUESTIONS 13–16

A 19-year-old man with a 7-year history of legal charges is admitted for treatment of phlebitis secondary to intravenous drug abuse. On the ward, he was initially quite charming to the staff but became irritable and aggressive when denied requests for more pain medication. He is demanding to be discharged. When changing his bed, staff found syringes and needles he had taken from the drug cart when a nurse was tending to another patient. When the nurse was reprimanded by her supervisor, the patient showed no remorse for the consequences of his action.

13. Which personality disorder diagnosis appears most appropriate?

[A] Antisocial
[B] Narcissistic
[C] Paranoid
[D] Schizoid
[E] Schizotypal

14. You expect this patient may act out in which of the following fashions when under stress in the hospital?

[A] Aloof; may want to leave against medical advice
[B] Strange behavior may put off caregivers
[C] Will likely be charming and fascinating; his sense of attractiveness may be threatened by illness
[D] Might suffer feelings of abandonment and helplessness
[E] Can be charming but in a manipulative fashion; resists rules — Ted Bundy

15. You might recommend which of the following interventions to the staff for the patient?

[A] Set firm limits and consider an antidepressant.
[B] Odd behavior may make staff uneasy, but avoid ridicule.
[C] Set firm limits; anticipate a demand for discharge against medical advice.
[D] Be straightforward, explain everything, and expect distrust.
[E] Share control with patient in as many ways as possible.

16. You would recommend which of the following courses of treatment for this patient after discharge?

[A] Treatment with benzodiazepines to reduce anxiety
[B] Individual therapy focusing on building a strong patient–therapist relationship
[C] Tell the patient there is no hope for treatment and you will not take his money
[D] Group therapy with a particular therapist and patients
[E] Volunteer work in a pain clinic to help develop more empathy

Answers and Explanations

1. The answer is D [*V C 2*]. Some diagnostic criteria for obsessive-compulsive personality disorder include preoccupation with details, perfectionism interfering with task completion, excessive devotion to work, scrupulousness, inability to discard collected belongings, reluctance to delegate, miserly spending style, rigidity, and stubbornness.

2. The answer is B [*V C 5*]. In the medical–surgical setting, persons with obsessive-compulsive personality disorder may become even more inflexible because the illness is perceived as a threat to their need for control.

3. The answer is E [*V C 5*]. In the medical treatment of persons with obsessive-compulsive personality disorder, sharing control with the patient may obviate the perceived threat to their need for control.

4. The answer is B [*IV B 2*]. Some diagnostic criteria for borderline personality disorder include impulsivity, recurrent suicidal or self-mutilating behavior, rapid mood swings, chronic feelings of emptiness, and possible paranoia when under stress.

5. The answer is D [*IV B 5 b*]. In the medical–surgical setting, persons with borderline personality disorder may use splitting as a defensive mechanism, sometimes resulting in dividing the staff, who might take sides.

6. The answer is C [*IV B 6*]. In the treatment of patients with borderline personality disorder, setting firm limits and providing structure can be therapeutic. Antidepressants can help some patients control impulsivity and self-injury while supporting mood.

7. The answer is D [*IV B 6 b (1)*]. Modern drugs such as fluoxetine and other serotonergic antidepressants have shown some efficacy in reducing behavioral impulsivity and self-injury in borderline patients. Benzodiazepines such as alprazolam and diazepam should be avoided because they may cause disinhibition or be abused. Antihistamines such as diphenhydramine are sometimes used for sedation but do not effect self-injury. Stimulants are contraindicated unless the patient has another condition for which stimulants would be appropriate.

8. The answer is E [*III B 2*]. Some diagnostic criteria for paranoid personality disorder include suspicion of being exploited or deceived, doubts about the loyalty of others, reluctance to confide in others, perceiving threats or attacks in benign remarks and actions, and angry reactions to perceived threats.

9. The answer is D [*III B 5*]. Patients with paranoid personality disorder may respond to treatment, but psychotherapy is preferred to pharmacotherapy. Low doses of antipsychotic medication can help at times, but side effects could be perceived as a threat. Individual psychotherapy is a better choice than referral straight to group therapy.

10. The answer is C [*IV D 2*]. Some diagnostic criteria for histrionic personality disorder include a need to be the center of attention, inappropriate seductive or provocative behavior, obsession with physical attractiveness, dramatic behavior and impressionistic speech, suggestibility, and exaggeration of the importance of relationships.

11. The answer is B [*IV D 5 a, b*]. In the medical–surgical setting, persons with histrionic personality disorder may give the impression of being charming and fascinating. The patient's dependence on his sense of attractiveness may be threatened by illness.

12. The answer is E [*IV D 5 c*]. In the treatment of persons with histrionic personality disorder, setting firm limits on patient and staff roles is critical. At the same time, staff should try to remain noncritical of behavior symptomatic of the disorder.

13. **The answer is A** [*IV A 2*]. Some diagnostic criteria for antisocial personality disorder include evidence of conduct disorder with onset before age 15 years, a pattern of disregard for or violation of the rights of others, irritable and aggressive behavior, deceitfulness, recklessness, and lack of remorse.

14. **The answer is E** [*IV A 5 a, b*]. In the medical–surgical setting, persons with antisocial personality disorder may give the impression of being quite charming but in a manipulative fashion. They may resist hospital rules and be noncompliant, and when challenged, they may leave treatment against medical advice.

15. **The answer is C** [*IV A 6 a*]. In the treatment of persons with antisocial personality disorder, setting firm limits is important but often triggers a demand to leave treatment against medical advice.

16. **The answer is D** [*IV A 6 b*]. Antisocial personality disorder can respond to treatment. Group psychotherapy can be effective, but an experienced therapist and a particular group of patients are needed. Controlled substances may be abused by some persons with antisocial personality disorder.

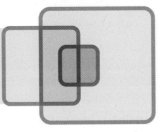

chapter 8

Somatoform and Dissociative Disorders

HARVEY L. CAUSEY III

I DEFINITIONS

A **Somatoform disorders** are a heterogeneous group characterized by symptoms suggestive of physical illness or injury, not explained by a general medical condition, or disproportionate to the symptoms expected from a general medical condition. To establish a somatoform disorder diagnosis, the clinician must take care to rule out physical illnesses or conditions, the effects of substance use, or other psychiatric disorders that might better explain the symptoms (e.g., a patient with major depressive illness who has a delusion of having a fatal cancer). The condition must cause clinically significant distress or be of sufficient severity to impair social, occupational, or other important areas of functioning. Presentations of symptoms where a somatoform diagnosis is considered can be broadly characterized as follows:

1. **Subjective symptoms unexplained by physical findings** (e.g., conversion disorder)

2. **Unusual attention to and/or preoccupation with symptoms, organs, and body parts** (e.g., body dysmorphic disorder)

3. **Psychological symptoms exacerbating a general medical condition.** General medical conditions exacerbated by psychological factors (such as stress) include some cardiovascular disorders, irritable bowel syndrome, psoriasis, and many other medical conditions.

4. **Psychiatric disorders presenting with primarily physical symptoms or presenting physical symptoms as an unusual/atypical form of the disorder.** This includes unusual presentations of familiar psychiatric disorders (e.g., a patient with depression who presents with headaches or malaise; a patient with panic disorder who presents with symptoms of a myocardial infarction).

5. **Psychiatric symptoms caused or exacerbated by a general medical condition.** Common examples include hypothyroidism mimicking depressive disorders, toxic delirium mimicking psychotic disorders, and paroxysmal atrial tachycardia resembling panic disorder.

6. **Physical symptoms incorrectly reported or created by patients for the purpose of gaining a specific benefit** (e.g., factitious disorder or malingering)

7. **Symptoms of a primarily medical nature mistaken for psychiatric conditions.** This mistake may lead to delayed or inappropriate treatment. Therefore, clinicians should note the formal diagnostic criteria for somatoform disorders to avoid this serious and costly mistake.

B **Factitious disorders** are characterized by the conscious fabrication of physical or psychological symptoms (e.g., a man putting blood from a fingerstick into his urine sample and complaining of flank pain) in order to assume the sick role. **See VII.**

C **Dissociative disorders** are characterized by disruption in the integration of consciousness, memory, identity, or perception. The disturbance may be sudden or gradual, transient or chronic. **See VI.**

II DIAGNOSIS

A Somatization disorder

1. **History.** Patients have **recurring, multiple physical complaints** beginning before age 30, occurring over several years, and resulting in treatment being sought, or significant impairment in social, occupational, or other important areas of functioning.

2. **Symptoms.** Each of the following criteria must be met, with individual symptoms occurring at any time during the course of the disturbance. The **symptoms are not intentionally produced or feigned** (e.g., as in factitious disorder or malingering).

   a. **Four pain symptoms.** History of pain related to at least four different locations (e.g., head, abdomen, back, joints, extremities, chest, rectum) or functions (e.g., menstruation, sexual intercourse, urination)

   b. **Two gastrointestinal symptoms.** History of at least two gastrointestinal symptoms other than pain (e.g., nausea, bloating, vomiting except during pregnancy, diarrhea, intolerance of several different foods)

   c. **One sexual symptom.** History of at least one sexual or reproductive symptom other than pain (e.g., sexual indifference, erectile or ejaculatory dysfunction, irregular menses, excessive menstrual bleeding, vomiting throughout pregnancy)

   d. **One pseudoneurologic symptom.** History of at least one symptom or deficit suggesting a neurologic condition not limited to pain such as conversion symptoms (e.g., impaired coordination or balance, paralysis or localized weakness, difficulty swallowing or lump in throat, aphonia, urinary retention, hallucinations, loss of touch or pain sensation, double vision, blindness, deafness, seizures) or dissociative symptoms (e.g., amnesia or loss of consciousness other than fainting)

3. **Other criteria.** Patients **have either of the following conditions:**

   a. After appropriate investigation, each of the symptoms described in II A 2 cannot be fully explained by a known general medical condition or the direct effects of a substance (e.g., a drug of abuse, a medication).

   b. If a related general medical condition is present, the physical complaints or resulting social or occupational impairment exceeds what would be expected from the history, physical examination, or laboratory findings.

B Undifferentiated somatoform disorder

1. Occurrence of one or more physical complaints (e.g., fatigue, loss of appetite, gastrointestinal or urinary problems)

2. **Occurrence of either of the following conditions:**

   a. After appropriate investigation, the **symptoms cannot be fully explained by a known general medical condition or the direct effects of a substance** (e.g., a drug of abuse, a medication).

   b. **If there is a related general medical condition,** the physical complaints or resulting social or occupational impairment **exceeds what would be expected** from the history, physical examination, or laboratory findings.

3. The **symptoms cause clinically significant distress or impairment** in social, occupational, or other important areas of functioning.

4. The **duration of the disturbance is at least 6 months.**

5. The **disturbance is not better explained by another mental disorder** (e.g., another somatoform disorder, sexual dysfunction, mood disorder, anxiety disorder, sleep disorder, psychotic disorder).

6. The **symptom is not intentionally produced** or feigned (e.g., as in factitious disorder or malingering).

C Conversion disorder

1. One or more symptoms **or deficits affecting voluntary motor or sensory function** suggest a neurologic or other general medical condition.

2. **Psychological factors are judged to be associated with the symptom or deficit** because the initiation or exacerbation of the symptom or deficit is preceded by conflicts or other stressors.

3. The symptom or deficit is not intentionally produced or feigned (e.g., factitious disorder and malingering).

4. The symptom or deficit cannot, after appropriate investigation, be fully explained by a general medical condition, by the direct effects of a substance, or as a culturally sanctioned behavior or experience.

5. The symptom or deficit causes clinically significant distress or impairment in social, occupational, or other important areas of functioning or warrants medical evaluation.

6. The symptoms or deficit is not limited to pain or sexual dysfunction, does not occur exclusively during the course of somatization disorder, and is not better accounted for by another mental disorder.

7. The *Diagnostic and Statistical Manual of Mental Disorders,* 4th edition, text revision (*DSM-IV-TR*), requires specification of the subtype of conversion disorder:
   a. **With motor symptoms or deficits** (e.g., impaired coordination or balance, paralysis or localized weakness, difficulty swallowing or "lump in throat," aphonia, urinary retention)
   b. **With sensory symptoms or deficits** (e.g., loss of touch or pain sensation, double vision, blindness, deafness, hallucinations)
   c. **With seizures or convulsions** (includes seizures or convulsions with voluntary motor or sensory components)
   d. **With mixed presentation** (symptoms are evident in more than one category)

D **Pain disorder**

1. Pain disorder is characterized by **pain in one or more anatomic sites** of sufficient severity to warrant clinical attention.

2. The pain causes **significant distress or impairment** in social, occupational, or other important areas of functioning.

3. **Psychological factors are judged to have an important role** in the onset, severity, exacerbation, or maintenance of the pain.

4. The symptoms or deficit is not intentionally produced or feigned (e.g., as in factitious disorder and malingering).

5. The pain is not better explained by a mood, anxiety, or psychotic disorder and does not meet criteria for dyspareunia.

6. **Subtypes** are defined as follows:
   a. **Pain disorder associated with psychological factors.** Psychological factors are judged to play a major role in the onset, severity, exacerbation, or maintenance of the pain. If a general medical condition is present, it does not play a major role in the onset, severity, exacerbation, or maintenance of the pain. This disorder is not diagnosed if criteria for somatization disorder are met. **Acute** or **chronic** duration should be specified.
   b. **Pain disorder associated with both psychological factors and a general medical condition.** Both psychological factors and a general medical condition are judged to have important roles in the onset, severity, exacerbation, or maintenance of the pain.
   c. **Pain disorder associated with a general medical condition.** A general medical condition has a major role in the onset, severity, exacerbation, or maintenance of the pain. This category is for medical conditions and for conditions in which the relationship between anatomic and psychological factors is not clearly established (e.g., low back pain). This subtype is *not* a mental disorder and is **coded on Axis III.**

E **Hypochondriasis**

1. Hypochondriasis is characterized by preoccupation with **fears of having (or the idea that one has) a serious disease due to a misinterpretation of bodily symptoms.**

2. The preoccupation persists despite appropriate medical evaluation and reassurance.

3. The belief in the serious disease is not of delusional intensity (e.g., as in delusional disorder, somatic type) and is not restricted to a circumscribed concern about appearance (e.g., as in body dysmorphic disorder).

4. The preoccupation causes clinically significant distress or impairment in social, occupational, or other important areas of functioning.

5. The duration of the disturbance is at least 6 months.

6. The preoccupation is not better explained by generalized anxiety disorder, obsessive-compulsive disorder (OCD), panic disorder, a major depressive episode (MDE), separation anxiety, or another somatoform disorder.

F Body dysmorphic disorder

1. Body dysmorphic disorder is a **preoccupation with an imagined defect in appearance,** or an excessive concern with a slight physical flaw.

2. The preoccupation causes clinically significant distress or impairment in social, occupational, or other important areas of functioning.

3. The preoccupation is not better explained by another mental disorder (e.g., dissatisfaction with body shape and size, as in anorexia nervosa).

G Somatoform disorder not otherwise specified   This category includes disorders with somatoform symptoms that do not meet the criteria for any specific somatoform disorder. Examples include:

1. **Pseudocyesis.** This false belief of being pregnant is associated with objective signs of pregnancy, which may include abdominal enlargement (although the umbilicus does not become everted), reduced menstrual flow, amenorrhea, subjective sensation of fetal movement, nausea, breast engorgement and secretions, and labor pains at the expected date of delivery. This condition cannot be explained by a general medical condition such as a hormone-secreting tumor.

2. A disorder involving nonpsychotic hypochondriacal symptoms of less than 6 months' duration

3. A disorder involving unexplained physical complaints that are of less than 6 months' duration and are not caused by another mental disorder

III ETIOLOGIC THEORIES

A Specificity theory   The theory of emotional specificity (i.e., the physiologic expression of blocked emotions) has led to personality studies of patients with peptic ulcers, coronary artery disease, and cancer. Although these studies have lent some support to the theory, it has generally lost favor as a comprehensive explanation.

1. **Sigmund Freud** and his followers studied somatic involvement in psychological conflict and were particularly interested in **conversion reactions,** in which a psychological problem is symbolically manifested physically, although physiologic tissue damage cannot be demonstrated.

2. **Flanders Dunbar** suggested that **specific conscious personality traits** cause specific psychosomatic diseases.

3. **Franz Alexander** theorized that **specific unconscious conflicts** cause specific illnesses in organs innervated by the autonomic nervous system. These illnesses occur because prolonged tension can produce physiologic disorders, leading to eventual pathology. Alexander also believed that constitutional predisposing factors are involved. His theory led to the concept of the **classic psychosomatic diseases,** including:
   a. Bronchial asthma
   b. Rheumatoid arthritis
   c. Ulcerative colitis
   d. Essential hypertension
   e. Neurodermatitis
   f. Thyrotoxicosis
   g. Peptic ulcers

B Stress response theories   Whatever event is perceived by patients as stressful can produce stress, whether it is the death of a loved one, divorce, financial loss, or illness. In each culture, different events may carry different "weights" as stressors. Within a culture, however, stressful life events can be assessed quantitatively for their risk of producing psychophysiologic illnesses in a large group of people. Psychological reactions to stress can alter neuroendocrine, immune, cardiovascular, and other physiologic parameters that can lead to a **nonspecific cause of disease.**

1. **Neurophysiologic reactions to stress** activate the pituitary–adrenal axis and are known as the **general adaptation syndrome.** The nonspecific systemic reactions of the body to stress include:
   a. **Alarm reaction** (shock)
   b. **Resistance** (adaptation to stress)
   c. **Exhaustion** (resistance to prolonged stress, which cannot be maintained)
2. **Physiologic reactions to stress** include the following:
   a. **Fight-or-flight response.** Arousal of the sympathetic nervous system results in increased production of epinephrine and norepinephrine (NE), with an increase in pulse and muscle tension. When an affected individual can neither fight nor flee, this state of arousal can lead to organic dysfunction.
   b. **Withdrawal and conservation.** George Engel and coworkers have shown that when an individual is threatened with loss (real or imagined), the metabolism can slow down. The individual withdraws, and this action conserves energy.
      (1) Pulse and body temperature decrease.
      (2) The individual may become susceptible to illness, particularly infection. Studies on the psychophysiologic effects of bereavement support the following hypothesis: morbidity and mortality rates are higher during the first year after death of a spouse in a bereaved group compared with those rates in an age-controlled, nonbereaved group. Elderly people removed from their homes and placed in nursing homes have an increased risk of death from cardiovascular causes.

C **Biopsychosocial model**   This model, proposed by George Engel, offers the interaction of biologic, psychological, and social events as the means for understanding the etiology, pathologic process, and treatment for psychiatric disorders as well as psychophysiologic conditions. This model is reciprocal rather than linear. In other words, a biologic event can alter psychological perceptions and cognitions set. These changes, in turn, can alter social behaviors. The social environment responds by treating the individual differently, and the response to that different treatment is an alteration in physiology.

1. **Biologic factors** reflect the physiologic, neurophysiologic, and pathophysiologic functioning of the individual.
   a. **Hereditary and congenital factors** include inherited risks for psychiatric disorders (e.g., affective and anxiety disorders), physiologic vulnerabilities (e.g., risks for heart disease or some cancers), and defects (e.g., malformations, biochemical abnormalities, differences in pain threshold).
   b. **Physical disease processes** can affect the functioning of the brain and other physiologic processes.
   c. **Environmental factors** (e.g., exposure to toxic substances, medications being prescribed, substances of abuse, amount of daylight, alterations of circadian rhythms related to a job) can affect the physiology of the brain and body.
   d. **Normal physiologic responses** to environmental events may place the individual at risk for a variety of additional physical and psychological events.
      (1) **Immune system compromise,** which is reflected in the increased risk of death after significant losses from causes such as infectious illnesses and some neoplasms
      (2) **Cardiovascular responses to stress,** which include hypertension and increased heart rate (which may unmask some arrhythmias)
      (3) **Neuroendocrine systems,** which are altered by environmental stressors, major mental illnesses, and many of the medications used to treat mental illnesses. Many of these abnormalities may reflect changes in hypothalamic–pituitary functioning modulated in the brain. Major systems involved include the following:
         (a) **Cortisol** is altered in relation to stress, anxiety, and depression.

(b) Prolactin is altered in a variety of psychiatric disorders as well as in normal stress responses. Interestingly, prolactin also may modulate T-lymphocyte function.

(c) Thyroid function is variably altered in major mental illnesses, particularly depression. Thyrotropin-releasing hormone (TRH) has been the focus of recent study, as has depression in mildly hypothyroid people.

(d) Other hormones such as growth hormone have been studied in relation to psychiatric disorders. Their role in stress response is less clear than the role of those factors just listed.

(4) **Neurohumoral factors** are reported to be altered in major mental illness and stress response. β-Endorphin and dynorphin abnormalities are associated with anxiety-related disorders. Somatostatin, corticotropin-releasing hormone, and TRH also appear to be altered with stress, as do dopamine, γ-aminobutyric acid (GABA), NE, and serotonin. These neurohumoral factors may be an intermediary mechanism by which stressful events are translated into longer-term alterations in brain function. However, any primary role for this function remains unclear.

2. **Psychological factors**

a. **Perception of pain or physiologic events** is the conscious registering of a stimulus or event. Perception of physical events has been shown to be altered by a number of factors such as a state of arousal, individual differences in threshold, mood, other stimuli, and physiologic events.

b. **Attention to the pain or physiologic event** is perhaps the best example of the conscious effect of the physical event on the person. For example, a patient with chronic pain notices the pain very frequently despite efforts to ignore it.

c. The **meaning or context of the symptom** determines how much attention it gets. For example, the literature contains many reports of broken legs and war wounds that go unnoticed by the injured person. In contrast, a patient who believes that a change in a physical symptom is the sign of a worsening or fatal illness pays a great deal of attention to the symptom.

d. **Primary gain from a physical symptom** is the abatement of a psychological symptom that results from the attention demanded by the physical symptom. For example, a broken leg takes attention away from worries about a relationship and may even be more "comfortable."

3. **Social factors** help determine the meaning of the physical symptom or pain and may serve to extinguish or perpetuate attention to the symptom. Some social factors that determine how a physical symptom is perceived are considered in the following discussion.

a. The **sick role** is defined by the culture, the family group, and the beliefs of the individual. The sick role can be understood as the expected behavior of the person as a result of illness. In some cultures, the sick role is very limited; a person, when sick, is allowed only to lie down and stop eating. In other cultures, the sick role may be highly elaborated on the basis of the type of sickness, chronicity, and supposed role of the individual in bringing on the illness. Some positive and negative aspects of the sick role include the following:

(1) **Secondary gain** results from the social benefits of the sick role. Individuals may be able to avoid work, gain financial rewards, avoid conflict, and gain sympathy.

(2) The sick role of some **"socially stigmatized" illnesses** such as HIV, mental illness, and epilepsy may preclude persons from working, finding housing, or enjoying social relationships, all of which are independent of concrete evidence contradicting the need for social isolation (e.g., actual contagiousness of HIV, low evidence of dangerousness).

(3) Some sick roles may create disability independent of or disproportionate to the disability associated with the illness. For example, in mental hospitals and tuberculosis sanitariums, **institutionalism** produced adaptation to the hospital culture, which was often more socially disabling than the condition itself.

b. **Interpersonal relationships are often altered by illness.**

(1) A family member (often a child) may be placed in the sick role to help the family avoid other major issues (e.g., substance abuse by a parent).

(2) Acutely, the sick role normally elicits caring responses from others. As the sick role becomes more chronic, it elicits increasing anger and rejection from others (including from unsophisticated physicians and caregivers).

(3) Development of socially stigmatized illnesses may elicit acute rejection from the social network (e.g., HIV, mental illness).

(4) Illness and the sick role may upset the power dynamics in a relationship. Individuals may seek to reestablish the power dynamics by precipitating another crisis.

(5) Communication between ill persons and others may become increasingly centered on the illness, creating a cycle in which exacerbation of symptoms becomes the mechanism for eliciting a response from others.

(6) Family communication style involving high levels of **expressed emotionality** is associated with many psychophysiologic disorders, as well as major mental illnesses (see Chapter 2: III C 2 c).

c. Health-related behaviors

(1) Social, educational, and psychological factors may contribute to the tendency of individuals to avoid or engage in behaviors that increase their risk of disease or injury (e.g., unprotected sex and HIV risk, smoking, substance abuse, motorcycle riding).

(2) Little is known about psychiatric comorbidity of many of these high-risk behaviors.

(3) Public health approaches to the reduction of high-risk behaviors have been largely educational and, in many cases, have been less effective than expected.

(4) Relatively little work has been done on altering lifestyle to reduce health risk using means other than education and substance abuse treatment.

IV COMORBIDITY AND DIFFERENTIAL DIAGNOSIS

Although somatoform disorders are presented as discrete diagnostic entities, in reality, there is a high degree of phenomenologic overlap between these disorders and other physical and psychological disorders. Furthermore, in contrast to other groups of psychiatric disorders such as schizophrenia and major affective disorders, relatively little phenomenologic and diagnostic work has been done. However, the costs of these patients to the health care system in excessive disability, needless diagnostic tests, and poorly justified surgery are enormous. Patients in this group usually have complex diagnostic and treatment pictures. Some of the diagnostic blurring in the *DSM-IV-TR* is intentional: it helps clinicians avoid dichotomous thinking about patients (e.g., "The patient has somatization disorder; now I can make a psychiatric referral and stop looking for physical disease.")

A Major illnesses with psychological factors

1. Gastrointestinal disorders. Emotional states have long been known to cause a reaction in the gastrointestinal tract. Vague complaints of nausea, indigestion, diarrhea, constipation, and abdominal pain are common in association with psychiatric disorders.

a. Peptic ulcers

(1) Etiology. Gastric, duodenal, and acute posttraumatic stress ulcers all have different etiologies. The Mirsky study of U.S. Army recruits showed that several factors are necessary for the development of ulcers, including high stress, high pepsinogen secretion, and psychological conflict (dependency). Although conflicts involving dependency are noticeable in some ulcer patients, not all individuals affected by these conflicts are prone to developing ulcers, nor are all ulcer patients psychologically distressed.

(2) Treatment. Patients who comply with good medical management do not usually require psychotherapy. Physicians should help patients identify the areas of their lives that seem to cause stress. Also, it may be useful to teach patients relaxation techniques in which the patient tenses all muscles, relaxes them in groups (e.g., arms, hands, legs, feet), and then notes the resultant feeling. Hypnotic techniques may also offer good relaxation for some patients. Antianxiety agents are occasionally indicated, as are antispasmodics.

b. Ulcerative colitis

(1) Etiology. A large proportion of cases of ulcerative colitis have a familial occurrence, which suggests a genetic cause. However, the exact etiology is unknown. It has been demonstrated that exacerbation of ulcerative colitis is associated with psychological stress and remission is associated with psychological support. Stress such as unresolved grief on the anniversary of a death can precipitate episodes of the disorder. Associated psychological features include:

(a) Immaturity

(b) Indecisiveness

(c) Conscientiousness

(d) Covertly demanding behavior

(e) Fear of loss of an important individual

(2) **Treatment.** Although psychotherapy cannot guarantee that the condition will not recur, it is useful when it focuses on helping patients develop mature ways of expressing needs, as well as helping them deal with unresolved losses.

c. **Irritable bowel syndrome** (also termed spastic colon and nervous diarrhea) is disordered bowel motility, including both hypermotility and hypomotility.

(1) **Etiology.** Although the syndrome is usually associated with environmental stress, patients tend to have other psychological symptoms such as anxiety and depression.

(2) **Treatment.** Brief psychotherapy to help patients identify environmental stress and effect changes usually aids in decreasing symptoms. Tricyclic antidepressants are also effective.

2. **Cardiovascular disorders.** Much evidence suggests that the cardiovascular system reacts to a patient's emotional state.

a. **Coronary artery disease** is the most common cause of death in the United States.

(1) **Etiology.** Multiple nonpsychiatric elements are implicated in the development of coronary artery disease, including genetics, diet, smoking, high blood pressure, obesity, and amount of physical activity. A personality type has also been implicated, according to some studies. The **type A behavior pattern** is only one risk factor out of many, and its exact role in the development of coronary artery disease is unclear. However, men who fall into this type of behavior pattern are at twice the risk for coronary artery disease as those who do not. Characteristics of the type A personality include:

(a) Competitiveness

(b) Ambition

(c) Drive for success

(d) Impatience

(e) A sense of time urgency

(f) Abruptness of speech and gesture

(g) Hostility

(2) **Treatment.** Behavioral methods designed to decrease environmental stress and modify lifestyle when mutable are increasingly common.

b. **Essential hypertension**

(1) **Etiology.** Causes are unknown, but psychological factors were initially thought to involve conflicts between passive-dependent and aggressive tendencies in patients who repressed their hostility. Unfortunately, no reliable evidence is available to support this theory. On the other hand, a common reaction to stress is elevation of blood pressure. Patients who have a biologic susceptibility to essential hypertension may react to stressful situations by exacerbating that hypertension rather than, for example, increasing gastrointestinal motility.

(2) **Treatment.** Therapy for hypertension may involve biofeedback, in which a patient is attached to a machine that provides information about ordinarily unnoticed biologic parameters. For example, a tone sounds when the patient's blood pressure rises. The patient then learns to relax to decrease the tone as well as the blood pressure. Biofeedback therapy, however, tends not to be long lasting and must be repeated to maintain the effect. Many antihypertensive agents have psychiatric effects, particularly that of producing depression. When treating depressed patients, care should be taken to avoid administering antihypertensive agents that cause depression.

c. **Arrhythmias**

(1) **Etiology.** Even in the absence of heart disease, psychological factors can influence the normal rhythm of the heartbeat. **Stress** may cause arrhythmias by arousing the sympathetic nervous system (as is evident in the fight-or-flight reaction). Sinus tachycardia,

paroxysmal atrial tachycardia, and ventricular ectopic beats are the most common arrhythmias to arise in reaction to stress. These reactions may be more common in patients who are already fearful of heart disease.

    (2) Treatment. Therapy involves questioning patients about unreasonable fears of heart disease and helping patients identify environmental stresses that precipitate the reaction. The condition may be part of either an anxiety disorder or a depression, which should be treated. Benzodiazepines may be useful for a limited time, as may β-blocking agents (e.g., propranolol). Contrary to a common belief among some physicians, effective treatment of depression with careful use of antidepressant medications (some of which have specific antiarrhythmic properties) may be safer than avoiding treatment for depressed patients with cardiac disease.

3. Respiratory disorders. Changes in respiration in normal individuals may correspond to an emotional state (e.g., the sigh of boredom, the gasp of surprise). The strongest psychological reactions associated with respiratory disease, however, are those that develop secondary to the illness. The panic associated with shortness of breath can be quite disabling.

  a. Hyperventilation syndrome

    (1) Etiology. This disorder is often associated with **anxiety,** particularly panic disorder (see Chapter 4: I B 1 a), which may cause an increased depth or rate of breathing. In turn, this response leads to **respiratory alkalosis** and then to lightheadedness, paresthesias, and carpopedal spasms. These symptoms increase the patient's anxiety, resulting in a vicious circle of increased hyperventilation and respiratory alkalosis. Hyperventilation may occur with the typical symptoms of shortness of breath; numbness of the fingers, nose, and lips; and lightheadedness.

    (2) Treatment. Educating patients about the syndrome after the acute event is past may be sufficient. However, if underlying anxieties continue to provoke the syndrome, psychotherapy is indicated. If patients satisfy the criteria for panic disorder, pharmacotherapy should be considered as well.

  b. Bronchial asthma

    (1) Etiology. Once thought to be caused by psychological factors, asthma attacks now are believed to be the result of a genetic vulnerability exacerbated by allergies and infections. Nevertheless, stress and an inconsistent relationship between an asthmatic child and an overly protective mother may be factors in the onset of specific episodes of illness. Overly dependent patients who react to any slight changes of symptoms and overly independent patients who deny symptoms are both at greater risk for hospitalization than are psychologically normal patients.

    (2) Treatment. Psychotherapy is usually indicated when anxiety, which may precipitate an asthma attack, is not relieved by the supportive care of a physician. Family therapy may be helpful in separation issues, which may also exacerbate asthma symptoms.

4. Migraine headache

  a. Etiology. More than 90% of chronic, recurrent headaches are migraine, tension, or mixed migraine–tension. Whereas muscle tension headaches (often with bilateral occipital or bitemporal distribution) represent muscle spasms, migraine headaches are usually unilateral and represent a period of vasoconstriction (aura) followed by vasodilatation (headache). Although anxiety and stress commonly precipitate all three types of headache, the theory that specific psychological dynamics (e.g., repressed hostility) lead to migraine headaches has not been proved. Many true migraine patients report development of headaches during a period of relaxation after a stressful period. Depression should be ruled out as a cause but treated if present.

  b. Treatment

    (1) Drug therapy

      (a) Serotonin receptor agonists (sumatriptan)

      (b) Ergot derivatives and combinations (ergotamine)

      (c) β-Adrenergic blocking agents (propranolol)

      (d) Tricyclic antidepressants

      (e) Divalproex sodium

      (f) Calcium channel blockers (e.g., verapamil)

(2) **Biofeedback**

(3) **Psychotherapy** in patients with chronic stress

(4) **Hypnosis** and **imagery** to increase peripheral blood flow (e.g., imagining that hand is in warm water) to abort progression from aura to headache

5. **Immune disorders.** Psychological states affect immune response in complex ways that are not yet fully understood. Stress may depress cell-mediated immune response (via T lymphocytes). Disorders of immune response may involve susceptibility to various conditions.

   a. **Autoimmune diseases**

     (1) Systemic lupus erythematosus (SLE)

     (2) Rheumatoid arthritis

     (3) Pernicious anemia

   b. **Allergic disorders**

   c. **Cancer.** Studies show that patients who react to stress with feelings of hopelessness or depression are at higher risk for cancer.

   d. **Immune system.** Although a controversial subject, increasing evidence suggests **immune system dysfunction** in disorders such as depression.

     (1) Evidence also suggests abnormal diurnal variation in circulating natural killer cell phenotypes and cytotoxic activity in patients with major depression.

     (2) Interleukin-1β is produced in increased amounts in patients with depression, which in turn may contribute to hypothalamic–pituitary axis dysregulation.

     (3) Mortality studies such as record linkage studies report increased mortality from physical illnesses that are at least indirectly associated with lack of full immunologic competence (e.g., deaths from infectious disease, neoplasms associated with major depression).

     (4) Clinicians have long noted that stresses, loss, and mental illness are associated with flare-ups in disorders usually kept in some control by the immune system (e.g., melanoma, tuberculosis).

B **General medical conditions presenting as somatoform disorders** In all of the somatoform disorders, patients may have an undiagnosed physical disorder with inconsistent, vague, or confusing symptoms. Several illnesses should be considered.

1. **SLE and several other autoimmune disorders.** These diseases, which are associated with multiple organ systems, are characterized by exacerbations and remissions. SLE typically begins in late adolescence or the early twenties, and women are nine times more likely to develop SLE than men. The onset may be vague, and psychiatric symptoms (e.g., mood disorders, schizophreniform disorder) may be present.

2. **Endocrine disorders**

   a. **Hyperthyroidism** (thyrotoxicosis) may be present, with complaints of fatigue, palpitations, dyspnea, and anxiety.

   b. **Hypothyroidism** may also manifest with fatigue and anxiety. Mood disorders, including depression, are possible. Menstrual problems are commonly seen and may be dismissed as a somatization problem.

   c. **Hyperparathyroidism** can manifest with severe anxiety, gastrointestinal symptoms, polyuria, and some pain.

3. **Neurologic disorders.** Any physical illness that begins early in life and is associated with an insidious or intermittent onset of symptoms should be considered in the differential diagnosis of somatoform disorder.

   a. **Multiple sclerosis** (MS) may have transient, remitting neurologic symptoms associated with dysphoric mood and anxiety. It often is misdiagnosed as a psychiatric illness early in its course.

   b. **Temporal lobe** or **complex partial seizures** may cause a distorted body image as well as mood disorders and changes in personality.

   c. **Acute intermittent porphyria** (AIP) is rare but may mimic somatization disorder with its gastrointestinal pain and neurologic complaints.

   d. **Other systemic diseases** and toxic or metabolic diseases can present physicians with confusing symptom pictures, particularly early in their course. They should not be dismissed as somatoform disorders, particularly if the symptoms do not fit the "classic" picture of the somatoform disorders.

4. **Psychiatric disorders**
   a. **Major depression** is perhaps the most common illness, with presenting complaints that are comorbid with or mistaken for somatoform disorders.
   b. **Acute adjustment reactions** can manifest as multiple somatic symptoms or preoccupation with symptoms.
   c. **Schizophrenia** occasionally manifests as multiple somatic complaints or delusions.
   d. **Panic disorder** can manifest as multiple somatic complaints and extreme preoccupation with symptoms.
   e. **Personality disorders** frequently coexist with somatoform disorder and should be differentiated from the somatoform disorder for purposes of treatment and diagnosis.

C Substance abuse

1. **Alcohol use disorders** remain the major comorbid substance use problem in various psychosomatic and psychophysiologic illnesses.

2. **Opioids** are probably underprescribed for acute pain (e.g., after surgery or acute physical trauma); however, their use in chronic pain in patients with somatization disorder, pain disorder, factitious disorder, or conversion disorder has less supportive evidence and presents a threat for addiction.

3. **Other substances** may be misused by vulnerable patients, including benzodiazepines, barbiturates, and psychomotor stimulants.

4. After a particular patient has become **habituated to a prescription** medication and uses it for relief of psychological as well as physical symptoms, **secondary drug-seeking behaviors** may develop (e.g., using multiple doctors simultaneously, magnifying or creating symptoms, and using other people's medications).

D Dissociative disorders (see VI)

1. **Significant association** is present among somatization disorder, conversion symptoms, and dissociation symptoms.
   a. An association between somatization disorder and dissociative symptoms is so frequent that they were considered to be in the same diagnostic class in previous editions of the *DSM* (i.e., "psychoneurotic reactions" in *DSM-I*, "hysterical neurosis" in *DSM-II*).
   b. Recent work demonstrates a strong association among somatization, dissociation, and a history of sexual abuse.

2. Clinically, dissociative symptoms are often found in patients with somatization disorder. Some odd symptoms (e.g., picking at skin, pulling own hair) may be mechanisms a particular individual has learned to prevent dissociation.

E Major depression

1. A strong tendency exists for **major depression** to present with **somatic complaints** in some cultures, with patients at the same time denying symptoms of depression (e.g., headaches, malaise, and abdominal pain in some Asian and Native American cultures). In most of these cases, patients respond well to treatment for major depression.

2. **Unipolar major depression** can manifest atypically, with symptoms resembling almost all of the somatoform disorders, particularly if psychotic and melancholic features are present.

3. In the United States, **hypochondriasis** and **body dysmorphic preoccupations** are not uncommon as features of a major depression.

4. For reasons that remain unclear, major depression is commonly missed and incorrectly treated in primary medical care settings.

5. **Depression concurrent with chronic pain** is very common. In some studies, up to 87% of patients with chronic pain suffer from major depression.

6. Somaticizing presentations seem to be more common in **unipolar depression** than in bipolar depression.

F Anxiety disorders

1. **Panic disorder** frequently occurs acutely, with symptoms resembling a myocardial infarction or a pulmonary embolus. Somatic preoccupations with heart disease, seizure disorders, and brain tumors are quite common and can become chronic, as patients grope for an explanation of their alarming symptoms.

   a. Some studies report that patients with panic disorder have comorbid rates of mitral valve prolapse on echocardiogram of between 10% and 20%. Other studies find no increase in prevalence of mitral valve prolapse compared with the general population.

   b. Cardiovascular causes of death increase the risk of premature death in patients with panic disorder.

2. Patients with **obsessive-compulsive disorder** frequently have health-related preoccupations and rituals that may involve contamination fears and excessive handwashing.

3. **Posttraumatic stress disorder** (PTSD) may involve physical health preoccupations, depending on the nature of the psychological trauma.

G Psychotic disorders

1. Occasionally, patients with **schizophrenia** and **schizophreniform disorder** may have primarily somatic hallucinations and delusions. These hallucinations tend to be bizarre enough to be distinguished easily from symptoms of somatoform disorders (e.g., one's organs are being squeezed by someone's telepathic powers).

2. **Mood-congruent hallucinations** and **delusions** involving the body rotting or having cancer are common in patients with psychotic depressions.

3. Distinguishing **folk beliefs** from psychotic and somatoform disorders may be difficult. If other members of the culture or subgroup share the belief system, beliefs should not be called "psychotic."

   a. **Culture-bound somatic syndromes** include **koro,** a syndrome primarily affecting Asian men, in which patients believe that the penis is shrinking into the body, with death as the expected result; and **dhat** in India, in which anxiety and concerns with the discharge of semen are associated with beliefs about weakness and exhaustion.

   b. In the United States, **health-related subcultures** have beliefs about such health topics as the cause of disease, nutrition, vitamin use, and crystals. On occasion, these beliefs lead to behaviors that can cause major health problems and even psychotic symptoms (e.g., fat-soluble vitamin overdose, scopolamine poisoning from too much herbal tea).

   c. Patients with limited information about health, physiology, and anatomy sometimes present with physical complaints that are grossly incorrect. This aspect should be seen as an educational problem rather than as a psychotic symptom in the absence of other symptoms of psychotic disorders.

4. Patients with **psychotic physical delusions** and **hallucinations** generally respond to the treatment of the specific psychotic disorder producing the symptom.

H Other psychiatric disorders

1. **Personality disorders** may manifest as a variety of physical preoccupations, concerns, and symptoms of a psychological etiology.

   a. Patients with **antisocial personality disorder** are likely to produce symptoms of malingering when legal cases promise substantial potential reward, when they can escape the legal consequences of their acts, or when they can otherwise experience profits through "secondary gain."

   b. Patients with **borderline personality disorder** may create injuries or harm themselves in ways that may resemble factitious disorder or malingering. However, the motivation does not appear to be adopting a sick role but rather relieving psychological distress through the self-mutilating act.

   c. Patients with **histrionic and narcissistic personality disorders** magnify symptoms of physical illnesses as a means of making themselves the center of attention and ensuring what they believe to be adequate commitment from the health care provider.

2. Patients with **social phobias** and/or **avoidant personality disorder** may avoid health care settings because of fears about having to disrobe and talk to a physician. They may even postpone treatment of very serious illnesses (e.g., myocardial infarctions, cancer).

V SPECIFIC SOMATOFORM DISORDERS

A Somatization disorder

1. **Epidemiology.** Approximately 1% of women have somatization disorder, and the ratio of women to men is 10:1. It is thought to be less common in individuals with higher education. Prevalence and incidence differ among cultures and ethnic groups.

2. **Etiology**
   a. Recent studies suggest a significant **genetic component** to somatization disorder. It has been linked to a high incidence of:
      (1) Alcoholism and other substance use disorders in first-degree male relatives
      (2) Antisocial personality disorder in first-degree male relatives
      (3) Somatization disorder in first-degree female relatives
   b. **Adoption studies** of female children of somatizing women showed a markedly increased rate of somatization disorder compared with control groups.
   c. **Environmental influences** are suggested by an increased rate of somatization disorder when children are raised in chaotic circumstances involving parental divorce, poverty, and alcoholism.
   d. Evidence of **dysfunction on neuropsychiatric tests** has led some investigators to hypothesize that patients have an impaired ability to screen out somatic sensations.
   e. **Secondary gains** of the sick role may provide a learned component of the disorder.

3. **Associated features**
   a. Excessive medical evaluations with frequent consultation with multiple physicians
   b. Unnecessary invasive diagnostic procedures and surgery
   c. Anxiety and depressive symptoms, which are common in this population
   d. A wide range of associated interpersonal difficulties, including marital and parenting problems
   e. Substance abuse, including prescribed medications
   f. Suicidal ideation, particularly in patients with substance abuse problems and depression
   g. Sexual function impairment (i.e., lack of interest in sex, specific sexual dysfunctions)

4. **Differential diagnosis.** Disorders to be ruled out include major depression, general medical conditions, schizophrenia, panic disorder, and hypochondriasis.

5. **Treatment.** Therapy is often frustrating for physicians, who should expect and accept their own feelings of frustration and anger when managing patients with this condition. Somatization disorder is best conceptualized as a lifelong disorder rather than a curable condition. Symptoms tend to fluctuate with stress in patients' lives. General principles of treatment include:
   a. **Regular appointments** so that patients are assured of an ongoing, supportive relationship with one physician. Appointments should focus on life stresses and the patient's functioning rather than on symptoms. Recent studies have shown that supportive treatment reduces use of health services (e.g., emergency department visits), hospital days, and physician charges. Periodic visits should include a limited but reasonable examination of new symptoms.
   b. **Consolidation of care with one physician** minimizes medication usage, reduces unnecessary surgery, and limits diagnostic evaluations to a reasonable level.
   c. **Avoidance of unnecessary surgery.** Surgical procedures should be considered only for clear indications. Physicians should thoughtfully consider the expected gains compared with the potential complications. Frequently, the initial surgery is followed by multiple subsequent surgeries for "adhesions."
   d. **Avoidance of habit-forming medications.** Little or no medication should be given for questionable indications.
   e. **Appropriate evaluation of new symptoms** when they occur. Patients with somatization disorder are still at risk for organic illness.

    f. Adequate use of antidepressant medications. Outcome studies demonstrate a much improved result for patients with somatization disorder who have depressive symptoms, in contrast to patients with the disorder but without depressive features.

    g. Use of monoamine oxidase (MAO) inhibitors. These agents are reported to be very effective in some patients with somatization disorder.

B Conversion disorder

1. **Clinical presentation**
   a. **Associated features.** Conversion disorder involves the unconscious "conversion of a psychological conflict" into a loss of physical functioning, which suggests a neurologic disease or other disease. The symptom is temporally related to a psychosocial stressor.
      (1) An **additional psychiatric diagnosis** (e.g., adjustment disorder, schizophrenia, personality disorder) can be made in 30% to 50% of patients.
      (2) Conversion disorders are also seen in patients with real organic physical illness.
      (3) *La belle indifference,* in which patients exhibit little concern over the symptoms, is sometimes present. However, it is not a reliable sign of conversion alone because patients with a physical illness may be stoic about their condition.
      (4) **Modeling** is common. Patients may unconsciously imitate the symptoms observed in important individuals in their lives.
   b. **Symptoms.** Although most conversion symptoms are transient, some can have a chronic course and result in a significant disability. Also, symptoms may be inconsistent with known pathophysiology such as a stocking-glove anesthesia. Patients classically present with an acute loss of function, which suggests neurologic disease. Symptoms may be bizarre or unusual, including:
      (1) Paresthesias and anesthesias
      (2) Gait disturbances (e.g., astasia, abasia)
      (3) Paralysis
      (4) Loss of consciousness and seizures
      (5) Aphonia
      (6) Vomiting
      (7) Fainting
      (8) Visual disturbances (e.g., blindness, tunnel vision)

2. **Epidemiology. Incidence and prevalence** are not known with certainty; however, conversion disorder seems to be less common now than in the past, and it may present with less classic symptomatology than was seen previously. Conversion disorder is seen more frequently in low socioeconomic classes, and some cultures have much greater rates of conversion disorder than others. Although the disorder occurs more commonly in women, it is seen in men as well. Onset is usually in adolescence through the twenties; however, it can occur at any age.

3. **Etiology.** Causes are thought to be psychological.
   a. **Two mechanisms** have been described that explain the gains experienced by patients with conversion disorder.
      (1) The **primary gain** is that the internal conflict is kept from consciousness.
      (2) The **secondary gain** is reinforcement from the environment (e.g., a patient who avoids unpleasant duties because of the symptoms). Some secondary gain is seen in almost all illnesses, however.
   b. **Other causes** that have been postulated include the following:
      (1) Less powerful individuals gain control over the environment by the elaboration of symptoms (i.e., the concern and attention of others are focused on the patient).
      (2) Symptoms are learned and are then reinforced by the reactions of those around patients.
      (3) Symptoms are seen more frequently in patients with brain injuries and other neurologic defects, which suggests a physiologic contribution.

4. **Differential diagnosis.** It is important to note that between 15% and 30% of patients diagnosed as having conversion disorder have an undiagnosed physical illness (e.g., MS, other neurologic conditions). Approximately 20% of cases initially diagnosed as conversion disorder have been later diagnosed as somatization disorder.

5. **Prognosis.** A good prognosis is associated with:
   a. Good premorbid functioning
   b. Acute onset
   c. An obvious stressful precipitant

6. **Treatment**
   a. **Attention to the possibility of organic disease is critical.** However, workups should be based only on objective findings. First, organic causes of the symptom must be considered and ruled out. If an organic condition such as intoxication with anticonvulsants is present, treatment of the organic condition may often lead to the resolution of the conversion symptom.
   b. Stressful events in patients' lives should be evaluated and appropriate intervention such as psychotherapy or family therapy should be provided. Associated psychiatric illness (e.g., depression) should be treated, which may involve pharmacologic approaches.
   c. The patients' symptoms have a psychological basis, but confronting patients with this fact is not helpful. Some patients come to understand the symbolic aspect of the symptom and gain conscious mastery of the conflict. However, most patients are receptive to the explanation that the disorder is a reaction to stress and to the reassurance that the condition will resolve over time. These interventions may allow patients to let go of symptoms without losing face.
   d. Suggestion during hypnosis or an amobarbital (Amytal) interview that the symptoms will improve can result in dramatic resolution. Symptom substitution, suggested in the psychodynamic literature, is relatively rare in actual practice.

C **Pain disorder**

1. **Clinical presentation.** Patients complain of pain for which there is no demonstrable physical cause or pain that is excessive given the known organic pathology. Generally, this disorder results in significant impairment and inability to function.
   a. **Clinical differentiation of pain disorder from chronic pain itself may be difficult,** and the distinction between pain disorder and chronic pain itself may not be terribly useful in daily practice. In both pain disorder and chronic pain, accepting the patient's pain is a good starting place for treatment. Individual differences in pain threshold, depressive and anxiety symptoms, and physical pathology that may have been missed dictate caution in making this diagnosis. As patients with pain disorder are followed over time, an organic cause of the pain becomes clear in a portion of the group.
   b. In some cases, **psychological factors** appear to play a role in the symptoms, such as:
      (1) Secondary gain because of financial compensation
      (2) Avoidance of objectionable work
      (3) Control of significant others
   c. In other cases, there is little indication of psychological factors.
   d. Most cases of chronic pain involve both physical and psychological contributions, which can lead to:
      (1) Problems with the physician–patient relationship
      (2) Multiple physical examinations
      (3) Unnecessary surgery
      (4) Substance abuse

2. **Epidemiology. Incidence and prevalence** are unknown. However, pain disorder is a common condition in primary care settings. The disorder occurs more frequently in women than in men.

3. **Etiology**
   a. **Psychological factors**
      (1) Patients may have learned as children to express emotions physically instead of verbally.
      (2) Patients may be unconsciously reinforced by the sick role.
      (3) When compensation for injury is an issue, patients may be consciously or unconsciously reinforced for illness behavior.
      (4) Many patients report histories of deprivation, neglect, or abuse, which may make them more vulnerable as adults.

(5) Many patients have a history of working at an early age, holding physically demanding jobs, and centering their lives around work.

b. Physical theories

(1) Endogenous opiate substances (endorphins) in the brain, which raise the pain threshold, may be altered genetically, developmentally, or secondarily to stress, making these individuals more prone to continued pain.

(2) Monoamine neurotransmitters (particularly serotonin) appear to be involved in pain inhibitory fibers in the brain stem. This neurotransmitter system may be altered genetically, developmentally, or secondarily to stress, which results in continued pain perception. This hypothesis is supported by patients' responsiveness to tricyclic antidepressants.

(3) A possible genetic component is suggested by the increased incidence of first-degree relatives with:

(a) Chronic pain

(b) Depression

(c) Alcohol dependence

(d) Substance abuse

4. Differential diagnosis (see IV E). This disorder requires a thorough diagnostic workup to rule out organic pathology. Other disorders to be ruled out include hypochondriasis, somatization, depression with somatic symptoms, and schizophrenia. When secondary gain (e.g., financial compensation) is evident, conscious simulation of the pain symptom (i.e., malingering) must be considered. When the assumption of the role of a patient is repeatedly the goal of the consciously produced symptom, factitious disorder must be considered. Also, personality and cultural attributes must be taken into consideration; for example, a dramatic, histrionic presentation of organic pain should not be confused with somatoform pain disorder.

5. Prognosis

a. Duration of illness. The longer the duration, the less likely the chance of functional recovery is. Very few patients with chronic pain of greater than 5 years' duration improve.

b. Age. The older the patient, the less likely the chance of recovery is.

c. Secondary gain. The more reinforcement (financial, social, or otherwise) for the symptom, the less likely the chance of recovery is. Many clinicians who treat patients with chronic pain refuse to treat patients with pending litigation because of the poor outcome under these circumstances.

d. Coexisting personality disorder is also a negative prognostic factor.

e. Prominent depressive features are considered a good prognostic feature if patients consent to treatment for the depression. (Surprisingly, few patients actually consent.)

6. Treatment. This condition is notoriously difficult to treat; although many patients can make significant improvements in functioning, few are cured.

a. Medications

(1) Chronic narcotic use, paradoxically, is not helpful in chronic pain because patients become habituated to the narcotics, which results in a loss of the analgesic effect and a vulnerability to withdrawal symptoms. Because of the peaks and valleys of short-acting narcotic blood levels, these agents can actually exacerbate chronic pain symptoms. Detoxification can improve pain symptoms. For a minority of patients with chronic pain who appear to require chronic narcotic treatment, a long-acting preparation such as methadone is preferable.

(2) Sedative-hypnotics depress the nervous system and increase pain perceptions as well as inactivity. Therefore, they should be avoided.

(3) Antidepressants may be useful. From 50% to 60% of patients report improvements in sleep, sense of well-being, and pain perception with tricyclic antidepressants (up to 87% in some studies). Some controversy exists in terms of what doses of antidepressants to use. Doses lower than antidepressant doses may be adequate for treatment of chronic pain (e.g., 75 to 125 mg/day amitriptyline or equivalent) versus an antidepressant dose (150 to 225 mg/day for adults). Antidepressant doses must be adjusted carefully because of the other medications these patients may be taking.

b. Therapies

(1) **Psychotherapy** may be useful. Supportive approaches are useful in helping patients deal with life stresses that may exacerbate pain symptoms. Cognitive and interpersonal therapy are indicated if patients have prominent depressive or anxiety symptoms.

(2) **Behavioral therapy** focuses on reinforcing wellness instead of sick role behavior. Although this approach may not affect patients' perception of pain, it is effective in improving the level of patient functioning. By reducing the secondary gain from the symptoms, patients may devote less attention to the pain.

(3) **Family therapy** is a useful adjunctive approach when family dynamics reinforce a patient's sick role and undermine attempts to improve functional capacity.

(4) **Group therapy,** where available, is a useful adjunct in supporting patients' efforts to improve functional capacity.

c. Multidisciplinary approaches, which are usually available in pain clinic settings, allow a comprehensive treatment plan, which some patients may need to maximize their functioning. It may involve the previously mentioned strategies, as well as:

(1) Physical therapy

(2) Occupational therapy

(3) Biofeedback training

(4) Relaxation techniques

(5) Hypnosis

(6) Acupuncture

(7) Neurosurgical ablation of pain tracts

(8) Transcutaneous electrical stimulation

7. Prevention

a. Information about preventing pain disorder is inadequate. However, some pain experts suggest that, paradoxically, inadequate treatment of acute pain may lead to the development of chronic pain. These experts suggest adequate prescription of narcotics after surgery or physical trauma, but they avoid chronic narcotic prescriptions.

b. Adequate screening and treatment of major depression and other psychiatric disorders are helpful in people whose pain complaints extend beyond the expected time or severity after surgery or trauma.

D Hypochondriasis

1. Clinical presentation. Patients are chronically preoccupied with fears that they have an illness despite thorough evaluation and reassurance from the physician that no organic problems can be found.

a. Normal physical sensations such as sweating and bowel movements **are misinterpreted. Minor ailments** such as cough or backache **are exaggerated.** Minor physical symptoms are interpreted as being of sinister health significance, and vigilance may become a form of auto-suggestion. The fear and misperception become a cyclic, self-reinforcing pattern. For example, patients may believe that a cough or a mole is cancerous, and close observation of the cough or mole convinces patients that the fear is realistic.

b. "Doctor shopping" is common and is a frustration for both patients and physicians. Simple reassurance that the feared symptom is not serious is interpreted by a particular patient as evidence that the treating physician is not taking the situation seriously. The patient then seeks another doctor.

c. Anxious and depressed mood as well as obsessive-compulsive features are commonly observed and suggest a good prognosis with treatment of the primary condition.

d. Impairment can be mild or so severe as to result in invalidism.

e. In general, these patients do not accept the idea that they have a psychiatric disorder.

2. Epidemiology

a. As many as 1% of the population may be hypochondriacal, and the condition is commonly seen in medical practice. Equal numbers of men and women are affected.

b. Usual age of onset is between age 20 and 30 years, but patients most commonly present to the physician in their forties and fifties.

3. **Etiology.** Patients with primary hypochondriasis may have been raised in homes with excessive concern about illness or little parental warmth except when children were ill. Hypochondriasis that occurs in the course of another psychiatric illness is thought to be a part of the familiar symptoms that develop in the primary illness (e.g., the foreboding of anxiety, the hopelessness of depression, or the delusional beliefs of schizophrenia). **Cognitive and behavioral theories** suggest the cyclic pattern of fear, vigilance, and distorted reasoning, which are also common to the development of phobias.

4. **Differential diagnosis.** Other conditions that must be ruled out are:
   a. Depression
   b. Panic attacks
   c. OCD
   d. Schizophrenia
   e. Somatization disorder
   f. Actual physical pathology
   g. Personality disorders (if comorbid condition, a poor prognostic feature)

5. **Treatment**
   a. **Physician reaction** to hypochondriacal patients is often negative. Physicians who are unaware of such feelings may act on them in an antitherapeutic way such as overprescribing medication or performing unnecessary diagnostic procedures.
   b. Physicians should acknowledge that patients are concerned and want assistance early in treatment. A sympathetic, educational approach to patients is ideal. As soon as rapport is established, screening for other conditions, particularly depression, anxiety, and OCD, should be undertaken. Regular follow-up appointments to evaluate new symptoms are often helpful and reassuring.
   c. It may be necessary to prescribe medication; however, patients should be told that it will help but not "cure" the ailment. Narcotics and other habit-forming drugs should not be prescribed in the absence of physical pathology (although hypochondriacal patients can also get broken legs, for example, which should be treated normally).
   d. **Pimozide** is reported to be dramatically effective in some patients with hypochondriasis of a delusional intensity, but this agent is not approved for this use in the United States. (It is approved in the United States only for the treatment of Tourette disorder.)

E **Body dysmorphic disorder**

1. **Clinical presentation.** The hallmark of this disorder is preoccupation with some imagined defect in the body, usually of the face. Usually a history shows frequent visits to doctors, especially dermatologists or plastic surgeons. Depressive mood and obsessive compulsive traits are common.

2. **Epidemiology. Incidence and etiology** are unknown. Even epidemiologic studies admit probable underestimation of the prevalence of the disorder because most of these patients have shame about reporting their symptoms.

3. **Differential diagnosis**
   a. If the symptom is of delusional intensity, it should be classified as a **delusional disorder, somatic subtype,** which may be responsive to antipsychotic medication.
   b. Major depression and schizophrenia should be ruled out. This process may be difficult if distorted ideas about the body reach delusional proportions. Many patients with body dysmorphic disorder have symptoms such as ideas of reference related to their symptoms.
   c. Recent evidence suggests strong links between OCD and body dysmorphic disorder, and suggests that they sometimes co-occur.
   d. Anorexia nervosa and body dysmorphic disorder should be differentiated.
   e. Personality disorders in the context of this disorder represent a poor prognostic feature.

4. **Treatment**
   a. Invasive diagnostic procedures or unnecessary surgery should be avoided. When reconstructive surgery is undertaken, patients are unlikely to be satisfied with the results.
   b. There are some reports of medication treatment with antidepressants (SSRIs and MAO inhibitors) and neuroleptics (pimozide) being therapeutic.

    c. There are anecdotal reports of behavior therapy and dynamic psychotherapy being effective; an educational–supportive approach has been reported to have some success.

F **Environmental illness** A relatively new phenomenon, environmental illness is a polysymptomatic disorder that some experts believe is associated with immune system dysfunction and allergy-like sensitivity to many compounds in food and air. Early studies suggest an association with increased somatic, mood, and anxiety symptoms indicative of personality disorders. Clinicians working with affected patients report very high levels of depression and anxiety in this population. This phenomenon may represent the emergence of a new culture-bound disorder in the United States and Europe, as was found with people who compulsively exercise to the point of physical damage.

VI DISSOCIATIVE DISORDERS

A **Diagnosis**

    1. Dissociative amnesia
      a. This disorder involves one or more episodes of **an inability to recall important personal information, usually of traumatic or stressful nature,** too extensive to be accounted for by ordinary forgetfulness.
      b. The disorder doesn't occur as a part of another dissociative disorder, acute or posttraumatic stress disorder, or somatization disorder, or due to substances or a general medical condition.
      c. The symptoms cause significant distress or impairment in functioning.

    2. Dissociative fugue
      a. Dissociative fugue is sudden, unexpected travel away from home or place of work, with an **inability to recall one's past, and confusion about personal identity or assumption of a new identity.**
      b. The disorder doesn't occur as a part of dissociative identity disorder and isn't due to substances or a general medical condition, and the symptoms cause life impairment or significant distress.

    3. Dissociative identity disorder
      a. Dissociative identity disorder involves the presence of **two or more distinct personalities or personality states,** which recurrently take control of the person's behavior.
      b. The patient has an inability to recall personal information too extensive to be explained by ordinary forgetfulness.
      c. The symptoms aren't due to substances or a general medical condition, and in children aren't attributable to fantasy or imaginary play.

    4. Depersonalization disorder
      a. Depersonalization disorder involves persistent or **recurrent experiences of detachment from one's body or mental processes** (like being an outside observer of oneself, or being in a dream).
      b. Despite the experience, reality testing is not impaired.
      c. The symptoms don't occur as part of a psychotic disorder, panic disorder, or another dissociative disorder, and aren't due to the effects of substances or a general medical condition.

    5. Dissociative disorder not otherwise specified
      a. This includes disorders with dissociative symptomatology that don't fit the criteria for any other disorder. Examples include:
        (1) Dissociate trance disorder, which covers a number of culturally bound syndromes of altered or selective conscious awareness such as *amok* or *latah*
        (2) Ganser syndrome, wherein people give approximate but incorrect answers to questions (e.g., "2 plus 2 equals 5") when not associated with dissociative amnesia or dissociative fugue, generally in the context of voluntary production of severe psychiatric symptoms (in which it might resemble factitious disorder)

B **Epidemiology and etiology** Generally, these disorders are uncommon, but their incidence is thought to increase in times of increased exposure to trauma, such as during war and natural disasters. Dissociative disorders tend to show a decreased incidence with age. Dissociative amnesia, dissociative identity disorder, and depersonalization disorder tend to occur more often in women than men. Dissociative amnesia, dissociative fugue, and dissociative identity disorder tend to occur after some traumatic event, for which these disorders are seen to arise as a defense against. Unlike repression, which creates a "horizontal" split in consciousness, dissociation creates a "vertical" split leading to a parallel consciousness of sorts. This defense is maladaptive in the sense that it delays "working through" the trauma.

C **Differential diagnosis** includes medical conditions that can create amnesia or altered consciousness (delirium, anoxia, cerebral neoplasms or infections, epilepsy, etc.), other psychiatric conditions (somatoform disorders, PTSD), and malingering.

D **Treatment** is limited for this group of disorders. Hypnosis and drug-assisted interviews with short-acting barbiturates (e.g., sodium amobarbital) may help recover lost memories. Psychotherapy may help to address issues surrounding the underlying events.

VII FACTITIOUS DISORDER

A **Clinical presentation**   Patients are in voluntary control of their symptoms, and although their behavior is deliberate, what precipitates this behavior is not.

1. **Symptoms.** Patients may complain of pain in a range of circumstances such as when they feel no pain or after self-inflicted infection such as that arising from self-injection with feces or saliva, which can develop into life-threatening illness. The medical knowledge of patients is often highly sophisticated. By complaining of bizarre or unusual symptoms, these patients may encourage invasive diagnostic procedures such as laparotomy or angiography. Patients may lie about any aspect of their history with a dramatic flair (**pseudologia fantastica**). Narcotic abuse and addiction are associated findings in about half of these patients.

2. **History.** At hospital admission, the patient's behavior is disruptive and demanding. Symptoms change as workups prove negative. Eventually, patients are confronted with evidence of faking, and they usually react angrily and leave against medical advice. This pattern of behavior can become chronic and involve multiple admissions to different hospitals.

B **Diagnosis**

1. **Factitious disorder** involves the intentional production or feigning of physical or psychological signs or symptoms. The motivation for the behavior is assumption of the sick role. External incentives for the behavior (e.g., profiting economically, avoiding legal responsibility, improving physical well-being, as in malingering) are absent. **Subtypes** include the following:
   a. With predominantly psychological signs and symptoms
   b. With predominantly physical signs and symptoms (Munchausen syndrome)
   c. With combined psychological and physical signs and symptoms

2. **Factitious disorder not otherwise specified,** which includes **Munchausen by proxy,** includes production of intentional symptoms in another individual such as a child for the purpose of having the other person assume the sick role.

C **Epidemiology**   The disorder may appear more common than it actually is because a single patient may interact with many physicians in different hospitals. It usually begins in adulthood and is a lifelong condition.

D **Etiology**   Although an illness or operation in early childhood may be a contributing factor, the disorder is considered to be entirely psychological. There may have been an experience with a physician in early life through a family relationship or through illness. A significant portion of these patients are employed in the health care field as paraprofessionals. Masochism has been considered an important feature in patients who seek unnecessary surgery. The illness has also been conceptualized as a variant of the borderline syndrome in that the physician becomes the perpetual object of transference; patients continually reenact with the physician the disordered relationship with their parents. Object loss or fear of loss is frequently reported as a precipitant of an episode. Studies indicate relatively frequent electroencephalogram (EEG) abnormalities in this group, suggesting some central nervous system (CNS) dysfunction.

E Differential diagnosis

1. **Physical illness.** A patient with a true physical disorder may present the symptoms with an unusual or dramatic flair that makes the physician suspicious of faking and that is more likely to occur if the patient also has a personality disorder, including one of the following types:
   a. Histrionic
   b. Borderline
   c. Schizotypal

2. **Somatization disorder.** The symptoms are not under patients' voluntary control, and patients do not usually insist on hospitalization. Conversion disorder may also be present.

3. **Hypochondriasis.** The essential feature of this disorder is the patient's preoccupation with the illness in general rather than with symptoms. The symptoms are not under the patient's voluntary control. Hypochondriasis starts later in life than factitious disorder, and patients with hypochondriasis are less likely to insist on hospital admission or submit to dangerous diagnostic procedures.

4. **Malingering.** Although it is difficult to differentiate between malingering and factitious disorder, the goals in malingering are clear to both patients and physicians, and the symptoms can be stopped when they no longer serve an end. In patients with factitious disorder, the goal of the behavior seems to be the patient role itself, in contrast to other secondary gain features of malingering.

F **Treatment** Patients with factitious disorder with physical symptoms rarely receive psychiatric treatment. The reactions of the treatment team are usually strongly negative, and this countertransference must be examined. Until patients are willing to face the reality of a psychiatric illness and agree to psychiatric hospitalization or treatment, the prognosis is likely to be poor. The therapeutic approach is one of management rather than cure, and unnecessary diagnostic procedures should be avoided. Patients should be confronted in a calm, nonjudgmental, indirect manner. There should be minimal expectation that patients admit the deception. Treatment must involve coordination with other treatment providers. The focus of therapy is usually underlying dynamic issues. When medication is used, it should target specific comorbid conditions and symptoms such as depression.

G **Factitious disorder by proxy (Munchausen by proxy)** This disorder is classified as factitious disorder not otherwise specified in the *DSM-IV-TR*. In this condition, intentional production of symptoms occurs in individuals who are under the care of other persons. Perpetrators desire to attain the sick role by proxy. There are *DSM-IV-TR* research criteria for the disorder.

VIII MALINGERING

A **Clinical presentation** Malingering is intentional production of false or grossly exaggerated physical or psychological symptoms and is motivated by external incentives (e.g., avoiding military duty, avoiding work, obtaining financial compensation, evading criminal prosecution, obtaining drugs).

B **Diagnosis** Malingering **is not considered a mental disorder or an illness.** Malingering is listed in the *DSM-IV-TR* as a "V" code. (A "V" code describes a condition that may be the focus of clinical attention.) Malingering should be strongly suspected if a combination of the following is noted:

1. Medicolegal context of presentation (e.g., the person is referred by an attorney to the clinician for examination)

2. Marked discrepancy between the person's claimed stress or disability and the objective findings

3. Lack of cooperation during the diagnostic evaluation and in complying with the prescribed treatment regimen

4. The presence of antisocial personality disorder

C **Epidemiology** True malingering is rarely seen. Physicians are more likely to misdiagnose this condition in patients with one of the somatoform disorders because they have a negative reaction to patients and are unable to see that patients are not consciously faking another disorder such as hypochondriasis.

D **Differential diagnosis**   In **factitious disorder,** the patient's goals cannot be clearly understood as they can in the case of malingering, even though the patient is voluntarily causing the symptoms of illness.

E **Treatment**   Because malingering is not an illness, it has **no medical** or **psychiatric treatment.**

IX   PLACEBO RESPONSE

A **Definition**   This condition has been defined as any effect attributable to a medication, procedure, or other form of therapy but not to the specific pharmacologic property of that therapy.

B **Epidemiology**   All medical treatments can show the effects of nonspecific curative factors, or placebo effects. For instance, 30% to 40% of patients in pain respond as well to placebos as they do to morphine. No particular personality type responds to a placebo (e.g., a histrionic patient is no more likely to have a placebo response than is any other patient).

C **Significance**   Physicians use the placebo response (mistakenly) to help differentiate "real" from "psychological" symptoms in their patients. The placebo response is a powerful aspect of most medical care. It operates commonly, even when the physician is unaware of it. However, **it does not differentiate physical from psychological symptoms.** Recent findings suggest that the placebo response to pain is a **physiologic phenomenon.** Placebo response can be blocked by a narcotic antagonist, naloxone, which suggests that the analgesic effect of a placebo may be based on the action of endorphins, the naturally occurring opioid substances in the brain, which increase the pain threshold.

BIBLIOGRAPHY

American Psychiatric Association: *Diagnostic and Statistical Manual of Mental Disorders,* 4th ed., text revision. Washington, DC, American Psychiatric Association Press, 2000.

DeLeon J, Bott A, Simpson GM: Dysmorphophobia: Body dysmorphic disorder or delusional disorder, somatic subtype? *Compr Psychiatry* 30:457–472, 1989.

Fallon BA, Schneir FR, Narshall R, et al: The pharmacotherapy of hypochondriasis. *Psychopharmacol Bull* 32:607–611, 1996.

Folks DG, Ford CW, Houck CA: Somatoform disorders, factitious disorders, and malingering. In *Clinical Psychiatry for Medical Students,* 3rd ed. Edited by Stoudemire A. Philadelphia, Lippincott-Raven, 1998, pp 343–381.

Jellinek MJ, Herzog DB: The somatoform disorders. In *Textbook of Child and Adolescent Psychiatry,* 2nd ed. Edited by Wiener JM. Washington, DC, American Psychiatric Press, 1997, pp 431–436.

Kent DA, Thomasson K, Coryell W: Course and outcome of conversion and somatization disorders. *Psychosomatics* 36:138–144, 1995.

Leamin MH, Plewes J: Factitious disorders and malingering. In *Essentials of Clinical Psychiatry,* 3rd ed. Edited by Hales RE, Yudofsky SC. Washington, DC, American Psychiatric Press, 1999, pp 439–451.

Martin RL, Yutzy SH: Somatoform disorders. In *Essentials of Clinical Psychiatry,* 3rd ed. Edited by Hales RE, Yudofsky SC. Washington, DC, American Psychiatric Press, 1999, pp 413–437.

Nernzer ED: Somatoform disorders. In *Child and Adolescent Psychiatry: A Comprehensive Textbook,* 2nd ed. Edited by Lewis M. Baltimore, Williams & Wilkins, 1996, pp 693–702.

Phillips KA: Body dysmorphic disorder: Diagnosis and treatment of imagined ugliness. *J Clin Psychiatry* 57(suppl):61–65, 1996.

Riding J, Munro A: Pimozide in the treatment of monosymptomatic hypochondriacal psychosis. *Acta Psychiatr Scand* 52:23–30, 1975.

Sadock BJ, Sadock VA: *Kaplan & Sadock's: Synopsis of Psychiatry,* 9th ed. Baltimore, Williams & Wilkins, 2003.

Weaver RC, Rodnick JE: Type A behavior: Clinical significance, evaluation, and management. *J Fam Pract* 23:255–261, 1986.

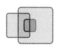

Study Questions

Directions: *Each of the numbered items or incomplete statements in this section is followed by answers or by completions of the statement. Select the ONE lettered answer or completion that is BEST in each case.*

1. A 53-year-old Asian man is brought to the clinic believing that his penis is shrinking into his body. He now has no energy. He thinks that he may eventually die from this problem. Which one of the following diagnoses is most appropriate?

- [A] Conversion disorder — *related to psychosocial stressor*
- [B] Major depression
- [C] Psychotic disorder not otherwise specified
- [D] Somatization disorder
- [E] Diagnosis deferred on Axis I

2. A 54-year-old mechanic has been unable to work for 2 years because of chronic back pain caused by lifting a heavy toolbox. Repeated neurologic and neuroradiologic examinations reveal muscle spasm and pain in the L4–L5 area, which occasionally is referred in the expected distribution. No herniations, tears, or fractures have been found. Which of the following interventions is **least** likely to be beneficial and presents additional risks?

- [A] Antidepressants
- [B] Anti-inflammatory agents
- [C] Appropriate exercise
- [D] Family therapy
- [E] Narcotic analgesics — > *NOT for chronic pain*

3. A 35-year-old woman is seen on a medical service for complaints of abdominal pain. The physician notes a 10-year history of poor health and multiple past somatic complaints. Which of the following is the best treatment strategy?

- [A] A trial of monoamine oxidase (MAO) inhibitors
- [B] Placement on long-term benzodiazepine medications
- [C] Immediate transfer to the psychiatry service
- [D] Appointments in the outpatient medicine clinic for periodic evaluations of the patient's symptoms by the same attending physician
- [E] A trial of neuroleptic medication to control the delusional aspects of the illness

4. Given the most probable diagnosis of the patient described in Question 3 above, which of the following is most likely?

- [A] There is a high incidence of a family history of alcoholism in male relatives in this disorder.
- [B] There is a high incidence of somatization disorder in female relatives in this disorder.
- [C] There is an increased rate of this disorder in persons raised in chaotic settings.
- [D] All of the above
- [E] None of the above

Somatization disorder

5. Patients who share the diagnosis of the patient in Question 3:

- [A] Are often underevaluated medically *(excessive medical attn)*
- [B] Have no need for evaluation of medical symptoms
- [C] Commonly experience anxiety and depressive symptoms
- [D] Often require use of benzodiazepines
- [E] Are rarely frustrating to treat

6. A 63-year-old man presents with a preoccupation with his bowel movements. He is convinced that this irregularity, which did not begin until during the past year, represents an occult cancer. Repeated examinations and a lower gastrointestinal series reveal no abnormalities. No occult blood is present in the stool. Which of the following is the most likely diagnosis?

- [A] Conversion disorder *usu neuro*
- [B] Hypochondriasis *2° to depression*
- [C] Major depression – *b/c prevalence, age, Sx*
- [D] Panic disorder
- [E] Somatization disorder *monoSx*

onset after age 35 is unusual

facing retirement?

7. A middle-aged man is brought in from a homeless shelter for evaluation due to his being unable to remember his name or any personal information. The man is subsequently discovered to be an executive from a neighboring state who had disappeared several weeks ago while out walking his dogs, which were later found roaming unattended. Other than the amnesia, psychiatric and medical workup is otherwise noncontributory. Which of the following diagnoses does this story best support?

- [A] Somatization disorder
- [B] Schizophrenia *younger, not as abrupt*
- [C] Dissociative fugue
- [D] Posttraumatic stress disorder
- [E] Factitious disorder

8. A 40-year-old woman sees her internist to be checked for colon cancer. She reports recent constipation and a family history of colon cancer. She denies other symptoms, and her organic workup is negative. She becomes irritated when she is reassured about her physical health and believes the evaluation was not complete. Which of the following statements about the patient is most likely to be correct?

- [A] Her disorder affects women more often than men. *♀ = ♂*
- [B] She perceives her bodily functions more acutely than others.
- [C] Medication will cure her disorder.
- [D] Narcotic analgesics are the treatment of choice.
- [E] It is unlikely that she will seek another medical opinion.

9. What should treatment of body dysmorphic disorder include?

- [A] Surgery
- [B] Selective serotonin reuptake inhibitors (SSRIs)
- [C] Long-term psychotherapy *(behavioral/dynamic therapy good)*
- [D] All of the above
- [E] None of the above

10. A 20-year-old woman presents with sudden loss of sensation and flaccid paralysis of her entire left arm. Which of the following is most likely to be her diagnosis?

- [A] Conversion disorder
- [B] Dissociative fugue
- [C] Dissociative identity disorder
- [D] General medical condition
- [E] Major depression

11. Many patients with the disorder described in Question 10 above:

- [A] Have comorbid body dysmorphic disorder
- [B] With an obvious stressful precipitant have a poor prognosis
- [C] Respond to benzodiazepines
- [D] Are later diagnosed with a physical illness that explains their symptoms
- [E] Intentionally produce their symptoms

12. In the patient described in Question 10, which of the following is a positive prognostic indicator?

- [A] Isolation to the left side
- [B] Acute onset
- [C] Female gender
- [D] All of the above
- [E] None of the above

13. In factitious disorder:

- [A] Symptoms are not under the patient's voluntary control.
- [B] The primary goal of the symptoms is secondary gain.
- [C] The physician may become the perpetual object of transference.
- [D] Substance addiction is rare.
- [E] None of the above

14. What does malingering involve?

- [A] Consciously faking an illness
- [B] The intent to deceive others
- [C] No medical or psychiatric treatment
- [D] All of the above
- [E] None of the above

15. The placebo response:

- [A] Helps to differentiate "real" from "psychological" symptoms in patients
- [B] To pain is a physiologic phenomenon
- [C] Is more likely to occur in a histrionic patient
- [D] Is a minimal part of most medical treatment

16. A 32-year-old woman with a history of childhood sexual abuse reports periods of "missing time" where she is unable to remember where she was or what she did, and having strangers call her by another name and act as if they know her. Which of the following is most likely to be this patient's diagnosis?

- [A] Panic disorder
- [B] Dissociative fugue
- [C] Dissociative identity disorder
- [D] Major depression
- [E] Somatization disorder

QUESTIONS 17–19

Match the following symptoms to the medical condition most likely to be associated with it.
- [A] Depressive symptoms
- [B] Schizophreniform disorder symptoms
- [C] Panic disorder symptoms

17. Paroxysmal atrial tachycardia *C*

18. Toxic delirium *B*

19. Hypothyroidism *A*

Answers and Explanations

1. The answer is E [*IV G 3 a*]. Without culture-specific information, the clinician has no idea whether this man's beliefs are associated with those of his culture. In this case, the culture-bound somatic syndrome, koro, accounts for his feelings. It is commonly assumed that his complaint is a symptom of psychosis and that treatment with a neuroleptic agent will be beneficial. Not only would this not help him, but it also exposes him to unnecessary additional risk. Although the patient may be depressed, his depression may have been triggered by his belief that he will die. The symptoms do not follow the pattern of a conversion or somatization disorder. In this case, the clinician's best choice is to defer the diagnosis and to seek consultation from another member of the culture, ideally a health care provider or traditional healer.

2. The answer is E [*V C 6*]. One would never treat a patient on the basis of such limited information or limit treatment to a single intervention. However, given the chronicity of the pain and the disproportionate level of disability, the worst choice of the group would be a narcotic analgesic. Although effective in the treatment of patients with acute pain, the role of narcotics in chronic pain is quite limited. The chances are that this patient would become habituated without long-term benefit from narcotics.

3. The answer is D [*V A 5 a*]. The best treatment strategy involves continuity of care as the most important aspect of patient care. At each scheduled visit, the physician conservatively evaluates new symptoms, attempts to keep the patient away from exploratory or unneeded surgery, and avoids giving the patient narcotics and other habituating medications. Any medication should be prescribed only in the context of an ongoing relationship with a single doctor to avoid "doctor shopping" and multiple prescriptions of habituating medications. Monoamine oxidase (MAO) inhibitors should be considered only with adequate informed consent after the physician knows the patient well. Benzodiazepines should be used with caution because of the propensity for patients with somatization disorder to become habituated and to use them in greater-than-prescribed amounts. Transfer to the psychiatry service will likely be opposed by the patient, who will view it as a rejection and evidence of lack of competence of the medical service. The patient is likely to try to get another doctor to diagnose and treat her condition adequately. Neuroleptic medications should be avoided because they are unlikely to produce substantial benefit, and they create a risk of producing tardive dyskinesia.

4. The answer is D [*II A; V A 1, 2*]. Given the onset before age 30 years, involvement of multiple organ systems, a long history of symptoms, and negative organic workups, the likely diagnosis is somatization disorder. Recent studies suggest both genetic (as in choices A and B) and environmental (as in choice C) components in somatization disorder.

5. The answer is C [*V A 2, 3, 4, 5*]. Patients with somatization disorder commonly experience symptoms of anxiety and depression. They often receive excessive medical evaluations with frequent consultations with multiple physicians. There should be appropriate medical evaluation done of any new symptoms. The physician should avoid prescribing habit-forming medications. Patients with somatization disorder are often frustrating for physicians to manage.

6. The answer is C [*IV B 4; V A, B, D*]. Major depression is the likely diagnosis on the basis of prevalence in the population, patient age, and patient symptoms. The most significant issue is the age of onset. For all of these disorders except major depression, onset beyond age 35 years is very unusual. It is likely that the patient is facing retirement, which may be a major stressor and a threat to his identity. Hypochondriasis is a possibility. However, if it is hypochondriasis, this condition is likely to be secondary to major depression, which receives diagnostic priority. Given the monosymptomatic nature of his presentation, somatization disorder is not possible. Conversion disorder is highly unlikely. Conversion symptoms are usually neurologic in focus and usually represent a sensory or motor loss. No evidence of a panic disorder is present, and the patient's age does not support this diagnosis.

7. The answer is C [*VI A 2*]. The combination of sudden, unexpected travel and inability to recall one's past are diagnostic features of dissociative fugue. The patient's age and the onset of the symptoms argue against schizophrenia. No criteria for somatization disorder are described. The amnesia of most personal information does fit posttraumatic stress disorder. Factitious disorder might be a consideration, but the patient does not seem to be making an effort to assume the sick role, which is a necessary component.

8. The answer is B [*V D 1*]. The patient most likely has hypochondriasis; she is preoccupied with a fear of cancer despite a thorough negative evaluation and reassurance by her physician. With hypochondriasis, normal physical sensations are often misinterpreted. Affected individuals seem to perceive their body functions more acutely than others and attribute their symptoms to serious disease. Men and women are equally affected. Medication does not "cure" hypochondriasis. Habit-forming medications such as narcotic analgesics should not be prescribed in the absence of physical pathology. Patients with hypochondriasis commonly "doctor shop."

9. The answer is B [*V E 1, 4*]. There are some reports of antidepressants (selective serotonin reuptake inhibitors) being effective in treating patients with body dysmorphic disorder. Surgery should be avoided. Patients are not usually satisfied with reconstructive surgery. There is no evidence for the use of long-term psychotherapy. Anecdotal reports show behavioral therapy, dynamic therapy, and educational–supportive therapy to be effective.

10. The answer is A [*V B*]. The sudden onset of a sensory and motor loss in the left arm could be caused by a neurologic illness (e.g., multiple sclerosis, stroke, cervical injury) but would be unlikely given the overlapping distribution of the sensory and motor losses, which do not follow more specific nerve distributions. There is no alteration of the patient's perceptions or consciousness necessary for any dissociative disorder. Likewise, no mood symptoms are mentioned, so major depression is unlikely.

11. The answer is D [*V B*]. Between 15% and 30% of patients diagnosed with conversion disorder have an underlying physical illness that is later diagnosed. Between 30% and 50% of patients with conversion disorder have a comorbid psychiatric diagnosis, but there is no specific association with body dysmorphic disorder. A good prognosis is associated with an obvious stressor, acute onset, and good premorbid functioning. There is no evidence to support the use of benzodiazepines in patients with conversion disorder. One criterion of conversion disorder is that the symptoms are not intentionally produced.

12. The answer is B [*V B 5*]. Acute onset is associated with a good prognosis in conversion disorder. Conversion is more common in women, but this doesn't predict prognosis. Anatomic location of the symptoms has no bearing on prognosis.

13. The answer is C [*VII A, C*]. The physician may become the perpetual transference object in factitious disorders. Symptoms are voluntarily produced by the patient for the primary goal of being in the patient role. Addiction occurs in about half of these patients.

14. The answer is D *[VIII A, D]*. By definition, malingering involves intentionally faking an illness or symptoms with the intent to deceive others for secondary gain. Because it is not an illness, malingering does not require any medical or psychiatric treatment.

15. The answer is B [*IX*]. Evidence suggests that the placebo response to pain is physiologically based. Physicians *mistakenly* think that the placebo response can differentiate real from psychological pain. No particular personality type is more likely to respond to a placebo. The placebo response is a powerful aspect of most medical care.

16. The answer is C [*VI A 3*]. The patient appears to have dissociative identity disorder, as there appears to be periods where another personality (using another name) takes control of her behavior and does things her primary personality doesn't recall. A history of trauma, particularly childhood physical or sexual abuse, is also common. The only other serious consideration of the available options would be dissociative fugue, but the lack of sudden, unexpected travel and the apparent contemporaneous existence of the other personality would argue against it.

17–19. The answers are 17-C, 18-B, and 19-A [*I A 5; IV*]. Medical conditions can cause psychiatric symptoms resembling almost any psychiatric disorder. Common examples are paroxysmal atrial tachycardia resembling panic disorder; toxic delirium mimicking schizophreniform disorder; and hypothyroidism mimicking depression.

chapter 9

Sexual and Gender Issues

R. GREGG DWYER • WILLIAM BURKE

I HEALTHY (NORMAL) SEXUAL RESPONSE

A General issues

1. Humans are naturally sexual as a function of their biology, psychology, and social interaction. The study of human sexuality has a long history; classic published works in the field date back to the 1900s, with many advances along the way but also much yet to be understood. This is in part due to the variety of expressions of human sexuality across time, among cultures, and for individuals during their life span. As with many human behaviors, sexual activity varies among persons and is influenced by social, political, religious, and cultural factors, which vary over time.

2. **Healthy sexual functioning** is a part of overall wellness and as such should be assessed as part of every comprehensive medical examination. Given the typically private nature of sexual thoughts, urges, desires, and behaviors, there is a natural tendency to avoid this line of inquiry. It is not uncommon for sexual topics to be avoided or given minimal attention because of personal anxiety, self-doubt about one's knowledge base, preconceptions about various behaviors, and unanswered questions or unresolved issues regarding one's own sexuality.

    Although components of sexual development and functioning are included in the curriculum of family practice, obstetrics/gynecology, pediatrics, and urology training programs, psychiatry addresses sexual development, thoughts, and behaviors across the life span. As a result, an understanding of the spectrum of healthy sexual development and functioning along with pathologic variations is required of psychiatrists. Having that knowledge will facilitate inquiry with patients and reduce the anxiety of low confidence and one's own questions typical of those making such inquiries.

    The field of human sexuality has vast breadth and depth, so this chapter will only focus on topics covering healthy sexual development and pathologic variations and at a level consistent with the educational expectations for medical students and the content of the *Diagnostic and Statistical Manual of Mental Disorders,* 4th edition, text revision (*DSM-IV-TR*).

B Stages of sexual response   To follow is a brief description of the sexual response cycles of men and women. The cycles of both sexes include the four phases of desire, excitement, orgasm, and resolution (1, 2).

1. **Phase I: Desire**
    a. The first phase begins with a primarily mental component in which there is a desire for and fantasies about engaging in sexual activity (1, 2).
    b. It is at this stage that an individual's personality, motives, and drives influence the sexual response (2).

2. **Phase II: Excitement**
    a. This stage includes the transition from subjective to objective arousal. The subjective fantasy or actual focus of sexual desire and/or physical stimulation lead to physiologic responses identified as sexual arousal (1, 2). This phase can last for minutes to hours for both sexes (2).
    b. **Physical arousal** can include not only the genitals but also the skin, breasts, cardiac and respiratory systems, and a variety of muscles.
    c. The characteristic features of this stage are penile tumescence, resulting in erection in men, and vaginal lubrication in women. The majority of women experience nipple erection, as do some

men. The woman's labia minora and clitoris become engorged with blood. Excitement can last seconds to hours. The duration for the height of excitement is seconds to minutes (2).

    d. Measurement of arousal. Physical arousal can be measured in men with the use of penile plethysmography, with either a penile strain gauge measuring changes in penile circumference or a vacuum chamber measuring changes in penile volume, thus capturing changes in both length and girth. Although less studied, photovaginal plethysmography can be used to measure female sexual arousal through measuring blood flow in the walls of the vagina.

  3. Phase III: Orgasm

    a. Both men and women. For men and women, orgasm occurs when sexual excitement reaches its peak and there is a release of the building tension, marked by loss of voluntary muscle control and rhythmic contractions of muscles in the genitalia and of the internal and external anal sphincter (2). Blood pressure and heart rate both increase.

    b. Men. Typically men experience a subjective indication of pending ejaculation followed by four to five rhythmic spasms of the prostate, seminal vesicles, vas, and urethra, causing the emission of semen (2). The force of ejaculation decreases with increasing age.

    c. Women. Women experience a series of three to 15 contractions of the labia minor and vagina (2). The origin of female emission of fluid during orgasm is controversial and debated regarding not only its content but also it being a female counterpart to the emission of male semen.

  4. Phase IV: Resolution

    a. Both men and women. For both men and women, this stage is characterized by a disgorgement of the genitalia. With orgasm, this usually takes 10 to 15 minutes, but without orgasm, it can last one-half to a full day (2). The mental facet of this stage is described as a relaxing and positive feeling (2).

    b. Men. The penis returns to its flaccid state. The refractory period begins, during which the penis cannot become erect for several minutes to several hours (2).

    c. Women. The labia and breasts return to their pre-excitement size. Vaginal blood pooling subsides and contractions cease (2). Women do not experience a refractory period and can immediately achieve another orgasm followed by a theoretically endless quantity of orgasms.

II   NORMAL SEXUAL FUNCTION AND GENDER IDENTITY DEVELOPMENT

A **Definitions**

  1. "Normal" can be defined as that which the majority of persons engage in and as such is statistically normal or mathematically average, or as what a given culture, religion, political entity, etc., perceive as acceptable during a given point in time. What is practiced by the majority varies both over time and across settings. For the purposes of this review, "normal" will refer to that which is healthy, nonabusive, consensual, and developmentally typical rather than what is linked to a particular sample of the population.

  2. Sexual identity refers to an individual's biologic composition including chromosome configuration, genitalia, hormone levels, and, after puberty, secondary sex characteristics (2).

  3. Gender identity is a person's self-identification as male or female, which usually occurs by the age of 2 or 3 years (2, 3). This is typically influenced by biologic characteristics and social interactions.

  4. Gender role is the external manifestation of being masculine, feminine, or androgynous in a social context (2, 3). It represents what society expects of each sex and thus to some extent is fluid across time and among cultures.

  5. Sexual orientation refers to the object of an individual's sexual desire and includes the typically reported variations: heterosexual, which is attraction to only the opposite sex; homosexual, which is attraction to only the same sex; and bisexual, which is attraction to both sexes. In addition, asexuality, which is a lack of sexual attraction to either men or women, has been reported.

  6. Sexual behavior describes all the activities employed in the expression of sexual desire including fantasy and physical interaction with self and others (2). It is a combination of both psychological and physiologic components driven by internal and external stimuli (2).

B **Sexual development**

1. Although everyone has a sexual drive, its strength and manifestation vary among people and across time and situations for each person (2). In addition, the sex drive is shaped and influenced by life experiences, especially during puberty, and life stage (2).

2. **Preadolescence** includes the building of a foundation of sexual behavior. Specifically, children experience and learn about the exchange of physical touch in a nonsexual manner, which satisfies needs and provides a sense of security (2). When such experiences are affirmative, a positive self-image of one's body develops, which is a component of healthy sexual development (2). This is also the time of initial genital exploration and self-stimulation, which again if managed in a healthy manner by the child's caregivers results in appropriate sexual attitudes and behaviors (2). Modeling by adults has a strong influence on the development of multiple behaviors during childhood, including intimacy (2). Children watch, listen, and learn from the interactions of the adults in their lives, so examples of equitable verbal exchanges and physical affection will shape their future behaviors (2).

   Likewise, unhealthy experiences during childhood can lead to poor sexual self-esteem and inappropriate behaviors. Children who are victimized sexually, including both contact and noncontact behaviors, by adults and adolescents can experience premature sexualization, sexual dysfunction during adulthood, psychiatric sequelae, general behavioral problems, and even delinquent activity (2).

3. **Adolescence** is most significant in terms of sexual development and is characterized by **puberty.** The increase in circulating sex hormones and presence of secondary sex characteristics increase their attention to sexual interests (2).

   A tension is built between what adolescents are now physically capable of and the social, religious, and cultural restraints imposed on their behaviors. This tension is reduced through masturbation, which now, unlike during childhood, includes fantasies involving coitus (2). These fantasies provide an opportunity for an exploration of sexual identity without risk (2). Further exploration occurs with physical contact between persons, who may be of the same sex, the opposite sex, or both sexes unrelated to their eventual adult sexual orientation (2). It is during this stage of development that one's self-concept of body image and the opinion of same- and opposite-sex peers influence a sense of sexual competence and identity (2).

4. **Early adulthood** is marked for most, but not all, by the establishment of relationships with a sexual component (2). The sex drive is part of the impetus for such relationships (2). Once there are routine opportunities for sexual relationships with others, people give more attention to engaging in such behaviors (2). The continued use of masturbation during a sexual relationship is not an indication of pathology unless it is preferred to sexual activity with a partner or becomes compulsive (2).

   a. **Middle age** is a time of divergence in sexual desire between men and women. Men may experience a reduction in sexual desire, which has been attributed by some to an increased focus on career development and consequently less time and energy for sexual activity (2). The idealized view of sexual arousal and exchange developed during adolescence doesn't always fit the reality of the routine and predictability found in long-term relationships (2). A positive outcome of a long-term sexual relationship is an increase in comfort levels and ability to know and use one another's arousal triggers (2). Women can display an increased interest in sexual activity during this time because of a stronger interpersonal bond during a long-term relationship (2). It is likely that career pursuits can impact the time and energy for sexual activity for women as well as men.

      As middle age progresses, the biologic component of the sex drive decreases with associated physiologic manifestations. Men require greater amounts of stimulation to obtain erections and their refractory periods lengthen. With changes in hormonal levels, women also require more stimulation for physiologic arousal. Despite these changes, the reduction in childrearing responsibilities typically found at this life stage and no fear of unplanned pregnancy for women in heterosexual relationships result in more sexual activity (2).

   b. Sexual activity during **old age** continues for both men and women at a rate proportional to that during their early adulthood periods unless they lack an available partner (2). Physiologic functioning is reduced with more time to erection, less firm erections, less forceful ejaculations, reduced vaginal lubrication, and atrophy of the vagina (2).

c. **Applicability** of these findings, which are based primarily on monogamous heterosexual relationships, to nondyadic relationships and other orientations is unclear.

III SEXUAL AND GENDER IDENTITY DISORDERS

The sexual and gender identity disorders chapter of the *DSM-IV-TR* is divided into the major category headings provided below. A brief description of each based on diagnostic criteria is included. Despite being a lengthy list, not every sexual dysfunction encountered in the clinical setting is addressed in the *DSM-IV-TR*.

(A) **Sexual dysfunctions** are conditions in which the sexual response cycle is disturbed or there is pain during coitus (1). Within this category are the sexual desire, sexual arousal, orgasmic, and sexual pain disorders as follows.

1. **Hypoactive sexual desire disorder** is characterized by either a persistent or recurrent deficiency, or lack, of sexual fantasies and desire for sexual activity (1). The clinician makes the determination with consideration given to the context of the symptoms. To receive this diagnosis there must be marked distress or interpersonal difficulty from the deficiency. The dysfunction cannot be from another nonsexual Axis I disorder, a general medical diagnosis, or substance effects including those of a medication or substance of abuse.

2. **Sexual aversion disorder** is characterized by either persisting or recurring aversion leading to avoiding almost all or all genital sexual contact with others that leads to marked distress or problems with interpersonal relationships (1). The symptoms cannot be the result of another nonsexual Axis I disorder.

3. **Female sexual arousal disorder** is diagnosed when there is a persisting or recurring lack of ability to achieve or sustain sexual excitement characterized by lubrication/swelling sufficient to complete sexual activity (1). There must be marked distress or problems with interpersonal relationships and no nonsexual Axis I diagnosis, general medical diagnosis, or use of a medication or illicit substance that could account for the same symptoms.

4. **Male erectile disorder** is the inability to achieve or sustain a penile erection sufficient to complete sexual activity, and the inability must be either persistent or recurring with the result of marked distress or problems with interpersonal relationships (1). The diagnosis does not apply if there is a nonsexual Axis I disorder, use of a medication, or use of another substance that could account for the symptoms.

5. **Female orgasmic disorder** is characterized by a pattern of recurring or persistent delayed or lack of orgasm after sexual excitement and results in marked distress or interpersonal relationship problems (1). The stimulation required to facilitate orgasm varies among women and this diagnosis requires a judgment by the clinician regarding whether the ability to reach orgasm is delayed or absent based on the stimulation provided in the context of the woman's age and experience (1). The diagnosis does not apply if there is a nonsexual Axis I disorder, use of a medication, or use of another substance that could account for the symptoms.

6. **Male orgasmic disorder** is characterized by a pattern of recurring or persistent delayed or lack of orgasm after sexual excitement and results in marked distress or interpersonal relationship problems (1). The clinician must judge whether the intensity and duration of sexual activity were sufficient to result in orgasm given the man's age (1). This diagnosis does not apply if there is a nonsexual Axis I disorder, use of a medication, or use of another substance that could account for the symptoms.

7. **Premature ejaculation** is diagnosed if there is a persistent or recurring pattern of ejaculation with minimal stimulation before, during, or within a short time after penetration; ejaculation occurs before desired; and there is subsequent marked distress or negative interpersonal consequences (1). Judgment of the clinician is required to account for age, uniqueness of the sexual partner or circumstance, and time since last sexual activity (1). The diagnosis does not apply if the symptoms are the result of substance use including medications and substances of abuse.

8. **Dyspareunia** is persisting or recurring genital pain in either men or women from sexual intercourse and causes marked distress or problems with interpersonal relationships (1). The diagnosis

does not apply if more accurately explained by vaginismus, no genital lubrication, another non-sexual Axis I diagnosis, a general medical diagnosis, a medication effect, or the effect of a substance of abuse (1).

9. **Vaginismus** is a recurring or persisting involuntary muscle spasm of the outer third of the vagina that disrupts vaginal intercourse and causes marked distress or interpersonal relationship problems (1). The diagnosis does not apply if there is a nonsexual Axis I disorder that could account for the symptoms.

10. Each of the aforementioned disorders can be further classified by the following subtypes (1):
    a. **Lifelong type** is defined as starting when sexual activity started.
    b. **Acquired type** begins after there has been a period of sexual activity without the disorder symptoms.
    c. **Generalized type** occurs during all types of sexual activity and is not limited to specific types of stimulation, specific situations, or specific partners.
    d. **Situational type** only occurs with specific types of stimulation, in specific situations, or with specific partners.
    e. **Due to psychological factors** applies when in the absence of a general medical diagnosis and substance use there is the presence of psychological issues that contribute to the initiation, intensity, exacerbation, or continuance of the symptoms.
    f. **Due to combined factors** refers to situations in which both psychological issues and a general medical diagnosis or effect of substance use contribute to the sexual dysfunction, but none on their own are sufficient causes.

11. **Sexual dysfunction caused by a general medical condition** is characterized by marked distress or interpersonal relationship problems and is caused by the physiologic effects of a general medical diagnosis as identified by patient history, physical examination, or laboratory results (1). The diagnosis does not apply if the symptoms are more accurately the result of a different mental health disorder. When making this diagnosis, both the sexual disorder's name and the general medical diagnosis are to be identified.

12. **Substance-induced sexual dysfunction** is characterized by marked distress or interpersonal relationship problems caused by substance use as identified by patient history, physical examination, or laboratory results and the symptoms began during or no more than a month after substance intoxication, or a medication is known to cause the sexual symptoms (1). This diagnosis does not apply if there is a sexual disorder that is more accurately the cause or the symptoms do not exceed those typical of intoxication with the given substance(s) resulting in a need for clinical intervention (1). When giving this diagnosis both the substance and the type of impairment from the following list are to be specified: impaired desire, arousal, or orgasm or sexual pain (1).

13. **Sexual dysfunction not otherwise specified** is used when the symptoms do not meet one of the aforementioned disorders or the criteria of a specific sexual disorder have been met but it is unclear if it is primary, secondary to a general medical condition, or the result of substance use (1).

B **Paraphilias** are characterized by recurring, intense, and sexually arousing fantasies, sexual urges, or behaviors that involve nonhuman objects or the suffering or humiliation of either oneself or someone else, or children or other nonconsenting persons (1). There is a requirement that the symptoms exist over a period of at least 6 months, but they can be episodic and either required or not for sexual arousal (1). Exhibitionism, frotteurism, pedophilia, and voyeurism can be diagnosed if the urges have led to paraphilic behaviors, and sexual sadism can be diagnosed if the urges have led to behaviors with nonconsenting persons (1). The preceding can also be diagnosed if the urges or fantasies led to marked distress or interpersonal relationship problems even without actual behaviors. All the remaining listed paraphilias are diagnosed if the urges, fantasies, or behaviors cause marked distress or interpersonal relationship problems. To follow are the diagnostic criteria unique to each of the specific paraphilias and the not otherwise specified category from the *DSM-IV-TR*.

1. **Exhibitionism** is characterized by exposure of one's own genitals to an unsuspecting stranger (1).

2. **Fetishism** is characterized by arousal from nonliving items, such as female undergarments (1). This diagnosis does not apply if the use of female undergarments is more appropriately a criterion

of transvestic fetishism or if the use is of items specifically designed for sexual arousal, such as vibrators (1).

3. **Frotteurism** is characterized by touching or rubbing against a nonconsenting person (1).

4. **Pedophilia** is characterized by arousal to a prepubescent child or children for a person who is at least 16 years of age and at least 5 years older than the aforementioned child or children (1). This diagnosis does not apply to late adolescence–aged persons involved in an ongoing sexual relationship with someone who is 12 or 13 years old (1). When making this diagnosis the following should be specified as appropriate for the symptoms: attraction to females, males, or both; limited to incest; and exclusive or nonexclusive type (1). The last refers to whether the person diagnosed is only sexually attracted to prepubescent children or is also attracted to pubescent persons.

5. **Sexual masochism** is characterized by the person experiencing real acts (not simulations) of humiliation, beating, being bound, or suffering in some other way (1). Refer back to the general paraphilia criteria regarding the requirement for marked distress or interpersonal relationship problems before this diagnosis applies.

6. **Sexual sadism** is characterized by the person being sexually aroused by real and not simulated acts in which another person suffers physically or psychologically (1). Refer back to the general paraphilia criteria regarding the requirement for either marked distress or interpersonal relationship problems or behaviors focused on a nonconsenting person before this diagnosis applies.

7. **Transvestic fetishism** applies only to heterosexual men and is characterized by cross-dressing. If the person also has persisting conflict with his gender role or identity, the phrase "with gender dysphoria" is specified (1). Refer back to the general paraphilia criteria regarding requirement for marked distress or interpersonal relationship problems before this diagnosis applies.

8. **Voyeurism** is characterized by observing an unsuspecting person naked, undressing, or engaged in sexual activity (1).

9. **Paraphilia not otherwise specified** is used for paraphilias other than those specifically listed and include but are not limited (there are hundreds of paraphilias described in the literature) to the following:
   a. **Coprophilia:** arousal from feces
   b. **Klismaphilia:** arousal from enemas
   c. **Necrophilia:** arousal from corpses
   d. **Partialism:** arousal restricted to a specific body part, such as feet
   e. **Telephone scatologia:** arousal from making obscene phone calls
   f. **Urophilia:** arousal from urine
   g. **Zoophilia:** arousal from nonhuman animals

C Gender identity disorders

1. **Gender identity disorder** is characterized by persisting identification with the other gender (cross-gender), not just for what is viewed as a culturally manifested gain by being the other gender; being uncomfortable with one's current sex or a belief that one's current gender role is incorrect; and lack of a physical manifestation of intersex, which together cause marked distress or impairment in social, employment, or other major aspects of life (1).
   a. Symptoms required for the diagnosis in children include the presence of at least four of the following (1):
      (1) Recurring statements of wanting to be or being the other sex
      (2) Dressing in the clothing or appearance of clothing stereotypically worn by the other sex
      (3) Persisting fantasies of being the other sex or taking the stereotypical role of the other sex during play
      (4) Pursuit of the stereotypical activities of the other sex
      (5) Preferring playmates of the other sex
   b. Symptoms in adolescents and adults include the following (1):
      (1) Verbalizing wanting to be the other sex
      (2) Portrayal as the other sex

(**3**) Wanting to live or be treated as the other sex

(**4**) Describing having the feelings and beliefs as someone of the other sex

   c. Discomfort with being one's current sex can include for prepubescent children a desire to have the genitalia of the other sex, not wanting the sex's secondary sex characteristics when puberty starts, and avoidance of activities, toys, and clothing stereotypical of the current biologic sex. Symptoms found among adolescents and adults include wanting to get rid of primary and secondary sex characteristics or the assertion of being born with the wrong physical sex (1). The diagnosis includes gender identity disorder in children, gender identity disorder in adolescents, and gender identity disorder in adults. When diagnosing persons who have completed puberty, their sexual attraction should be specified as one of the following: to males, to females, to both, or to neither (1).

  2. **Gender identity disorder not otherwise specified** is used for gender identity disorder symptoms that do not meet the criteria of one of the specific disorders, including intersex conditions with gender dysphoria; transient, stress-related cross-dressing; and persisting obsession with being castrated or having a penectomy, but no accompanying wish for the sexual characteristics of the other sex (1).

D **Sexual disorder not otherwise specified** is used when there is a sexual issue focus that does not meet the criteria of a specific sexual disorder and is not a sexual dysfunction or paraphilia (1).

E **Diagnosis of sexual dysfunction and sexual disorders**

  1. **The sexual complaint** may be the chief complaint or discovered during elicitation of a sexual history. As with all health complaints, the following basic information should be sought:

   a. Time of onset of symptom(s)

   b. Duration of symptom(s)

   c. Frequency of symptom(s)

   d. Context of symptom(s)

   e. Mitigating factors

   f. Aggravating factors

   g. Co-occurring symptom(s)

   h. Impact on functioning

   i. Previous occurrence(s) of the symptom(s)

  2. **Sexual history** taking should be conducted during all complete history and physical examinations, during initial psychiatric evaluations, and whenever there is a complaint directly or potentially related to sexual functioning. A thorough sexual history should also be conducted in the presence of specific medical conditions in which the sequelae of the illness or side-effect profile for the treatment can result in sexual dysfunction. Topical areas for a sexual history include:

   a. Whether in a current relationship and, if yes, describe (age and sex; duration; cohabitating or not) and, if no, if there ever has been, and then the same information for each with a reason(s) for termination of the relationship(s)

   b. Biologic sex (male, female, intersex, transgender)

   c. Gender identity

   d. Sexual orientation: autosexual (self only), asexual (no drive/desire), bisexual (both same and opposite sex), heterosexual (opposite sex only), homosexual (same sex only)

   e. Age first provided with sex education information, if ever; who provided it; what was provided; reaction to the experience

   f. Onset age of puberty; first sign(s); for females, menstruation onset age; reaction

   g. Age at first sexual fantasies/thoughts; reaction; current frequency

   h. Age of onset of masturbation; highest ever frequency and at what age and duration; current frequency; ever experienced injury from masturbation

   i. Religious/cultural/other reasons against or in favor of masturbation

   j. Sexually active consensually with other(s) (any behavior); and if no, ever been sexually active; age first time; age of first-time partner; sex of first-time partner

   k. Current frequency of sexual activity with another person/other persons; desired frequency

   l. Total number of consensual sex partners; number of each sex

    m. Duration of longest sexual relationship; sex of the other person

    n. Total number of one-night stands/short-term encounters/casual sex encounters; number of each sex

    o. Current marital, partnership, committed relationship status

    p. Ever unfaithful in a committed monogamous relationship; if yes, how often; how many different partners; if partner discovered, what was his or her reaction

    q. Ever had a sexually transmitted infection (STI)/sexually transmitted disease (STD); if yes, which one(s), treatment, current status

    r. Pain during sexual activity to include masturbation and orgasm

    s. Satisfaction with current sexual functioning

    t. Satisfaction with current sexual activity frequency, content, and partner(s)

    u. Sexual dysfunction related to general medical or mental health diagnosis

    v. Sexual dysfunction from medication use, including over-the-counter and prescription medications; sexual dysfunction from substances of abuse

    w. Past treatment of sexual dysfunction or difficulty to include self-treatment and professional intervention

    x. Use of the Internet for sexual purposes: chat rooms; viewing of photographs/videos; exchange of sexual material; meeting partners; cybersex

    y. Sexual behavior resulting in difficulties socially, with relationships, with employment, and with the legal system

    z. Engagement in paraphilic fantasy and/or behavior; if yes, type(s), frequency, age of onset, impact on functioning

    aa. Engagement in consensual and/or nonconsensual violence, coercion, or manipulation; if yes, type, age of onset, frequency, impact on relationship(s), legal conflict, effect on functioning

    bb. Experienced sexual abuse, nonconsensual sexual activity, sexual coercion and/or sexual violence; if yes, frequency, age of first such experience, relationship to perpetrator(s) of abuse, legal system involvement, counseling for the abuse

    cc. Desired change in current sex life and/or sexuality

  3. Sexual history can be reviewed as a follow-up to a sexual chief complaint, as a category of questions, and as part of the review of systems in the context of the genitourinary system.

F Etiology and differential diagnosis

  1. Medications prescribed and obtained over the counter or home-made can cause sexual dysfunction or improve sexual function.

    a. Adrenergic antagonists such as those used to treat angina, arrhythmias, and hypertension can prevent penile erection, reduce ejaculation volume, cause retrograde ejaculation (into the bladder), and decrease libido for both men and women (2). For those with premature ejaculation, a usually negative side effect could prove beneficial.

    b. Anticholinergics such as benztropine can cause vaginal dryness and penile erection dysfunction (2).

    c. Antihistamines such as diphenhydramine can be sexually inhibiting because of their hypnotic side effect (2).

    d. Antianxiety medications such as benzodiazepines can improve performance anxiety but require caution given their effects on short-term memory, cognition, and motor control (2).

    e. Antipsychotic medications can have antiadrenergic and anticholinergic effects as previously described (2). Second-generation antipsychotics are less likely to cause such effects (2). Some first- and second-generation antipsychotics also pose the rare but serious side effect of priapism.

    f. Lithium, used to treat bipolar disorder, has been known to cause erectile dysfunction (2).

    g. Monoamine oxidase inhibitors (MAOIs), used to treat depression, can pose the risk of erectile dysfunction, retrograde ejaculation, delayed ejaculation, vaginal dryness, and anorgasmy (2).

    h. Psychostimulants, used to treat attention deficit hyperactivity disorder (ADHD), can increase libido for the short term and decrease libido and penile erections with long-term use (2).

    i. **Selective serotonin reuptake inhibitors (SSRIs),** used as antidepressants, can decrease libido and delay orgasm for both men and women (2).

    j. **Tetracyclic antidepressants** can cause erectile dysfunction and delayed ejaculation due to anticholinergic effects (2).

    k. **Tricyclic antidepressants** can cause erectile dysfunction and delayed ejaculation due to anticholinergic effects (2). Painful ejaculation has been reported as has increased sex drive for individual medications in this class (2).

2. **Substances of abuse** vary in their effects, with some causing only sexual dysfunction, others enhancing sexual experiences, and some causing both effects.

    a. **Alcohol** has a depressant effect on the central nervous system, thus impairing penile erections; with long-term use estrogen metabolism is decreased, leading to male feminization (2). In small quantities, it can increase testosterone levels in women, which can in turn increase libido (2).

    b. **Barbiturates** can improve sexual functioning for those with performance anxiety but pose life-threatening risk when combined with other central nervous system depressants or alcohol (2).

    c. **Benzodiazepines** are prescribed to relieve anxiety. See antianxiety medication effects in the previous section of this chapter for impact on sexual functioning.

    d. **Cannabis** can reportedly increase sexual pleasure for some, but long-term use decreases testosterone levels (2).

    e. **Hallucinogens** such as lysergic acid diethylamide (LSD), phencyclidine (PCP), and mescaline (peyote) have reportedly enhanced sexual pleasure for some and resulted in the opposite for others due to delirium and psychotic symptoms (2).

    f. **Opioids** such as heroin cause impotence and decreased libido for some and because of changes in consciousness reportedly improve sexual experiences for others (2).

3. **General medical conditions** resulting in sexual dysfunction include every major system and account for 50% to 80% of male sexual dysfunction. For men, conditions causing erectile dysfunction include mumps, atherosclerotic disease, cardiac failure, Peyronie disease, chronic renal failure, cirrhosis, respiratory failure, Klinefelter syndrome, malnutrition, vitamin deficiencies, diabetes mellitus, hyperthyroidism, multiple sclerosis, Parkinson disease, temporal lobe epilepsy, peripheral neuropathy, lead poisoning, and prostatectomy (2). Women's sexual functioning is affected by surgeries and major illness, including ones affecting body image (2). Included are hypothyroidism, diabetes mellitus, primary hyperprolactinemia, hysterectomy, and mastectomy (2).

4. **Psychiatric disorders** that are routinely associated with sexual dysfunction or performance problems include mood disorders, anxiety disorders, personality disorders, and schizophrenia (2).

G **Treatment**

1. **Sexual dysfunctions**

    a. **Evaluation** is the first, most critical step in devising a treatment plan. A complete physical examination and, if appropriate, urologic or gynecologic examinations are indicated. Substance abuse and psychiatric screening examinations are the next steps in the evaluation.

    b. **Education** may be among the most effective available treatments for general sexual dysfunctions. The clinician should gently assess the patient's knowledge of sexual function and beliefs about sex. Interventions should be tailored to the information deficits identified.

        (1) Patients may need to learn the stages of sexual arousal to solve misinterpretation problems.

        (2) A couple may need to be taught details of sexual activity to eliminate the cause of their sexual "dysfunction."

        (3) Teaching each partner about the sexual responses of both sexes often is a major step in helping couples deal with sexual dysfunction.

        (4) Desensitizing the discussion of sexual issues for individuals and couples by teaching language for discussing sex is a useful communication tool for sexual partners or for the therapist and patient.

        (5) Specific physiologic and anatomic education may be helpful for some patients. For example, some patients may not know that most women cannot have an orgasm without some clitoral stimulation. These patients can be taught that in some women, sexual positions that pull down on the labia minora can provide strong, indirect stimulation of the clitoris. Often, this type of simple suggestion solves much of a patient's or couple's sexual dysfunction.

c. **Communication training** of the couple to enable them to talk about sex and about their own wishes and needs can lead to greater intimacy. Getting both partners to agree to tell the other what they enjoy and what they find unpleasant is a critical step in working with the couple (if they can agree to express needs and wishes in a nonthreatening manner and learn to accept feedback nondefensively). Steps to better communication include the following:

(1) Exploration of cultural and religious beliefs

(2) Examination of the "goals" of sex, which can lead to a productive renegotiation of these goals

(3) Teaching the couple to talk during sex, which is often a major step in resolving minor difficulties

d. **Behavioral therapy** is another effective group of techniques for "simple" sexual dysfunctions. Behavioral interventions usually involve education and a behavioral technique designed to address a specific problem.

(1) **Relaxation training** may be helpful for both men and women whose dysfunction is related to anxiety.

(2) **Sensate focus (male).** Couples are instructed to explore noncoital caressing, focusing on the discovery and enjoyment of sensual feelings. These exercises should have a pleasuring quality rather than a demanding quality. This allows rediscovery of sensual feelings, which may have been suppressed by the sexual problem.

(a) **Managing anxiety.** Fear of failure and pressure to perform are common in men with erectile dysfunction. Prohibition of intercourse during sensate focus sessions removes this anxiety and allows the patient a feeling of success in enjoying arousal.

(b) **Regaining confidence.** As sensate focus exercises continue, the stop–start technique may be used. After the erection has occurred, the couple ceases the sexual stimulation and allows the erection to subside. They then continue the pleasurable activity, which allows recurrence of the erection. With this technique, the man gains a sense of control of his own arousal level.

(c) **Gradual resumption of coitus.** As the couple feels more confident, gradual approximation of coitus can occur. The man first achieves vaginal containment of the penis but then withdraws so that anxiety is managed and the sense of success can continue. As the couple feels confident, active thrusting can be added with stopping and starting as needed to control anxiety.

(3) **Sensate focus (female).** Exercises initially are used for the woman to explore her own sensuality. The activities are designed to progress at the patient's own rate and to be nondemanding.

(a) The woman starts by touching her skin, breasts, and genitals and noticing the pleasurable sensations. She then progresses to caressing her genitals while noting pleasurable sensations. She is then encouraged to explore clitoral and vaginal sensations and masturbation. A vibrator may be used to provide a high level of stimulation and assist in the experience of orgasm.

(b) **Anxiety management.** Prohibiting orgasm during sensate focus exercises reduces performance anxiety. Relaxation techniques, hypnosis, and, occasionally, antianxiety agents may be used.

(c) **Strengthening the pubococcygeal muscles** is associated with a high rate of orgasmic competence. This is accomplished by having the woman consciously tighten the pelvic floor muscles several times a day.

(d) **Experiencing orgasm with a partner.** After the woman has gained confidence in her ability to experience orgasm by herself, she then learns to experience it with a partner. The woman is encouraged to educate her partner about activities that she finds stimulating. She is thus given permission to obtain pleasure for herself in the relationship.

e. **Combined educational and behavioral techniques.** Most physicians use the **P-LI-SS-IT model** developed by Jack Annon for the treatment of sexual dysfunction. For several sexual dysfunctions, these techniques may be effective in approximately 90% of cases.

(1) **Permission (P).** The physician's relaxed manner and interest facilitate the discussion of sexual concerns, normalizing these concerns and providing permission to discuss them.

Approval and permission for enjoyment of sexual activity should be conveyed. The authority of the physician's role contributes to the effectiveness of this approach.

(2) **Limited information (LI).** In the many cases of sexual dysfunction that result from lack of information or misinformation about sex, the physician can reassure as well as educate the patient about "normality" by providing limited information about anatomy and physiology.

(3) **Specific suggestions (SS).** This type of intervention requires physician skill, and the level of intervention depends on the complexity of the problem. Masters and Johnson, among others, have developed therapy programs for couples that use short-term behavior approaches. After an extensive history is taken and physical and laboratory examinations are conducted, the couple is taught sensate focusing.

(4) **Intensive therapy (IT).** Patients who do not respond to the basic therapy described in permission, limited information, and specific suggestions may require psychotherapy and should be referred accordingly. In these cases, there usually are more complex problems in the relationship or associated psychopathology.

   (a) **Relationship problems** may be addressed for the individual patient through **interpersonal therapy** or **psychodynamic therapy.** Trouble with sexual relationships usually extends to other nonsexual relationships in the patient's life (e.g., a fear of abandonment may infiltrate relationships with coworkers, friends, and extended family).

   (i) The therapist may focus on overcoming the fear of abandonment by exploring past relationships, exploring feelings about current relationships, and testing the reality of assumptions about these relationships.

   (ii) Psychodynamic approaches may focus on the patient's fears and feelings about the therapist to illustrate the patient's relationship problems with people in general.

   (b) **Cognitive therapy** may be particularly useful for anxious and depressed patients, whose routine styles of thinking create a pattern of incorrect interpretations of events and expectations.

f. **Couples therapy (conjoint therapy).** As with individual psychotherapy, couples therapy has a long history of use in the treatment of sexual dysfunctions, starting with Masters and Johnson. Some of the issues that may be dealt with in couple's therapy include the following:

(1) Communication problems

(2) Conflict management, in which rules for productive arguing are set

(3) Power and control issues, which are solved by power-sharing arrangements or, if needed, individual psychotherapy

g. **Group therapy** is reported to be effective for people with sexual dysfunctions. People with similar problems gain a great deal from sharing with each other.

h. **Medications.** The section of this chapter includes reference to the use of some medications for their side-effect profile, including causing ejaculatory delay for the treatment of premature ejaculation. Other medications are used for their primary effects, which are in some cases by design.

(1) **Alprostadil** contains prostaglandin E, which is a vasodilator that relaxes penile vasculature, thus improving blood flow and in turn erection (2). Alprostadil is injected directly into the penis when an erection is planned (2).

(2) **Dopaminergic** medications such as L-dopa, bromocriptine, bupropion, and selegiline can increase libido (2).

(3) **Estrogen** replacement decreases the onset of vaginal atrophy and aids vaginal lubrication (2).

(4) **Gonadotrophin-releasing hormone (GnRH)** such as **luteinizing hormone–releasing hormone (LHRH)** causes an increase in testosterone production, which can benefit either sex when testosterone levels are low (2).

(5) **Testosterone** is used with postmenopausal women and women with otherwise low testosterone levels (2). The effect of testosterone supplementation for women and men with low levels is typically an increase in libido (2). As with most medications, caution is warranted. For men there is a risk of hypertension and prostate hypertrophy, and for women there is a risk of irreversible virilization. For both, hepatotoxicity is possible (2).

(6) Yohimbine, an α_2 antagonist, has been found to dilate the penile artery and aid erections (2).

2. **Gender identity disorders**
   a. **Psychotherapy.** Pervasive identity problems can sometimes cause confusion and doubt about sexual and gender roles.
      (1) For example, patients with borderline personality disorder may have histories of a variety of paraphilic-like behaviors and sexual dysfunctions.
      (2) In other cases, the patient may experience specific conflicts about sexuality (e.g., patients whose parents had rigid morals and condemned sex, and patients with homosexual desires who try to perform heterosexually).
      (3) In patients with **secondary gender identity disorder,** the fluctuations in the patient's dissatisfaction with his or her assigned sex allows the clinician to get a sense of the permanent versus temporary issues of the patient's gender identity.
         (a) For example, the patient may be most rejecting of his or her gender in relation to conflicts with a significant person or as a result of a depressive illness.
         (b) In such cases, helping the patient to cope better with relationships or treating the depression may give the clinician a better sense of the stable versus unstable parts of the patient's gender identity issues.
   b. **Behavioral therapies for children with primary gender identity disorder** involve a number of methods of reinforcing desired gender-specific behaviors without reinforcing nondesired behaviors.
      (1) Techniques range from therapeutic communities to specific rewards for desired behaviors.
      (2) Many of these techniques are highly effective for modifying patterns of gender-specific play and behavior. Critics argue that they may not alter "core identity" as a person of the other sex. There is little evidence that psychotherapy, pharmacotherapy, or other psychiatric interventions can reverse established patterns of gender dysphoria in people with primary gender identity disorder.
      (3) Long-term outcome data for these approaches are sparse.
   c. **Psychodynamic and psychoanalytic approaches for children with gender identity disorder** are no longer considered the preferred interventions. As noted above, the World Professional Organization for Transgender Health (4), formally known as the Harry Benjamin International Gender Dysphoria Association, provides the most widely accepted approaches to treatment.
   d. **Medication treatment** for adults with protracted gender dysphoria has not proven to be effective, and in some cases reassignment surgery is an appropriate option (2). An evaluation by a gender identity clinic and a Real Life Test of 1 to 2 years are considered requirements before such surgery is given consideration (2).
   e. **Sex reassignment surgery** is an option for some with gender identity disorder after a Real Life Test.
      (1) **Real Life Test** refers to a 1- to 2-year period of living as the opposite sex in all aspects of life (2). A period of hormonal treatment lasting at least 1 year is included, as is at least 1 year of employment or full-time student status (2). The latter ensures the ability to function as the other sex among the general public.
      (2) The literature on the postoperative adjustments of those who undergo reassignment surgery is limited by sample size and control groups. The data supporting success are greater than those describing regret, although the latter does occur (2).
      (3) The psychiatrist's role can be one of ensuring that a competent and informed decision is made free of the effects of a psychiatric illness comorbid with the gender identity disorder. In addition, there is a role for the psychiatrist in assessing the likelihood of a positive adjustment outcome, preparation for the risks of side effects from hormonal treatment, and management of those persons who only want or can only afford to undergo the hormonal treatment phase of the reassignment process.

3. **Paraphilias.** Treatment success varies with the intensity of the behavior, effort of the patient to engage in treatment, and treatment modalities employed.
   a. **Psychodynamic and psychoanalytic approaches** do not seem to provide significant results in patients with paraphilias.

b. **Behavioral therapies** consisting of aversive conditioning (i.e., pairing a noxious odor with a deviant stimulus), satiation therapy (i.e., overstimulation of deviant stimuli until exhaustion), and covert sensitization (i.e., matching early cues with severe consequences) are the predominant methods.

c. **Cognitive therapies** focus on changing thought processes and patterns that lead to paraphilic behavior (5).

d. **The Relapse Prevention Model** and similar approaches have resulted in effective therapy and lowered recidivism rates (6–9). There has been considerable debate as to the effectiveness of this method (10, 11).

e. **The Good Lives Model** is an approach that is more comprehensive in scope by including the assessment and subsequent treatment of coterminous personal deficits (i.e., socialization skills, intimacy deficits, decision-making skills, excellence in work and play) (12).

f. **Objective measures** including penile plethysmography, which is the measurement of penile engorgement during auditory and/or visual stimuli representing healthy versus abusive sexual and/or violent behaviors (13), and visual reaction time, which is the covert measurement of viewing time per categories of static visual stimuli (14), facilitate the determination of sexual arousal patterns and interests. For women, vaginal photoplethysmography involves the use of light to measure vaginal blood flow as a measure of sexual arousal. It is typically only utilized in research settings. Viewing time measurement can also be used with women.

g. **Pharmacologic treatments** currently employed include antiandrogens, antigonadotropics, and SSRIs.

   (1) **Antiandrogens** decrease androgen levels at their target sites (15, 16) and block the action of androgens (16). The effects are a reduction to complete cessation of sexual fantasies and decreased sperm synthesis, ejaculate, and penile erections (15). Pure antiandrogens include cyproterone (17) and flutamide (15), and major antigonadotropics include cyproterone acetate (CPA) (16, 18–21) and medroxyprogesterone acetate (MPA) (15, 16, 19, 21). CPA is not available in the United States. MPA, a synthetic progestin (22), increases testosterone-A-reductase activity (15) and in turn decreases testosterone blood levels (22).

   (2) **GnRH agonists** (15, 19–21) such as **LHRH agonists** (15, 20, 21) are also employed. LHRH ethylamide, which interferes with the hypothalamic–pituitary axis by blocking secretion of gonadotropins, decreases sexual desire and in turn sexual intercourse (15). Leuprolide acetate, a synthetic analog of LHRH used to treat prostate cancer, decreases pituitary–gonadal function and testicular steroidogenesis, thus lowering testosterone level (24).

   (3) **SSRIs** have also been used to treat paraphilic behavior, but with less success and significantly less supporting scientific literature. Efficacy has been difficult to determine from published studies because of heterogeneous samples, small sample sizes, and varied outcome measures. SSRIs have been recommended for use with compulsive sexual behaviors and suggested to be avoided in cases of sexual sadism and pedophilia (25). The data supporting SSRI use for treatment of paraphilias are retrospective and minimal (21).

h. **Multimodal treatment** currently is the treatment of choice for patients with paraphilias.

   (1) The Standards of Care as established by the Association for the Treatment of Sexual Abusers is considered the most effective approach for the treatment of paraphilic behaviors (26).

   (2) There are services available for persons with paraphilias who have not offended or been arrested through organizations that support primary prevention strategies, defined as treatment and support before an offense occurs (27, 28).

   (3) Treatment should be multimodal and address comorbid psychiatric diagnoses and lack of social skills and provide empathy training, cognitive restructuring, and supportive group therapies.

   (4) Treatment outcomes are difficult to assess because data collected for recidivism often have only a single source (i.e., documented criminal reoffending) and there are differing definitions of recidivism depending on the study.

   (5) Although there is overlap, the treatment for adolescents differs considerably from treatment for adults and is beyond the scope of this chapter (29).

<table>
<tr><td>**IV**</td><td>**CRITERIA SETS UNDER STUDY IN THE *DSM-IV-TR*
AND DIAGNOSES BEING CONSIDERED FOR THE *DSM-V***</td></tr>
</table>

A **Premenstrual dysphoric disorder** is among those symptom sets included for further study at the time the *DSM-IV-TR* was completed. The following symptoms occur during the last week of the luteal phase and the symptoms are gone by the week after menses for most menstrual cycles during a year (1).

1. Premenstrual dysphoric disorder is characterized by at least one of the following symptoms:
   a. Depressed mood, sense of hopelessness, or self-deprecation
   b. Anxiety or tension
   c. Labile affect
   d. Persisting anger or irritability

2. At least four (or less if more than one of the preceding is present) of the following symptoms are present:
   a. Reduced interest in typical activities
   b. Poor concentration by self-report
   c. Low energy level
   d. Overeating or food cravings
   e. Sleep disturbed by hypersomnia or insomnia
   f. Feeling overwhelmed
   g. Physical symptoms such as breast tenderness, breast swelling, headache, weight gain, bloating sensation, joint pain, or muscle pain

3. The symptoms interfere with work, school, social activity, or interpersonal relationships and are not symptoms of another disorder (1). To render the diagnosis, data must be collected prospectively on a daily basis for a minimum of two consecutive cycles with symptoms (1).

B **Diagnoses under consideration for the *Diagnostic and Statistical Manual of Mental Disorders*, fifth edition (*DSM-V*),** include changes to several existing diagnoses and the following new ones:

1. **Hypersexual disorder** is proposed to be characterized by the same basic *DSM-IV-TR* paraphilia criteria of 6 months of recurring and intense sexual fantasies, urges, or behaviors, which result in marked distress or impaired life functioning and are associated with three out of five of the following, which are recurring: time engaged in the aforementioned interferes with nonsexual responsibilities; fantasies, urges, or behaviors are a reaction to a dysphoric mood or life stressor; there have been repeated failed attempts to reduce the fantasies, urges, or behaviors; and one ignores physical or emotional risk to self or others (30). This diagnosis will not apply if the aforementioned are secondary to a medication or substance of abuse. If this becomes an official diagnosis, it will also require one of the following to be specified (30):
   a. Masturbation
   b. Pornography
   c. Sexual behavior with consenting adults
   d. Cybersex
   e. Telephone sex
   f. Strip clubs
   g. Other

2. **Coercive paraphilic disorder** has been proposed to be characterized as recurring, intense, sexually arousing fantasies or urges about sexual coercion, occurring during a period of at least 6 months, which results in distress or impairment, or the person being diagnosed has pursued sexual arousal by forcing sexual activity on three or more persons during separate incidents (31). This diagnosis will not apply if the person to be diagnosed meets criteria for a sexual sadism diagnosis (31). A variation is for coercive paraphilia to be a specifier of sexual sadism (31).

BIBLIOGRAPHY

1. American Psychiatric Association Task Force on DSM-IV: *Diagnostic and Statistical Manual of Mental Disorders,* 4th ed., text revision. Washington, DC, American Psychiatric Association, 2000.
2. Sadock VA: Normal human sexuality and sexual and gender identity disorders. In *Kaplan & Sadock's: Comprehensive Textbook of Psychiatry,* Vol I, 8th ed. Philadelphia, Lippincott Williams & Wilkins, 2005, pp 1902–2001.
3. Yates A: Childhood sexuality. In *Child and Adolescent Psychiatry: A Comprehensive Textbook.* Edited by Lewis M. Philadelphia, Lippincott Williams & Wilkins, 2002, pp 274–286.
4. WPATH: Standards of care, 1998. Available at: http://www.wpath.org. Accessed May 30, 2010.
5. Laws DR, Marshall WL: A brief history of behavioral and cognitive behavioral approaches to sexual offender treatment: Part 1. Early developments. *Sex Abuse* 15:75–92, 2003.
6. Andrews D, Bonta J: *The Psychology of Criminal Conduct,* 2nd ed. Cincinnati, Anderson Publishing, 1998.
7. Hanson RK, Gordon A, Harris AJR, et al: First report of the collaborative outcome data project on the effectiveness of psychological treatment for sex offenders. *Sex Abuse* 14:169–194, 2002.
8. Hollin CR: Treatment programs for offenders: Meta-analysis, "what works" and beyond. *Int J Law Psychiatry* 22:361–372, 1999.
9. McGuire J: Criminal sanctions versus psychologically-based interventions with offenders: A comparative empirical analysis. *Psychology Crime Law* 8:183–208, 2002.
10. Hanson RK, Gordon A, Harris AJR, et al: First report of the collaborative outcome data project on the effectiveness of psychological treatment for sex offenders. *Sex Abuse* 14:169–194, 2002.
11. Dowden C, Antonowicz D, Andrews D: The effectiveness of relapse prevention with offenders: A meta-analysis. *Int J Offender Ther Comp Criminol* 47(5):516–528, 2003.
12. Ward T, Mann RE, Gannon TA: The good lives model of offender rehabilitation: Clinical implications. *Aggression Violent Behav* 12:87–107, 2007.
13. Marshall WL, Fernandez YM: Phallometry in forensic practice. *J Forensic Psychol Pract* 1(2):77–87, 2001.
14. Abel G, Lawry S, Karlstrom E, et al: Screening test for pedophilia. *Crim Justice Behav* 21:115–131; 1994.
15. American Psychiatric Association Task Force on Sexually Dangerous Offenders: *Dangerous Sex Offenders: A Task Force Report of the American Psychiatric Association.* Washington, DC, American Psychiatric Association, 1999.
16. Freund K: Therapeutic sex drive reduction. *Acta Psychiatr Scand* 287(suppl, 62):1–39, 1980.
17. Bradford J, Pawlak A: Double-blind placebo crossover study of cyproterone acetate in the treatment of the paraphilias. *Arch Sex Behav* 22(5):383–403, 1993.
18. Bancroft J, Tennent G, Loucas K, et al: The control of deviant sexual behaviour by drugs: I. Behavioural changes following oestrogens and anti-androgens. *Br J Psychiatry* 125:310–315, 1974.
19. Bradford J: Treatment of men with paraphilia. *N Engl J Med* 338(7):464–465, 1998.
20. Grossman LS, Martis B, Fichtner CG: Are sex offenders treatable? A research overview. *Psychiatr Serv* 50(3): 349–361, 1999.
21. Saleh FM, Grudzinskas Jr AJ, Bradford JM, Brodsky DJ. Eds. Sex offenders identification, risk assessment, treatment and legal issues. New York, NY, Oxford Press. 2009.
22. Berlin F, Schaerf F: Laboratory assessment of the paraphilias and their treatment with antiandrogenic medication. In *Handbook of Psychiatric Diagnostic Procedures,* Vol 2. Edited by Hall R, Beresford T. Hicksville, NY, Spectrum Publications, Inc., 1985.
23. Miethe T, McCorkle R: *Crime Profiles,* 2nd ed. Los Angeles, Roxbury Publishing Co., 2001.
24. Gratzer T: Treatment of sex offenders with leuprolide acetate. *American Academy of Psychiatry and the Law Newsletter* 28(2):10–11, 2003.
25. Saleh FM: Serotonin reuptake inhibitors and the paraphilias. *American Academy of Psychiatry and the Law Newsletter* 29(3):12–13, 2004.
26. Association for the Treatment of Sexual Abusers: *Association for the Treatment of Sexual Abusers: Standards of Care.* Beaverton, OR, Association for the Treatment of Sexual Abusers, 2001.
27. *Stop It Now!* Available at: http://www.Stopitnow.com. Accessed May 30, 2010.
28. *Texas Association Against Sexual Assault.* Available at: http://www.TAASA.org. Accessed May 30, 2010.
29. Ryan G, Lane S: *Juvenile Sexual Offending: Causes, Consequences, and Correction.* Hoboken, NJ, John Wiley & Sons, 1997.
30. Kafka MP. Hypersexual disorder: A proposed diagnosis for DSM-V. *Arch Sex Behav* 39:377–400, 2010.
31. Thornton D: Evidence regarding the need for a diagnostic category for a coercive paraphilia. *Arch Sex Behav* 39:411–418, 2010.

Study Questions

Directions: *Each of the numbered items or incomplete statements in this section is followed by answers or by completions of the statement. Select the ONE lettered answer or completion that is BEST in each case.*

1. A 38-year-old man presents to his family physician complaining that he has had no interest in sex for the past 4 months. There have been no significant changes in his life circumstances in the past year (e.g., divorce, death in the family, loss of job). With no additional information, what is the most likely cause of this patient's loss of interest in sex?

[A] Generalized anxiety disorder
[B] Major depressive episode
[C] Paranoid schizophrenia
[D] Personality disorder
[E] Sexual aversion disorder   *must r/o Axis I first*

2. A 47-year-old woman presents to her primary care physician complaining of pain during intercourse. The pain has become increasingly problematic over the last 6 months. What should be the first item in the differential diagnosis?

[A] Atrophic vaginitis
[B] Dyspareunia
[C] Major depression
[D] Somatization disorder
[E] Vaginismus

3. A 25-year-old man is brought to the emergency room by the police. He has been rubbing his penis against unsuspecting young women in the subway. He was apprehended by the police, admitted this was not the first occasion during the last year, and became suicidal, saying that his arrest would ruin his job and his relationship with his family. What is the most likely diagnosis?

[A] Frotteurism
[B] Major depression
[C] Paraphilia not otherwise specified
[D] Pedophilia
[E] Voyeurism - *no physical contact*

4. A 30-year-old man presents with a 15-year history of dressing in women's clothing in order to become sexually aroused. He reports being comfortable with his male gender identity. What is the most likely diagnosis?

[A] Gender dysphoria
[B] Gender identity disorder
[C] Paraphilia
[D] Transsexualism
[E] Transvestic fetishism

5. Which one of the following reactions is associated with the resolution phase of sexual response?

[A] Erection of the penis begins.
[B] The refractory period occurs.
[C] The clitoris becomes engorged with blood.
[D] Vaginal lubrication begins.
[E] The vaginal walls contract.

QUESTIONS 6–10

Match each of the possible effects with the corresponding medication or other substance most likely responsible for the effect.

- [A] Alcohol
- [B] Benztropine
- [C] Antihypertensive
- [D] Selective serotonin reuptake inhibitor
- [E] Antipsychotic

6. Increased time to ejaculation ~~B~~ D

7. Vaginal dryness B ← *weird b/c I thought Benz's made vaginal wetness...*

8. Priapism E

9. Decrease libido C

10. Decreased erectile function in males ~~D~~ A   *whiskey dick*

QUESTIONS 11–15

11. Providing treatment and intervention for persons with paraphilias <u>before</u> they commit a sexual crime is known as:

- [A] Relapse prevention
- [B] Primary prevention
- [C] Group therapy
- [D] The Good Lives Model

12. Which of the following objective measures is not typically utilized outside of research studies?

- [A] Penile plethysmography
- [B] Vaginal photoplethysmography
- [C] Viewing time measures
- [D] Polygraphy

13. Aversion therapy involves:

- [A] Showing the patient videos depicting the negative consequences of paraphilic behavior
- [B] Overstimulation of deviant stimuli until exhaustive satiation
- [C] Matching a noxious odor with a deviant stimulus
- [D] None of the above

14. Which of the following treatment interventions is considered the <u>least</u> <u>effective</u> in the treatment of paraphilic behavior?

- [A] Covert sensitization
- [B] Aversion therapy
- [C] Psychodynamic therapy
- [D] Cognitive therapy

15. An adult male patient reports that he has always felt like he should have been a woman. He frequently dresses in women's clothes and reports feeling considerably better when he does so. Which organization would be the best choice to refer him to for treatment guidelines?

- [A] World Professional Organization for Transgender Health
- [B] The Harry Benjamin International Gender Dysphoria Association
- [C] The Association for the Treatment of Sexual Abusers
- [D] Stop It Now!

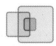

Answers and Explanations

1. The answer is B [*III A 2*]. A major depressive episode is the most likely etiology for reduced libido given the recent onset and no major life events. Sexual aversion disorder cannot be diagnosed until other Axis I disorders are ruled out.

2. The answer is A [*III A 8–9*]. Given the population frequency and the patient's age, menopause is a likely diagnosis as an etiology for the woman's decreased circulating estrogen causing atrophic vaginitis. A pelvic examination will be required before making a definitive diagnosis because a neoplasm or other disease process could also cause pain. Dyspareunia and vaginismus require exclusion of general medical conditions prior to final diagnosis. Dyspareunia can be a symptom of somatization disorder but is unlikely to be a late-onset symptom, and there are no data supporting the multiple physical complaints found with somatization disorder.

3. The answer is A [*III B 3*]. This case most closely describes the diagnosis of frotteurism. Voyeurism involves watching unsuspecting persons and does not involve physical contact. A major depressive disorder is an unlikely etiology given the lack of depression symptoms prior to the behavior and subsequent arrest. His suicidal ideations are likely the result of his perception of the legal and social consequences, but nevertheless must be addressed as life threatening.

4. The answer is E [*III B 7*]. Transvestic fetishism typically begins with the onset of puberty and includes sexual fantasies and urges to dress in stereotypical female clothing. Transvestic fetishism is a paraphilia and as such requires a minimum 6-month period during which symptoms occur, but of the choices this is the most likely diagnosis. Gender identity disorder and gender dysphoria are incorrect because there is no discomfort with gender identity. Transsexualism is incorrect because there is no desire to be female.

5. The answer is B [*I B 4*]. The refractory period begins for males after orgasm. Penile erection and engorgement of the clitoris with blood begin during the excitement phase. The vaginal walls contract during the orgasm phase.

6–10. The answers are 6-D, 7-B, 8-E, 9-C, and 10-A [*III F*]. Selective serotonin reuptake inhibitor can increase time to ejaculation through their serotonergic effects. Vaginal dryness has been reported with benztropine, and priapism has been reported with some antipsychotic medications. Use of antihypertensive medications can lead to decreased libido. Alcohol use can cause erectile dysfunction through its depressant effect on the central nervous system.

11–15. The answers are 11-B, 12-B, 13-C [*III B*]**, 14-C, and 15-A** [*III G*].

chapter 10

Eating Disorders

NIOAKA N. CAMPBELL

Eating disorders are defined as severe disturbances in eating behavior in the *Diagnostic and Statistical Manual of Mental Disorders,* 4th edition, text revision (*DSM-IV-TR*), and include anorexia nervosa, bulimia nervosa, and eating disorder not otherwise specified (1).

I   **ANOREXIA NERVOSA**

Anorexia nervosa is an eating disorder characterized by a refusal to maintain a minimally normal body weight, fears and preoccupations with gaining weight, and a disturbance of body image.

A **Diagnostic criteria (Table 10–1)**

B **Epidemiology**

1. **Onset.** The average age of onset of the illness is 17 years in women and 18 years in men, with the most common age being between 15 and 19 years. The onset may be preceded by a period of mild obesity or mild dieting (2).

2. **Incidence and prevalence.** Anorexia is estimated to occur in 1% of adolescent girls. Recent community-based studies show a prevalence ratio of 2:1 or 3:1 for women to men, a much narrower margin than the 20:1 previously reported in clinical trials. It is more frequent in developed countries. Whites tend to have the highest rate of occurrence. The disorder is more often found in higher socioeconomic classes and among young women in professions such as modeling and dance that require thinness (3).

C **Clinical features and associated findings**

1. **Behavioral features** are varied but commonly include:
   a. Overactivity
   b. Obsessions and rituals connected with food and food preparation
   c. Purging (self-induced vomiting), diuretic or laxative abuse
   d. Secretiveness
   e. Extreme behavioral rigidity and inflexibility
   f. Preoccupations and distortions regarding body image and weight (4)

2. **Associated findings** that accompany the illness are listed in Table 10–2. In general, these findings reflect metabolic slowing, fluid and electrolyte disturbances, alterations in multiple endocrinologic axes, and organic brain symptoms (3–4).

3. **Comorbidity** with other psychiatric disorders is common with anorexia nervosa.
   a. **Depression** is associated in approximately 60% to 65% of patients with anorexia.
   b. **Phobic disorders** are associated in approximately 43% of cases.
   c. **Anxiety disorders** are associated in up to 65% of cases.
   d. **Obsessive-compulsive disorder (OCD)** is associated with 14% of the restrictive and 56% of the binge/purge types of anorexia nervosa, respectively. Perfectionistic traits in other areas of life may overlap with compulsivity in eating behavior as well (3).

TABLE 10–1 *DSM-IV-TR* Diagnostic Criteria for Anorexia Nervosa

Refusal to maintain weight at or above minimal weight for age and height (85% of ideal body weight or developmentally expected body weight)

Fear of gaining weight or becoming obese, even when significantly underweight

Disturbed body image, such that appropriate body weight is perceived as excessive or low body weight is perceived as appropriate

Amenorrhea in postmenarchal women (absence of at least three consecutive menstrual cycles)

Two distinct types:

Restricting: Weight maintained largely by caloric restriction

Bingeing/purging: Both binge eating and purging (vomiting; use of laxatives, diuretics, enemas) occur during the current episode

Reprinted with permission from the Diagnostic and Statistical Manual of Mental Disorders, Fourth Edition, Text Revision, (Copyright 2000). American Psychiatric Association.

4. **Clinical subtypes.** There are two identifiable subtypes recognized by the *DSM-IV-TR*, both with specific historic and clinical features.

   a. The **binge eating–purging type** exists in up to 50% of individuals with anorexia nervosa. These individuals may have a history of a heavier body weight as well as family members who are obese. Patients may be more extroverted or present with the disorder later in life. This type is more likely to be associated with substance use, impulse control, and personality disorders. **Suicide** is higher in these patients than in the restricting subtype. Some patients may purge without binge eating.

   b. The **restricting** subtype is characterized by strict self-starvation and calorie restriction. Obsessive-compulsive traits may often be associated with food and preparation. Individuals with both subtypes may exercise excessively (1, 3–5).

5. **Medical complications.** See Table 10–3.

D **Etiology and pathogenesis**   Although no single cause is known, biologic and psychosocial factors are implicated in the etiology of anorexia nervosa.

1. **Biologic factors** include comorbidities with certain mental disorders, neuroendocrine abnormalities, and genetic factors. Dieting itself is a biologic vulnerability relating to the results of undernutrition.

   a. **Mental illnesses** such as unipolar and bipolar mood disorders occur at an increased rate in anorectic patients. These illnesses tend to occur later in life and are not causative of anorexia nervosa. As already noted (1 C 4 a), there is a higher rate of suicide in specific subtypes of anorexia.

   b. **Neuroendocrine dysfunction**

      (1) **Alterations in catecholamine activity** within the central nervous system (CNS) may account for some of the clinical features of the illness. Because most of these changes normalize after weight gain, causality is difficult to determine.

      (2) **Hypothalamic–pituitary axis dysfunction** may account for some of the endocrine abnormalities that occur in individuals with anorexia. Serotonin, dopamine, and norepinephrine are neurotransmitters involved in the hypothalamus associated with eating behaviors.

TABLE 10–2 Associated Findings in Anorexia Nervosa

Peripheral edema

Lanugo hair development

Skin changes (dryness, scaling, yellow tinge caused by carotinemia)

Lowered metabolic rate (bradycardia, hypotension, hypothermia)

Normal thyroid-stimulating hormone levels; low triiodothyronine (T_3) syndrome

Normal or overstimulated adrenal axis; possible loss of diurnal variation in cortisol

Normal serum protein and albumin concentrations

Impaired regulation in growth hormone levels; increased basal levels

Decreased total brain volume/increased ventricular size on imaging

TABLE 10–3	Medical Complications of Anorexia Nervosa

Organic brain symptoms (cognitive slowing, apathy, dysphoria)
Gastric dilatation and rupture if bingeing and purging
Constipation, bloating, abdominal pain
Hematologic changes (anemia, leukopenia)
Endocrinologic changes, cold intolerance
Menstrual irregularities, amenorrhea
Electrocardiogram changes
Osteoporosis
Cachexia (loss of fat and muscle mass, inability to maintain core temperature)

(3) **Other factors** that may be involved include corticotrophin-releasing factor (CRF), neuropeptide Y, thyroid-stimulating hormone, and gonadotropin-releasing hormone.

c. **Genetic studies** involving twin pairs suggest heritability in the transmission of anorexia nervosa. A review of clinic-based samples revealed concordance rates of 50% to 80% in monozygotic twins. The ratio of monozygotic to dizygotic twins is 3:1. Molecular genetic research shows initial promise in the importance of serotonin mechanisms and gene polymorphisms. Population studies show that genetics contributes 50% to the appearance of eating disorders (3, 5).

2. **Psychological factors** include proposed theories in the etiology of anorexia nervosa.

a. **Fear of sexuality** is a classic theory that holds that anorectic patients fear impregnation and fantasize that impregnation may occur orally. Therefore, they defend themselves by not eating. A corollary with this theory is that affected adolescents starve themselves to remain prepubertal for fear of sexuality, menarche, and pregnancy.

b. **Mood and anxiety disorders** and perfectionist personality traits are vulnerability factors in the development of anorexia nervosa. **Temperament** is a factor that may be associated in the etiology of anorexia. Many anorectics are high achievers with above-average intelligence. They may tend toward rigid self-control and affective constriction. Interpersonal conflict is more likely expressed through passive-aggressive modalities than through direct confrontation.

c. **Dysfunctional family** dynamics may involve the **family system model** that considers parent–child interactions and asserts that family systems seek to maintain equilibrium. Changes in any part of the system cause disequilibrium and require compensatory changes elsewhere. An adolescent's attempt to begin the process of separation and emancipation in an overinvolved family or to exert developmentally appropriate autonomy and self-control in a rigid, autocratic family is seen as disrupting the family system. Therefore, the regression of the child from normal adolescent strivings to a preadolescent developmental posture (through the symptoms of anorexia nervosa) represents an accommodation within the family system. The influence of a specific family functioning style as a predisposing risk factor is controversial. However, nonspecific stresses, such as negative blame or criticism, may add to vulnerability.

d. **Media** and **societal roles** may psychologically contribute to overvaluation of thinness and dieting. Whether these factors influence the prevalence of eating disorders remains controversial (3, 5).

3. **Racial/ethnic factors** offer no protection or predisposition to anorexia nervosa except within subgroups who historically promote weight loss or change. Gay men have been shown to be predisposed to anorexia while lesbian women may be slightly protected from the illness. This is not because of their sexual orientation per se, but because of the norms for slimness within these groups (3).

E Differential diagnosis

1. **Medical conditions.** The differential diagnosis for unexplained weight loss in adolescence includes several medical conditions. An adequate medical assessment for illnesses that may account for weight loss must include consideration of the following:

a. **Addison disease** may present as weight loss, anorexia (loss of appetite), vomiting, and electrolyte and endocrine abnormalities (low sodium concentration, high potassium concentration, and suppressed serum cortisol levels). Listlessness and depression are common findings, in contrast to the hyperactivity of anorexia nervosa.

    b. **Hypothyroidism** may present as intolerance to cold, constipation, bradycardia, low blood pressure, and skin changes similar to those seen in anorexia nervosa (i.e., dry, scaling skin). Obsessional food handling, weight loss (and accompanying fear of weight gain), and hyperactivity are not usual, however.

    c. **Hyperthyroidism** presents as elevated vital signs, hyperactivity, and sometimes weight loss. However, patients with hyperthyroidism are usually not obsessive about food.

    d. **Any chronic illness** (e.g., Crohn disease, ulcerative colitis, rheumatoid arthritis, tuberculosis) can cause progressive weight loss but should be readily identifiable as a physical disorder.

    e. **Neoplasms, especially CNS tumors** (e.g., tumors of the hypothalamus or third ventricle), can cause endocrine malfunction with accompanying weight loss of either a primary or secondary nature. Other symptoms of the tumor, such as visual disturbances or panhypopituitarism, should be evident.

    f. **Superior mesenteric artery syndrome** can cause vomiting and anorexia. The mechanism apparently involves compression of the duodenum by the superior mesenteric artery, particularly when the patient is supine and especially in individuals who are thin. When found concomitantly with anorexia nervosa, it is often difficult to ascertain whether superior mesenteric artery syndrome is primary (causative) or secondary to the weight loss of anorexia nervosa (4, 5).

2. **Psychiatric conditions**

    a. **Schizophrenia.** Although individuals with schizophrenia may be delusional about food, the delusions are more bizarre than those seen in individuals with anorexia (e.g., "There's poison in this" versus "This will make me fat"). Other features of schizophrenia should be present.

    b. **Bulimia nervosa** involves binge eating, usually followed by some form of purging, in a patient who otherwise maintains a normative weight. Patients with bulimia rarely lose 15% of their body weight.

    c. **Depression** often is accompanied by anorexia. In this case, the anorexia is a so-called "vegetative" sign of depression, and a depressed mood is usually pronounced.

    d. **Anxiety disorders** can be present before or after the occurrence of an eating disorder. **OCD** comorbidity occurs in 15% to 25% of patients with anorexia, but can also be a separate disorder. The symptomatology of OCD involves ego-dystonic thoughts or behaviors that create anxiety if resisted.

    e. **Substance use disorders** can lead to significant weight loss. The use of stimulants or other substances should be assessed as part of the differential diagnosis (3).

F Treatment

1. **Medical assessment** and treatment of the anorectic patient must consider the potentially lethal complications of starvation such as metabolic disturbances, fluid and electrolyte disturbances, and cardiac arrhythmias. Management should always begin with the assessment and treatment of these potentially life-threatening medical complications. Only when medical stability has been attained does treatment for the underlying psychological disorder begin. Outcomes are shown to be better for patients treated in specialty eating disorder units. **Weight restoration** is the initial short-term goal, with the ideal being a weight in which normal sexual physiology and function returns. Supervised refeeding and the cessation of compulsive exercising or other detrimental behaviors are treatment strategies (3–8).

2. **Screening tools** have been developed, including the Eating Attitudes Test (EAT) and the SCOFF (acronym based on questions). These tools have shown some success in epidemiologic studies regarding identification and assessment (3–8).

3. **Psychotherapeutic modalities**

    a. **Individual psychotherapy** is a useful adjunct to other treatment modalities but is rarely effective alone. **Psychoanalysis** can be particularly ineffective in patients with anorexia nervosa. Such therapies can foster a regression in patients, which, in treatment, is useful only when the patient has the ability and strength to pull out of the regression at the end of the session.

       (1) Initially, therapeutic work should be aimed at forming an alliance with the patient to work on particular problems. The focus need not include weight or eating habits as long as physiologic stability is maintained.

(2) Gaps in the patient's ego should be clarified. For example, when the patient is obviously angry about something but is unaware of this, the isolation of affect may be addressed.

(3) Transference reactions should be interpreted if and when they interfere with the patient's ability to work out and talk about problems.

(4) An empathic stance should be maintained with the patient at the same time that issues of physiologic stability and compliance with medical treatment are treated as nonnegotiable. A close partnership must be maintained among the patient, the psychiatrist, and the primary care physician in the collaborative management of these patients.

b. Cognitive behavioral therapy (CBT) as an adjunct can be used in the treatment of anorexia nervosa, although no large sample size studies have yet shown effectiveness in this illness. Monitoring feelings of food, intake, feelings, emotions, relationships, and behaviors is essential. Cognitive restructuring identifies automatic thoughts and core beliefs, and behavioral problem solving for coping strategies replaces former maladaptive patterns.

c. Group therapy. Peer interaction and feedback should be sought and emphasized because adolescents often pay more attention to their peers than to adults. Adolescents respond to peers with more trust and less suspicion, such that the perception of empathy is enhanced. In addition, the realization that others share the same symptoms helps adolescents feel less isolated.

d. Family therapy. Some form of **family intervention is nearly always indicated,** especially for adolescents. Styles of family interaction should be clarified and family members' roles in addressing the patient's symptoms should be interpreted and restructured. Individual therapy for either or both of the parents may be indicated; when marital issues contribute to the symptomatology of the child, marital therapy for the parents may also be indicated. Parent education concerning the normal developmental tasks and transitions of adolescence may be necessary. In general, the family should be allied with the staff, working toward patient improvement (3–9).

e. Hospitalization. In some cases, the patient cannot be treated effectively within the home environment and adequate, less restrictive alternatives are not available. **Out-of-home placement** is indicated if the patient loses weight despite outpatient intervention, if the patient is suicidal, or if vomiting and purging is causing serious medical complications.

(1) Therapeutic approach reflects the understanding that individuals with anorexia have a propensity to deny and conceal the severity of their condition.

(a) Careful attention must be paid to the **accuracy of weight measurements.** Serial weights should be obtained at the same time of day, on the same scale, in the same garb (preferably a hospital gown only), and after voiding. Attempts to pad weight artificially by drinking large quantities or concealing objects on the body are typical.

(b) Splitting (pitting one staff member against another) and manipulations concerning eating are common and should be discussed at staff meetings and with the patient. Flexibility among members of the treatment team with regard to the treatment plan is important.

(2) Behavioral techniques may be necessary with refractory adolescents.

(a) The patient should be **weighed every other day.** Urine should be **monitored regularly for ketones,** sometimes as often as daily before every meal.

(b) Supervised refeeding or alimentation should be provided, even by a nasogastric tube if the patient steadfastly refuses to eat, and should be readministered if the food is vomited. **Hyperalimentation** may be provided through a central intravenous line if these measures fail.

(c) Patient privileges (e.g., freedom to leave the ward versus confinement in a locked unit) should be tied to the behavioral approach and commensurate with the patient's ability to regulate activity and eating. Such a program may take the following form:

(i) The patient's weight should be the target symptom. Reinforcers should be tied to weight fluctuation.

(ii) As soon as the patient is stable medically and has some weight reserve, urine can be monitored for ketones before every meal as part of a behavioral treatment approach. Monitoring ketones provides information about starvation state, provides the patient with immediate feedback, and offers the opportunity to alter the starvation state immediately. If the patient's urine contains ketones, activities and privileges should be completely restricted until urine reverts to normal (3–8).

f. Medications. There is no pharmacologic treatment established for anorexia nervosa. Medications may be useful therapeutic adjuncts, but only when targeted at specific, underlying symptoms.

(1) **Cyproheptadine** may be of value due to appetite-stimulating properties.

(2) **Antidepressants** may be beneficial when depressive symptoms are prominent. Fluoxetine has been shown to reduce relapse and maintain weight, but only after weight is restored. Further studies are needed in this area.

(3) Prominent anxiety symptoms should be treated with **anxiolytics.**

(4) When eating and food preparation are excessively ritualized or other symptoms of OCD are present, medications to target these symptoms may prove beneficial.

(5) Because of potentially severe side effects, **antipsychotic medication** should be used only when the patient suffers from a psychotic illness.

(6) In cases of anorexia associated with major depression, some studies have shown improvement with electroconvulsive therapy (ECT) (3–8).

G Prognosis On average, 30% of patients will have a relatively complete recovery; 30% will demonstrate partial improvement; 30% will continue to demonstrate a chronic disease course; and 10% will die. About half of patients will have some symptoms of bulimia during their illness.

1. **Positive prognostic indicators** include onset in the early teens to midteens, decreased denial of a problem, attainment of a normal weight posthospitalization, participation in intensive follow-up treatment, and less psychiatric comorbidity.

2. **Negative prognostic indicators** include a long disease course, high rates of psychiatric comorbidities, family conflict, and very young onset or onset before age 25 years.

3. **Mortality rates** are reported in up to 19% of patients who receive little follow-up. Death is often caused by electrolyte abnormalities, suicide, cardiac arrhythmias, or sudden rehydration and weight gain complications (3–8).

II BULIMIA NERVOSA

Bulimia nervosa is an eating disorder characterized by ravenous overeating while feeling out of control, followed by guilt, depression, and anger at oneself. Recurrent compensatory behaviors such as purging accompany the overeating. Additionally, a body weight within the normal range is maintained.

A Diagnostic criteria are listed in Table 10–4. Bulimia nervosa patients fall into two distinct categories:

1. Patients with the **purging type** engage in regular vomiting and use of diuretics or cathartics.

2. Patients with the **nonpurging type** compensate for high-calorie binges with subsequent caloric restriction or exercise; they do not regularly purge (1).

B Epidemiology

1. **Onset** of bulimia nervosa is often later in adolescence than in anorexia nervosa, with the highest incidence rates between 20 and 24 years of age (2).

TABLE 10–4 *DSM-IV-TR* Criteria for Bulimia Nervosa

Two distinct types ("purging" and "nonpurging")
Recurrent episodes of bingeing, characterized by:
- Consumption of a quantity of food that exceeds what a normal person would eat during a given time period, under similar circumstances
- A feeling of not having control over eating during the episode

Recurrent inappropriate weight-controlling behavior (e.g., self-induced vomiting, use of cathartics, excessive exercise)
Bingeing and inappropriate weight-controlling behavior, both at least twice weekly for 3 months
Self-evaluation unduly influenced by body shape and weight
Disturbance does not occur exclusively during episodes of anorexia nervosa

Reprinted with permission from the Diagnostic and Statistical Manual of Mental Disorders, Fourth Edition, Text Revision, (Copyright 2000). American Psychiatric Association.

TABLE 10–5   Associated Findings in Bulimia Nervosa

Ingestion of high-calorie food
Bingeing episodes occur in secret
Wide fluctuations in weight
Persistent overconcern with weight and body shape
Attempts to lose weight (through dieting, exercise, or use of cathartics, diuretics, or enemas)
Bingeing episodes terminated by sleep, abdominal pain, social interruption, or self-induced vomiting
Lengthy phases of normal eating

---

2. **Incidence and prevalence.** Bulimia nervosa is very common, existing in gradations from mild (perhaps a variant of normal) to severe. Prevalence is 2% to 4% in industrialized countries. It is more common than anorexia nervosa and may be present in up to 20% of college-age females. The disorder is more common in females than in males. It is equally present in all socioeconomic classes (3).

C **Clinical features and associated findings**

1. **Behavioral features.** Individuals with bulimia nervosa have an increased frequency of mood and anxiety symptoms, substance use disorders, and personality disorders. Other symptoms of impulsivity, such as stealing, are common. Stealing may be necessary to support an expensive eating habit.

2. **Associated findings** are listed in Table 10–5.

3. **Medical complications** are listed in Table 10–6 (3, 4).

D **Etiology**   The exact etiology of the disorder is unknown, although biologic, psychological, and social factors are considered.

1. **Psychological theories**
   a. Factors may involve an unconscious desire to take in something orally, perhaps as a substitution for some degree of maternal deprivation. Conflict concerning separation from a maternal figure may be played out in ambivalence toward food. Generally, this ambivalence is egodystonic for the patient.
   b. Patients with bulimia nervosa may have histories of difficulty separating from caretakers and may use their own bodies as transitional objects.
   c. Bulimia may be a disorder of self-regulation. There are high rates of coexistent substance use disorders, impulsivity, and stealing. Up to 15% have multiple comorbid impulsive disorders (3–5).

2. **Biologic factors** may include similar neurotransmitters as in anorexia nervosa, such as serotonin and norepinephrine, which are linked to satiety in the hypothalamus. Elevated endorphins have been identified in some patients after purging that may relate to reported feelings of satisfaction after the behavior. Genetic studies demonstrate 50% to 80% concordance rates for eating disorders combined, and population studies show a genetic contribution of 50% in the appearance of bulimia nervosa (3).

TABLE 10–6   Medical Complications of Bulimia Nervosa

Metabolic abnormalities (e.g., hypokalemia, hypochloremic alkalosis)
Parotid gland swelling
Dental erosion and caries
Menstrual irregularities
Gastric dilatation and rupture
Chronic sore throats and esophagitis
Anemia
Neuropsychiatric symptoms (seizures, neuropathies)

E **Differential diagnosis**

1. **Prader-Willi syndrome** is characterized by continuous overeating, obesity, mental retardation, hypogonadism, hypotonia, and diabetes mellitus.

2. **Klüver-Bucy syndrome.** Objects are examined by mouth, and hypersexuality and hyperphagia are characteristic. Visual agnosia, compulsive licking and biting, and hypersensitivity to stimuli are common as well. The condition may result from temporal lobe dysfunction.

3. **Kleine-Levin syndrome** manifests as hyperphagia and hypersomnia, both of which occur in spurts of 2 to 3 weeks at a frequency of two or three cycles per year. Loss of sexual inhibitions may occur as part of the syndrome. This disorder is more common in men and may represent a limbic or hypothalamic dysfunction.

4. **Hypothalamic lesions** or other **CNS tumors** should be considered.

5. **Anorexia nervosa.** Binge eating and purging cannot occur solely during the episodes of anorexia nervosa. This would fall under a subtype of anorexia.

6. **Binge eating in obesity** represents a pattern of overeating that is not terminated by purging and is not accompanied by a preoccupation with body shape (3–5).

F **Treatment**   Patients with bulimia nervosa are more amenable to outpatient treatment than are those with anorexia nervosa.

1. **Individual psychotherapies** of psychodynamic, behavioral, and cognitive orientations have been used in the treatment of this population with some success. However, a specific form of **CBT** is identified as the benchmark and most effective primary treatment for this illness. It has been effective in both individual and group forms, with short-term abstinence achieved in 40% to 50% and higher rates of symptom reduction. The efficacy data are based on 18 to 20 strictly manual-based sessions over a 6-month period. The goals of these sessions focus on:
   a. Educating patients about the illness and identifying and interrupting the binge–purge cycle of behavior
   b. Addressing the patient's distorted and dysfunctional thoughts regarding food, weight, behaviors, and self-image while instituting a change in these beliefs (3, 8, 10)

2. **Antidepressant medications,** including selective serotonin reuptake inhibitors (SSRIs) and tricyclic antidepressants (TCAs), have been shown to be effective, with up to 60% showing symptom reduction. Combination treatment with CBT and antidepressants has been shown to be the most effective modality. Fluoxetine at higher doses of 60 and 80 mg/day has been the most extensively studied medication that has demonstrated effectiveness (3, 10).

3. **Hospitalization** is indicated for the management of serious medical complications, for relentless bingeing and purging (several times daily), and for severely depressed or suicidal bulimic patients.

G **Prognosis**   Bulimia nervosa tends to result in better outcomes than anorexia nervosa. Patients participating in treatment programs have better outcomes. A 10-year follow-up showed that of those participating in treatment programs, only 30% continued to engage in binge–purge behaviors. Bulimia is a chronic illness, with a varied course and differing prognostic outcomes. Those patients with comorbid impulsive or borderline personality disorders have less likelihood of recovery (3, 10).

III   EATING DISORDER NOT OTHERWISE SPECIFIED

Eating disorder not otherwise specified is the *DSM-IV-TR* category for disorders of eating that do not meet criteria for any specific eating disorder. This category includes patients with some but not all criteria for anorexia nervosa or bulimia nervosa. Binge-eating disorder, without inappropriate compensatory behaviors, is also included in this category. This disorder and nonpurging bulimia nervosa overlap. Treatment recommendations for binge eating currently include medications such as SSRIs and psychotherapy such as CBT (3, 11).

BIBLIOGRAPHY

1. American Psychiatric Association: *Diagnostic and Statistical Manual of Mental Disorders,* 4th ed., text revision. Washington, DC, American Psychiatric Association, 2000.
2. Favaro A, Caregaro L, Tenconi E, et al: Time trends in age at onset of anorexia nervosa and bulimia nervosa. *J Clin Psychiatry* 70(12):1715–1721, 2009.
3. Anderson AE, Yager J: Eating disorders. In *Kaplan and Sadock's Comprehensive Textbook of Psychiatry,* vol 1, 8th ed. Edited by Sadock BJ, Sadock VA. Philadelphia, Lippincott Williams & Wilkins, 2005, pp 2002–2021.
4. American Academy of Pediatrics, Committee on Adolescence, Policy Statement: Identifying and treating eating disorders. *Pediatrics* 111(1):204–211, 2003.
5. Keel PK, Herzog DB: Long-term outcome, course of illness, and mortality in anorexia nervosa, bulimia nervosa, and binge eating disorder. In *Clinical Handbook of Eating Disorders, An Integrated Approach.* Edited by Brewerton TD. New York, Marcel Dekker, 2004, pp 97–116.
6. American Psychiatric Association, Work Group on Eating Disorders: Practice guideline for the treatment of patients with eating disorders (revision). *Am J Psychiatry* 157(1 suppl):1–39, 2000.
7. Bulik CM, Berkman ND, Brownley KA, et al: Anorexia nervosa treatment: A systematic review of randomized controlled trials. *Int J Eat Disord* 40(4):310–320, 2007.
8. Agras WS, Robinson AH: Forty years of progress in the treatment of the eating disorders. *Nord J Psychiatry* 62(Suppl 47):19–24, 2008.
9. Lock J, Fitzpatrick KK: Advances in psychotherapy for children and adolescents with eating disorders. *Am J Psychother* 63(4):287–303, 2009.
10. Shapiro JR, Berkman ND, Brownley KA, et al: Bulimia nervosa treatment: A systematic review of randomized controlled trials. *Int J Eat Disord* 40(4):321–336, 2007.
11. Brownley KA, Berkman ND, Sedway JA, et al: Binge eating disorder treatment: A systematic review of randomized controlled trials. *Int J Eat Disord* 40(4):337–348, 2007.

Study Questions

Directions: *Each of the numbered items or incomplete statements in this section is followed by answers or by completions of the statement. Select the ONE lettered answer or completion that is BEST in each case.*

1. A 15-year-old girl presents to the emergency room with severe weight loss. On physical examination, she is cachectic, with a weight of 68 pounds. Her heart rate is 36 bpm, and her blood pressure is 72/50 mm Hg. Her height is 5 feet 3 inches. What should be the first intervention?

- A Evaluate the family to determine the family's dynamics.
- B Immediately administer a high-protein and high-carbohydrate diet via a nasogastric tube.
- C Draw blood for a serum electrolyte determination and then start refeeding.
- D Arrange to have the patient admitted to the psychiatric service.
- E Arrange for electroconvulsive therapy.

2. The Prader-Willi syndrome is characterized by which constellation of symptoms?

- A Overeating, mental retardation, and stealing food
- B Hypersexuality, overeating, and mouthing objects
- C Binge eating interspersed among lengthy phases of normal eating
- D Overeating and hypersomnia
- E Overeating, weight loss, and heat intolerance

3. Which is FALSE regarding treatment for anorexia nervosa?

- A There is clear evidence for pharmacologic treatment.
- B Medical assessment and management are priorities.
- C The primary goal is weight restoration.
- D Family therapy has shown effectiveness, specifically in adolescents.
- E None of the above

4. A 17-year-old young woman is referred by her dentist for evaluation after she was found to have severe caries and bilateral parotitis. She is 5 feet 5 inches tall and weighs 116 pounds. She is a talented gymnast and a straight-A student. Her serum potassium is 3.1 mEq/L. What is the most likely diagnosis?

- A Addison disease
- B Anorexia nervosa
- C Bulimia nervosa
- D Rumination disorder
- E Superior mesenteric artery syndrome

5. Which symptom of bulimia nervosa must be invariably present to establish diagnosis?

- A Episodic purging behaviors
- B Periods of binge eating
- C Periods of excessive exercising
- D Periods of fasting
- E Wide fluctuations in weight

6. What percentage of weight loss below ideal body weight is necessary to diagnose anorexia nervosa?

- A 10%
- B 15%
- C 20%
- D 25%
- E 30%

7. What mortality rate for anorexia nervosa has been reported in most studies?
   A. 1% to 8%
   B. 5% to 19%
   C. 20% to 25%
   D. 25% to 35%
   E. >35%

8. Which of the following is not associated with bulimia nervosa?
   A. Mood symptoms, anxiety symptoms, substance use, or personality disorders
   B. Cognitive behavioral therapy is the current treatment of choice, alone or in combination with medication management
   C. Parotid gland enlargement
   D. Highest mortality rate of eating disorders (AN)
   E. Metabolic alkalosis

9. All of the following are characteristics of anorexia nervosa EXCEPT:
   A. Onset is most common in the midteens.
   B. Prevalence is 20:1 in females versus males based on community studies. (more narrow ratio)
   C. Race and ethnicity offer no protection or predisposition as a risk factor.
   D. It is more prevalent in developed countries.
   E. It is often associated with professions that require thinness.

10. Which of the following factors may be associated with the etiology of anorexia nervosa?
   A. Comorbidity of other mental illnesses
   B. Genetic predisposition
   C. Neurobiologic factors
   D. Family dysfunction
   E. All of the above

Answers and Explanations

1. The answer is C [*I F 1, G 3*]. Anorexia nervosa may be a life-threatening illness. Significant mortality accompanies this condition, most commonly caused by the metabolic or cardiac complications secondary to starvation. The first intervention with anorectic patients should always be an assessment of the medical state by drawing blood for serum electrolyte determination, followed by supportive or emergency medical intervention, such as starting refeeding or intravenous feeding. Too-rapid hydration or weight gain should be avoided because it may lead to further complications and even death. A high-protein and high-carbohydrate diet administered by nasogastric tube would not correct fluid and electrolyte problems quickly. Evaluation and treatment of the individual and family dynamics are always secondary to emergency medical management.

2. The answer is A [*II E 1–3*]. The Prader-Willi syndrome is characterized by ravenous overeating and is accompanied by obesity, mental retardation, and hypotonia. It is probably caused by a hypothalamic lesion. Examining objects by mouth, hypersexuality, and hyperphagia are attributed to the Klüver-Bucy syndrome, and overeating and hypersomnia are associated with the Kleine-Levin syndrome. Binge eating interspersed with lengthy phases of normal eating may be seen in individuals with bulimia nervosa and may be associated with wide fluctuations in weight. The constellation of increased appetite, weight loss, and heat intolerance suggests hyperthyroidism.

3. The answer is A [*I F*].

4. The answer is C [*Table 10–6, I E*]. Frequent exposure of the teeth, parotid salivary gland, and esophagus to gastric acid (as occurs in the purging type of bulimia nervosa) can result in irritation, inflammation, and damage to each of these tissues. Individuals with Addison disease may present with weight loss, but it occurs in conjunction with hyperkalemia rather than hypokalemia. Superior mesenteric artery syndrome can cause vomiting and anorexia, but this usually occurs after substantial weight loss. Anorexia nervosa cannot be diagnosed until weight is at or below 85% of ideal body weight. Rumination disorder, in which food is repeatedly regurgitated and rechewed, is an uncommon disorder of infancy and early childhood that rarely progresses into adulthood except in individuals with mental retardation or pervasive developmental disorders.

5. The answer is B [*Table 10–4*]. The diagnosis of bulimia nervosa requires both recurrent episodes of binge eating and recurrent, inappropriate, compensatory behaviors aimed at preventing weight gain. Prevention of weight gain may be achieved by fasting, excessive exercise, or purging behaviors such as self-induced vomiting or laxative or diuretic abuse. Individuals with bulimia nervosa vary according to which weight management method they use. Wide fluctuations in weight are common but not invariable.

6. The answer is B [*Table 10–1*]. Refusal or inability to maintain weight at or above 85% of ideal body weight is necessary for the diagnosis of anorexia nervosa.

7. The answer is B [*I G 3*]. Most studies report mortality rates ranging from 5% to 19%.

8. The answer is D [*Table 10–5, Table 10–6, II G*]. Bulimia nervosa tends to result in better outcomes than in anorexia nervosa, with more than half of patients who are in treatment reporting improvement in binge eating and purging. Associated findings do include parotid gland enlargement, metabolic alkalosis, and increased comorbidity with other Axis I and Axis II disorders.

9. The answer is B [*I B 1, D 3*]. Racial/ethnic factors offer no protection or predisposition to anorexia nervosa except within subgroups who historically promote weight loss or change. Community studies reveal a more narrow ratio of females to males with anorexia than previously reported in clinical trials.

10. The answer is E [*I D 1–3*]. Although no single cause is known, various biologic and psychosocial factors are implicated in the etiology of anorexia nervosa.

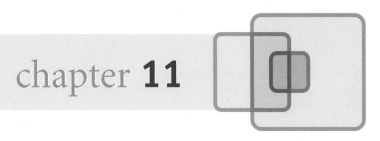

chapter 11

Emergency Psychiatry

RACHEL A. HOUCHINS · LESLIE FRINKS

I OVERVIEW

Emergency psychiatry is the clinical and academic use of psychiatry in emergency settings. The demand for emergency psychiatric services is already high and continues to increase due to a number of factors including deinstitutionalization, urbanization, and overcrowding of psychiatric hospitals and the prison system. This has resulted in the development of psychiatric emergency services (PES) that may be community or hospital based to provide emergent evaluation of psychiatric concerns (1).

A The **most common reasons for emergency psychiatric evaluation** are:

1. **Suicidal or parasuicidal** thoughts or behavior
2. **Homicidal** threats, thoughts, or behavior
3. **Psychotic or disorganized** behavior or verbalizations
4. **Inability to perform self-care** such as not bathing or eating, neglecting medical needs, or putting oneself in immediate danger
5. **Altered mental status** or impaired cognitive functioning
6. **Substance intoxication** and **withdrawal**

A **psychiatric emergency** or **crisis** can be a response to stress or an exacerbation of the patient's chronic condition that endangers the affected individual or others or significantly disrupts the functioning of the individual.

B **Evolution of a crisis** **Stressors** from any source can create a problem for an individual. In a crisis, the normal **coping mechanisms** of the individual are insufficient, and the individual is overwhelmed. A dynamic interplay occurs among the stressor, the affected individual, and the social system that influences the individual's response.

1. **Stressors.** Although stressors depend on the interplay between individual and social factors, they are predominantly either internal or external.
   a. **Internal stressors** occur when individuals face a normal developmental task for which they are not prepared. Examples include an anxious adolescent who becomes disorganized when she leaves her family to attend college, or an aging, lonely woman who becomes suicidal after her cat dies.
   b. **External stressors** result from a life event that is normally recognized as a significant source of stress. Common examples include:
      (1) Death of a loved one
      (2) End of a relationship
      (3) Having a child (childbirth or adoption)
      (4) Serious medical illness in oneself or a loved one
      (5) Financial crises
      (6) Assault, including domestic violence and rape
      (7) Changing or losing jobs
      (8) Moving
      (9) Natural disasters

2. **Psychosocial support,** and the availability of this, helps determine the effect of a stressor for any individual. Some individuals have many supportive resources that facilitate an adaptive resolution to a crisis, while others have very little support.

3. **Increased anxiety and disorganization** may follow the stressor and may further impair the individual's functional and problem-solving capacity.

4. **Failure of adaptation** may cause an increasing sense of helplessness and disorganization. Healthy individuals may resolve a crisis in an adaptive, growth-promoting fashion; however:
   a. **Healthy individuals** may become so overwhelmed by stress that they have a pathologic adaptation. They are then more vulnerable to future stress.
   b. **Individuals with significant disorders** may decompensate with even minor environmental stress.

5. **Impulsive and maladaptive attempts by the individual to regain control** are likely in this situation. These attempts may help the individual cope and reduce distress but may still be ultimately detrimental. For example, an individual may use alcohol to lower anxiety and reduce the frequency of nightmares after a traumatic event. However, medical, social, and occupational complications may eventually result from excessive alcohol use.

6. **A request for help** may occur at any time during this cycle, depending on the individual's response to the crisis and the social context. **An individual with any psychiatric diagnosis or an individual with no preexisting disorder can have a psychiatric emergency.**

II EVALUATION AND MANAGEMENT OF PSYCHIATRIC EMERGENCIES

Multiple psychiatric conditions including depression, psychosis, anxiety, and substance use may cause patients to present to the emergency room (ER), but patients presenting for emergency evaluation also have a high prevalence of combined general medical and psychiatric impairment (1). A critical role of the ER psychiatrist is to differentiate organic or medical presentations from behavioral or psychiatric ones, and to then determine what type of treatment is needed: medical, psychiatric, or both. The initial step in this determination is a thorough assessment.

A **Medical assessment of an ER patient with psychiatric symptoms** The medical evaluation of an ER patient with psychiatric symptoms should include a thorough medical history, a complete review of systems, the assessment of vital signs, a physical examination, and laboratory tests when indicated. Patients who present for emergency psychiatric evaluation should also be questioned about intravenous drug use, homelessness, recent physical or sexual assault, and unprotected sexual activity because a positive history of these may indicate the need for further medical workup.

1. **Medical evaluation of psychiatric patients in the ER should include:**
   a. **Chief complaint and history of present illness,** which may be psychiatric in nature; medical concerns may not be elicited until the medical review of systems
   b. **Complete medical review of systems**
   c. **Medical history** including chronic medical problems, any acute diagnoses, and history of surgeries and hospitalizations
   d. **Physical examination including vital signs,** which should include documentation of the patient's physical status and a description of the patient's appearance and ability to cooperate with the exam, which will be helpful in formulating the patient's mental status
   e. **Complete blood count** if concerns are present about infection, such as fever with altered mental status or depressive symptoms consistent with anemia, or if the patient is treated with medications that may affect blood count values, such as clozapine or valproic acid
   f. **Electrolytes,** because alterations in sodium, potassium, creatinine, and glucose can present with alterations in mental status
   g. **Liver function tests** if there are concerns about alcohol use or hepatic effects of psychiatric drugs such as valproic acid
   h. **Pregnancy test**
   i. **Thyroid-stimulating hormone,** because hypothyroidism can present with depression and anxiety is characteristic of hyperthyroid states
   j. **Urine drug screen (UDS) and blood alcohol level**

k. Electrocardiogram (ECG) as indicated by history or if patient is on medications known to alter patterns such as antipsychotics, lithium, and tricyclic antidepressants

l. HIV screen and **hepatitis** or other blood-borne disease panels as indicated by history

m. Medication levels including valproic acid, other anticonvulsants, lithium, and tricyclic antidepressant levels

n. Computed tomography (CT) of the head if patient presents with new-onset psychosis or acute altered mental status, to rule out hemorrhage, trauma, or mass lesion; rarely magnetic resonance imaging (MRI) may be indicated if presentation suggests vascular lesions or a brain mass or if there is concern for subtle changes

o. Electroencephalogram (EEG) if seizure disorder is a possible differential diagnosis

p. Lumbar puncture if patient has symptoms of infection and other sites have been ruled out or if intracranial hemorrhage is a consideration

q. Vitamin B$_{12}$ and folate if patient presents with dementia or cognitive status changes (2, 3)

2. **Psychiatric assessment of an ER patient with psychiatric symptoms.** The psychiatric assessment of an ER patient is a focused evaluation with the goals of making a differential diagnosis, managing acute symptoms, considering comorbid medical concerns, completing a risk assessment, and determining the patient's disposition to the appropriate level of care. The initial history should focus on the symptoms or events that brought the patient in for care, the current mental status examination, the process of how the patient arrived at the current evaluation, stressors affecting the current presentation, current medical concerns, and recent substance use. Further information from family, treatment providers, and outside agencies (police, EMS) is important to obtain when time and acuity allow. In a cooperative patient, when time allows, the following should be included in the psychiatric evaluation:

   a. Chief complaint

   b. History of present illness including symptoms and their duration, what led up to the patient's presentation, mechanism of the patient's presentation to the ER (via EMS, police, family, or voluntary), and any stressors influencing symptoms

   c. Psychiatric review of systems including screening questions about each major diagnostic category such as anxiety, depression, mania, and psychosis. **Every psychiatric patient in the ER should also be asked about suicidal and homicidal ideation, plan, or intent.**

   d. Substance use including specific substances used, duration of use, amount used, most recent use, and history of withdrawal symptoms and treatment

   e. Mental status examination including the mini-mental state examination if concerns about cognitive function exist

   f. Psychiatric history including past hospitalizations, diagnoses, current or recent treatment, and history of treatment compliance or noncompliance

   g. Medical history including current diagnoses, chronic medical conditions, and surgeries

   h. Current medications and drug allergies

   i. Family history of psychiatric illnesses including family history of psychiatric disorders, suicide, and substance use

   j. Psychosocial history including current living situation, relationship status, educational history, work history, abuse history if not obtained in the review of systems or history of present illness (HPI), and current stressors if not elicited in the HPI. This information is very helpful in determining the patient's baseline ability to function.

   k. Collateral information from family, friends, treating physicians, and past records as available (1, 3)

III SPECIFIC PSYCHIATRIC EMERGENCIES

A Suicidality

1. **Clinical presentation.** Suicide was the 11th leading cause of death in the United States in 2006 (4). It is the quintessential emergency of all mental health personnel.

   a. Overt

   (1) Suicidal behavior. Patients may attempt suicide by overdosing on drugs or medications, cutting their wrists, or jumping from a high place, among many other ways. These particular patients may require medical and/or surgical intervention (e.g., gastric lavage, activated charcoal, or suturing) due to the seriousness of the attempt prior to a psychiatric evaluation. Patients should be considered acutely suicidal until proven otherwise. Careful observation is needed to prevent another suicide attempt and to prevent the patient from leaving the emergency department.

(2) Suicidal ideation. The patient may be obviously depressed, expressing concerns with little prompting and experiencing considerable pain and distress. The patient may ask for help in the control of suicidal impulses and for relief from depression.

b. Covert

(1) Suicidal behavior. Although patients may minimize or deny the implications of their behavior, they may have accidents that range from suspicious to obviously suicidal. A patient who is unconscious of these self-destructive impulses may still be highly suicidal. A similar type of patient is one who appears homicidal or assaultive but whose behavior is primarily an attempt to provoke others, such as the police, to kill them.

(2) Suicidal ideation. Patients may seek medical evaluation of a minor or severe somatic symptom. They may appear depressed or may disguise distress. Empathic questioning may prompt patients to reveal their feelings. Patients may show distress that is out of proportion to objective findings or may visit the emergency department many times over a short period. Although hoping to obtain help, patients may take the medication given for a somatic symptom in a suicide attempt.

c. Chronic suicidal ideation and behavior. The patient repeatedly calls or visits the emergency department for suicidal ideation and attempts. Self-destructive behavior may be a means by which the patient attempts to manipulate the environment or relieve internal distress. The patient evokes frustration and hostility in caregivers and is at great risk to be ignored or actively rejected. Because this type of patient is also at great risk for suicide by design, miscalculation, or impulsiveness, careful evaluation is required.

2. Risk factors

a. Demographics

(1) The suicide rate in men is four times higher than in women. However, women attempt suicide three times as often (5).

(2) Whites and Native Americans have much higher suicide rates than blacks and Hispanics. Recent studies have shown that the suicide rate is rising in blacks (6).

(3) Divorced, widowed, and separated individuals have higher suicide rates than married people.

(4) Men 75 years of age and older have the highest suicide rate.

(5) Suicide patterns have shifted over the past few years, with the overall suicide rate being highest in persons (this includes both males and females) ages 45 to 54 in 2006 and 2007, as opposed to the previous pattern of the highest rate being in persons ages 80 years or older (7).

(6) The suicide rate among adolescent boys has risen significantly in recent years.

(7) The elderly account for 12.6% of the American population and 18.1% of suicides.

(8) Physicians have higher suicide rates than other professionals.

b. Psychopathology. Psychiatric illness is present in almost all people who commit suicide. Comorbidity (i.e., multiple psychiatric illnesses) is common.

(1) Mood disorder. Major depression is the most common disorder and is present in approximately half of people who commit suicide.

(2) Substance abuse–related disorder. Depression and substance-related disorders are present in two-thirds of all suicides. Alcohol is implicated in more than 25% of suicides. Other drugs such as cocaine and marijuana are seen in younger victims.

(3) Schizophrenia. Patients with a diagnosis of schizophrenia have a 4% lifetime risk of suicide. About 10% of individuals with schizophrenia attempt suicide. Individuals with schizophrenia have approximately the same risk for suicide as those with major depression.

(4) Delirium, dementia, and other cognitive disorders. These disorders, as primary diagnoses, are found in 4% of people who commit suicide. Another psychiatric diagnosis is usually present as well.

(5) Panic disorder. The diagnosis of panic disorder is statistically correlated with an increased incidence of suicide attempts. Researchers believe that the presence of comorbid mental disorders such as depression and substance abuse–related disorder in patients with panic disorder is more important in predicting suicidal behavior than the diagnosis of panic disorder itself.

(6) **Personality disorders.** Borderline and antisocial personality disorders occur in patients with suicidal behavior. Other psychiatric illnesses, especially substance abuse disorders, are usually present as well.

c. **Medical illness.** Poor health in the past 6 months increases the risk of suicide. Terminal illness accounts for fewer suicides than the media suggests.

d. **Genetics.** Most family studies involve mood disorders in which suicide is a factor, rather than suicide alone. Suicide risk is increased in families with psychiatric illness.

(1) One study of twins showed a concordance rate of 13.2% in monozygotic pairs and 0.7% in dizygotic pairs for suicide (8).

(2) There appears to be a genetic risk of suicide that is independent of the risk of psychiatric illness.

3. **Assessment of lethality (suicide risk)**

a. **Episodic suicidal ideation and behavior.** Suicidal behavior may remit and relapse in response to patients' changing internal emotional and cognitive states and their environment.

b. **Ambivalence of the suicidal patient.** The balance between the patient's wish to live and wish to die must be evaluated, including the factors that tip the balance one way or the other. Most patients who eventually commit suicide give some warning of their intentions.

c. **Risk factors (predictors).** In many cases, the patient's ambivalence and the episodic nature of suicidal behavior permit the behavior to be identified and prevented.

(1) **Demographic indicators** are older age and male gender.

(2) **Historical indicators.** A recent loss or a change in the patient's current status may precipitate a crisis, with the patient experiencing anxiety and depression.

(a) **Current illness.** Patients who report hopelessness, helplessness, loneliness, and exhaustion are worrisome. An unexpected change in behavior, such as giving away possessions, or an unexpected change in attitude, such as calmness or resignation in the midst of a distressing situation, should be investigated. Overt or indirect talk of death should be followed up with specific and direct questions regarding fantasies, wishes, plans, and means. In a patient who makes an unsuccessful suicide attempt, the following additional issues are important:

(i) The patient's perception of lethality of the attempt, expectations of rescue, and relief or disappointment at being alive are often more important than the objective dangerousness of the attempt, particularly in cases of apparent imminent danger.

(ii) The extent to which the precipitating crisis is resolved or is being resolved may influence a patient's wish to remain alive and his or her attitude toward the future.

(b) **History of suicide attempts.** A history of previous attempts increases the risk of suicide, particularly if many attempts have been made. The circumstances and lethality of the previous attempts should be determined. Forty percent of depressed patients who commit suicide have made a previous attempt.

(c) **Medical history.** A history of chronic illness or an acute change in physical health increases the risk of suicide.

(d) **Family history.** A family history of suicide is important both in terms of the patient's identification with the individual who died and the possibility of inheritance of an affective disorder. The patient may experience stress at the anniversary of the death or when he or she reaches the age of the person who died.

(3) **Diagnostic indicators.** Depression, thought disorder, and impairment of impulse control, especially secondary to alcohol or drug abuse, are diagnostic indicators.

(4) **Mental status.** The physician should assess the severity of depression, the presence of psychosis (especially command hallucinations), and any problems with impulse control. In addition, the physician should be aware of the patient's response to the interview (e.g., whether the patient feels understood; experiences some relief; and expresses more hopefulness or remains angry, pessimistic, and desperate).

(5) Resources. The availability and support of family and friends are crucial. In addition, the physician must be confident of their support and willingness to assume some responsibility for the patient. In particular, the physician must ascertain that there is no collusion with or covert encouragement of the patient's suicidal behavior.

4. **Countertransference reactions to suicidal patients.** Countertransference refers to the physician's emotional reactions to the patient. These reactions may be unconscious or only vaguely conscious. They may have a powerful effect on the physician's attitude toward the patient, approach to the patient, and even clinical judgment.
   a. **Physician attitudes.** Physicians have their own attitudes toward suicide and death, their own set of personal and clinical experiences, and conflicts about their own aggressive or self-destructive impulses. Unless physicians are aware of these reactions, they may minimize or distort patients' clinical data to accommodate their personal feelings or beliefs. Physicians may even fear that they will encourage patients to commit suicide by talking about it.
   b. **Feelings of caregivers.** The patient's behaviors may produce frustration, anger, and helplessness in most caregivers. A patient may evoke so much hostility that the physician may wish that the patient were dead. This reaction is serious because others in the patient's environment may feel similarly.

5. **Principles of emergency treatment**
   a. The patient must be protected.
   b. A psychiatric consultation must be sought if there is any question about the patient's lethality.
   c. Treatment must be considered. Treatment options include the following:
      (1) Hospitalization. Patients should be hospitalized if the lethality of their ideation or behavior is high. A greater degree of lethality may be due to the persistence of the patient's wish to die, the severity of concurrent psychopathology, or the absence of reliable sources of support in the patient's social environment.
         (a) Patients can be hospitalized voluntarily if they agree with the need for inpatient treatment.
         (b) Suicidal patients can also be hospitalized involuntarily if they refuse voluntarily hospitalization. Severely suicidal patients who resist treatment may require one-on-one observation to prevent escape or self-injury.
      (2) Outpatient treatment. Less-restrictive treatment is indicated in patients who have some crisis resolution, mild concurrent psychopathology, supportive environmental resources, and a therapeutic response to the interview. Somatic treatment can be initiated on an outpatient basis, but limited quantities of medication should be dispensed because of the potential for overdose.

B **Agitation**   In an emergency room setting, patients are in a situation that is not under their control. Agitation is often a manifestation of the patient's anxiety and fear within the context of this situation. Agitation can be the result of many psychiatric issues, such as substance intoxication or withdrawal, an acute psychotic state with hallucinations and/or delusions, anxiety/panic, hypervigilance, acute mania, or personality pathology. Agitated patients can assault staff and may require restraints or rapid tranquilization to stabilize a volatile situation.

1. **Nonpharmacologic interventions.** Not all agitated patients are psychotic; these patients may only require verbal intervention and supportive reassurances from staff and/or counselors (3).
   a. It is best to start with the least restrictive form of treatment (i.e., talking with the patient, establishing a therapeutic alliance to put the patient at ease).
   b. If the patient does not respond to verbal intervention and is becoming a danger to him- or herself or others present, a show of force may be needed to reinforce boundaries.
   c. Soft restraints can be used for agitated patients and are not as invasive as intramuscular medications. Patients should be closely monitored while restrained, and if possible, should not be restrained physically if they are medically unstable.

2. **Pharmacologic interventions**
   a. In severely agitated patients, rapid tranquilization may be necessary to prevent harm. The administration of oral or intramuscular medications to treat agitation, anxiety, or hostility can be helpful despite the underlying diagnosis for these symptoms.

TABLE 11–1   Treatment of Acute Agitation

Medication	Dose/Route	Routine	Maximum Dose
Haloperidol	2–5 mg PO/IM	q1–8h	100 mg/day
Chlorpromazine	50–100 mg PO/IM	q1–6h	2,000 mg/day
Ziprasidone	10–20 mg IM	q2–4h	40 mg/day
Olanzapine	5–10 mg PO/IM	q2–6h	30 mg/day
Aripiprazole	9.75 mg IM	q2–8h	30 mg/day
Lorazepam	2–4 mg PO/IM	q1–6h	10 mg/day
Benztropine	1–2 mg PO/IM	q1–6h	6 mg/day

   b. Oral medications can be offered in an effort to help patients maintain some control. However, intramuscular medications are used more often in the emergency setting for the advantage of quicker absorption and increased bioavailability (9).

   c. Both typical and atypical antipsychotics are used for rapid tranquilization and can be given in combination or alternately with benzodiazepines.

   d. Medications commonly used in the emergency setting for acute agitation are haloperidol, ziprasidone, olanzapine, aripiprazole, chlorpromazine, and lorazepam (Table 11–1).

   e. Atypical antipsychotics may be preferred for the decreased incidence of akathisia and dystonic reactions. High doses of typical antipsychotics are more likely to cause akathisia and dystonia, especially in young males. Benztropine can be used to treat acute dystonic reactions (Table 11–1).

   f. The administration of benzodiazepines alone may be sufficient for alleviating agitation in nonpsychotic patients. Lorazepam can be given orally, intramuscularly, or intravenously and is therefore often used (Table 11–1).

   g. It is essential that agitation be treated in the emergency setting as it may proceed to violence if left untreated.

C Violence/homicidality

1. **Etiology.** Violent behavior is a result of the interplay between innate psychobiologic factors and the external environment.

   a. Biologic factors. Serotonin metabolism is thought to be involved in violent behavior much as it is in suicidal behavior. There is a clear association between alcohol intoxication and violent behavior. Alcohol decreases impulse control and inhibition and impairs judgment. Other drugs that have a similar effect on the brain and behavior include amphetamines, cocaine, phencyclidine (PCP), and sedative-hypnotic drugs.

   b. Psychosocial factors. Patients who were abused as children have an increased risk of becoming abusive adults. Witnessing abuse in childhood is also associated with increased violent behavior. Spousal abuse and family violence, even if not directed at the child, can influence the individual's later behavior.

   c. Socioeconomic factors. Severe poverty and marital disruption are more related to violence than race or economic inequality. Factors that disrupt the family structure also appear to increase the risk of aggression and violence of affected families.

   d. Guns. The number of deaths and injuries caused by firearms continues to increase. Guns are now the leading cause of death of adolescent males, replacing the automobile.

2. **Differential diagnosis.** Certain diagnoses are more likely to be associated with violence, although all patients may be potentially dangerous.

   a. Bipolar disorder: manic type

   b. Schizophrenia. Individuals with schizophrenia who refuse to take medication, who have a history of violence, and who have command hallucinations are particularly at risk for violent behavior. Hallucinations may command patients to hurt others. More commonly, patients with paranoid schizophrenia exhibit violence as they feel the need to defend themselves.

    c. **Delusional disorders**

    d. **Intermittent explosive disorder**

    e. **Posttraumatic stress disorder.** Explosions of aggressive behavior may be unpredictable and may be associated with flashbacks or triggered by something environmental. This situation is often complicated by drug and alcohol use.

    f. **Personality disorders.** Substance abuse increases the likelihood of acting-out behavior in persons with any type of personality disorder, including:

        (1) Borderline personality disorder

        (2) Antisocial personality disorder

        (3) Paranoid personality disorder

    g. **Substance abuse**

        (1) Alcohol intoxication

        (2) Other drugs that are associated with violence include sedative-hypnotics such as barbiturates and benzodiazepines, as well as stimulants such as cocaine, amphetamines, and PCP. Glue sniffing and steroid use also increase violent behavior.

        (3) Physicians should evaluate patients for dysarthria, nystagmus, unsteady gait, and tremors.

        (4) Patients with PCP intoxication often exhibit confusion, disorientation, rage, horizontal and vertical nystagmus, and violent behavior.

    h. **Central nervous system (CNS) disorders.** Traumatic brain injuries are associated with violent behavior. Minor injuries and organic insults, as well as seizure disorders, can also affect behavior.

    i. **Attention deficit hyperactivity disorder**

  3. **Assessment of dangerousness**

    a. Future violence is difficult to predict, and an overall assessment of imminent and ongoing dangerousness is necessary.

        (1) Certain combinations of internal and external factors may produce an assaultive crisis.

        (2) Important factors to keep in mind are the patient's perception of external danger, whether real or imagined, and the need for self-protection.

    b. **Risk factors**

        (1) Males ages 16 to 25 are at high risk for violent behavior.

        (2) History of violence (fighting, assaults, and arrests) is the most reliable predictor of future violence.

        (3) Use of substances increases risk of violence.

        (4) A recent major life change may lead to internal tension and frustration.

        (5) A history of impulsive or self-destructive behavior (i.e., accidents, arrests for speeding or reckless driving, self-mutilation) increases risk.

        (6) A history of neglect or abuse in childhood (witnessed or experienced) increases the likelihood of abuse and brutality directed toward the patient's children.

        (7) A childhood history of cruelty to animals is associated with continued aggressiveness.

    c. **Diagnostic factors.** The common diagnostic denominator is the degree to which the patient's thoughts are impaired in the contexts of hostility, irritability, and distorted perceptions of reality.

    d. **Mental status.** Fluctuations of the patient's level of agitation throughout the interview should be noted. The patient's impulse control and judgment during the examination may contradict the content of his or her speech. Command hallucinations to hurt others are particularly worrisome, as are escalating delusional perceptions of external danger because these perceptions may be accompanied by frantic attempts at self-preservation. Sometimes delusional thinking places others in danger in the guise of protecting them. Any evidence of confusion or an organic mental disorder is significant because it suggests impairment of impulse control and judgment.

    e. **Social system.** The thoughts of the patient's family and friends concerning the patient's potential for violence should be sought in separate interviews, especially if these individuals are potential victims. The family may provide reliable information about the patient's access to weapons.

    f. **Physician feelings.** Persistent feelings of fear or unease on the part of the physician may be an important clue that further investigation and evaluation are necessary.

4. **Countertransference reactions toward violent patients**
   a. **Physician reaction.** Angry, agitated, threatening patients are likely to frighten physicians.
   b. **Consequences.** Intense, unacknowledged countertransference reactions can interfere with clinical judgment and treatment.
5. **Principles of managing a violent patient**
   a. **Safety.** An adequate number of trained staff members must be available to restrain the patient physically if necessary. Staff members should treat the patient firmly but compassionately.
   b. **Behavioral techniques**
      (1) It is important to act calmly.
      (2) Clinicians and staff should speak softly in a nonauthoritarian way.
      (3) Both the patient and the examiner should sit during the interview.
      (4) Offering food and drink or other comfort measures can often diffuse a tense situation.
      (5) Staff should check for the presence of weapons and confiscate these.
      (6) The exam room should provide immediate access to an exit for the patient and clinicians.
      (7) Seclusion and restraint can be used to prevent harm to staff or the patient.
   c. **Psychopharmacologic approach**
      (1) **Neuroleptics** are the most commonly used medication in emergency situations. Neuroleptics should be avoided in patients who are experiencing alcohol or drug toxicity or withdrawal (Table 11–1).
      (2) **Benzodiazepines** may be used with neuroleptics and in cases of withdrawal. It is important to note that in some patients, benzodiazepines disinhibit violent behavior.
   d. **Responsibility to warn and protect others**
      (1) Information provided to a physician is considered confidential. However, as a result of the *Tarasoff* decision (*Tarasoff v. Regents of University of California,* 1976) and other legal cases involving attacks on third parties, clinicians are now expected to weigh the need for confidentiality against the need to protect others.
      (2) If the patient makes a credible threat to harm a specific person, the clinician has a duty to warn that person. Good medical practice may also require involuntary treatment of the patient.

D **Delirium** Approximately 4% to 10% of ER patients may present with altered mental status (10). In the *Diagnostic and Statistical Manual of Mental Disorders,* fourth edition, text revision (*DSM-IV-TR*), delirium is characterized by a fluctuating course of disturbance of consciousness and change in cognition that is the direct effect of a general medical condition or a substance intoxication/withdrawal. Delirium is associated with an increased mortality and morbidity rate. In a study by Han et al, 76% of delirium cases in older adults went undiagnosed in the ER (11).

1. **Presentation.** Patients can present agitated and irritable or hypoactive and sluggish.
2. **Diagnosis.** A thorough history and physical examination should be taken in the emergency department to properly diagnose delirium. This may require contacting family or caretakers if the patient is too obtunded to give a coherent history.
3. **Course.** Delirium develops over a short period of time and is characterized by a change from the patient's baseline of functioning.
4. **Treatment.** Haloperidol is used most often, but atypical antipsychotics have also been used. Benzodiazepines have not been found to be helpful except in the case of alcohol or benzodiazepine withdrawal.
5. **Differential diagnosis.** Some common causes of delirium are neurologic problems (stroke), substance withdrawal, overdoses, trauma, metabolic abnormalities, and infections.
6. **Risk factors** include elderly age, male gender, poor premorbid functioning, dementia, and a prior episode of delirium.
7. **Goals** are to diagnose and treat the underlying cause of the delirium, reduce the associated morbidity and mortality, and, if possible, help the patient return to the previous level of functioning.

E **Toxicity and withdrawal syndromes** Toxicity and withdrawal syndromes are common in the ER setting. These syndromes may be the result of intentional or unintentional overdose or exposure. Patients with toxicity and withdrawal syndromes can be especially difficult to treat given that they are often unable to give an accurate history due to decreased mental status. Initial treatment of these syndromes should focus on minimizing the effects of exposure and providing medical support, with secondary treatment of psychiatric intervention after medical stabilization. Table 11–2 summarizes some of the most common toxicity and withdrawal syndromes and their management (12).

F Neuroleptic malignant syndrome, serotonin syndrome, and hypertensive crisis

1. **Neuroleptic malignant syndrome** (NMS) is a psychiatric emergency that is rare but has the potential for a fatal outcome. It is associated with the administration of neuroleptic medications

TABLE 11–2   Management of Toxicity and Withdrawal Syndromes

Substance	Clinical Presentation	Treatment
Acetaminophen	Abdominal pain, nausea, vomiting, anorexia, jaundice, liver failure	N-Acetylcysteine
Alcohol	Decreased mental status, sedation, ataxia, anesthesia, coma	Supportive measures Airway protection
Amphetamines	Agitation, tachycardia, hypertension, dilated pupils, hyperthermia	Supportive measures Benzodiazepines
Anticholinergics	Tachycardia, dilated pupils, fever, agitation, delirium, dry skin and dry mucous membranes	Physostigmine
Barbiturates	Sedation, coma, hypotension, decreased respirations, hypothermia	Supportive measures Airway protection Charcoal if within 60 minutes
Benzodiazepines	Coma, sedation, decreased reflexes, mild hypotension or bradycardia, decreased respirations	Supportive measures Airway protection Flumazenil (controversial because of possible induction of seizures)
β-Blockers	Hypotension, CNS depression	Glucagon Cardiac pacing
Cocaine	Agitation, tachycardia, hypertension, dilated pupils	Supportive measures Benzodiazepines
Carbon monoxide	Shortness of breath, headache, dizziness, nausea, confusion, tachycardia, "cherry red" skin is rare	Supportive measures 100% O_2 Hyperbaric oxygen
Lithium	Decreased mental status, hyperreflexia, nausea, vomiting, polyuria, tremor, seizures, coma	Hydration Supportive measures Hemodialysis
Opiates	Miosis, decreased respirations, hypotension, coma	Supportive measures Airway protection Naloxone
Organophosphates and cholinergics	Bradycardia, constricted pupils, salivation, lacrimation, diarrhea	Atropine
PCP	Agitation, aggression, altered perception, hypertension, ataxia, nystagmus and mydriasis, amnesia	Supportive measures Benzodiazepines
Salicylates	Hyperventilation, flushing, hyperthermia, tinnitus, nausea and vomiting	Charcoal if within 60 minutes Urinary alkalinization
Tricyclic antidepressants	Decreased mental status, tachycardia, hyperreflexia, cardiac conduction delays, seizures	Supportive measures Charcoal if within 60 minutes Blood alkalinization Cardiac monitoring

CNS, central nervous system; PCP, phencyclidine.

but can also be seen with the use of antiemetic medications and sedatives or the abrupt withdrawal of antiparkinsonian agents.

  a. **Prevalence** is estimated to be 0.02% to 2.4% of patients exposed to dopamine receptor antagonists (3). The incidence of NMS in patients treated with antipsychotic medications is estimated to be 0.01% to 0.02% (13).

  b. **Presentation.** Patients often present with altered mental status, muscle rigidity, hyperthermia, diaphoresis, tachycardia, and elevated blood pressure. Other symptoms noted in the presentation of NMS are dysphagia, incontinence, mutism, and tremor.

  c. **Diagnosis and course.** The onset of NMS can occur at any time while the patient is taking neuroleptic medications, may occur rapidly, and may progress quickly. The first step is to recognize this syndrome and then immediately discontinue the offending agent. Laboratory measures will likely reveal elevated creatine phosphokinase (CPK) and leukocytosis.

  d. **Treatment**
    (1) Vital signs should be monitored closely and intravenous fluids administered.
    (2) Cooling blankets or antipyretics may used for temperature control.
    (3) Dantrolene may be used alone or in combination with benzodiazepines or dopamine agonists (e.g., amantadine or bromocriptine) to treat the symptoms of NMS.
    (4) If pharmacotherapy fails, a trial of electroconvulsive therapy (ECT) may be successful.

  e. **Prognosis.** NMS has an estimated mortality rate of 10% to 30%. Associated complications that are more likely to result in death are renal failure due to rhabdomyolysis, respiratory arrest, hyperpyrexia, liver failure, and cardiovascular collapse (3).

  f. **Risk factors** associated with an increased likelihood of developing NMS are catatonia, dehydration, use of neuroleptics with anticholinergic side effects, rapid titration of high-potency neuroleptics, concurrent administration of lithium, male gender, younger age, agitation, and a prior episode of NMS.

2. **Serotonin syndrome** is a result of excessive serotonin in the central nervous system, usually secondary to the administration of multiple serotonergic agents.

  a. **Presentation.** Patients can present with myoclonus, mental status changes, akathisia, diaphoresis, tremor, hyperreflexia, mydriasis, diarrhea, headache, and autonomic instabilities.

  b. **Diagnosis.** Laboratory results yield no conclusive findings for diagnosis; therefore, the physical examination is paramount to diagnosis. Important findings on physical examination are clonus, hyperreflexia, increased bowel sounds, sialorrhea, and pupil dilation. Deep tendon reflexes are noted to be increased, especially those of the lower extremities (i.e., patellar reflex).

  c. **Course.** The onset is rapid, but once the causative agents are discontinued and treatment started, most cases resolve within 24 hours (14). Severe cases can lead to admission to the intensive care unit and intubation. Complications that can result in death are disseminated intravascular coagulation, rhabdomyolysis, and acute organ failure.

  d. **Treatment.** After diagnosis, the serotonergic agents should be discontinued and supportive care instituted. Vital signs should be monitored closely. Intravenous fluids may be given as well as medications or treatment for hyperthermia.
    (1) Agitation can be controlled with benzodiazepines.
    (2) Cyproheptadine is given in moderate cases to treat symptoms, at an initial dose of 12 mg and then 2 mg every 2 hours, with a maximum dose of 20 to 32 mg in 24 hours.

  e. **Drug interactions.** Agents likely to cause serotonin syndrome in combination include monoamine oxidase inhibitors, tricyclic antidepressants, selective serotonin reuptake inhibitors, opiate analgesics, over-the-counter cough medicines, antimigraine medications, antibiotics, herbal products, and certain drugs of abuse (14).

  f. **Differential diagnosis.** Other syndromes to rule out when serotonin syndrome is suspected are NMS, malignant hyperthermia, and anticholinergic poisoning.

3. **Hypertensive crisis** is a tyramine-induced adverse side effect of irreversible monoamine oxidase inhibitors (MAOIs).

  a. **Mechanism.** MAOIs prevent the metabolism of tyramine in the gut by inhibiting monoamine oxidase A (MAO-A).

  b. **Precautions.** Patients taking an MAOI should be careful of ingesting foods rich in tyramine (e.g., red wine, certain types of cheeses, beer, fava beans). Patients should also be cautious when using over-the-counter medicines that may interact with MAOIs (e.g., pseudoephedrine, dextromethorphan. and ephedrine).

c. Presentation. Patients may present with headache, severely elevated blood pressure, sweating, tachycardia, and vomiting.

d. Treatment. Phentolamine 5 mg intramuscularly or intravenously in a single dose is usually effective. Also used in hypertensive crisis are nifedipine for hypertension, propranolol for tachycardia, and Lasix for fluid retention.

BIBLIOGRAPHY

1. American Psychiatric Association: *APA Practice Guideline: Psychiatric Evaluation of Adults,* 2nd ed. Washington, DC, American Psychiatric Publishing, Inc., 2006.

2. Park JM, Park L, Prager LM: Emergency psychiatry. In *Mass General Hospital Comprehensive Clinical Psychiatry.* Edited by Stern TA, Rosenbaum JF. St. Louis, MO, Mosby, 2008.

3. Slaby AE, Dubin WR, Baron DA: Other psychiatric emergencies. In *Kaplan & Sadock's Comprehensive Textbook of Psychiatry,* 8th ed. Edited by Sadock BJ, Sadock VA. Philadelphia, Lippincott Williams & Wilkins, 2005, pp 2453–2471.

4. Centers for Disease Control and Prevention: *FastStats.* Available at: http://www.cdc.gov/nchs/fastats/suicide.htm. Accessed May 18, 2010.

5. American Psychiatric Association: *Practice Guidelines for the Treatment of Psychiatric Disorders,* Compendium 2006. Arlington, VA, American Psychiatric Association, 2006.

6. Joe S, Baser RE, Breeden G, et al: Prevalence of and risk factors for lifetime suicide attempts among blacks in the United States. *JAMA* 296:2112–2123, 2006.

7. Karch DL, Dahlberg LL, Patel N: Centers for Disease Control and Prevention: Surveillance for violent deaths – National Violent Death Reporting System, 16 states, 2007. *MMWR Surveill Summ* 59(No. SS-4), 2010.

8. Sudak HS. Suicide. In *Kaplan & Sadock's Comprehensive Textbook of Psychiatry,* 8th ed. Edited by Sadock BJ, Sadock VA. Philadelphia, Lippincott Williams & Wilkins, 2005, pp 2442–2452.

9. Schatzberg AF, Cole JO, DeBattista C, eds. *Manual of Clinical Psychopharmacology,* 6th ed. Arlington, VA, American Psychiatric Publishing, 2007.

10. Kanich W, Brady WJ, Huff JS, et al: Altered mental status: Evaluation and etiology in the ED. *Am J Emerg Med* 20:613–617, 2002.

11. Han CH, Kim YK: A double-blind trial of risperidone and Haldol for the treatment of delirium. *Psychosomatics* 45:297–301, 2004.

12. Zimmerman JL: Poisonings and overdoses. In *11th Critical Care Reader.* Edited by Szalados JE. Society of Critical Care Medicine, Mount Prospect, Illinois, 2007, pp 73–83.

13. Strawn JR, Keck PE, Caroff SN: Neuroleptic malignant syndrome. *Am J Psychiatry* 164:870–876, 2007.

14. Boyer EW, Shannon M: The serotonin syndrome. *N Engl J Med* 352:1112–1120, 2005.

Study Questions

QUESTIONS 1 AND 2

You are working in the emergency room when a Jane Doe is brought in by EMS secondary to being "found down in the field." On examination she is arousable only to painful stimuli, her pupils are constricted bilaterally, and she has an irregular respiratory rate of 6. Her skin is dusky and lips are blue. She is hypothermic.

1. After the above initial survey the first step should be to:
    - [A] Administer naloxone
    - [B] Administer naltrexone
    - [C] Control the airway
    - [D] Order a urine drug screen (UDS)
    - [E] Call a code

2. Jane Doe is admitted to the hospital and found to have pneumonia with diffuse bilateral infiltrates, diffuse lymphadenopathy on physical examination, an increased lactate dehydrogenase (LDH) level, and generalized wasting. What further laboratory test would you want to obtain?
    - [A] Hepatitis panel
    - [B] Magnetic resonance image of the chest
    - [C] HIV screen
    - [D] Thyroid function
    - [E] Serum glucose

QUESTIONS 3–5

A 31-year-old man is brought into the emergency room by his wife due to night sweats, fever, and confusion. His wife says that this started about 2 days ago and has quickly grown worse. She reports no one else in the family has been sick. His medical history is positive only for bipolar disorder and he has been on "some new medicine" for about 4 weeks.

On examination his temperature is 104°F, blood pressure is 160/108, pulse is 105, and respirations are 18. He is sweaty and responds to questions with "yeah I know" or "whatever." He is disoriented and unable to follow commands. His chest is clear to auscultation, and he shows full range of motion of his neck without any complaint. His abdomen is soft and nontender. Complete blood count (CBC) shows normal hemoglobin. The white blood cell (WBC) count is 15,200. Urinalysis is negative for bacteria, leukocyte esterase (LE), nitrite, and glucose but dark in appearance and positive for myoglobinuria. Lumbar puncture is normal, and chest radiograph is normal.

NMS

3. What would be the next diagnostic test indicated?
    - [A] Electrocardiogram (ECG)
    - [B] Electroencephalogram (EEG)
    - [C] Computed tomography (CT) scan of the head
    - [D] Liver function tests
    - [E] Creatine phosphokinase (CPK)

4. What type of medication is the patient most likely to have been started on 4 weeks ago?
    - [A] Stimulant
    - [B] Antipsychotic → NMS
    - [C] Mood stabilizer
    - [D] Antidepressant
    - [E] Sedative-hypnotic

5. What is the most common cause of death in patients with this syndrome?

[A] Cardiac ischemia
[B] Pulmonary edema
[C] Liver failure
[D] Renal failure → myoglobinuria from rhabdomyolysis
[E] Secondary infection

6. A 29-year-old man is brought into the emergency room (ER) via EMS after cutting himself with a broken glass at a busy nightclub. He reports, "Life isn't worth living if my girlfriend doesn't love me anymore." He reports that they were at the club when he saw her talking to another man and they then got into an argument. He endorses multiple previous cutting episodes in the past, stating, "It usually makes me feel better." Social history is notable for many past relationships but none lasting for more than 6 months. He continues to study in college but has changed fields of study multiple times. He states, "I just can't seem to figure out who I am." During the course of the ER stay his affect is noted to change from anger and sadness to later flirting with some of the ER nurses caring for him. What is the patient's most likely diagnosis?

[A] Borderline personality disorder   Unstable sense of self!
[B] Dysthymia
[C] Avoidant personality disorder
[D] Bipolar disorder
[E] Posttraumatic stress disorder

QUESTIONS 7–9

A John Doe arrives in the emergency room (ER) by EMS after ingesting an unknown number of pills. He called 911 shortly after taking the overdose. He is unconscious upon arrival in the ER but family reported to EMS a long history of depression that has been worsening recently. They report that he is on "several depression medicines." On examination he is unconscious but breathing spontaneously. His pupils are dilated. His temperature is 99.0°F, blood pressure is 150/90, pulse is 108, and respirations are 15. Electrocardiography shows QRS prolongation of 115 milliseconds.

7. What drug was the patient most likely to have overdosed on?

[A] Sertraline
[B] Lithium
[C] Benzodiazepines
[D] Amitriptyline   TCA = QT prolong
[E] Acetaminophen

8. After initial stabilization and airway management in the emergency room, what setting should this patient be treated in?

[A] Inpatient psychiatric
[B] Intensive outpatient psychiatric
[C] Inpatient general medical
[D] Inpatient telemetry or intensive care unit → arrhythmia risk
[E] Discharged home with outpatient follow-up with primary care and psychiatry

9. Which of the following psychiatric illnesses is most common in patients who successfully commit suicide?

[A] Generalized anxiety disorder
[B] Major depressive disorder
[C] Schizophrenia
[D] Borderline personality disorder
[E] Alcohol dependence

QUESTIONS 10 AND 11

A 19-year-old man presents to the emergency room with a complaint of a headache that has worsened over the past 3 days. Additionally, his partner has been concerned because of some "strange behavior," including calling their daughter by an incorrect name several times and staying up "all hours of the night." On examination his temperature is 101.2°F and the remainder of his vital signs are normal. His physical examination reveals a normal heart, lung, head, neck, and abdominal exam. His medical history is significant only for hepatitis C, for which he was treated in the distant past. Complete blood count showed a left shift with a white blood cell count of 16.5.

10. What would be the next diagnostic exam to order for this patient?

- [A] Lumbar puncture
- [B] Peripheral smear
- [C] HIV screen
- [D] Liver function tests (LFTs)
- [E] Computed tomography (CT) scan of the head

11. You are asked to evaluate the patient while he is still in the emergency room (ER) because he is exhibiting disorganized behavior and confusion. During your exam he starts taking out his IV lines and attempting to leave the ER. He reports to you that he is "just following my dog over there," pointing to an IV pole in the corner of the room. What medication would be most helpful for the patient's current condition?

- [A] Risperidone → agitation, confusion, psychotic sx in delirium
- [B] Benztropine
- [C] Lorazepam
- [D] Phenobarbital
- [E] Amitriptyline

Answers and Explanations

1. The answer is C. [*III E*] The patient's respiratory distress, constricted pupils, and hypothermia raise concern about opiate overdose. While administering naloxone is ultimately the treatment of choice for opiate overdose, initial management of any patient in respiratory distress should be to control the airway.

2. The answer is C. [*II A 1 l*] The pattern of patchy bilateral infiltrates with diffuse lymphadenopathy and increased lactate dehydrogenase (LDH) suggests *Pneumocystis* pneumonia. This, combined with concern about IV drug use and generalized wasting, suggests the need for an HIV screen.

3. The answer is E. [*III F 1 c*] The patient has some autonomic abnormalities, an altered mental state, and leukocytosis. His urine is dark and positive for myoglobinuria. This patient likely has neuroleptic malignant syndrome. A creatine phosphokinase (CPK) is the next diagnostic test indicated in this case and should be elevated.

4. The answer is B. [*III F 1 c*] The patient was most likely started on a neuroleptic for mood stabilization. This is the most probable cause of the patient's symptoms of neuroleptic malignant syndrome.

5. The answer is D. [*III F 1 e*] Patients with neuroleptic malignant syndrome are most likely to die from renal failure secondary to rhabdomyolysis and subsequent myoglobinuria.

6. The answer is A. [*III A 2 b (6)*] The patient has a history of self-injurious behaviors, unstable relationships, affect instability, and an unstable sense of self. These are all symptoms found in the *DSM-IV-TR* criteria for borderline personality disorder.

7. The answer is D. [*III E*] The tachycardia with QRS prolongation combined with dilated pupils and a known history of being on multiple antidepressants makes tricyclic antidepressant overdose likely for this patient. Benzodiazepines would cause bradycardia and respiratory depression. Lithium, sertraline, and acetaminophen would be much more likely to present with gastrointestinal symptoms and altered mental status.

8. The answer is D. [*III E*] Because of the patient's overdose on a tricyclic antidepressant, possible cardiac arrhythmias should be a concern. This patient, who already has QRS prolongation, should be monitored in an inpatient medical setting with the availability of telemetry.

9. The answer is B. [*III A 1 b (1)*] Major depressive disorder is the most common psychiatric illness seen in patients who commit suicide. Substance use and depression are present in over half of suicides. Patients with generalized anxiety disorder, schizophrenia, and borderline personality disorder are at risk for suicide, although less so than patients with major depressive disorder and substance use disorders.

10. The answer is E. [*II A 1 n*] This patient has a negative physical examination with the exception of a fever and leukocytosis. He has a history of hepatitis C but no other significant history. He presents with altered mental status and disorientation. He does not have a history of psychiatric illness and therefore should have a complete medical workup to reveal any medical causes. The next most appropriate diagnostic test for this patient is a computed tomography (CT) scan of the head to rule out an acute intracranial process.

11. The answer is A. [*III D 4*] The patient is hallucinating and is likely delirious. An antipsychotic medication, typical or atypical, is indicated for the treatment of agitation, confusion, and psychotic symptoms in delirium. Anticholinergic agents such as benztropine are likely to increase confusion in patients with delirium. Benzodiazepines can disinhibit patients further and have not been found to be useful except in cases of alcohol and benzodiazepine withdrawal.

chapter 12

Child Psychiatry

CRAIG STUCK

I INTRODUCTION

Child and adolescent psychiatry is the study and treatment of the mental, developmental, and behavioral problems of children.

A **Overview of childhood psychopathology**

1. **Psychopathology is usually the result of an interaction between genetic predisposition and the child's environment.** Development of mental health problems is best viewed from a **multifactorial model (biopsychosocial/spiritual/cultural)** in which genetically determined capacities, individual differences in temperament, physiologic variables, and environmental interactions all contribute. Protective biologic factors include intelligence and physical attractiveness. Protective environmental factors include having physical and emotional needs met; being intellectually stimulated; feeling loved and appreciated; having opportunities to achieve success in various endeavors (academics/athletics/arts); and having opportunities to form healthy peer relations. The absence of protective factors or the presence of biologic risk factors, such as genetic predisposition to mental illness, or environmental risk factors, such as loss or trauma, increase the probability that the child will develop mental illness.

B **Approach to the child and adolescent patient**

1. **The physician must be an advocate for the child** rather than for the parents. To do otherwise is to subject the child to the parents' wishes, even when they are unrealistic, inappropriate, or detrimental to the child. Nevertheless, child psychiatrists must deal respectfully and attempt to develop a working relationship with the parents. Often, the effectiveness of the work with the child is measured by the effectiveness of the work with the parents. Ineffective work with the parents may substantially limit the therapeutic progress of the child.
    a. In general, parents should be seen frequently, especially at the beginning of treatment.
    b. Preadolescents should usually be seen alone, but in most cases, after the parents have been seen.
    c. An attempt should be made to communicate with the child patient by talking. If this is difficult, a small assortment of toys, including a dollhouse, paper and crayons, games, puppets, modeling clay, and building materials, can help a child communicate through play.
    d. Adolescents should usually be seen alone. Often, their emerging and developmentally appropriate autonomy should be supported by seeing them before their parents are seen. Use of unnatural slang to bridge the "generation gap" should be avoided. An attitude of sincerity and concern for the adolescent usually establishes rapport with the patient.

2. **The following should be observed during the patient interview:**
    a. The child's reaction to separation from the parents
    b. The child's behavior toward the interviewer (e.g., anxious, very open, shy)
    c. The child's perception of people in general (e.g., trustworthy or dangerous, reliable or neglectful, kind or hostile)
    d. The choice of verbal versus play communication
    e. The clarity of the child's thought processes
    f. The child's level of development (i.e., social, language, motor, psychosexual, cognitive, moral) and its appropriateness to the child's age

      g. The ability of the child to identify different affective states and to discharge these states in an age-appropriate manner

      h. The ability of the child to tolerate frustration and to control impulses (In most cases, this may be observed through naturalistic circumstances such as setting a limit on an inappropriate behavior, declining an inappropriate request, announcing the end of a session, or requiring the child's assistance in cleaning up toys.)

      i. The child's perception of him- or herself (e.g., competent or ineffectual, master or victim) and the relative strength of his or her self-esteem

      j. The child's reaction to rejoining the parents after the interview

  3. Gathering information from the child can be facilitated by requesting that the child:

      a. Make three wishes and elaborate on each wish.

      b. Make drawings and elaborate on each drawing. (Drawings of people and families are especially helpful.)

      c. Describe his or her family.

      d. Describe important nonfamily members.

      e. Describe favorite television shows, movies, and musicians, noting with whom the child identifies.

      f. Describe the problem that initiated therapy and how the family told the child of the appointment.

      g. Describe hopes and wishes for the future.

II   NORMAL DEVELOPMENT

(A) Definitions

  1. Bonding describes the **parent's affective relationship with the child.** Bonding develops over time. There appears to be no critical phase of bonding in humans such as that described in animal studies. Bonding likely commences long before the birth of the child and is apparent in the parents' attitudes, fantasies, and wishes for the child.

  2. Attachment describes the **child's affective relationship with the parents.** Attachment, like bonding, develops over time. There is no critical phase for the development of attachment relationships, which may be formed at any time throughout the life cycle.

(B) Assessment of bonding

  1. The parents should be asked **when and how a name was chosen** for the child. This may suggest when they began planning for the new arrival. The name may also have special meaning. It may indicate how the family perceives the child or suggest attributions made to the child. For example, a son who is named after his father may be dealt with harshly by his mother when an acrimonious relationship exists between the parents.

  2. It is important to determine what sort of **dreams and fantasies the parents had** about the child **during pregnancy.** Frequent, realistic, and hopeful reflection about the baby enhances the outcome related to bonding and attachment.

  3. Likewise, it is important to determine **how the parents' relationship toward each other changed during the pregnancy.** The husband often assumes a maternal role toward his wife when she is pregnant. If, however, he begins abusing her, has affairs, or grows distant or uninvolved, a more difficult relationship between the parents and the new baby is likely. In addition, at this time, the parents' own unmet or inadequately met dependency needs and needs for nurture from childhood may complicate their relationships with each other and with their new child.

  4. Parents should be questioned regarding their **early reactions to the child in the delivery room and in the nursery.** Ambivalence of the parents concerning their child may be communicated behaviorally. It is important, however, to distinguish ambivalence from uncertainty, anxiety, and lack of confidence, all of which are normal reactions to childbirth and are particularly common to first-time parents.

  5. The parents should be asked **of whom the child reminds them.** This question assesses for transferences and preconceived attitudes about the infant. Inappropriate attributions to the child must be identified, clarified, disconnected from the child, and reconnected with the original object of attribution.

6. **The mental health of the parents** should be investigated. Depression, psychosis, personality disorders, and drug abuse are examples of problems that can distort the way the parent perceives, responds to, and interacts with the child.

7. **Special problems** are posed if the newborn spends extra time in the nursery because of illness (e.g., a child born 3 months premature who spends his first 2 months of life in a neonatal intensive care unit). A family with a child in the critical care nursery should be evaluated before discharge to ensure that the child will receive adequate care.

C Developmental screening

1. Parents should be asked about the child's achievement of **early milestones, such as sitting up, walking, development of speech, fine and gross motor skills, and potty training.**

2. It is important to gather information about the child's relationships with primary caregivers, other relatives, siblings, and peers.

III FEEDING AND EATING DISORDERS OF INFANCY AND EARLY CHILDHOOD

A **Pica** involves the persistent (for a period of at least 1 month) eating of nonfood products (e.g., dirt, clay, paper, plaster). This behavior is developmentally inappropriate and must be differentiated from the practice of mouthing inanimate objects, which is normal between 6 and 12 months of age.

1. **Epidemiology.** Pica may be more common in lower socioeconomic groups.

2. **Etiology**
   a. Pica is a heterogeneous disorder.
   b. Children with **mental retardation** mouth objects more than normal children.
   c. **Nutritional deficiencies** may play a role in some cases. Deficiencies of both vitamins and minerals have been suggested. In particular, iron deficiency can cause a craving for ice and nonfood items.
   d. **Parental psychopathology and environmental deprivation** are common in cases of children eating paint chips.
   e. By definition in the *Diagnostic and Statistical Manual of Mental Disorders*, fourth edition, text revision (*DSM-IV-TR*), pica is not sanctioned by the culture. **Cultural factors** play a role in the ingestion of some nonnutritive substances, such as the ingestion of religious clay tablets in some areas of Latin America.

3. **Complications** include **bezoars**, parasitic infestations, nutritional deficiencies, and heavy metal poisoning. **Lead poisoning** is extremely dangerous and is more common in older homes with lead-based paint. Lead poisoning should be suspected in any child who has an encephalopathy or who exhibits unusual behavior (e.g., irritability, anorexia, decreased activity).

4. **Treatment** for younger children involves appropriate supervision and removal of toxic substances from the child's environment. Nutritional deficiencies should be corrected. Behavioral interventions are preferred, especially for youths who are developmentally delayed or mentally retarded.

B **Rumination disorder** is a potentially fatal disorder that is characterized by the regurgitation of previously ingested food followed by rechewing of the food. Onset is typically in the first year of life, but in mentally retarded individuals the onset may be delayed until adulthood.

1. **Epidemiology.** Rumination disorder is rare.

2. **Etiology.** It has been suggested that individuals with rumination disorder have an underlying predisposition to regurgitate food and the process becomes habitual when it is learned that the regurgitating and chewing of food provides relief from emotional distress or is soothing.

3. **Treatment**
   a. **Dyad (parent–child) interactions should be observed.** Cues that the parent gives the child to encourage regurgitation should be interpreted and eradicated.
   b. **In-depth psychotherapy of one or both parents** is often needed.
   c. The **infant's nutritional status** should be followed closely.
   d. **Behavioral interventions** are the primary means of treatment among retarded individuals.
   e. There is a high rate of association of **gastroesophageal reflux** with rumination and it should be appropriately evaluated and treated.

C Feeding disorder of infancy or early childhood (failure to thrive) is diagnosed when a child **fails to gain or maintain weight at age-appropriate norms** and has **delayed development of social and behavioral milestones.** Usually, the third percentile for weight for age group is considered the threshold. Failure to grow in height sometimes accompanies this, but failure of head circumference growth occurs only in severe cases. It is common, accounting for 1% to 5% of inpatient pediatric admissions. The growth deceleration occurs because of inadequate caloric intake, which is compounded by the reduced interest the infant has in feeding. The delays in development are related to emotional deprivation in the environment.

1. **Failure to thrive is a syndrome.** A variety of terms have been used to describe it. **Hospitalism** emphasizes the extreme failure of any affective relationship to develop when an infant was institutionalized. **Anaclitic depression** describes failure to thrive in infants who were abruptly removed from their mothers between 9 and 12 months of age. Other terms include psychosocial deprivation, dwarfism, and nonorganic failure to thrive.

2. **Etiology**
   a. Failure to thrive as a **psychiatric condition** has numerous causes and manifestations. Irene Chatnoor has proposed seven categories of infant feeding disorders.
      1. **Feeding disorder of caregiver–infant reciprocity** develops when the caregiver is either depressed or has psychopathology such as borderline personality disorder. The mother often experienced her own mother as rejecting. The infant usually requires hospitalization and treatment requires a multidisciplinary team.
      2. **Feeding disorder of state regulation** describes the infant who has difficulty reaching a state of calm alertness to feed. The infant may be too sleepy or agitated. Treatments include treating the mother if necessary (anxiety/depression), helping the mother to read the infant's cues, and modifying the environment.
      3. **Infantile anorexia** begins between 9 and 18 months of age, when the child is beginning to self-feed. It is theorized to be related to issues of control. Cognitive development is normal.
      4. **Sensory food aversions** occur when a child refuses to eat foods with specific tastes, textures, or smells. It is more often associated with nutritional problems and infrequently severe enough to cause weight loss.
      5. **Posttraumatic feeding disorder** begins with an episode such as choking, severe vomiting, or a medical procedure that triggers severe distress in the infant/child and causes extreme fear of eating.
      6. **Feeding disorder associated with a concurrent medical illness** occurs when the caloric intake is inadequate because the infant has physical distress, such as reflux or respiratory distress, related to a medical problem.
      7. **Organic failure to thrive.** Several medical conditions can cause failure to thrive. These include cystic fibrosis, infectious diseases such as tuberculosis, endocrine disorders such as diabetes mellitus, and malabsorption syndromes. Medical workup should be guided by the history and examination. Any underlying medical disorders must be treated. Parent–child interactions should be evaluated carefully.
   b. When parental neglect is present, **child protective agencies** must be involved, to ensure that the child receives adequate care and that the services necessary to correct parental deficits are available. At times, custody of the child must be taken from the parents, and the child must be placed outside the home.

IV   REACTIVE ATTACHMENT DISORDER

A **Definition**   Beginning before age 5, the child has impaired social interactions that are due to pathologic parenting and not due to an autism spectrum disorder. In the **inhibited type,** the child does not initiate or respond appropriately socially, and may avoid contact or approach and then avoid contact. In the **disinhibited type,** children are overly familiar with strangers. Deficiencies in physical growth and behavioral development (failure to thrive) may co-occur.

B **Incidence** in community populations is not known. The **highest rates are reported among institutionalized children** (22%–56%), followed by children in foster care and homeless children.

C **Etiology** by definition is related to pathologic care involving neglect of the child's emotional and physical needs and/or multiple changes of caregivers. For youths reared in institutions, longer duration of institutionalization and deficiencies in the quality of care increase the severity of symptoms.

D **Treatment** is focused on having the child's physical and emotional needs met in a nurturing environment with a consistent caregiver. If the child is in foster care, a therapeutic foster home is preferred. Psychotherapy focuses on working with the infant–parent dyad. Caregivers should be advised to avoid unproven treatments that have documented risk, such as "holding" and "rebirthing." Treatment of the anxiety, mood, and disruptive behavior disorders that are frequently comorbid is important.

V AUTISM SPECTRUM DISORDERS (ASDs)

A **Autistic disorder**

1. **Clinical data.** Autistic disorder is an illness in which the child is relatively unresponsive to other human beings, demonstrates bizarre responses to the environment, and has unusual language development. Autistic disorder most commonly begins before age 3 years. Autism is a symptom of several disorders (e.g., schizophrenia). As a symptom, autism refers to a preoccupation with the internal world of the individual to the exclusion of external reactivity.
   a. Autistic children often treat other individuals indifferently, almost as though they are inanimate objects.
   b. Language abnormalities include echolalia, pronoun reversals (e.g., use of the pronoun "you" when "I" is correct), mutism, qualitative abnormalities (e.g., a sing-song or monotonous quality), and general language delays.
   c. Autistic children have a great need for consistency in their environment and may decompensate if, for example, furniture is rearranged. The cause of this need for sameness is unknown.
   d. Social development is invariably abnormal.

2. **Diagnostic criteria** (Table 12–1)

3. **Epidemiology.** Although the disorder has an even socioeconomic distribution, it is more common in boys.

4. **Etiology.** Autism is a strongly genetic disorder with a concordance rate of 60% to 90% among monozygotic twins. Several candidate genes have been identified and it is likely that there are multiple genes involved.

TABLE 12–1 Diagnostic Criteria for Autistic Disorder

Social interactional deficits, such as impairment in:
- Nonverbal communicative behaviors
- Peer relationships
- Taking the initiative in social interactions
- Interpersonal reciprocity within relationships

Communicative deficits, such as:
- Impairment in language development
- Impairment in conversational skills
- Use of repetitive or idiosyncratic language
- Impairment in the development of imaginative or imitative play

Behavioral deficits, such as:
- Consuming preoccupation with one or a few idiosyncratic areas of interest; otherwise, restricted breadth of interest in the surrounding environment
- Excessive need for routine; ritualized behaviors; inordinate resistance to change
- Stereotyped motor movements (e.g., hand flapping, rocking)
- Preoccupation with parts of objects

Reprinted with permission from the Diagnostic and Statistical Manual of Mental Disorders, Fourth Edition, Text Revision, (Copyright 2000). American Psychiatric Association.

5. Associated findings

    a. Recurrent seizures occur in 20% of individuals with autism.

    b. Associated genetic abnormalities may include **fragile X syndrome, tuberous sclerosis, and phenylketonuria.**

    c. Infants with ASD experience an acceleration of head growth after birth; **brain size of toddlers is larger than normal.**

    d. Neurobiologic studies have demonstrated that autistic individuals tend to engage in looking at objects rather than people, and when engaging people tend to **fixate on the mouth** rather than the eyes.

    e. During face perception tasks functional neuroimaging has consistently demonstrated decreased activity in the fusiform face area (FFA) of the temporal lobe.

    f. Mental retardation is often comorbid. Only 23% of individuals with autism have intelligence quotients (IQs) above 70; 50% fall between IQs of 50 and 70; and 27% have IQs below 50.

6. Differential diagnosis

    a. Hearing deficits

    b. Visual deficits

    c. Mental retardation accompanied by global developmental delays (not focal social and language distortions and delays as in autism)

    d. Organic mental disorders (e.g., hepatic encephalopathy and congenital cytomegalovirus), which can mimic autism

    e. Tourette disorder

    f. Childhood schizophrenia

    g. Obsessive-compulsive disorder (OCD)

    h. Selective mutism

    i. Other pervasive developmental disorders (e.g., Rett disorder, childhood disintegrative disorder, Asperger disorder)

7. Treatment

    a. A **highly structured classroom setting** is important to help autistic children focus their attention on learning and communication tasks. Pragmatics, daily living skills, and a functional curriculum may take precedence over conventional academics. Precautions should be taken to ensure that the environment remains stable (e.g., predictable schedules, routines, personnel, and materials).

    b. Behavioral modification, such as Applied Behavioral Analysis (ABA), may help to increase appropriate behavior and decrease inappropriate behaviors. Early interventions should also foster social skills. **Developmental, Individual Differences (DIR)** is an approach that develops social interaction by building on activities that are of interest to the child. It has not been evaluated in controlled studies. **Social stories** are used to convey information about specific social situations to help the child understand issues such as social cues and exchanges.

    c. Medication is rarely of value unless a specific indication is present.

        (1) Some hyperactive autistic children may benefit from stimulant medication (e.g., methylphenidate).

        (2) Obsessional features may respond to selective serotonin reuptake inhibitors (SSRIs) such as fluvoxamine.

        (3) Mood instability may be improved with **mood stabilizers** such as lithium, valproic acid, and carbamazepine.

        (4) Self-stimulating behaviors may improve with **opioid antagonists** such as naltrexone.

        (5) Atypical antipsychotics, such as risperidone, are occasionally indicated for acute stabilization of aggressive, self-injurious, or severely out-of-control behaviors.

    d. Adjunctive therapies, such as speech and language therapy, occupational therapy, and physical therapy, are often indicated.

8. Prognosis. Many autistic children develop grand mal seizures before adolescence. However, the prognosis for autistic disorder is better if the child has:

    a. A high intelligence quotient

    b. Reasonable language development

    c. Relatively mild symptomatology

VI LEARNING DISORDERS

A **Clinical data**   A wide range of disorders can interfere with a child's ability to perform certain intellectual functions. Children may suffer from specific reading, processing, writing, mathematical, and language disabilities (e.g., developmental dyslexia).

1. These disorders must be distinguished from both mental retardation and pervasive developmental disorders.

2. **Diagnosis** is established by documenting a mismatch between the child's performance on standardized measures of the skill in question and his or her intellectual capacity as measured by IQ testing.

3. The *DSM-IV-TR* includes the following **categories and specific disorders:**
   a. **Learning disorders**
      (1) Reading disorder
      (2) Mathematics disorder
      (3) Disorder of written expression
   b. **Motor skills disorder** (developmental coordination disorder)
   c. **Communication disorders**
      (1) Expressive language disorder
      (2) Mixed receptive–expressive language disorder
      (3) Phonologic disorder
      (4) Stuttering

B **Differential diagnosis** of specific developmental problems includes a variety of psychiatric conditions:

1. **Depression**
2. **Attention deficit hyperactivity disorder**
3. **Anxiety**
4. **Childhood psychosis**
5. **An interaction problem with the teacher**
6. **Pervasive developmental disorders**
7. **Mental retardation**

C **Treatment** is aimed at the underlying dysfunction. Learning disorders require academic remediation. The spectrum of services in this domain ranges from extra tutoring focused on the problematic academic skill (e.g., phonics tutoring for children with dyslexia) to placement in self-contained, special education classrooms for those with learning disorders.

1. **Motor skills disorder** may require occupational or physical therapy.

2. **Communication disorders** usually require intensive speech and language therapy.

VII ATTENTION DEFICIT HYPERACTIVITY DISORDER (ADHD)

A **Clinical data**   Key symptoms of ADHD include a short attention span, difficulty concentrating, impulsivity, distractibility, excitability, and hyperactivity.

1. **Hyperactivity** is defined subjectively as an increase in motor activity to a level that interferes with the child's functioning at school, at home, or socially.

2. It is important to note, however, that symptoms of **attention deficit disorder may exist with or without hyperactivity.**

3. The *DSM-IV-TR* distinguishes **three subtypes** of the disorder based on this differentiation:
   a. ADHD, predominantly inattentive type
   b. ADHD, predominantly hyperactive-impulsive type
   c. ADHD, combined type

TABLE 12–2 Diagnostic Criteria for Attention Deficit Hyperactivity Disorder

Symptoms of inattention, such as:
- Lack of attention to details
- Difficulty sustaining attention for prolonged periods
- Not listening
- Difficulty following through or completing tasks
- Disorganization
- Avoidance of activities that require sustained attention
- Tendency to lose personal belongings
- Marked distractibility
- Forgetfulness

Symptoms of hyperactivity, such as:
- Fidgetiness or squirminess
- Difficulty remaining in seat, or sitting quietly
- Developmentally excessive activity level
- Difficulty engaging in nonaction activities
- Talking excessively

Symptoms of impulsivity, such as:
- Blurting out answers without raising hand or waiting for the end of the question
- Difficulty with "turn-taking" activities
- Frequent interruption or intrusion into others' conversations or activities
Presence of some symptoms before age 7 years
Significant functional impairment as a result of the symptoms

Reprinted with permission from the Diagnostic and Statistical Manual of Mental Disorders, Fourth Edition, Text Revision, (Copyright 2000). American Psychiatric Association.

B **Diagnostic criteria**   (Table 12–2)

C **Differential, comorbidity and etiology**

1. **Medication.** Sedative-hypnotics paradoxically cause hyperactivity in some children.

2. **Depression.** Sad feelings may be expressed by means of increased activity.

3. **Anxiety**

4. **Severe CNS disease.** A grossly abnormal CNS or a history of significant head trauma may cause hyperactivity.

5. **Constitutional hyperactivity.** Some children have a hyperactive temperament that is present from birth.

6. **An intolerant parent, teacher, or supervisor** may bring about factitious hyperactivity (i.e., the child is not truly suffering from increased motor activity).

7. **Specific learning disabilities** may be associated with hyperactivity.

8. Severe **language disorders**

9. There is an increased incidence of ADHD among children with **Tourette disorder.**

10. ADHD is a strongly genetic disorder.

D **Treatment**   Any underlying disorder should be treated (e.g., depression should be treated by means of psychotherapy, possibly in conjunction with antidepressant medication).

1. **Medications**
    a. **Stimulant medications** are the most studied and most effective treatment. Choices include **methylphenidate, dextroamphetamine,** and **dexmethylphenidate,** which have sustained-release preparations that provide more even blood levels and once-in-the-morning dosing. Growth curves should be followed on all children taking stimulant medications because appetite and growth suppression are the most common side effects. Blood pressure and pulse should be followed.
    b. **Clonidine** and **guanfacine** have been shown to be effective alternatives to psychostimulants in many children. They may also be used effectively to augment psychostimulants in certain

refractory cases. Aggression, hyperactivity, and impulsivity are more responsive than are the symptoms of inattention.

    c. Atomoxetine, a norepinephrine reuptake inhibitor, is less effective than the psychostimulants but has no abuse potential.

    d. Antidepressants such as **bupropion** have been effective alternative agents in some children.

2. **Diet.** An alteration in the child's diet may be helpful, presumably because the emphasis on food alters a parent's relationship with a child in some meaningful way.

    a. Many parents of hyperactive children report that reducing the child's sugar intake reduces the hyperactivity.

      (1) These parents may pay more attention to their child, feel more in control of the problem, and spend more time with the child at mealtime as a result of changing the child's diet.

      (2) All of these secondary effects can be beneficial.

    b. No direct effects of diet on either the etiology or treatment of ADHD have been demonstrated, however.

3. **Behavior modification programs** are often beneficial. Despite the ADHD symptomatic deficits, children with this disorder must still be held accountable for their behavior and its consequences.

4. Although **psychotherapy** is not the mainstay of treatment in this disorder, it may be a useful adjunct to a comprehensive treatment plan in certain children.

5. **Environmental engineering** is of great benefit in ADHD. Because children with ADHD do not readily adapt to change or function well within highly stimulating environments, the environment around them should be constructed to minimize these distractions.

    a. Within the classroom, children with ADHD attend and concentrate better in the front row than in the rear.

    b. Study carrels are helpful because they block distracting stimuli.

    c. Children with ADHD function better with one-on-one instruction and in small groups rather than in larger groups.

VIII   DISRUPTIVE BEHAVIOR DISORDERS

A   Conduct disorder (CD)

1. **Definition.** The *DSM-IV-TR* describes conduct disorder as a pervasive and repetitive pattern of behaviors that violate the rights of others or violate social rules. At least three of the 15 criteria must be present. **The criteria include physical aggression toward people or animals, property destruction, stealing, lying, truancy, and running away from home. Childhood onset** describes those with at least one symptom of conduct disorder before age 10. This group tends to be male, have comorbid ADHD, and have a greater risk of adult antisocial personality disorder. **Adolescent-onset** conduct disorder usually carries a better prognosis.

2. **Epidemiology.** Conduct disorder is predominately a male disorder, with a male:female ratio of 3:1 to 4:1. Common comorbid disorders include ADHD, learning disorders, mood disorders, and substance abuse. Anxiety disorders, especially posttraumatic stress disorder (PTSD), are more common in females with conduct disorder.

3. **Etiology. Untreated or inadequately treated ADHD** contributes to disruptive behavior in many juveniles. These youths often have difficult temperaments and are novelty seeking. **Aversive parenting is often present;** the parent(s) may be inconsistent, abusive, or neglectful. There is an increased incidence of parents with mental illness and substance abuse problems. As youths experience a lack of academic success and rejection, they tend to associate with other similar peers and may affiliate with gangs.

4. **Treatment. There is a lack of evidence-based treatments for adolescents.** The emphasis should be on early intervention. Assessment of the child should identify any comorbid disorders, with comprehensive treatment including family, behavioral, pharmacologic, and educational interventions. An assessment of the family should include a history of the parenting practices, any involvement of child protective services, the family's mental health history, and current social stressors. Older youths may require inpatient treatment, residential treatment, intensive in-home

interventions such as Multi-Systemic Therapy (MST), or incarceration. Predictors of positive outcomes include adolescent onset, higher verbal IQ, and higher socioeconomic status. **Lower IQ, more severe conduct disorder symptoms, and parental antisocial personality disorder increase the likelihood that youths will meet criteria for antisocial personality disorder in adulthood.**

B **Oppositional defiant disorder (ODD)**

1. **Definition.** Youths with this disorder have problems with **anger, irritability, and defiance.** If criteria for conduct disorder are met, then this diagnosis is not given.

2. **Epidemiology. Lifetime prevalence for ODD is 10%.**

3. **Etiology. It is frequently comorbid with ADHD.** Studies have shown that when children with ODD are **excited by possible reward and are less concerned about possible punishment than controls.**

4. **Treatment.**

   a. Psychopharmacologic treatments should address symptoms of comorbid ADHD. **Stimulants, clonidine, and atomoxetine can decrease oppositional behavior in children with ADHD.**

   b. **Behavioral treatments with proven efficacy include parent management training and problem-solving training for the child.**

IX TOURETTE DISORDER

A **Clinical data** Tourette disorder consists of motor tics (sudden, recurrent, nonrhythmic motor movements) and vocal tics (e.g., coprolalia, barking, and grunting), not necessarily occurring at the same time. Psychological stress exacerbates the symptoms, but the cause, although unknown, is probably organic. Both ADHD and OCD occur with increased frequency among patients with Tourette disorder.

B **Diagnostic criteria** (Table 12–3)

C **Epidemiology** Tourette disorder is three times more common in boys than girls. Onset is before the age of 21 years and often occurs in early childhood. Lifetime prevalence is 0.4% to 1.8%. There is a spectrum of symptom severity, and previously undiagnosed individuals with more mild symptoms are now being appropriately diagnosed.

D **Treatment**

1. **Education** about the nature and course of the disorder for both the patient and the family is essential.

2. **Habit reversal training,** a type of behavioral therapy that teaches the child to use a competing response, has been shown to be useful.

3. **Medical treatment** can be used to reduce tics. It includes the use of the following agents:

   a. Dopamine-blocking agents such as **haloperidol, pimozide, and risperidone can reduce tics. Side effects are common, and with pimozide, there is a risk of QTc prolongation, which can lead to cardiac arrhythmias.** The typical antipsychotics have an increased risk of tardive dyskinesia.

   b. **Clonidine** has proved to be effective in some cases of Tourette disorder. Although highly sedating, clonidine does not have the dystonic and dyskinetic side effects of the neuroleptics. **Guanfacine** is a similar but less sedating alternative to clonidine.

TABLE 12–3 Diagnostic Criteria for Tourette Disorder
Multiple tics, including both motor and vocal tics
Frequent tics, nearly daily, for a year or more, with no asymptomatic period of more than 3 months
Emotional distress or functional impairment as a result of the tics
Onset before age 18 years

Reprinted with permission from the Diagnostic and Statistical Manual of Mental Disorders, Fourth Edition, Text Revision, (Copyright 2000). American Psychiatric Association.

X   **MOOD DISORDERS**

A **Major depressive disorder (MDD)**

1. **Epidemiology.** The prevalence is 2% in children and 4% to 8% among adolescents.

2. **Diagnostic criteria.** *DSM-IV-TR* criteria are the same for children as for adults (see Table 3–1). Depressed **preschool children** often demonstrate behavioral difficulties, such as hyperactivity and aggression, more than older children. In children and adolescents, the depressive mood is commonly expressed as **marked irritability. Adolescents** may also demonstrate the usual signs of depression, especially a pervasive sense of boredom and lack of future orientation. The incidence of depressive disorders increases in adolescence, with girls affected more often than boys.

3. **Treatment**

   a. **Psychotherapy. Cognitive behavioral models** aimed at correcting cognitive distortions and reversing pervasive patterns of negativistic thinking have been successful, but it may take up to 12 weeks for more severe depressive symptoms to improve. Most studies demonstrate a 60% response among treated youths. **Interpersonal psychotherapy** also has demonstrated efficacy.

   b. **Medication**

      (1) For youths with MDD treated with SSRIs, about 60% have a positive response. When combined with cognitive behavioral therapy, SSRIs help produce a more rapid response.

      (2) SSRIs such as fluoxetine, sertraline, and escitalopram are considered the first-line medications of choice.

      (3) In 2004, the **U.S. Food and Drug Administration (FDA) issued a black-box warning** that "antidepressants increased the risk of suicidal thinking and behavior (suicidality) in short-term studies of children and adolescents with major depressive disorder and other psychiatric disorders." Analyses of data showed that children and adolescents receiving antidepressants were two times more likely to show suicidal thinking and behavior during the first few months of treatment. No completed suicides occurred in any of the clinical trials. It is important to balance the FDA warning against the potential therapeutic benefit and risk of untreated psychiatric illness. Children and adolescents taking antidepressants should be closely monitored for clinical worsening, suicidality, and unusual changes in behavior.

      (4) Parents must take responsibility for administering the medication and for safeguarding the child and siblings from an inadvertent overdose.

B **Dysthymic disorder**

1. **Epidemiology.** The prevalence is about 1% in children and 2% to 8% in adolescents.

2. **Diagnostic criteria.** Compared with the *DSM-IV-TR* criteria in adults, the duration of mood change required is at least 1 year and the mood can be irritable.

3. **The treatment approaches are the same as those used for MDD.**

C **Bipolar disorder**

1. Of youths with depression, 20% to 40% will develop **bipolar disorder.** *DSM-IV-TR* criteria are the same for children as for adults (see Table 3–2).

2. **Risk factors include family history of bipolar disorder, psychotic depression, and experiencing mania that is induced by antidepressant medications.**

3. **Treatment. Lithium, valproic acid, carbamazepine, lamotrigine, and atypical antipsychotics** have been used effectively in children and adolescents. Psychoeducation and psychosocial interventions are recommended.

D **Suicide** may be a complication of a mood disorder in children and adolescents, as well as in later developmental stages.

1. **Suicide is the third leading cause of death among adolescents and young adults.**

2. **Male children and adolescents are more likely to complete suicide. Female children and adolescents are more likely to attempt suicide.**

3. Conduct disorder and substance abuse increase the risk of suicide.

4. **Treatment.** Depressed children should be carefully evaluated for suicidal ideation. When suicidal ideation is found, the child may require psychiatric hospitalization for acute clinical stabilization and his or her own safety. **Parents should be advised to take measures to decrease the risk of suicide by removing all firearms and other weapons from the home and removing or locking up all medications and poisons.**

XI ANXIETY DISORDERS

A Specific phobias

1. **Epidemiology.** Five percent of children and adolescents have specific phobias.

2. **Clinical data.** Most phobias are triggered by an inciting event and perpetuated by patterns of avoidance.

3. **Treatment. Behavioral treatments such as systematic desensitization are effective.** Flooding approaches are less preferred. **For blood/needle/injury phobias,** the use of **applied tension** is beneficial. This technique involves tensing the muscles of the arms, legs, and abdomen to help counter the hypotensive response that commonly precedes the fainting associated with this type of phobia.

B Obsessive-compulsive disorder

1. **Epidemiology. One percent of children and adolescents have OCD.** Contamination obsessions and compulsions are most common; other typical presentations include checking and symmetry compulsions. Children may hide the behavior from adults. Adults may misinterpret compulsive questioning as defiant behavior.

2. **Differential.** If there is abrupt onset in early childhood, **PANDAS** (pediatric autoimmune neuropsychiatric disorders associated with streptococcal group A infections) **should be considered. A throat culture should be performed and appropriate antibiotic treatment used.** Studies to date have not demonstrated efficacy for antibiotic prophylaxis.

3. **Treatment. Cognitive behavioral therapy should be the initial treatment.** Major components include psychoeducation and **exposure and response prevention.** The child learns to rate the degree of anxiety experienced with the obsessions and practices tolerating the anxiety without performing the compulsive behaviors previously employed. A hierarchy is used to progressively address all symptoms. SSRIs may be used as an adjunctive treatment, and comparatively higher doses may be required.

C Generalized anxiety disorder (GAD)

1. Previously described as "overanxious disorder of childhood," the current *DSM-IV-TR* terminology uses the same criteria as for adult GAD. The fears are excessive and cause marked distress or psychosocial impairment.

2. **Epidemiology.** Prevalence is 2% to 4%. It is more common in females.

3. **Treatment. Cognitive behavioral therapy and SSRIs are beneficial.**

D Posttraumatic stress disorder

1. The *DSM-IV-TR* criteria describe the different ways symptoms may present in younger children. For example, **young children** may have nightmares but not report the content. They **may not describe intrusive recollections but instead play out traumatic themes repeatedly.** Aggression in response to triggers and dissociative symptoms may be misinterpreted by adults. **PTSD in youths can occur as a result of physical abuse, sexual abuse, accidents, and natural disasters. It also can result from observing life-threatening trauma (e.g., a young child witnessing domestic violence).** It is important to assess youths' perception of risk, particularly as younger children may overestimate the risk of bodily harm or death from traffic accidents.

2. **Risks.** Youths exposed to trauma do not always develop PTSD. Other possible outcomes include depression and resilience. Previous psychopathology and lack of maternal support predict greater risk of developing PTSD.

3. **Therapy. Cognitive behavioral therapy** has the most evidence for efficacy. Components include relaxation therapy, establishing a hierarchy, gradual exposure, creating a trauma narrative, and addressing distorted cognitions.

E Separation anxiety disorder

1. **This disorder is characterized by excessive fear of separation from home or the primary caregivers. Refusal to attend school is the most common presentation.** Legitimate causes of fear should be evaluated for and eliminated when present. **The child should usually be sent back to school immediately** so that school avoidance is not reinforced by staying home.

2. **Desensitization and other behavior therapy** modalities may be of benefit.

3. **Parental therapy** is necessary when the child is acting out the parent's anxiety about separating from the child.

4. **Anxiolytic medications** such as the SSRIs and, occasionally, benzodiazepines may be beneficial.

XII CHILDHOOD AND EARLY-ONSET SCHIZOPHRENIA

A The differential for psychotic symptoms in children and adolescents includes:

1. **Anxiety disorders (PTSD, OCD)**

2. **Mood disorders (depression with psychotic features; mania)**

3. **Substance abuse (hallucinogens, anticholinergics, stimulants)**

4. **Psychosis due to a medical disorder**

B Childhood schizophrenia and early-onset schizophrenia

1. **Clinical data**
   a. **Early-onset schizophrenia refers to onset before age 18.**
      (1) The presentation is comparable to adult presentations, with **an initial prodromal period. Visual hallucinations are more common in youths** and delusions are less common.
   b. **Childhood schizophrenia refers to onset before age 13 and is extremely rare.**
      (1) **Affected children have a history of poor premorbid functioning;** problem areas include learning, language, behavior, and socialization.
      (2) **The psychotic symptoms tend to be severe and persistent; outcomes are poor.**

2. **Diagnostic criteria.** *DSM-IV-TR* criteria are the same for children as for adults (see Table 2–1).

3. **Etiology**
   a. Studies continue to demonstrate a **genetic component** to the development of schizophrenia. The concordance among monozygotic twins is 40% to 60%. Heredity alone, however, does not account for the etiology.
   b. Association with advanced paternal age has been proposed but remains unproven.
   c. In utero exposure to maternal famine is a risk factor.
   d. The loss of gray matter has been demonstrated in neuroanatomic studies.

4. **Treatment**
   a. **Treatment with antipsychotic medications** is mostly based on studies of adults. Risperidone and aripiprazole have been FDA approved for adolescents with schizophrenia.
   b. **Psychiatric day treatment** may be indicated when the child's symptoms preclude his or her ability to function adequately in a public school environment.
   c. Psychotherapy addresses issues such as medication compliance, family functioning, and interpersonal skills.

5. **Prognosis**
   a. It is likely that early-onset schizophrenia is a more severe variant as compared to adult-onset schizophrenia.
   b. **A poorer prognosis is associated with the duration of untreated psychosis and the degree of severity of the negative symptoms.**

XIII   SLEEP DISORDERS

A **Parasomnias** are much more prevalent in children than adults.

1. **Somnambulism** (sleepwalking)
   a. **Somnambulism** is exacerbated by psychological stress in some people but is normal much of the time.
   b. **Epidemiology.** Sleepwalking is common, with an estimated prevalence of 40%, though only 2% of these sleepwalk more than once a month. **Onset is typically between the ages of 4 and 8 and incidence peaks at age 12.**
   c. **Treatment.** Most sleepwalking resolves, but may persist up to the age of 15 years. It is important to promote regular sleep schedules. Youths are at risk of injury and parents should take precautions such as locking doors and windows. While medications such as imipramine and benzodiazepines have been used, symptoms tend to recur when the medication is discontinued.

2. **Somniloquy** (sleep talking) has little clinical significance; however, if somniloquy is present, more significant parasomnias may also be present.

3. **Night terrors**
   a. **Clinical data.** Night terrors occur during non–rapid eye movement (NREM) stage 4 sleep just before the point of change to rapid eye movement (REM) sleep. They occur during the first third of the night, about 90 to 120 minutes after the onset of sleep. The child suddenly becomes agitated, screams, appears terrified, and stares. This is accompanied by autonomic arousal with sweating, tachycardia, hyperventilation, and pupil dilatation. The typical episode lasts 3 to 5 minutes. **Night terrors should be distinguished from nightmares,** which occur during REM sleep and whose content is remembered as a bad dream. Night terrors are characterized by:
      (1) Inconsolability of the child during the event
      (2) Absence of recall of the content of the dream
      (3) Absence of recall of the event the following morning
   b. **Epidemiology.** Night terrors are more common in boys and typically occur between the ages of 3 and 6.
   c. **Treatment.** Education of the parents with reassurance is important, as sleep terrors do not require any specific treatment and will resolve without intervention. Regular sleep habits are important. Awakening the child before the usual time of onset of the sleep terrors may help to abort attacks. Benzodiazepines have been used in severe cases, but the parasomnia typically recurs when they are withdrawn.

4. **Nightmares.** Dreams are reported by children beginning at the age of 4. Nightmares are frightening dreams that can be related to typical childhood fears, such as monsters, or can occur as part of anxiety disorders, such as separation anxiety or posttraumatic stress disorder. **Nightmares usually occur in the early morning hours, when the proportion of REM sleep in the REM–NREM sleep cycle is greater.**

B **Dyssomnias**

1. **Narcolepsy**
   a. **Clinical data. Narcolepsy begins during adolescence** and early adulthood. REM sleep suddenly intrudes on wakefulness, causing **excessive daytime drowsiness and sleep attacks.** Symptoms include the following:
      (1) **Cataplexy,** a classic symptom of narcolepsy, is the loss of motor tone in response to an emotion (e.g., anger or excitement).
      (2) On awakening, the patient may be transiently but completely paralyzed (**sleep paralysis**).
      (3) **Hypnagogic hallucinations** are vivid auditory and visual hallucinations that occur at the onset of sleep.
   b. **Epidemiology. It has a prevalence of 0.04%.**
   c. **Treatment.** The excessive daytime sleepiness may be treated with traditional stimulant medications as well as **modafinil,** an α_1-adrenergic receptor agonist that reduces the number of sleep attacks. Regular scheduled sleep times are important, including naps of 20 to 30 minutes two to three times a day. For the **treatment of cataplexy,** tricyclic antidepressants such as **clomipramine** may be used.

2. **Primary insomnia**
   a. **Clinical data.** This disorder includes problems with children **protesting bedtime, prolonged sleep latency, and nocturnal awakenings.**
   b. **Epidemiology**. Primary insomnia occurs in 25% to 35% of preschool-aged children.
   c. **Treatment. Behavioral treatment interventions are preferred;** these include emphasizing bedtime routines, limit setting on reunions, having the child sleep in his or her own bed (instead of sleeping with the parent), sleep hygiene measures, and cognitive behavioral interventions. There are no FDA-approved medications for pediatric insomnia. Antihistamines such as hydroxyzine may be used, but they have the adverse potential to cause daytime drowsiness and anticholinergic side effects. Melatonin has been used for initial insomnia, but it is not helpful for sleep maintenance insomnia.

XIV ELIMINATION DISORDERS

A Enuresis

1. **Clinical data.** Children with enuresis continue to urinate at inappropriate times and places after the time when they should have been toilet trained (i.e., between the ages of 2 and 4 years). **The prevalence in 5-year-olds is 5% to 10% and decreases to 3% to 5% by the age of 10.** The disorder is much more common in boys.
   a. **Primary enuresis** is that which has never been interrupted by a period of good bladder control.
      (1) **Nocturnal enuresis** is a parasomnia that occurs during stages 3 and 4 of sleep.
      (2) **Diurnal enuresis** occurs during the waking hours.
   b. **Secondary enuresis** develops after at least 1 year of good bladder control. As in primary enuresis, the disorder may occur during both the sleeping and waking hours.
   c. The *DSM-IV-TR* specifies that episodes occur at least twice weekly for 3 months or more or cause significant distress or psychosocial impairment. In addition, the condition is not diagnosed before the chronologic age (or in developmentally impaired children, the developmental age) of 5 years.

2. **Etiology**
   a. **Organic disorders** may cause enuresis. These include:
      (1) **Systemic illnesses,** such as:
         (a) Juvenile-onset diabetes mellitus
         (b) Sickle cell anemia or sickle cell trait
         (c) Diabetes insipidus
      (2) **CNS disorders,** such as:
         (a) Frontal lobe tumor
         (b) Spinal cord lesion (e.g., spina bifida or spina bifida occulta)
         (c) Peripheral nerve damage
      (3) **Anatomic disorders,** such as:
         (a) Posterior urethral valvular dysfunction
         (b) Proximal genitourinary malformations
      (4) **Urinary tract infections**
   b. **Psychological factors** account for most cases of secondary enuresis.
      (1) **Acute stress** can cause enuresis (e.g., the birth of a sibling, a family move, starting kindergarten).
      (2) **Hostility** can be expressed through the symptom of enuresis. Such an expression of hostility is nearly always unconscious.
      (3) **Family reaction** to the enuresis sometimes causes more psychopathology than the psychological causes of the enuresis. The family may encourage enuresis unconsciously. The parents may take vicarious pleasure in the child's enuresis.
      (4) **Preoccupation.** Children who are too busy or preoccupied to remember to use the bathroom may suffer from enuresis.

3. **Treatment** may be necessary only sporadically. Because enuresis is a self-limited disorder, sometimes the best treatment is no treatment. Parents should be reassured that the disorder is a time-limited,

normal developmental variant (especially the primary nocturnal pattern) that will ultimately be outgrown.

    a. Probing diagnostic procedures to search for an organic etiology, unless the preponderance of evidence points to such, **should be avoided.**

    b. The parents should be assured that the child is not purposefully wetting (enuresis is usually beyond the child's control). **Remedial measures** include:

        (1) Use of special feedback devices that set off an alarm upon urination in bed have a success rate of 75%, and has been associated with increased bladder capacity.

        (2) Other approaches that may be beneficial but are less effective than alarm systems include reduction of fluid intake after dinner, awakening the child to urinate after 1 to 2 hours of sleep, and bladder exercises (having the child hold urine during the day for progressively longer periods of time).

    c. Medication is not considered first-line treatment.

        (1) DDAVP (Desmopressin), a synthetic antidiuretic hormone that may be administered either orally or as a nasal spray, may offer symptomatic improvement.

        (2) Because of the time-limited nature of the disorder, drug holidays should be instituted at least every 6 months to assess the need for continuing pharmacologic intervention.

B **Encopresis**

    1. Clinical data. Encopresis is fecal incontinence beyond the period when bowel control should normally have developed. Most encopresis is unconscious and involuntary; only occasionally does it occur deliberately.

    a. Primary encopresis has occurred continuously throughout the child's life.

    b. Secondary encopresis develops after at least 1 year of good bowel control.

    c. The *DSM-IV-TR* delineates two additional **subtypes:**

        (1) With constipation and overflow incontinence

        (2) Without constipation and overflow incontinence

    2. Etiology

    a. Medical causes

        (1) In the encopresis variant with constipation and overflow incontinence, the encopresis results from children avoiding evacuating their bowels and retaining feces.

            (a) This results in a fecal impaction that is readily identifiable within the rectal vault.

            (b) In these children, stool is passed around the impaction, often in small amounts.

            (c) Causes of constipation include an inherent physiologic predisposition to become constipated (present in more than 50% of children with encopresis), diet, and avoiding defecation because of pain (anal fissures or traumatic injuries) or fears (toilet phobias).

        (2) In Hirschsprung disease, the functional obstruction is proximal to the rectal vault so that no fecal obstruction is palpable on digital examination.

    b. Psychological factors

        (1) Encopresis without constipation and overflow incontinence, also referred to as nonretentive encopresis, has not been comprehensively studied. In case studies problems identified have included the following:

            (a) Unresolved anger at a parent is sometimes expressed unconsciously through fecal incontinence.

            (b) Regressive wishes may be expressed by soiling in undernurtured and emotionally deprived children.

            (c) Fecal smearing may be a **psychotic symptom,** especially if the child is older than 4 or 5 years of age.

        (2) As is true with enuresis, parents can get vicarious pleasure from their child's symptoms.

    3. Treatment

    a. Correction of fecal impaction is necessary. A bowel regimen that consists of periodic cathartic administration to ensure that no impaction develops and to help regulate bowel control (e.g., administration of a bisacodyl suppository daily at the same time, immediately followed by placing the child on the toilet) may be beneficial. Polyethylene glycol is an osmotic agent that can help promote soft bowel movements in children predisposed to constipation.

b. Behavior modification that reinforces continence is effective in some children (e.g., rewarding a child after a day of good bowel control or after evacuation in the toilet).

c. Psychotherapy may be indicated. Occasionally, encopresis is a symptom of psychosis. The underlying disease should then be treated.

d. Family therapy also is often indicated.

XV CHILD ABUSE

Child abuse occurs when the individuals in a child's environment retard the child's development by hurting him or her.

A Epidemiology

1. Child abuse may be **physical, sexual,** or **emotional. Significant neglect** should be considered equivalent to abuse.

2. Approximately **15% of children who come to the emergency room with obvious trauma** have been abused. Children are unlikely to spontaneously report sexual abuse and should be specifically asked about the possibility of abuse. Behaviors that are strongly correlated with sexual victimization include masturbating with an object and placing objects into the rectum or vagina.

3. **Most abusive parents were maltreated as children.** However, most abused children do not subsequently become abusive parents. It is estimated that two-thirds of individuals who were abused as children do not perpetuate abusive behavior with their children.

4. Parents who are not overtly abusive may be **silently participating** in the abuse by failing to protect the child from the abusive parent (e.g., a mother who is physically present in the home yet is "unaware" of years of ongoing stepfather–daughter incest).

5. **Premature infants** are abused more often than full-term infants, probably at least partly because of poor bonding.

6. **Abuse of infants** occurs more frequently because their parents are emotionally needy and feel that the infant is taking attention away from them.
   a. In this case, role reversal is also common. That is, the parent feels it is the duty of the child to meet the parent's emotional needs—to make the parent feel whole and good about him- or herself.
   b. When the infant "demands" that his or her needs for basic care or nurture be met, conflict with the reciprocal "demand" by the parent results, and a potentially abusive situation ensues.
   c. Likewise, when the parents' self-esteem is threatened by the perception that they are not good or effective parents (e.g., when the child cries), they are at increased risk for abusing the child.
   d. Therefore, periods of normal infant fussiness (e.g., when hungry, sleepy, in need of diapering) or times when the infant is physically ill are potential crisis points for abusive parents and their infants.

7. **Children with physical or developmental disorders** are at increased risk for abuse and neglect.

8. The abused child often is the **scapegoat** for the individual pathology of other family members or for family pathology.

9. It is **unusual for child abuse to begin after the age of 6 years,** with the exception of sexual abuse.

10. Abuse occurs in **all socioeconomic** groups but is more common among those who are poor.

11. **Parental substance abuse** and **domestic violence** are often are associated with child abuse.

B Effects on the child

1. Occasionally, **emotional development may be precocious.**
   a. The expectation that a child function as "a parent" (role reversal) causes some children to develop quickly.

     b. Fear of being abused for mistakes can also lead to precocious development and to **perfectionism** as a personality trait.

       (1) The precocity, however, tends to be superficial and defensive.

       (2) The underlying desire to be validated as a child for age-appropriate attributes is also usually apparent.

  2. Conversely, in some children, **development may be retarded** if the abuse is severe or enduring. In these cases, the destructive and deleterious impact of the abuse outweighs the child's ability to mount adaptive defenses against it.

  3. **Physical injuries** are a constant risk.

  4. **Emotional injuries** are an equally significant and consistent risk.

     a. Higher rates of **posttraumatic stress disorder** and **depressive disorders** occur.

     b. Other possible outcomes include reactive attachment disorder, self-destructive behavior, eating disorders, and substance abuse disorders.

     c. Sexually inappropriate behaviors are more common.

  5. **Exposure to chronic violence** can increase aggression and antisocial behavior in abused children.

C Treatment

  1. **Suspected abuse must be reported** to the county protective services. If the child's health or life is in jeopardy, he or she should be removed from the abusive environment. If there is no improvement within 1 to 2 years after diagnosis, termination of parental rights should be considered.

  2. **Most abused children need psychotherapy.** Ultimately, the goal is to break what is often a multigenerational pattern of abuse in a family and to allow the child to grow into an adult who is capable of empathy, intimacy, and relational reciprocity in ways the previous generations were not. At times, the therapeutic relationship may be the first adult–child relationship that models a nonexploitative, noncontingent, emotionally available, and empathically attuned focus on the needs and well-being of the child.

  3. **Parents almost always need intensive, individual psychotherapy,** and often **marital therapy** as well. When appropriate, substance abuse treatment should be provided. Parents may also benefit from **parent training classes** that educate them about normal development, appropriate limits and boundaries, and nonexploitative techniques for discipline and behavioral management.

BIBLIOGRAPHY

American Psychiatric Association: *Diagnostic and Statistical Manual of Mental Disorders,* 4th ed., text revision. Washington, DC, American Psychiatric Association, 2000.

Chatoor I: Feeding disorders in infants and toddlers: Diagnosis and treatment. *Child Adolesc Psychiatr Clin N Am* 11(2):163–183, 2002.

Dulcan M (ed): *Dulcan's Textbook of Child and Adolescent Psychiatry.* Arlington, VA, American Psychiatric Publishing, 2010.

Dulcan M, Martini R, Lake M: *Concise Guide to Child and Adolescent Psychiatry,* 3rd ed. Arlington, VA: American Psychiatric Publishing, 2003.

Emde RN, Harmon RJ, Good WV: Depressive feelings in children: A transactional model for research. In *Depression in Children: Developmental Perspectives.* Edited by Rutter M, Izard D, Reed P. New York, Guilford Press, 1986, pp 135–160.

Garfinkle BD, Carlson GA, Weller EB (eds): *Psychiatric Disorders in Children and Adolescents.* Philadelphia, WB Saunders, 1990.

Klaus MH, Kendall JH: *Parent-Infant Bonding.* St. Louis, CV Mosby, 1982.

Martin A, Volkmar F (eds): *Lewis's Child and Adolescent Psychiatry: A Comprehensive Textbook,* 4th ed. Philadelphia, Lippincott Williams & Wilkins, 2007.

Sadock BJ, Sadock VA: *Kaplan & Sadock's Synopsis of Psychiatry,* 9th ed. Baltimore, Williams & Wilkins, 2003.

Spitz RA: Hospitalism: An inquiry into the genesis of psychiatric conditions in early childhood. *Psychoanal Study Child* 1:53–74, 1945.

Steele BF, Pollock CB: A psychiatric study of parents who abuse infants and small children. In *The Battered Child.* Edited by Helfer RE, Kempe CH. Chicago, University of Chicago Press, 1968, pp 103–145.

U.S. Food and Drug Administration, Public Health Advisory: *FDA Launches Multi-Pronged Strategy to Strengthen Safeguards for Children Treated with Antidepressant Medications,* Washington, DC, October 15, 2004.

Study Questions

Directions: *Each of the numbered items or incomplete statements in this section is followed by answers or by completions of the statement. Select the ONE numbered answer or completion that is BEST in each case.*

1. A 22-year-old woman has just delivered her first child, a healthy boy, by cesarean section under general anesthesia. When she awakens, she is frantic because she did not have the opportunity to "bond to her child." The physician's best course of action is to:

[A] Reassure the patient that bonding is a lengthy process.
[B] Suggest that the mother breastfeed in order to offset the effects of poor postnatal bonding.
[C] Return in 1 day to see if the patient's concerns have dissipated.
[D] Recommend psychiatric counseling aimed at helping the patient bond to her child.
[E] Dismiss her concern as expectable, new-parent anxiety.

2. The etiology of conduct disorder is most accurately described as:

[A] Developmental
[B] Environmental
[C] Familial
[D] Genetic
[E] Multifactorial

3. An evidence-based treatment for autism is: *depression/anxiety*

[A] Cognitive behavioral therapy, such as Exposure/Response Prevention
[B] Behavioral therapy, such as Applied Behavioral Therapy
[C] Family therapy
[D] Pharmacologic treatment
[E] Gluten-free diet

— bowel incontinence

4. Which of the following statements about the etiology of encopresis is most accurate? The symptoms often:

[A] Are conscious and deliberate
[B] Derive from delayed nervous system maturation
[C] Indicate underlying gastrointestinal pathology
[D] Derive from an underlying psychotic disorder
[E] Derive from constipation and fecal impaction — *MC results in overflow soiling*

5. Which of the following statements regarding diagnostic criteria for learning disorders is most accurate?

[A] They are usually associated with low-average intelligence.
[B] It is an equivalent but less pejorative term than mental retardation.
[C] Achievement testing and intelligence testing reflect differential profiles among individuals with these disorders.   *cognitive potential*

academic performance

[D] They fall within the broader spectrum of pervasive developmental disorders.
[E] Subtypes of the disorder include reading, writing, mathematics, history, and humanities.

QUESTIONS 6–8

A 7-year-old boy is brought to a child psychiatrist by his parents on a referral by the school where the child is in the second grade. The boy does not have a discipline problem, but he frequently answers questions without being called on and is often out of his seat without permission. His schoolwork is adequate, but the teacher believes he is capable of better. He has difficulty completing tasks and appears to spend much of the class time daydreaming.

6. Which additional piece of information would support the most likely etiology for his symptoms?
   - [A] A history of head injuries
   - [B] A history of neurologic symptoms
   - [C] A history of tics
   - [D] His medication history
   - [E] Family psychiatric history

7. The most likely diagnosis is:
   - [A] Attention deficit hyperactivity disorder (ADHD)
   - [B] Conduct disorder
   - [C] Impulse control disorder
   - [D] Learning disorder
   - [E] Receptive language disorder

8. Regarding treatment, the best advice to the family would be that:
   - [A] He has a diagnosable disorder, so he should not be held accountable for his symptoms.
   - [B] They should alter his diet immediately.
   - [C] He needs intensive, probably long-term psychotherapy.
   - [D] Medications might be helpful.
   - [E] They should probably not discuss his diagnosis with his teacher because it might be stigmatizing.

QUESTIONS 9–11

A 4-year-old girl is brought to the emergency department by her mother with a swollen and discolored forearm. Radiographs reveal an ulnar fracture. Her mother reports that the child had been jumping on the bed, lost her balance, and fell. The physician observes that the mother is apparently in her seventh or eighth month of pregnancy. He also observes that the child is quite thin and somewhat disheveled in appearance, and her hygiene is poor. When he asks if anyone else lives in their home, the mother acknowledges that her boyfriend does and then hastens to state, "But he wasn't even home when this happened."

9. After the radiographs, the physician's most appropriate next step is to:
   - [A] Obtain a detailed developmental history from the mother.
   - [B] Insist that the mother's boyfriend come in to be interviewed.
   - [C] Interview the child separate from her mother.
   - [D] Examine the child's genitalia for signs of sexual abuse.
   - [E] Ask the hospital's child protection team to investigate.

10. Which statement best describes the physician's obligation to report the incident to the local child protective service agency?
   - [A] If the physician suspects that the injuries might derive from abuse, then the incident must be reported.
   - [B] If the physician finds additional evidence of deprivation and neglect, then he must report it.
   - [C] If the physician finds additional evidence of physical abuse, then he must report it.
   - [D] If the physician finds additional evidence of sexual abuse, then he must report it.
   - [E] If in addition to the physician's findings, the child alleges abuse, then he must report it.

11. It is ultimately determined that the child's injury was inflicted by her mother's boyfriend. At this time, the most appropriate intervention with regard to the mother is to:

- A Remove the child from her care and place her in a foster home.
- B Leave the child in her care as long as the perpetrator is not in the home.
- C Insist on parenting classes as part of a court-ordered treatment plan.
- D Evaluate her ability to effectively parent her yet unborn child.
- E Be certain that her potential "silent" participation in the abuse is investigated.

12. The etiology of autistic disorder is best understood to be:

- A Infectious
- B Neurologic
- C Psychogenic
- D Psychological
- E Toxicologic

13. Which of the following antidepressant medications would be the best second-line treatment for the symptoms of attention deficit hyperactivity disorder (ADHD)?

- A Bupropion
- B Fluoxetine
- C Fluvoxamine
- D Sertraline
- E Escitalopram

Answers and Explanations

1. The answer is A [*II A, B*]. Bonding and attachment are processes that occur over a lengthy period. Although many parents worry that a cesarean section interferes with this process, simple reassurance is usually helpful. Breastfeeding would not necessarily offset any sort of aberration in bonding and attachment. At first, many new mothers feel that their infants do not belong to them. This feeling can last several days. Returning to see the patient is a good idea but should be done 3 to 4 days later; however, conditions can warrant returning sooner. When the mother is severely depressed, anxious, or psychotic, she should be evaluated for psychiatric treatment and follow-up. Sincere parental concerns should almost never be dismissed without discussion.

2. The answer is E [*VIII A 3, 4*]. Conduct disorder is best understood from an interaction of biologic, psychological, and social factors. Biologic factors include untreated or inadequately treated attention deficit hyperactivity disorder (ADHD) and low intelligence quotient (IQ). Learning disorders are often present. Parenting is often inconsistent, abusive, or neglectful. Parents are more likely to have mental illness and antisocial personality disorder. Youths tend to associate with other peers with behavioral problems, further increasing their risk for antisocial behaviors such as truancy and substance abuse.

3. The answer is B [*V A 7*]. Cognitive behavioral therapies are indicated for depression and anxiety disorders in youths. While many treatments are used for autism, behavioral interventions such as Applied Behavioral Analysis have demonstrated efficacy. In some cases family therapy may be beneficial as an adjunct for addressing issues such as parenting, education about autism, and caregiver stress. Pharmacologic interventions do not reverse the core symptoms of autism, but can be used selectively to target specific symptoms such as aggression or comorbid anxiety. Families often use modified diets, such as a gluten-free diet, but these dietary modifications have not been demonstrated to impact the symptoms of autism.

4. The answer is E [*XIV B*]. Soiling is only variably deliberate and is usually self-limited. Whereas enuresis often derives from delayed nervous system maturation, this is not true for encopresis, and it does not usually signify underlying gastrointestinal pathology. Although it may signify an underlying psychotic disorder within the child, this is not typically the case. The most common form of encopresis is in a child who retains feces, develops an impaction within the rectal vault, and experiences "overflow" soiling around the impaction.

5. The answer is C [*VI A*]. The three subtypes of learning disorders are in reading, writing, and mathematics. Although mental retardation is often euphemistically referred to as a learning disorder, the term is used inaccurately in that context. The presence of a learning disorder does not suggest below-average intelligence. Although learning disorders fall broadly among the developmental disorders, they are not subsumed within the pervasive developmental disorders, which are characterized by pervasive developmental deficits in language, social relatedness, and behavior. Diagnosis of learning disorders is established by documenting a mismatch between cognitive potential (as demonstrated on intelligence tests) and academic performance (as demonstrated on standardized achievement tests).

6–8. The answers are 6-E, 7-A, and 8-D [*VII C–D*]. Although both major (grossly abnormal central nervous system or history of significant head trauma) and minor (e.g., "soft" neurologic signs or nonspecific electrocardiographic changes) nervous system dysfunction may underlie the symptoms of attention deficit hyperactivity disorder (ADHD) in certain children, the most common etiology is a "constitutional" ADHD in the presence of a normal nervous system, often with a family history. A history of tics is important, both because Tourette disorder and ADHD can be comorbid conditions and because tics may be a side effect from stimulant medications that are commonly used to treat ADHD. Most children with ADHD do not have comorbid Tourette disorder, however, nor do they develop tics as a side effect of treatment. Certain medications, particularly sedative-hypnotics, may result in paradoxic excitation, which causes hyperactivity in some children, but these medications are seldom used chronically in children.

ADHD is characterized by variable levels of hyperactivity along with impulsivity, distractibility, and attention and concentration deficits. Learning deficits secondary to inattention may be present; however, no primary learning deficits are derived from ADHD. Attentional difficulties are not characteristic of learning disorders. Conduct disorder may co-occur with ADHD, but it involves the repetitive and serious violation of multiple age-appropriate behavioral norms. Receptive language deficits do interfere with learning, but the learning difficulty derives from an inability to understand spoken language rather than from attentional deficits. Children with ADHD are behaviorally impulsive; this is to be distinguished, however, from impulse control disorders that are characterized by impulse disinhibition in discrete domains such as eating, substance use or abuse, gambling, stealing, fire setting, and violent outbursts.

Although the child has a diagnosable disorder, he still must be held accountable for his behavior and its consequences. Although many parents believe to the contrary, there is little empiric support for the notion that diet plays a role in this disorder, either etiologically or in terms of its treatment. Likewise, uncomplicated ADHD probably does not require psychotherapy, other than occasional behavioral interventions. Although stigmatization is always a risk of psychiatric diagnosis, the school would ideally be a partner in the therapeutic process, both to implement behavioral programs and to monitor overall therapeutic efficacy. Most children with ADHD are most effectively managed with medications, used at least adjunctively.

9–11. The answers are 9-C, 10-A, and 11-E [*XV C*]. Although the child's injury might have been sustained exactly as described by her mother, the physician must wonder whether nonaccidental trauma is involved. An interview with the child is essential. This should occur separate from the parent, and the child should be asked the source of her injuries. Questions should be otherwise nonleading and in language appropriate to her developmental level. Likewise, the responses of the child should be assessed in terms of their appropriateness to her developmental level. Developmental history may be important, insofar as there often is a history of problematic bonding between abused children and their parents. Likewise, children who physically or developmentally deviate from the norm are at increased risk for abuse. Nonetheless, obtaining a detailed developmental history is less urgent than hearing the child's own story. Although the physician must be sensitive to the potential for sexual abuse, a genital examination should be deferred until after the child is interviewed because it might not be indicated. A physician would not typically "investigate" a suspected perpetrator such as the mother's boyfriend. If that appeared necessary, it should be referred to the appropriate investigative agency (i.e., child protective services).

Reporting laws across the United States require that reasonable suspicions of abuse and neglect must be reported. Physicians are mandated to report under these circumstances and are civilly liable for failing to follow these reporting guidelines. Proof of abuse is not necessary, and neither is an inordinately high level of suspicion or direct allegations made by the child. Rather, any reasonable level of suspicion must be reported.

Abuse and neglect must always be viewed as reflecting adult pathology. The role of the perpetrator in the abuse is obvious. The role of other adults in the abused child's life is less obvious, however. At the very least, the "nonabusive" parent failed to protect the child from the perpetrator. In cases in which the abuse was known by the "nonabusive" parent or when the circumstances of the abuse were so obvious as to be impossible to miss, the "nonabusive" parent must be recognized as a silent and passive but equal participant in the abuse of the child. The child's immediate safety is the issue of first importance. Whether the child needs to be placed outside of her mother's care depends on her mother's "participation" in the abuse. Whether the mother needs a court-ordered treatment plan or needs to be evaluated in terms of her capacity to parent are issues to be addressed after the more immediate issues of current safety are addressed.

12. The answer is B [*V A 1*]. Autistic disorder is a neuropathic disorder that commences in early childhood (before age 3 years) in which the child demonstrates disturbed relatedness to other human beings, inappropriate responses to the environment, and delays and oddities in language development. Findings that support the neurologic etiology of this condition include 20% incidence of seizures, decreased activity in the fusiform face area (FFA) of the temporal lobe, and a high incidence of comorbid mental retardation. Only occasionally are toxicologic agents (e.g., heavy metals) or infectious etiologies (congenital infections) suspected. *facial recognition*

13. The answer is A [*VII D 1*]. Bupropion, which is an antidepressant that may produce central nervous system stimulant effects, has also been demonstrated to be of some therapeutic benefit, particularly in individuals with attention deficit hyperactivity disorder (ADHD) and depressive symptoms. Fluoxetine, fluvoxamine, sertraline, and escitalopram are all antidepressants of the selective serotonin reuptake inhibitor family. Although these medications are effective antidepressants and anxiolytics, they generally offer little benefit in the treatment of children with ADHD.

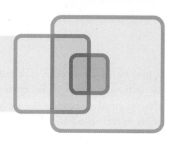

chapter **13**

Geriatric Psychiatry

SHILPA SRINIVASAN • JAMES G. BOUKNIGHT

I   INTRODUCTION

Although psychiatrists have always treated the elderly, the specialty of geriatric psychiatry is relatively new. Recently the Centers for Medicare and Medicaid Services (CMS) recognized the specialty of geriatric psychiatry with a separate code to identify care provided by physicians in this specialty. At exactly what age a person becomes "geriatric" is open to interpretation. The age of 65 is the age at which most U.S. citizens qualify for Medicare benefits, so it is commonly used as the threshold for becoming a geriatric patient. Other ways to group the geriatric population include the "young old" (65–74 years), the "old" (75–84 years), and the "old old" (85 and older). In the twenty-first century, geriatric psychiatry will become an increasingly more important specialty of psychiatry because of the growth in the numbers of elderly in the United States and other developed countries. The geriatric population is not equally distributed between males and females: in the population over 85 years there are more than double the number of women compared to men.

The geriatric patient differs from the adult patient in more than age. As an individual ages, changes occur in body composition, renal and hepatic function, blood protein level, and gastric and hepatic enzyme levels. The elderly have proportionately more fat and less muscle (thus less water) than a middle-aged adult. The elderly typically have a decreased renal clearance of drugs and a decrease in hepatic metabolism. All of these changes have implications for medication tolerance, safety, and efficacy.

II   PSYCHIATRIC DISORDERS

These include cognitive disorders, mood disorders, anxiety disorders, psychotic disorders, and substance abuse disorders. These disorders are coded on Axis I in the *Diagnostic and Statistical Manual of Mental Disorders,* fourth edition, text revision (*DSM-IV-TR*).

A **Cognitive disorders**

1. **Alzheimer dementia.** First described by Dr. Alois Alzheimer in 1917, Alzheimer disease (AD) is the most common type of dementia, contributing to over 60% of dementia cases. It is a chronic, insidious, and acquired decline in memory accompanied by impairment in at least one other cognitive function: aphasia, apraxia, agnosia, and executive function. This impairment affects day-to-day functioning. Although it is more commonly diagnosed in individuals over the age of 65, AD can develop in those younger than 65 as well (often referred to as "early-onset AD"). A small percentage of cases are familial, usually involving mutations of chromosome 21, which codes for **amyloid precursor protein** (APP), the precursor to amyloid in plaques.

   a. **Prevalence.** Approximately 5.3 million individuals in America have Alzheimer disease, including 5.1 million people aged 65 and older (1) and 200,000 individuals under the age of 65 who have early-onset AD (2). Prevalence is less than 1% for individuals 60 to 64 years old. This rises exponentially with age such that prevalence increases to 25% to 33% among those aged 85 years or older. It is estimated that 7.7 million people over the age of 65 will have AD in 2030—representing a 50% increase from the 5.1 million people aged 65 and older currently affected. By 2050, this number is projected to be between 11 million and 16 million. Therefore, by 2050, more than 60% of AD sufferers will be aged 85 or older (1).

b. Risk factors. Risk factors for the development of AD include nonmodifiable factors such as age and mutations in APP. Modifiable factors include low level of education, cardiovascular status, smoking, obesity, sedentary lifestyle, and diet (3, 4).

c. Etiology and pathogenesis. In AD, insoluble β-amyloid (Ab42) accumulates, leading to the formation of plaques. In addition, hyperphosphorylation of τ protein leads to the formation of **neurofibrillary tangles.** Plaques and tangles represent the pathologic hallmarks of AD. They cause neuronal death and neurotransmitter deficits in areas of the brain, most prominently in the cholinergic system. **Apolipoprotein E4 allele** expression (genetic factor for late-onset AD), oxidative cell damage, and inflammatory changes in the brain are also implicated in AD. While the **hippocampus is most affected by AD,** atrophy of the parietal and temporal lobes is also found.

d. Diagnosis. The diagnosis of AD remains a clinical one, although definitive diagnosis at autopsy entails finding the characteristic lesions of plaques and tangles in the brain. Clinically, diagnosis is based on history provided by the patient and family members, thorough physical and neurologic examinations, functional assessments of day-to-day activities, cognitive assessments (including formal neurocognitive testing), laboratory and neuroimaging results to rule out reversible or other causes (such as vitamin B_{12} deficiency, hypothyroidism, cerebrovascular accident [CVA], etc.). According to the *DSM-IV-TR*, **memory impairment along with either aphasia, apraxia, agnosia, or executive function impairment** and a concomitant impact on day-to-day functioning is necessary to make a diagnosis of dementia (5). Early detection of dementia is important to the extent that early therapy may delay disease progression. However, AD remains an insidiously progressive disease. Early diagnosis can lead to enhanced early safety monitoring in areas including medicine administration, use of tools and appliances, and driving. The goals of early family education include improved caregiver satisfaction and decreased caregiver burden; intensive outpatient care programs can delay nursing home placement.

(1) **Formal neuropsychological assessments** are time consuming, resource intensive, and not readily available to all patients.

(2) **Office-based, readily available cognitive screening tools** are often used in the clinical setting. These include:

(a) **SLUMS** (Saint Louis University Mental Status Examination) (6)

(b) **MMSE** (mini-mental state examination) (7)

(c) **Mini-Cog:** Three-item recall plus clock draw

(i) Three of three items correct = no dementia

(ii) Zero of three items correct = dementia

(iii) One to two out of three items correct PLUS abnormal clock = dementia

(d) **Animal fluency test:** The patient names as many animals as he or she can in 1 minute. Scores less than 15 are considered positive tests (8, 9).

(3) **Neuroimaging,** including computed tomography (CT), magnetic resonance imaging (MRI), and positron emission tomography (PET) scans, is also used to aid in the clinical diagnosis.

e. Clinical features. Disease severity is characterized by mild, moderate, and severe stages. The SLUMS and MMSE are screening tools often used clinically to aid in characterizing disease severity (both are scored out of a maximum of 30 points, with lower scores indicating cognitive impairment). However, a clinical and functional assessment incorporating basic and instrumental **activities of daily living** (ADLs) is an essential component of disease severity monitoring. Basic ADLs include feeding and toileting, while instrumental ADLs include more complex but nevertheless day-to-day tasks such as cooking, using the telephone, etc.

(1) **Mild cognitive impairment** (MCI) is an early form of memory loss, which may lead to AD in 15% to 20% of cases annually. In this condition, the patient reports memory loss, but there is no functional impairment and ADLs are independently performed. SLUMS scores range from 20 to 26 (education dependent) and MMSE scores range from 26 to 28. The early stage of AD usually lasts 1 to 3 years from symptom onset. Symptoms include:

(a) Disorientation for date/time

(b) Naming difficulties

(c) Social withdrawal

    (d) Problems managing finances

    (e) Recent memory and recall problems

    (f) Irritability or mood change

(2) As the disease progresses (with progressing atrophy, neuronal loss, and neurotransmitter deficits) over 2 to 8 years from symptom onset, **moderate-severity characteristics** include:

    (a) Disorientation to date and place

    (b) Comprehension difficulties

    (c) Getting lost in familiar areas

    (d) Delusions, agitation, aggression

    (e) Restlessness, anxiousness, depression

    (f) Problems with dressing, grooming

    (g) Impaired new learning and calculating skills

    (h) Impairment in instrumental ADLs (e.g., not able to cook, shop, handle finances)

(3) The **late or severe stage of AD** occurs 6 to 12 years from symptom onset and includes the following symptoms:

    (a) Nearly unintelligible verbal output

    (b) Incontinence (bowel, bladder, or both)

    (c) Impaired remote memory

    (d) Motor and/or verbal agitation

At this point individuals are usually in a nursing-home level of care, with total dependence on others for their daily needs, including feeding (10). In 2006, Alzheimer disease was the seventh leading cause of death across all ages in the United States and the fifth leading cause of death for those aged 65 and older (11). **Complications of severe/end-stage dementia** include immobility, swallowing apraxias, and malnutrition. At this stage, individuals with severe AD are at significantly greater risk of developing pneumonia, which has been found in several studies to be the most commonly identified cause of death among elderly people with AD.

  f. **Pharmacologic treatment.** There is no cure for AD at the present time. Available pharmacotherapies are symptomatic treatments; that is, they are initiated once symptoms appear. Medications currently approved by the U.S. Food and Drug Administration (FDA) for AD address cognitive symptoms by targeting either the **cholinergic neurotransmitter system** (acetylcholinesterase inhibitors) or the **glutamate system** (*N*-methyl-D-aspartate [NMDA] receptor antagonists). Side effects include gastrointestinal concerns such as nausea, diarrhea, and decreased appetite. However, given the cholinomimetic nature of these agents, it is also important to be aware of bradycardia, increased gastric acid secretion, and syncope as potential side effects. Currently available FDA-approved pharmacologic treatments for AD are listed in Table 13–1.

  g. **Behavioral management.** Approximately 60% to 90% of individuals with AD develop behavioral and psychiatric symptoms along the course of their disease. Symptoms include agitation, psychosis, depression, anxiety, irritability, pacing, and restlessness, which cause significant distress to both patients and caregivers. They may at times be the determining factor for long-term care placement. **Strategies for management** include a thorough medical examination to rule out underlying organic causes (such as urinary tract infections, iatrogenesis, or pain) as

TABLE 13–1   **FDA-Approved Pharmacologic Treatments for Alzheimer Dementia (AD)**

Generic Name	Approved	AD Stage Indication	Dose (mg)
Tacrine	Sept. 1993	Mild–moderate	N/A
Donepezil	Nov. 1996	Mild–severe	5–10 (PO qd)
Rivastigmine	April 2000	Mild–moderate	1.5, 3, 4.5, 6 (PO bid)
Galantamine	Feb. 2001	Mild–moderate	4, 8, 12 (PO bid)
Galantamine ER	Dec. 2004	Mild–moderate	8, 16, 24 (PO qd)
Rivastigmine transdermal	July 2007	Mild–moderate	4.6, 9.5 (q24h)
Memantine	Oct. 2003	Moderate–severe	5, 10 (PO bid)

well as environmental approaches. Medications may be considered after nonpharmacologic strategies have been employed. In addition to treating cognitive and behavioral symptoms, patients and their caregivers should be counseled about the importance of initiating health care directives and decisions, especially while the patient still has the cognitive capacity to do so. This may prevent conflicts related to medical decision making and ease the burden for the family as the disease progresses.

2. **Vascular dementia.** While Alzheimer dementia is the most common type of dementia in the Western world, vascular dementia is considered by some to be the second most common type. The spectrum of vascular dementia subtypes include **multi-infarct dementia,** vascular dementia due to a strategic single infarct, vascular dementia due to lacunar lesions (subcortical), vascular dementia due to hemorrhagic lesions, **Binswanger disease** (subcortical leukoencephalopathy), Alzheimer disease with cerebrovascular features (previously known as mixed dementia), and cerebral autosomal dominant arteriopathy with subcortical infarcts and leukoencephalopathy (CADASIL), a rare autosomal dominant condition localized to chromosome arm 19q12 that affects small vessels supplying the deep white matter. Pathologically, multiple small infarcts are observed in the white matter, thalamus, basal ganglia, and pons.

Vascular dementia can have cortical or subcortical variants. However, **the three most common mechanisms of vascular dementia are multiple cortical infarcts, a strategic single infarct, or small vessel disease.**

   a. **Prevalence.** Vascular dementia is the **second most common cause of dementia** in the United States and Europe. However, in some parts of Asia, vascular dementia is the most common form of dementia. In contrast to the prevalence rate of 1.5% in Western countries, rates approximating 2.2% are seen in Japan. Patients who have had a stroke have a nine times higher prevalence rate of dementia than controls. One year after a stroke, 25% of patients develop new-onset dementia (12).

   b. **Risk factors.** Risk factors for vascular dementia include cardiovascular and cerebrovascular disease, hypertension, smoking, hypercholesterolemia, and diabetes mellitus. After a stroke, the incidence of vascular dementia can be influenced by many factors. These include:

      (1) Advanced age
      (2) Lower education level
      (3) Positive family history of dementia
      (4) Left-sided lesions
      (5) Periventricular white matter ischemic lesions
      (6) Strokes in thalamic artery territory, inferomedian temporal lobes, or hippocampus
      (7) Watershed infarcts involving superior frontal and parietal regions (13)

   c. **Clinical features.** A pattern of patchy cognitive impairment, often with focal neurologic signs and symptoms, is seen in vascular dementia. While the onset may be abrupt, it is usually associated with a **stepwise clinical decline. Subcortical signs** include **balance problems**, **gait problems**, and **urinary incontinence.** In order to make the diagnosis of vascular dementia, the presence of focal neurologic signs, evidence of cerebrovascular disease on neuroimaging, and a temporal relationship between the onset of focal neurologic signs and dementia (usually 3 months), along with a stepwise deterioration, are required (14).

   d. **Treatment.** There are no FDA-approved medications for the treatment of vascular dementia. Prevention of new strokes is at the core of disease management. This includes antiplatelet agents and controlling major vascular risk factors.

3. **Dementia with Lewy bodies (DLB).** In 1914, Frederick Lewy first described **Lewy bodies** (LBs), cytoplasmic inclusions found in cells of the substantia nigra in patients with idiopathic Parkinson disease. Lewy bodies are **round inclusions composed of α-synuclein,** found intracellularly in substantia nigra cells and in the locus ceruleus, nucleus basalis of Meynert, dorsal raphe nuclei, and dorsal motor nucleus of cranial nerve X. They are also found in the nonpyramidal cells in layers V and VI of the limbic and transitional cortex.

   a. **Prevalence.** Studies suggest that DLB accounts for 10% to 20% of dementias. However, patients with Parkinson disease and Alzheimer disease also have LBs found on autopsy (LB variant of Alzheimer disease [LBV-AD]). There are no good epidemiologic data on incidence or prevalence of DLB (15). Subsequently, Lewy body disorders are thought to exist along a spectrum.

     b. Clinical features. DLB is a **progressive degenerative dementia.** Clinical features include:
       (1) Fluctuations in cognitive function with fluctuations in levels of alertness and attention (e.g., daytime drowsiness, lethargy, disorganized speech, staring into space)
       (2) Visual hallucinations
       (3) Parkinsonian motor features (rigidity, bradykinesia, tremors)
       (4) Depression is also frequently seen in LDB [16].

     c. Treatment. Although the acetylcholinesterase inhibitors have been investigated, there are no FDA-approved medications for the treatment of LBD. Dopamine agonists including levodopa/carbidopa may improve motor function in some patients with DLB; however, these agents may also worsen confusion and psychosis. Hallucinations and agitation are challenging in LBD. Benefits of treatment must outweigh the risks, especially given that patients with LBD have a heightened sensitivity to neuroleptics, with the propensity for worsening extrapyramidal symptoms (EPSs). If the psychotic symptoms do not pose a danger to the patient or others and are not distressing to the patient, no medical treatment may be necessary. Atypical neuroleptics may have a role when acetylcholinesterase inhibitors are ineffective [17]. Conventional neuroleptics (such as haloperidol) should be avoided because of neuroleptic sensitivity [18].

  4. Parkinson dementia. Parkinson disease (PD) is a **progressive neurodegenerative illness** caused by **loss of dopaminergic neurons in the substantia nigra.** Classic symptoms include resting tremor, rigidity, bradykinesia, and postural instability. Depression, dementia, and psychosis are commonly seen as the disease progresses. Histopathologically, α-synuclein is the predominant pathologic protein, being found in the Lewy bodies and Lewy neurites of Parkinson disease, Parkinson disease dementia, and DLB [19].

     a. Prevalence and risk factors. Cognitive impairment occurs in 30% to 40% of people with PD, while another 40% develop dementia [20]. Risk factors for the development of dementia in PD include:
       (1) Longer duration of PD
       (2) Greater disability
       (3) Male gender
       (4) Age at onset older than 60 years
       (5) Akinetic rigid disease
       (6) Postural instability
       (7) Lower education
       (8) Presence of psychotic symptoms
       (9) Depression and sleep disturbance [21, 22]

     b. Clinical features. Dementia in Parkinson disease is typically **frontal-subcortical** with moderate levels of visuospatial deficits and executive dysfunction. Difficulties in generating, maintaining, and shifting sets characterize executive function disorders, which manifest clinically as mental rigidity. Fluctuation in attention can also occur [23]. The combination of progressive dopaminergic disruption in the nigrostriatal pathways and subsequent cholinergic and frontal-subcortical loop dysregulation as the disease progresses leads to cognitive impairment [24].

     c. Treatment. In June 2006, the FDA approved rivastigmine for the treatment of mild to moderate Parkinson dementia in dose ranges of 3 to 12 mg total daily (administered with food twice daily). In 2007, the FDA also approved the rivastigmine transdermal patch (skin patch) for mild to moderate Parkinson dementia. The dose ranges and titration are the same as that for Alzheimer dementia. In addition to cognitive enhancers, it is also important to treat the symptoms of depression that are also common in Parkinson disease.

  5. Infectious causes of dementia
     a. HIV. This is the **most common cause of dementia due to infection.** While the elderly represent a relatively small portion of patients with HIV dementia at present, these numbers will grow as HIV-infected patients live longer due to antiviral medications. **HIV-associated dementia** (HAD) patients present with a **subacute decline in cognitive functioning.** It is estimated that as many as 25% of AIDS patients may be affected by HAD. Symptoms include cognitive slowing, apathy, slowed movements, and psychomotor slowing. Because HAD is a subcortical dementia, there are usually parkinsonian symptoms associated with the dementia. Treatment is with antiviral agents, which reduce the viral load in the central nervous system (CNS) [25].

Although there are no large-scale studies of the use of cognitive enhancers in HAD, many clinicians employ cholinesterase inhibitors and a glutamate modulator in the treatment of these patients.

    b. **Prion diseases,** also called **transmissible spongiform encephalopathies** (TSEs), are rare neurodegenerative disorders that are believed to be caused by prions. Prions are transmissible agents that induce brain damage, which is always fatal. There are no treatments for TSEs. The diseases in this group include **Creutzfeldt-Jakob disease**, **Gerstmann-Straussler-Scheinker syndrome,** and **kuru** (26).

    c. **Dementia due to neurosyphilis** is much less common since the advent of penicillin and other antibiotics but is still seen. At one time neurosyphilis, or "general paresis of the insane," accounted for 4% to 10% of all admissions to mental hospitals. There has been a resurgence of neurosyphilis because of immunocompromised patients who have HIV. In general, dementia due to neurosyphilis occurs after many years of meningitis due to syphilis. It is characterized by memory deficits, changes in conduct, impaired reasoning, and a disheveled appearance. If the disease is allowed to progress, the patient develops the typical signs and symptoms of dementia: memory loss, aphasia, apraxia, and agnosia. Serologic tests for syphilis include nonspecific reagin tests, which indicate exposure to the organism. A large percentage of serum reagin tests are negative in patients with advanced disease. The FTA-ABS test is a fluorescent treponemal antibody absorption test that identifies treponemal antigens. The cerebrospinal fluid (CSF) usually shows an increase in cells, protein content, and γ-globulin. Treatment of neurosyphilis is penicillin G IV in a dosage of 18 to 24 million units daily for 14 days. Patients with a penicillin allergy may be treated with erythromycin or tetracycline. If the CSF remains abnormal after 6 months, additional treatment is recommended (27).

6. **Frontotemporal dementia (FTD).** Frontotemporal dementia is a term used to describe a non–Alzheimer-type dementia characterized by **progressive behavioral, cognitive, and language changes that have an insidious onset.** This syndrome was first described by Arnold Pick, a neurologist at the University of Prague in 1892; thus, the term **Pick disease** is sometimes used for this syndrome. There are various ways to classify subgroups of frontotemporal dementia, including a behavioral subgroup, semantic dementia, and nonfluent aphasia. All are characterized by degeneration of the temporal and frontal lobes of the brain. In some cases there are histologic findings of τ-positive neuronal cytoplasmic inclusions, called Pick bodies (28).

    a. **Prevalence.** Many epidemiologic studies of dementia exclude younger patients, so the prevalence of FTD is often underestimated because patients as young as 40 may be victims of the disease. It mainly occurs in patients aged 50 to 65 years. FTD is reported to be the **most common cause of dementia in patients younger than 65 years.**

    b. **Risk factors.** Risk factors for frontotemporal dementia are not well understood. There seem to be hereditary factors, at least in North American and European samples. Data from Japan do not show a familial risk factor. Some studies indicate that men are more likely than women to be diagnosed, but these are not consistent findings (29).

    c. **Clinical features.** Patients with frontotemporal dementia present with memory loss but the **most concerning symptoms are behavioral changes.** Patients may display disinhibition, loss of insight, compulsive behaviors, sexually inappropriate behaviors, apathy, and abnormal eating behaviors. This disease places a tremendous burden on caregivers, whether in an institutional setting or in the home.

    d. **Treatment.** There is no FDA-approved treatment for frontotemporal dementia, and there are few studies of medications for this disease. No drug has been shown to alter the course of the disease, and for many patients drug therapy has a modest impact on the troubling symptoms of FTD. Caregivers require support, encouragement, and assistance in providing care for these challenging patients.

B **Other psychiatric disorders**

1. **Depression in late life.** Depression in the elderly is a serious health challenge and a significant cause of suffering in older adults. It is often underdiagnosed, misdiagnosed, and undertreated. At one time, depression in late life was thought to be an expected response to loss and change associated with aging. We now know, however, that depression in the elderly is as much a disorder as that

TABLE 13–2 Depressive Syndromes
Major depression • Single episode • Recurrent • Psychotic • Atypical • Melancholic • With seasonal pattern Dysthymia Bipolar I/II disorder—most recent episode depressed Mood disorder secondary to a general medical condition Substance-induced mood disorder Depressive disorder not otherwise specified

Adapted from American Psychiatric Association: *Diagnostic and Statistical Manual of Mental Disorders*, 4th ed., text revision. Washington, DC, American Psychiatric Association, 2000.

in younger adults. It is associated with increased medical morbidity and disability and is a leading cause of suicide among the elderly. According to the World Health Organization, by the year 2020, "Depression will be second only to heart disease as cause of disability and premature death" (30).

Table 13–2 lists the depressive syndromes found in the *DSM-IV-TR.*

a. **Etiology.** As is the case with most major psychiatric conditions, depression is best conceptualized with the biopsychosocial model. Neurobiologic explanations of depression include the catecholamine theory, with serotonin and norepinephrine dysfunction as a major causal association.

   (1) **Biologic factors** predisposing to depression in the elderly include:
      (a) Medications
      (b) Genetic predisposition (depression in a first-degree relative confers a two to three times higher risk)
      (c) Comorbid medical illness
      (d) Vascular factors (cerebrovascular or coronary artery disease)
      (e) Striatofrontal dysfunction
      (f) Cognitive illness

   Certain medical conditions are highly comorbid with depression in the elderly. These include hypothyroidism (50%), myocardial infarction (45%), macular degeneration (30%), and diabetes (20%). Comorbid CNS diseases associated with depression in the older adult include Parkinson disease, multiple sclerosis, cerebrovascular infarctions, Alzheimer disease, and Huntington disease (31).

   (2) **Psychosocial factors.** The "state versus trait" schema identifies innate vulnerabilities and defenses, as opposed to life circumstances (e.g., grief, caregiver stress), as contributors to depression.

b. **Prevalence.** The prevalence of late-life depression varies by health and independence status. Up to 25% of community-dwelling older adults have reported mild depressive symptoms, while the prevalence rate of major depression in these individuals approximates that reported by younger adults (1%–9%) (32). However, the rates of major depression rise significantly with medical illness and institutionalization. Prevalence rates of 10% to 15% have been reported in the elderly in acute medical–surgical settings, and rates in the nursing home setting range from 12% to 16% (33).

c. **Impact.** Depression in older adults has far-reaching physical and psychological consequences. It can cause functional decline, cognitive dysfunction (also known as **pseudodementia**), amplified physical symptoms and disability, failure to thrive, pain, and poor outcome with cardiovascular disease and stroke. When compared to chronic medical illnesses such as diabetes, chronic obstructive pulmonary disease (COPD), and arthritis, depression is second only to heart disease in its impairment in functioning and disability.

   Among causes of mortality, suicide remains a significant factor with depression in late life. **Older adults are disproportionately likely to die by suicide.** Comprising only 13% of the U.S. population, individuals aged 65 and older accounted for 18% of all suicide deaths in 2000. Among the highest rates (when categorized by gender and race) were white men aged 85 and older: 59 deaths per 100,000 persons, more than five times the national U.S. rate of 10.6 per 100,000.

Risk factors for suicide in the elderly include:

(1) Depression
(2) Previous suicide attempt
(3) Comorbid physical illness
(4) Living alone
(5) Death of spouse
(6) Lacking a confidant
(7) Hopelessness
(8) Male gender
(9) Stressful life event
(10) Access to firearms
(11) Alcoholism
(12) Family history of suicide
(13) Lack of access to treatment

d. **Assessments.** A thorough assessment with history-taking and screening for comorbidities is the cornerstone of accurate diagnosis. **Depression in the elderly can manifest with atypical features,** with prominent neurovegetative signs and symptoms. Core features include apathy or anhedonia, sleep disturbance (often hypersomnia), social withdrawal, loss of appetite, and psychomotor retardation. Patients may complain about memory problems, and it is important to distinguish "pseudodementia" or memory symptoms occurring solely in the context of depression from other degenerative neurocognitive illnesses such as dementia. **Older adults also do not tend to emphasize emotional complaints;** rather, they focus on medical "aches and pains"; as a result, depressive symptoms may be overlooked during a brief office visit. While the *DSM-IV-TR* criteria for major depressive episode and disorder apply to depression in the elderly as well (see Chapter 3), clues to depression in the primary care setting include persistent "somatic" complaints (pain, headache, fatigue, insomnia, nonspecific gastrointestinal symptoms, malaise). Unfortunately, as many as 50% of depressed patients may be undiagnosed in primary care settings (34).

In addition to a comprehensive history and physical examination to rule out underlying medical causes, screening questionnaires can be useful adjuncts in the office setting. In the clinical setting, some **useful questions to ask when evaluating older adults for depression** include the following:

(1) Are you feeling sad?
(2) Are you sleeping poorly?
(3) Have you lost interest or pleasure in doing things?
(4) Have you felt that life is not worth living?

A positive response to such questions requires further evaluation.

e. **Differential diagnosis.** When evaluating an older adult for depression, it is important to rule out other conditions that may mimic the symptoms of major depression, including:

(1) Bipolar mood disorder (screen for any history of manic or hypomanic symptoms)
(2) Dysthymic disorder
(3) Mood disorder due to a general medical condition
(4) Substance-induced mood disorder
(5) Bereavement

f. **Management.** The effective treatment of late-life depression can result in improved quality of life, reduced mortality, improved function, and better outcomes with comorbid medical conditions (35). While medications are the mainstay of treatment in primary care settings, other validated, evidence-based treatments such as structured psychotherapies should be considered as well as family therapy and electroconvulsive therapy (ECT). It is important to customize treatment approaches for late-life depression by factoring in the patient's preferences, prior treatment history (including treatments that have been helpful or have failed in the past), and comorbid medical and psychiatric conditions. Treatment availability and cost are important considerations. A discussion about side effects with informed consent can help avoid premature medication cessation and address noncompliance issues. Patients' fears about antidepressants causing dependence or blunting of normal emotional responses such as bereavement should be allayed through active listening, psychoeducation, and reassurance (36).

(1) Psychotherapy. Evidence-based forms of psychotherapy shown to be effective for depression in the elderly include:

   (a) Cognitive behavioral therapy (CBT) helps patients become aware of and correct cognitive distortions, such as negative thinking associated with depression.

   (b) Interpersonal psychotherapy (IPT)

   (c) Problem-solving therapy (PST). Patients work through strategies for managing day-to-day problems associated with depression. These treatment modalities can be delivered by trained therapists in brief (six to 12) sessions in mental health or primary care settings. They should be considered as monotherapy or adjunctive to antidepressant treatment as the clinical condition warrants. In some studies, psychotherapy has been shown to be as effective as antidepressant treatment (37, 38).

(2) Pharmacotherapy. Among the various FDA-approved antidepressants for treating depression, selective serotonin reuptake inhibitors (SSRIs) are common first-line agents. Dosing should be customized to the physiology of the older adult, with the adage "start low, go slow." Among other antidepressant classes, tricyclic antidepressants (TCAs) and monoamine oxidase inhibitors (MAOIs) require extreme caution in the elderly and are generally NOT considered first-line treatment because of their side-effect profile, which includes anticholinergic, arrhythmogenic, and hypertensive effects.

Dosing guidelines by class are outlined in Table 13–3.

TABLE 13–3   Antidepressants for Major Depression

Medication	Starting Dose (mg/day)	Target Dose (mg/day)	Common Side Effects
Selective Serotonin Reuptake Inhibitors			
Citalopram	10	20–60	Gastrointestinal (diarrhea, nausea), weight gain, tremors, sexual dysfunction, hyponatremia (SIADH), serotonin syndrome
Escitalopram	10	10–20	
Fluoxetine	10	10–60	
Paroxetine	20	20–60	
Paroxetine CR	12.5–25	25–62.5	
Sertraline	25	50–200	
Serotonin-Norepinephrine Reuptake Inhibitors			
Venlafaxine	25	25–150 (bid)	Hypertension
Venlafaxine XR	37.5	75–300	
Duloxetine	30	20–60	
Norepinephrine-Dopamine Reuptake Inhibitors*			
Bupropion	75	75–200 (bid)	Insomnia, jitteriness
Bupropion SR	100	100–400	Less likely to cause sexual side effects or weight gain
Bupropion XL	150	150–450	
Serotonin Modulators			
Mirtazapine	15	15–45	Sedation, weight gain
Tricyclic Antidepressants†			
Nortriptyline	10	75–125	Sedation, dry mouth, anticholinergic, orthostasis, cardiac arrhythmia
Desipramine	25	100–200	

SIADH, syndrome of inappropriate antidiuretic hormone secretion.

*Contraindicated in patients at increased risk for seizures.

†Contraindicated in individuals with recent history of myocardial infarction, cardiac conduction problems, or narrow-angle glaucoma. Potential of lethality in overdose. Not used first line for depression in elderly.

Adapted from Adams SR: *Unnecessary Drugs in the Elderly, Including the Psychotropic Utilization Protocol: Establishing Compliance with the OBRA Regulations Concerning Unnecessary Drugs.* Dayton, OH, Med-Pass, 1999; and Unutzer J: Late-life depression. *N Engl J Med* 357:2269–2276, 2007.

2. **Bipolar disorder in the geriatric population.** The prevalence of bipolar affective disorder in the geriatric population (those older than age 65 years) ranges from 0.1% to 0.4%. It accounts for 10% to 20% of all geriatric patients with mood disorders (5). Most of these patients were diagnosed early in life with bipolar disorder, but **as many as 10% develop the illness after age 50** (41). Women tend to outnumber men in the geriatric population diagnosed with bipolar disorder, partially because there are more older women than older men. The frequency of psychotic features among older patients with bipolar disorder is similar to that of middle-aged samples (42). The **treatment** of bipolar disorder in the geriatric population is similar to that of younger patients, but the physiologic changes that affect drug tolerance and clearance in the geriatric population must be kept in mind. Lithium carbonate remains the "gold standard" for the treatment of bipolar disorder, but it is a drug that requires careful monitoring and that can be fatal in overdose. Lithium may cause impairment of renal function and can be toxic to the thyroid. Because lithium carbonate is metabolized by the kidney, there can be a deadly feedback loop in which lithium causes renal impairment, which leads to decreased renal clearance of lithium, which causes increased blood levels of lithium and thus further damage to the kidneys. Alternatives to lithium include antiseizure medications and some of the newer antipsychotic medications.

3. **Anxiety disorders in the elderly.** It was long held that the elderly had a lower prevalence of anxiety disorders than younger patients, in part because available data were limited and often not comparable due to different definitions of "elderly," differing time frames, and differences in assessment instruments. **Recent estimates indicate that anxiety disorders may surpass mood disorders in this age group.** Important comorbidities include mood disorders and cognitive impairment (43). The elderly may be diagnosed with any of the *DSM-IV-TR* anxiety disorders, including panic disorder (with and without agoraphobia), agoraphobia without panic disorder, specific phobia, social phobia, obsessive-compulsive disorder, posttraumatic stress disorder, acute stress disorder, generalized anxiety disorder, anxiety disorder due to a medical condition, substance-induced anxiety disorder, and anxiety disorder not otherwise specified (5).

   a. **Prevalence.** Anxiety disorders have an estimated lifetime prevalence of up to 15.3% in the elderly (43). Generalized anxiety disorder and panic disorder are common in the elderly, with a prevalence rate about the same as that for young and middle-aged adults. Rates of obsessive-compulsive disorder are comparable to middle-aged adults but lower than rates for adults aged 18 to 44 years. Finally, specific phobia and posttraumatic stress disorder are less common than in adults aged 18 to 65 years. There is considerable comorbidity in the geriatric population between anxiety disorders and mood disorders and anxiety disorders and cognitive impairment (44).

   b. **Risk factors.** There is a familial pattern for most of the anxiety disorders, but there is no clear link to a specific genetic marker at this time. The risk factors for developing an anxiety disorder in older patients are not well understood (5).

   c. **Clinical features.** Just as in younger patients, anxiety disorders cause distress and dysfunction in the lives of older patients as well. Elderly patients may become fearful of routine life events to such an extent that they become isolated. Obsessive worry may accompany decisions that are not stressful for most individuals. In extreme cases, full-blown panic attacks may incapacitate the patient and present with signs and symptoms of cardiac events. Medication side effects and invasive evaluation procedures mean that anxiety disorders often impact the physical health of these distressed patients (44).

   d. **Treatment.** Anxiety disorders in the elderly may be treated with pharmacologic and nonpharmacologic interventions (or a combination). The available data points to a benefit from cognitive behavioral therapy, particularly for generalized anxiety disorder. Pharmacologic treatment includes treatment with anxiolytics (usually benzodiazepines) and antidepressants. Benzodiazepines are not preferred for long-term use in the elderly because they can increase risk of falls, increase confusion, and be addicting. Sedating antihistamines should be avoided because of their anticholinergic action, which can affect cognition. Most physicians prefer antidepressant medications for the treatment of anxiety disorders. Most practitioners avoid TCAs and MAOIs because of their side effects in the elderly. SSRIs and combination norepinephrine/serotonin medications are preferred (45).

4. **Late-onset schizophrenia.** The *DSM-IV-TR* identifies a type of schizophrenia that begins later in life, late-onset schizophrenia. The diagnostic criteria for late-onset schizophrenia are no different from those detailed in Chapter 2. This type of schizophrenia strikes more women than men; individuals affected are more likely to have been married but they remain isolated from friends and family. Positive symptoms predominate in this type of schizophrenia, and patients often experience persecutory delusions and hallucinations. The *DSM-IV-TR* also mentions that patients who experience the onset of schizophrenia after age 60 experience auditory and vision loss at a higher frequency than the general population. There is no determination of a causal relationship between these losses and the development of schizophrenia in the elderly.

5. **Substance abuse in the geriatric population.** In the past, substance abuse in the geriatric population was limited to tobacco and alcohol. The baby boom generation has displayed striking changes in the quantity and number of substances abused by this age group. The cohort of individuals born in 1930 have a lifetime rate of illicit drug use of 10%. For the cohort born in 1960, the rate of lifetime use of illicit drugs is 75% (46). Mortality rates are higher for individuals who abuse substances, so young substance abusers sometimes do not live long enough to become geriatric substance abusers.

   Alcohol remains the substance most abused by the geriatric age group. The division between alcohol use and alcohol abuse/dependence is important and may be influenced by cultural factors. According to the 10th Special Report to the U.S. Congress on Alcohol and Health, the guidelines for alcohol use in individuals older than 65 years is one standard drink or less per day. A standard drink is defined as 0.5 ounces or 15 grams of alcohol (12 ounces of beer, 5 ounces of wine, or 1.5 ounces of 80-proof distilled spirits). Changes in the body with age may increase the negative impact of alcohol. For instance, the liver's ability to metabolize alcohol typically diminishes with age, so even moderate amounts of alcohol may have pronounced effects. As the population ages, alcohol abuse and dependence may be expected to grow. The prevalence of alcohol abuse and dependence among the age group older than 65 years is 1% to 3% of the general population, 5% to 10% of primary care outpatients, 7% to 22% of medical inpatients, and 10% to 15% of elderly patients presenting to hospital emergency rooms (47).

6. **Alcohol-induced disorders in geriatric patients.** Older patients are vulnerable to all of the alcohol-induced disorders that affect younger patients: alcohol intoxication, alcohol withdrawal, alcohol intoxication delirium, alcohol withdrawal delirium, alcohol-induced persisting dementia, alcohol-induced persisting amnestic disorder, alcohol-induced psychotic disorder with delusions, alcohol-induced psychotic disorder with hallucinations, alcohol-induced mood disorder, alcohol-induced anxiety disorder, alcohol-induced sexual dysfunction, and alcohol-induced sleep disorder. **Alcohol-induced persisting dementia is worthy of particular attention in the geriatric population.** Patients with this type of dementia may display many of the same symptoms as other patients with dementia, but there will also be the signs and symptoms of alcohol dependence/abuse. Patients may undergo alcohol withdrawal, which can be life threatening. They also will often display peripheral neuropathy and ataxia from chronic alcohol use. Laboratory tests may reveal abnormal liver function tests, macrocytic anemia, and an elevated mean cellular volume (MCV).

   Treatment of alcoholic dementia in the elderly consists of managing acute withdrawal, nutritional supplementation (folic acid and thiamine), and referral to a substance abuse treatment facility. Unlike other forms of dementia, which are usually relentlessly progressive, a patient with alcohol-induced persisting dementia usually does not become more demented if he or she remains sober. In fact, cognition often improves after a period of sobriety (48).

   Alcohol will likely continue to be the main drug of abuse in the future, but baby boomers also abuse marijuana, cocaine, and prescription medications more than past generations. The Substance Abuse and Mental Health Services Administration (SAMHSA) predicts that the number of substance abusers older than age 50 will increase by 150% from 2001 to 2020 (46).

C **Delirium** Delirium is a clinical syndrome characterized by an acute disturbance in attention and concentration that is common and potentially life threatening in the older adult. Whereas dementia is usually chronic, delirium is an acute confusional state. **Almost all cases of delirium have an identifiable medical cause that should be identified and addressed.**

1. The *DSM-IV-TR* criteria characterize delirium according to the following features:
   a. Disturbance of consciousness (ranging from drowsiness, lethargy, or stupor to agitation)
   b. Decreased ability to attend, focus, or shift attention
   c. Acute onset with fluctuation during the course of the day
   d. Causal association with a general medical condition (5)

2. **Etiology and risk factors.** Delirium occurs because of global brain dysfunction that is initiated by some event—either infectious, iatrogenic, or multifactorial. Predisposing and precipitating factors in the vulnerable individual increase the likelihood of delirium. Various neurotransmitters have been implicated including the cholinergic, dopaminergic, and glutamate systems (49). The saying "Mad as a hatter, dry as a bone, red as a beet, hot as a hare" is a helpful aid to remembering the symptoms of anticholinergic toxicity. The cognitive disturbance associated with anticholinergic agents can induce delirium (50).

    The etiologies and risk factors for delirium often overlap.
    a. **Risk (predisposing) factors** include:
       (1) Age older than 65 (elderly individuals are at higher risk)
       (2) Cognitive impairment (higher risk in those with dementia, depression)
       (3) Previous history of delirium
       (4) Sensory impairment (vision, hearing)
       (5) Poor nutritional status (dehydration, malnutrition)
       (6) Iatrogenesis and polypharmacy (especially with psychoactive agents and narcotics)
       (7) High medical comorbidities (e.g., congestive heart failure, renal or pulmonary insufficiency, liver disease, hepatic encephalopathy)
       (8) Severe illness
       (9) Neurologic disorders (including stroke and seizures)
    b. **Etiologic or precipitating factors** include (51, 52):
       (1) Infections
          (a) Urinary tract infections
          (b) Pneumonia
          (c) Meningitis or encephalitis
          (d) HIV
       (2) Comorbid illnesses
          (a) Severe acute illness
          (b) Hypoxia
          (c) Shock
          (d) Fever or hypothermia
          (e) Anemia
          (f) Dehydration
          (g) Protein-calorie malnutrition, low serum albumin level
          (h) Terminal illness
       (3) Metabolic dysfunction
          (a) Hypo-/hyperglycemia, hypothyroidism
          (b) Electrolyte/acid-base imbalance
       (4) Drugs
          (a) Anticholinergic agents
          (b) Sedative-hypnotics
          (c) Narcotics analgesics
          (d) Polypharmacy
          (e) Iatrogenic complications
       (5) Alcohol or substance withdrawal
       (6) Trauma or orthopedic injury
          (a) Burns
          (b) Head trauma
       (7) Environmental factors
          (a) Intensive care unit status (ICU psychosis)
          (b) Use of restraints (physical or chemical)

TABLE 13–4 Prevalence of Delirium	
Clinical Setting	**Prevalence Rates (%)**
Community dwelling	1–2 (14% in those older than age 85)
At admission	14–24
During hospitalization	6–56
Postoperatively	15–53
Intensive care unit	70–87
Nursing home and rehabilitation	60

Adapted from Agostini JV, Inouye SK: Delirium. In *Principles of Geriatric Medicine and Gerontology,* 5th ed. Edited by Hazzard WR, Blass JP, Halter JB. New York, McGraw-Hill, 2003, pp 1503–1515; Pisani MA, McNicoll L, Inouye SK: Cognitive impairment in the intensive care unit. *Clin Chest Med* 24:727–737, 2003; and Kiely DK, Bergmann MA, Jones RN, et al: Characteristics associated with delirium persistence among newly admitted postacute facility patients. *J Gerontol A Biol Sci Med Sci* 59:344–349, 2004.

      (c) Urinary catheterization
      (d) Pain
  (8) Surgical or postoperative states
      (a) Orthopedic surgery
      (b) Cardiac surgery
      (c) Prolonged cardiopulmonary bypass
      (d) Noncardiac surgery (especially hip)
  (9) Neurologic diseases
      (a) Stroke, particularly nondominant hemispheric
      (b) Intracranial bleeding

3. Prevalence. While delirium is most prevalent among older patients in the hospital setting, rates vary depending on the patients' comorbidities and medical setting as outlined in Table 13–4.

    Delirium is associated with a high degree of mortality, with rates of 22% to 75% in hospitalized patients. Studies suggest that up to 25% of patients with delirium die within months and 35% to 40% die within 1 year (55–57).

4. Clinical features and diagnosis. While the clinical presentation of delirium varies, **three subtypes are often seen based on psychomotor activity: hypoactive, hyperactive, and mixed (58). Hyperactive delirium** manifests with restlessness, agitation, hyperarousal, and psychosis (visual, tactile, or auditory hallucinations and delusions). In contrast, patients with **hypoactive delirium** present with lethargy, somnolence, and psychomotor retardation (slow speech and slow movements). Although the hypoactive form is more common in the elderly, these patients are often underdiagnosed or misdiagnosed as having depression or dementia. Patients with **mixed delirium** show symptoms of both hyperactive and hypoactive forms. Delirium may be difficult to recognize in certain settings such as the intensive care unit (ICU), where patients may not be able to verbally respond to standard tests of attention (e.g., if they are intubated).

    Screening tools such as cognitive tests of attention include digit span or asking the patient for the months of the year backwards. Other screening tools available for use in the ICU setting (especially for patients who are unable to verbally communicate) include the Intensive Care Delirium Screening Checklist and the Confusion Assessment method for the ICU(59, 60). A thorough medical workup is paramount in the evaluation of a patient with delirium, which, in many elderly patients with or without underlying cognitive impairment, can be the initial presentation of a new serious condition. Because delirium can be overlooked during routine examination, a brief cognitive assessment should be part of the workup of patients at risk for delirium. The Confusion Assessment method is one example of a standardized instrument that provides a diagnostic algorithm for the identification of delirium (61).

    Once a diagnosis of delirium has been established, the **underlying cause must be determined.** Delirium should be considered to be a medical emergency until proven otherwise.

Neuroimaging may be helpful in certain cases to exclude focal abnormalities such as an acute stroke, while an electroencephalogram (which usually shows generalized slowing in delirium) may be helpful to rule out seizures that might mimic delirium in their presentation. However, the diagnostic yield of these tests can be quite low (62).

5. **Treatment.** Nearly a third of delirium cases are estimated to be preventable, so prevention should be the primary strategy to minimize the occurrence of delirium (63). Iatrogenic agents and known precipitants should be avoided, including benzodiazepines and anticholinergic agents. Environmental modulation and staff education strategies have been found helpful. These include regularly orienting patients to their surroundings during their hospitalization; adequately meeting nutrition, hydration, and sleep parameters; promoting mobility (when feasible while respecting the limitations of the patient's physical condition); and providing visual and hearing aids for patients with sensory impairments (64, 65).

   a. **Nonpharmacologic treatment strategies** are similarly multifactorial. These include:
      (1) Environmental modulation: Avoid loud noises and provide calm, soothing milieu
      (2) Cues to reorient the patient (calendar and clock in the room, leave blinds open during the day when comfortable to do so)
      (3) Frequent one-to-one support: Using sitters in the hospital setting or placing the delirious patient in a room closer to the nurses' station
      (4) Maintaining diurnal rhythm
      (5) Avoiding restraints
      (6) Avoiding pharmacologic sleep aids (nonpharmacologic methods, including soothing music; herbal, noncaffeinated teas or milk; and massage)

   b. **Pharmacotherapies for the management of delirium** are primarily symptomatic, and there is limited evidence-based support for many of these agents. Antipsychotic agents, cholinesterase inhibitors, and benzodiazepines are among the psychotropic medications studied in delirium. However, such agents may further compromise not only the patient's mental status but also the ongoing evaluation of the course of the mental status change. Medications to treat delirium should be started at the lowest dose and used as briefly as possible. Neuroleptics have been used for agitation in delirium. Among these, haloperidol (available orally and parenterally) has been the most widely used with efficacy demonstrated in randomized controlled clinical trials (66, 67). However, **extrapyramidal side effects** and **acute dystonias** are known side-effect concerns with haloperidol and conventional neuroleptics. Although these side effects are less common with atypical antipsychotics, these agents are not without their inherent risks. Among the atypical antipsychotics, risperidone, olanzapine, and quetiapine have shown comparable efficacy to haloperidol in controlled trials (68, 69). However, all the antipsychotics, including the atypicals and haloperidol, carry an increased risk of stroke in elderly patients with dementia and can result in cardiac dysrhythmias with QTc interval prolongation. Benzodiazepines as first-line agents should be avoided due to their potential to worsen confusion and add to sedation and fall risks.

III ELDER ABUSE

Like the definition of "geriatric," elder abuse is open to some interpretation. Every state has laws against the abuse of the elderly, but there are differences among states in the definition of "elderly" and what constitutes abuse. In general, physical abuse, sexual abuse, neglect, and financial abuse are illegal in every state in the United States. Some states include self-neglect as a form of elder abuse. An important national study was the 2004 Survey of State Adult Protective Services, which tallied reports of elder abuse from all 50 states. The results of this survey reveal that women are more likely to be the victims of abuse and neglect (67.7%), the majority of the victims (77.1%) were white, and the perpetrators were more likely to be female (52.7%) and younger than 60 (75.1%). Most of the perpetrators were family members (65.4%). The most common form of abuse was self-neglect (37.2%), with caregiver neglect second (20.4%) and financial exploitation third (14.7%).

Defining sexual abuse can be challenging since there are no clear guidelines regarding when an elderly patient with a physical illness or dementia is able to give consent for sexual relations. In every state, medical providers of care are required to report suspected elder abuse (70).

BIBLIOGRAPHY

1. Hebert LE, Scherr PA, Bienias JL, et al: Alzheimer's disease in the U.S. population: Prevalence estimates using the 2000 census. *Arch Neurol* 60:1119–1122, 2003.

2. Alzheimer's Association: *Early-Onset Dementia: A National Challenge, A Future Crisis.* Washington, DC, Alzheimer's Association, June 2006. Available at: www.alz.org.

3. Evans DA, Hebert LE, Beckett LA, et al: Education and other measures of socioeconomic status and risk of incident Alzheimer's disease in a defined population of older persons. *Arch Neurol* 54(11):1399–1405, 1997.

4. Solomon A, Kivipelto M, Wolozin B, et al: Midlife serum cholesterol and increased risk of Alzheimer's and vascular dementia three decades later. *Dement Geriatr Disord* 28:75–80, 2009.

5. American Psychiatric Association: *Diagnostic and Statistical Manual of Mental Disorders,* 4th ed., text revision. Washington, DC, American Psychiatric Association, 2000.

6. Tariq SH, Tumosa N, Chibnall JT, et al: The Saint Louis University Mental Status (SLUMS) examination for detecting mild cognitive impairment and dementia is more sensitive than the mimi-mental state examination (MMSE): A pilot study. *Am J Geriatr Psychiatry* 14:900–910, 2006.

7. Folstein MF, Folstein SE, McHugh PR: "Mini-mental state": A practical method for grading the cognitive state of patients for the clinician. *J Psychiatr Res* 12(3):189–198, 1975.

8. Holsinger T, Deveau D, Boustani M, et al: Does this patient have dementia? *JAMA* 297(21):2391–2404, 2007. (doi:10.1001/jama.297.21.2391.)

9. Canning SJ, Leach L, Stuss D, et al: Diagnostic utility of abbreviated fluency measures in Alzheimer disease and vascular dementia. *Neurology* 62:556–562, 2004.

10. Feldman H, Gracon S: Alzheimer's disease: Symptomatic drugs under development. In *Clinical Diagnosis and Management of Alzheimer's Disease.* Edited by Gauthier S. London, Martin Dunitz Ltd., 1996, pp 239–259.

11. Heron MP, Hoyert DL, Xu J, et al: Deaths: Preliminary data for 2006. In *National Vital Statistics Reports,* vol. 56, no. 16. Hyattsville, MD, National Center for Health Statistics, 2008.

12. Alagiakrishnan K, Masaki K. Vascular dementia. Available at: http://emedicine.medscape.com/article/292105-overview. Accessed April 5, 2010.

13. Roman GC: The epidemiology of vascular dementia. In *Handbook of Clinical Neurology,* vol. 89, 3rd series. New York City, NY, Wiley Interscience, 2008, pp 639–658.

14. Roman GC, Tatemichi TK, Erkinjuntti T, et al: Vascular dementia: Diagnostic criteria for research studies. Report of the NINDS-AIREN International Workshop. *Neurology* 43:250–260, 1993.

15. Crystal HA: Dementia with Lewy bodies. Available at: http://emedicine.medscape.com/article/1135041-overview. Accessed April 5, 2010.

16. National Institute of Neurological Disorders and Stroke: Dementia with Lewy bodies information page. Available at: http://www.ninds.nih.gov/disorders/dementiawithlewybodies/dementiawithlewybodies.htm. Accessed April 5, 2010.

17. Fernandez HH, Wu CK, Ott BR: Pharmacotherapy of dementia with Lewy bodies. *Expert Opin Pharmacother* 4(11):2027–2037, 2003.

18. Ballard C, Grace J, Homes C: Neuroleptic sensitivity in dementia with Lewy bodies and Alzheimer's disease. *Lancet* 351(4):1032–1033, 1998.

19. Goldmann Gross R, Siderowf A, Hurtig HI: Cognitive impairment in Parkinson's disease and dementia with Lewy bodies: A spectrum of disease. *Neuro-Signals* 16(1):24–34, 2008.

20. Liang T-W, Horn S: Parkinson's disease. In *Principles and Practice of Geriatric Psychiatry.* Edited by Agronin ME, Maletta GJ. Philadelphia, Lippincott Williams & Wilkins, 2006, p 621.

21. Galvin JE, Pollack J, Morris JC: Clinical phenotype of Parkinson disease dementia. *Neurology* 67(9):1605–1611, 2006.

22. Aarsland D, Anderson K, Larsen JP, et al: Prevalence and characteristics of dementia in Parkinson's disease: An 8-year prospective study. *Arch Neurol* 60:387–392, 2003.

23. Swanberg MM, Kalapatapu RK: Parkinson disease dementia. Available at: http://emedicine.medscape.com/article/289595-overview. Accessed April 5, 2010.

24. Sakauye KM: Cognitive disorders: Differential diagnosis and treatment. In *Geriatric Psychiatry Basics.* New York, W.W. Norton and Company, Inc., 2008, p 73.

25. Rachford JN, Rumbaugh J, Venkataramana A: Dementia, HIV-associated. Online Johns Hopkins Point-of-Care Information Technology, August 17, 2009.

26. Centers for Disease Control Website. Prion Diseases. Available at: www.cdc.gov/ncidod/dvrd/prios/ Accessed Februarey 19, 2010.

27. Ropper A, Brown R: *Adams and Victor's Principles of Neurology.* New York, McGraw-Hill, 2005, pp 614–619.

28. Wittenberg D, Possin K, Raskovsky K, et al: The early neuropsychological and behavioral characteristics of frontotemporal dementia. *Neuropsychol Rev* 18:91–102, 2008.

29. Shinagawa S, Toyota Y, Ishikawa T, et al: Cognitive function and psychiatric symptoms in early- and late-onset frontotemporal dementia. *Dement Geriatr Cogn Disord* 25:439–444, 2008.

30. Murray CJL, Lopez AD: Alternative visions of the future: Projecting mortality and disability, 1990–2020. In *The Global Burden of Disease*. Edited by Murray CJL, Lopez AD. Cambridge, MA, Harvard University Press, 1996, pp 325–397.

31. Raj A: Depression in the elderly: Tailoring medical therapy to their special needs. *Postgrad Med* 115(6): 26–42, 2004.

32. Steffens DC, Skoog I, Norton MC, et al: Prevalence of depression and its treatment in an elderly population: The Cache County Study. *Arch Gen Psychiatry* 57:601–607, 2000.

33. Mulsant BH, Ganguly M: Epidemiology and diagnosis of depression in late life. *J Clin Psychiatry* 60(suppl 20):9–15, 1999.

34. Simon GE, VonKorff M: Recognition, management, and outcomes of depression in primary care. *Arch Fam Med* 4:99–105, 1995.

35. Unützer J, Katon W, Callahan CM, et al: Collaborative care management of late life depression in the primary care setting: A randomized controlled trial. *JAMA* 288:2836–2845, 2002.

36. Givens JL, Datto CJ, Ruckdeschel K, et al: Older patients' aversion to antidepressants: A qualitative study. *J Gen Intern Med* 21:146–151, 2006.

37. Pinquart M, Duberstein PR, Lyness JM: Treatments for later-life depressive conditions: A meta-analytic comparison of pharmacotherapy and psychotherapy. *Am J Psychiatry* 163:1493–1501, 2006.

38. Cuijpers P, van Straten A, Smit F: Psychological treatment of late-life depression: A meta-analysis of randomized controlled trials. *Int J Geriatr Psychiatry* 21:1139–1149, 2006.

39. Adams SR: *Unnecessary Drugs in the Elderly, Including the Psychotropic Utilization Protocol: Establishing Compliance with the OBRA Regulations Concerning Unnecessary Drugs.* Dayton, OH, Med-Pass, 1999.

40. Unutzer J: Late-life depression. *N Engl J Med* 357:2269–2276, 2007.

41. Sajatovic M. Treatment of bipolar disorder in older adults. *Int J Geriatr Psychiatry* 17:865–873, 2002.

42. Depp CA, Jeste DV: Bipolar disorder in older adults: A critical review. *Bipolar Disord* 6:343–367, 2004.

43. Beaudreau SA, Ohara R: Late-life anxiety and cognitive impairment: A review. *Am J Geriatr Psychiatry* 16: 790–803, 2008.

44. Lauderdale SA, Kelly K, Sheikh JI: Anxiety disorders in the elderly. In *Principles and Practices of Geriatric Psychiatry*. Edited by Agronin A, Maletta G. Philadelphia, Lippincott Williams & Wilkins, 2006, pp 429–448.

45. Wetherell JL, Lenze EJ, Stanley MA: Evidence-based treatment of geriatric anxiety disorders. *Psychiatr Clin N Am* 28:871–896, 2005.

46. Substance Abuse and Mental Health Services Administration. (2007). Results from the 2006 National Survey on Drug Use and Health: National Findings (Office of Applied Studies, NSDUH Series H-32, DHHS Publication No. SMA 07-4293). Rockville, MD.

47. Holbert KR, Tueth MJ: Alcohol abuse and dependence: A clinical update on alcoholism in the older population. *Geriatrics* 59:38–40, 2004.

48. American Psychiatric Association: *Diagnostic and Statistical Manual of Mental Disorders*, 4th ed., text revision. Washington, DC, American Psychiatric Association, 2000, pp 212–213.

49. Roche V: Etiology and management of delirium. *Am J Med Sci* 325:20–30, 2003.

50. Stead LG, Stead SM, Kaufman MS: *First Aid for the Emergency Medicine Clerkship,* 2nd ed. New York, McGraw-Hill, 2006, pp 395–396.

51. Inouye SK: Delirium in older persons. *N Engl J Med* 354:1157–1165, 2006.

52. Raskind MA, Bonner LT, Peskind ER: Cognitive disorders. In *Textbook of Geriatric Psychiatry,* 3rd ed. Edited by Blazer DG, Steffens DC, Busse EW. Arlington, VA, American Psychiatric Publishing, 2004, pp 222–223.

53. Agostini JV, Inouye SK: Delirium. In *Principles of Geriatric Medicine and Gerontology,* 5th ed. Edited by Hazzard WR, Blass JP, Halter JB. New York, McGraw-Hill, 2003, pp 1503–1515.

54. Pisani MA, McNicoll L, Inouye SK: Cognitive impairment in the intensive care unit. *Clin Chest Med* 24:727–737, 2003.

55. Kiely DK, Bergmann MA, Jones RN, et al: Characteristics associated with delirium persistence among newly admitted postacute facility patients. *J Gerontol A Biol Sci Med Sci* 59:344–349, 2004.

56. American Psychiatric Association: *Practice Guideline for the Treatment of Psychiatric Disorders Compendium.* Washington, DC, American Psychiatric Association, 2006, pp 65–100.

57. Trzepacz P, Teague G, Lipowski Z: Delirium and other organic mental disorders in a general hospital. *Gen Hosp Psychiatry* 7:101–106, 1985.

58. Moran JA, Dorevitch MI: Delirium in the hospitalized elderly. *Aust J Hosp Pharm* 31:35–40, 2001.

59. Lipowski ZJ: Transient cognitive disorders (delirium, acute confusional states) in the elderly. *Am J Psychiatry* 140:1426–1436, 1983.

60. Ely EW, Margolin R, Francis J, et al: Evaluation of delirium in critically ill patients: Validation of the Confusion Assessment Method for the Intensive Care Unit (CAM-ICU). *Crit Care Med* 29:1370–1379, 2001.

61. Bergeron N, Dubois MJ, Dumont M, et al: Intensive care delirium screening checklist: Evaluation of a new screening tool. *Intensive Care Med* 27:859–864, 2001.

62. Wei LA, Fearing MA, Sternberg EJ, et al: The Confusion Assessment Method: A systematic review of current usage. *J Am Geriatr Soc* 56:823–830, 2008.

63. Fong TG, Tulebaev SR, Inouye SK: Delirium in elderly adults: Diagnosis, prevention and treatment. *Nat Rev Neurol* 5:210–220, 2009.

64. Siddiqi N, House AO, Holmes JD: Occurrence and outcome of delirium in medical in-patients: A systematic literature review. *Age Ageing* 35:350–364, 2006.

65. The Hospital Elder Life Program (HELP). Available at: http://www.hospitalelderlifeprogram.org. Accessed April 5, 2010.

66. Inouye SK, Bogardus ST Jr, Charpentier PA, et al: A multicomponent intervention to prevent delirium in hospitalized older patients. *N Engl J Med* 340:669–676, 1990.

67. Breitbart W, Marotta R, Platt MM, et al: A double-blind trial of haloperidol, chlorpromazine, and lorazepam in the treatment of delirium in hospitalized AIDS patients. *Am J Psychiatry* 153:231–237, 1996.

68. Hu H, Deng W, Yang H, et al: Olanzapine and haloperidol for senile delirium: A randomized controlled observation. *Chin J Clin Rehab* 10:188–190, 2006.

69. Han CS, Kim YK: A double-blind trial of risperidone and haloperidol for the treatment of delirium. *Psychosomatics* 45:297–301, 2004.

70. National Center on Elder Abuse: *2004 Survey of Adult Protective Services.* Washington, DC, National Center on Elder Abuse, 2004.

Study Questions

Directions: *Each of the numbered items or incomplete statements is followed by answers or completions of the statement. Select the ONE lettered answer or completion that is BEST in each case.*

1. Examination of population trends in the United States indicates that in the next 40 years:
   - A. The number of U.S. citizens older than the age of 65 will decline.
   - B. There will be almost double the number of women compared to men in the age group older than 85.
   - C. The age group 65 to 84 will grow more rapidly than the age group older than 85.
   - D. The number of patients diagnosed with dementia will decrease.

2. HIV-associated dementia (HAD) is:
   - A. A subcortical dementia
   - B. An inevitable result of HIV infection for all patients
   - C. A type of Alzheimer disease that afflicts patients with HIV infection
   - D. Treated with antipsychotic medications

3. As the baby boomers age, physicians can expect:
   - A. To see less alcohol abuse or dependence
   - B. To observe a decline in the number of patients reaching the age of 85 because of substance abuse and dependence
   - C. To see increased rates of abuse and dependence for all substances of abuse including alcohol
   - D. To see increased rates of alcohol abuse and dependence but a decreased rate of abuse of marijuana

4. A 68-year-old woman presents on referral with a 10-day history of poor sleep, agitation, and hyper-sexuality. She believes she is an angel sent from heaven to destroy wickedness and populate earth with only righteous people. A medical workup does not reveal any physical disorder. This patient's most likely diagnosis:
   - A. Usually is first diagnosed in patients age 65 or older
   - B. In the geriatric age group is more common in women than in men   *Bipolar I*
   - C. Is usually treated with antidepressant medications
   - D. Cannot be diagnosed in patients older than 50

5. Three times in the past month, a 73-year-old woman has presented to the emergency room with complaints of sudden onset of chest pain, shortness of breath, palpitations, dizziness, and numbness in her hands. On each occasion she has received a complete medical evaluation without any organic findings to justify her symptoms. This patient's most likely diagnosis:
   - A. Is uncommon in the elderly
   - B. Can be debilitating for elderly patients
   - C. Cannot be diagnosed in a patient who has Alzheimer disease
   - D. Is usually treated with sedating antihistamines

6. Mrs. Jones, a 78-year-old woman with no prior psychiatric history, who resides at a local assisted-living facility, is brought to the emergency room after being found on the floor in her bathroom. She is confused and distracted and picks at her skin, crying, "They are trying to get into my body!" She has diabetes, hypertension, and a history of stroke. Staff from the facility supervise and administer all her medications, including metoprolol, aspirin, and glipizide, with which she has been compliant. She is incontinent of foul-smelling urine. All of the following diagnoses are likely in this patient's case EXCEPT:
   - A. Urinary tract infection (UTI)
   - B. Delirium
   - C. Cerebrovascular accident (CVA)
   - D. Delusional disorder
     → *usually have a clear sensorium*

7. A 72-year-old woman with no previous psychiatric history is brought to her internist by her concerned son, who reports that she has not been eating well for the past 2 to 3 months and appears to have lost a considerable amount of weight. The woman appears apathetic and answers questions in a flat voice with few words. She complains of profound fatigue and having no appetite. She falls asleep with no difficulty but wakes after 4 to 5 hours and cannot go back to sleep. This patient's most likely diagnosis is:

[A] Primarily due to bereavement

[B] A normal part of aging   *Depression*

[C] Not associated with suicide risk factors

[D] Associated with functional impairment

8. A 67-year-old woman with a history of diabetes and hypertension is seen in the emergency department after being found by a neighbor unresponsive in her home. She is now alert but seems disoriented and is having some difficulty forming words properly partly because of a pronounced facial droop. She does not remember what happened to her prior to passing out. Her symptoms are characteristic of which of the following dementias?

[A] HIV dementia

[B] Pick disease – *Personality Δ*

[C] Vascular dementia

[D] Parkinson dementia

9. A 67-year-old man is brought in by his son to see his family practitioner. The son is worried that his father seems more forgetful than usual. He believes the problem began 6 or 7 months ago. On examination the patient is alert and oriented. He makes an obvious effort to answer the physician's questions, but tends to give answers that are close, but not exactly right. Which of the following substances is found in senile plaques associated with this patient's most likely illness?

[A] α-Synuclein – *in Lewy Bodies*

[B] Amyloid precursor protein – *precursor to amyloid in senile plaques*

[C] β-Amyloid protein

[D] Hyperphosphorylated τ protein – *neurofibrillary tangles*

10. Mr. A is a 69-year-old white man who has lived alone since his male partner died of HIV/AIDS 5 years ago. Mr. A is HIV positive but has been treated by an infectious disease specialist with antiretroviral medications. However, he missed his last appointment because "he forgot." His only close relative is a niece who sees him once or twice a month. She notes that he has seemed "down" lately, worries about his alcohol use, and feels that he is not keeping his home or himself clean. Mr. A maintains that he drinks no more than he did 10 years ago but does admit that he forgets to take his medications "sometimes." All of the following should be included in the differential diagnosis of Mr. A EXCEPT:

[A] HIV-associated dementia

[B] Generalized anxiety disorder

[C] Alcohol-induced mood disorder

[D] Major depressive disorder

Answers and Explanations

1. The answer is B [*I*]. The geriatric population is not equally distributed between men and women. The number of Americans older than the age of 65 will continue to increase, and thus, so will the number of patients diagnosed with dementia.

2. The answer is A [*II A 5 a*]. Not all patients with HIV develop HIV-associated dementia (HAD). HAD is treated with antiviral agents.

3. The answer is C [*II B 5–6*]. As the geriatric population increases, so will the rates of abuse and dependence for all substances including alcohol. While many young substance abusers do not live to old age, this is not significant enough to cause a decrease in individuals reaching the age of 85.

4. The answer is B [*II B 2*]. Bipolar disorder is usually diagnosed early in life, but can be diagnosed after the age of 50. First-line treatment is with a mood stabilizer such as lithium.

5. The answer is B [*II B 3*]. Anxiety disorders are common in the elderly, and a diagnosis of Alzheimer disease does not preclude the diagnosis. Treatment includes anxiolytics and antidepressants; sedating antihistamines should be avoided because of their anticholinergic side effects.

6. The answer is D [*II C 2 b*]. Given this patient's medical history and symptoms, a number of diagnoses would be in the differential, including a urinary tract infection (UTI), a cerebrovascular accident (CVA), and delirium. Patients with delusional disorder usually present with a clear sensorium.

7. The answer is D [*II B 1*]. Depression in the elderly is not a normal part of aging or primarily due to bereavement. Older adults are at significant risk for suicide.

8. The answer is C [*II A 2 b, c*]. This patient's medical illnesses and symptoms of a cerebrovascular accident (CVA) are most characteristic of vascular dementia. There is no evidence of HIV infection, personality changes, or tremor.

9. The answer is C [*II A 1 c*]. This patient's most likely diagnosis is Alzheimer disease. α-Synuclein is found in Lewy bodies. Amyloid precursor protein is a precursor to amyloid in senile plaques. Hyperphosphorylated τ protein is found in neurofibrillary tangles.

10. The answer is B [*II A 5 a; B 1, 3, 6*]. This patient's symptoms could be stemming from the development of an HIV-associated dementia, his alcohol use, and/or major depression. There is no indication of significant anxiety that would meet the criteria for generalized anxiety disorder.

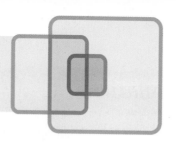

chapter 14

Legal Issues and Forensic Psychiatry

RICHARD L. FRIERSON

I · INTRODUCTION

Legal issues pervade psychiatric practice to such an extent that forensic psychiatry has emerged as a subspecialty. Forensic psychiatrists engage in clinical practice and research in areas where psychiatry and the legal system interact. They routinely evaluate persons alleged to be mentally ill and provide court testimony related to criminal and civil issues. They also provide consultation to general psychiatrists about the numerous legal issues that arise in general psychiatric practice. These issues are divided into three areas: the legal regulation of psychiatry, criminal law, and civil law.

A · Dual agency Dual agency is serving both as a treating physician and an evaluator of a patient who is involved in a legal proceeding. Psychiatrists frequently encounter problems when their patients become involved in legal disputes, especially when patients or their attorneys seek to have a psychiatrist testify about the patient's condition and give an opinion related to the legal issue. For example, a psychiatrist treating a man who is involved in a divorce proceeding might be asked to testify about the patient's illness as it relates to child custody and give an opinion about the fitness of the man as a parent. These situations can be very damaging to the therapeutic alliance and the physician–patient relationship because an undesirable legal outcome for a patient can lead to feelings of distrust toward the treating psychiatrist. For this reason, dual agency situations should be avoided. In general, a psychiatrist should not be involved in both treatment of a patient and evaluation of that same patient for a court or attorney.

B · Psychiatrists in court When psychiatrists are subpoenaed to court, they should clarify their role before they appear to testify. They may assume the role of one of the two types of court witnesses: fact witnesses and expert witnesses.

1. **Fact witnesses** testify to events. For example, a psychiatrist called as a fact witness might testify to dates and type of treatment and medical record documentation. Fact witnesses are not allowed to give expert opinions about a patient's mental illness as it relates to a legal issue.

2. **Expert witnesses** testify to issues outside the knowledge of an average layperson. These witnesses must be qualified by a judge as experts after the judge reviews their credentials. Expert witnesses may testify about the reasoning behind a diagnosis, a patient's prognosis, and how a patient's mental illness relates to the legal issue in dispute. For example, a psychiatrist called as an expert witness may be used to establish the standard of care in a malpractice suit or to determine a defendant's legal sanity in a criminal trial.

II · LEGAL REGULATION OF PSYCHIATRIC PRACTICE

The practice of psychiatry is regulated by both statutory and case law. Therefore, psychiatrists must be familiar with basic laws applicable to psychiatric practice in their jurisdiction. Although statutes vary from state to state, they are based in core legal principles.

A **Involuntary psychiatric hospitalization**   The first civil commitment law was passed in New York in 1788 and involuntary hospitalization statutes now exist in all 50 states. Because the U.S. Constitution provides individuals with "life, liberty, and the pursuit of happiness," denial of these freedoms requires due process and legal oversight. Commitment laws establish the criteria by which individuals may be involuntarily committed to a psychiatric hospital and the procedural safeguards to be used in this process. In most states, patients who are hospitalized involuntarily are afforded a formal hearing before or shortly after they are hospitalized. During this hearing, a judge (or jury) determines whether commitment criteria have been met based on the testimony of clinicians who have examined the person suspected of needing involuntary treatment. Almost all commitment statutes require that individuals be suffering from a *treatable* mental illness. The criteria used to determine whether involuntary psychiatric commitment is appropriate are based on one of the following two legal doctrines:

1. **Police powers.** This emergency commitment model, based in the government's authority to protect public safety, allows for hospitalization of patients if they are mentally ill *and* represent a danger to themselves or others. A mentally ill person who is acutely suicidal or homicidal would be committable using this model. This is the most common basis for psychiatric commitment laws in the United States. In most states, a physician, psychiatrist, or mental health professional determines if a patient meets commitment criteria, and the patient may be detained until a hearing is conducted in front of a judge or designated judicial reviewer. The reviewer ultimately decides if the patient is to remain hospitalized.

2. *Parens patriae.* Some jurisdictions also allow for commitment under a *parens patriae* model. Literally, *parens patriae* translates as "father of the country" and refers to the government's role to protect individuals who are mentally ill and who cannot take care of themselves or provide themselves with basic necessities. Imminent dangerousness to themselves or others is not required for involuntary treatment using this model. For example, psychotic individuals who are so disorganized in their thinking that they are having some difficulty managing their need for food or shelter could possibly meet commitment criteria under this model, even if this person is not acutely suicidal or dangerous to others. However, case law has established that hospitalization in such a case must represent the *least restrictive alternative* for treatment.

B **Informed consent**   Many medical procedures, including psychiatric treatment with neuroleptic (i.e., typical antipsychotic) medications and electroconvulsive therapy (ECT), require written informed consent. Informed consent has three basic elements: information disclosure, patient competence, and voluntariness.

1. **Information disclosure.** The amount of information to be disclosed to patients during the informed consent process depends on the risk associated with the treatment and the risk associated with the illness if it is left untreated. In general, the riskier the treatment, the more information patients should be given.
   a. Table 14–1 lists the types of information disclosed. Patients should always be afforded an opportunity to ask questions about the information presented to them.
   b. In more than half of the states, the standard for information disclosure is the **reasonable professional standard,** which means that the amount of information disclosed should be the amount that the majority of physicians practicing in that jurisdiction would normally disclose. An increasing number of other states have adopted a "materiality of the information" or **reasonable person standard,** meaning the amount of information disclosed should be the amount that any reasonable person would want to know before consenting to or declining treatment.

TABLE 14–1 Information Given to Patients When Obtaining Informed Consent

Description of the proposed procedure or treatment
Expected benefits of the procedure or treatment
Risks and side effects associated with the procedure or treatment
Advantages and risks associated with the absence of treatment
Available alternatives to the proposed treatment
Advantages and risks associated with alternative treatment options

TABLE 14–2 Elements of Competency in Informed Consent
The patient can communicate a choice. The patient applies rational reasoning in making the choice. The patient has the ability to understand the information presented by the clinician. The patient understands the information, as evidenced by an ability to answer questions correctly about the information presented.

2. **Competency to consent.** Most adult patients are presumed to be competent to consent to treatment, and most minors are presumed incompetent, which means that they lack the ability to understand the information presented in the informed consent process. However, major mental illness can affect patients' ability to make informed decisions. This concern frequently arises in psychotic patients and elderly patients with dementia. Many clinicians question patients' competency when they refuse treatment. However, patients can just as incompetently consent to a medical procedure as they can refuse it.

   a. The elements of competency involved in informed consent are outlined in Table 14–2. Failure to consider patient competency may increase a clinician's liability, especially if a patient incompetently consents to a procedure that ends with a poor clinical outcome.

   b. If a patient is incompetent to consent to medical treatment, a substitute decision maker is usually required. If the patient does not have a legally appointed guardian, most jurisdictions allow the closest relative to give informed consent. A small minority of jurisdictions require a judge to order treatment, especially when the treatment involves involuntary psychiatric medications.

3. **Voluntariness.** Informed consent must be given freely and voluntarily. Often the distinction between coercion and persuasion can be difficult. For example, if a clinician has withheld visitation or recreational privileges for an institutionalized patient because he refused to consent, the clinician would be coercive. The use of justified encouragement to a patient to accept treatment would not be considered coercive on the part of the clinician.

4. **Exceptions to informed consent**

   a. In **emergency situations** in which a delay in treatment could jeopardize the life of the patient or others, informed consent is not necessary. Although these situations are more common in other medical specialties, they do occur in psychiatry. For example, an acutely psychotic patient who is assaulting others may be medicated acutely or restrained without obtaining consent.

   b. **Therapeutic privilege** allows for withholding informed consent if the clinician believes that the information disclosed would be harmful to the patient or significantly worsen the patient's condition. This exception has a high potential for abuse by clinicians and should be used very rarely. Note that withholding information because a clinician believes a patient would refuse treatment is *not* therapeutic privilege.

   c. A **waiver** of informed consent occurs if the patient indicates that he or she does not want to be told information related to the procedure or wants the clinician to make the decision for him or her. A patient waiver should be initially challenged by the clinician and clearly documented in the medical record.

C **Confidentiality and privilege**

1. **Confidentiality.** The physician–patient relationship is based on trust, and many patients routinely reveal intimate details of their lives to their treating clinicians. Confidentiality is the clinician's duty to prevent the communications received in the physician–patient relationship from being divulged to third parties. It is the clinician's obligation to maintain confidentiality, and courts have found clinicians liable for revealing patient information without the expressed written consent of the patient. This applies to information released to family members, other nontreating physicians, insurers and managed care companies, and medical researchers. Confidentiality also survives death.

   a. However, **exceptions to confidentiality** include:

      (1) **Emergencies.** In certain situations, release of confidential information to other health care providers may be necessary to guarantee a patient's immediate welfare. These cases are the

most widely recognized exception to patient confidentiality, and physicians are unlikely to be held liable if they genuinely believe they are acting in the patient's best interest.

   (2) **Voluntary or involuntary hospital admissions.** Psychiatrists may release information to a receiving hospital at the time of hospital admission.

   (3) **Certain infectious diseases, child abuse, and abuse of elderly and mentally or physically disabled individuals.** Most states have requirements mandating the reporting of certain diseases and child abuse. In addition, some states have passed legislation mandating the reporting of abuse of elderly or disabled individuals.

   (4) **Ancillary medical personnel.** Patient information can also be released to a physician's supervisor or other medical personnel involved in the direct care of a patient on a hospital ward. However, these ancillary staff members are bound by the same confidentiality expectations as the primary clinician.

   b. In some jurisdictions, **failure to abide by the reporting laws** [listed in *II E 1 a (3)*] **can lead to criminal charges against psychiatrists.** In general, previous crimes revealed by patients do not have to be reported.

2. **Privilege.** The patient's right to prevent a physician from testifying in a legal proceeding about material gained from the therapeutic relationship is known as privilege. If a psychiatrist receives a subpoena for records (i.e., a subpoena *duces tecum*), he or she should contact the patient and, with the patient's permission, the patient's attorney. If the patient does not want the records released, the psychiatrist should notify the attorney who sent the subpoena that the patient has invoked privilege, and the records cannot be released without a court order. It is ultimately up to the judge to decide whether the material subpoenaed is privileged or admissible. In the case of a deceased or gravely disabled patient, the psychiatrist may be obligated to claim privilege for the patient. Usually, if a patient places his or her mental status at issue in a legal proceeding (e.g., a patient sues a former psychiatrist), the patient cannot claim privilege.

D Duty to third parties Throughout the United States, courts are holding psychiatrists liable for damages to third parties as a result of acts on the part of their patients that led to injury to persons or property. Psychiatrists have been held liable for physical assaults by their patients, automobile accidents in which their patients were drivers, and "false memories" of childhood abuse uncovered in psychotherapy that led to subsequent disruption of family relationships.

1. A psychiatrist's liability toward a nonpatient (i.e., a third party not in treatment with the psychiatrist) was first created in the 1976 California Supreme Court case of *Tarasoff v. Regents of the University of California.* This case involved a college student who had told a university psychologist that he planned to kill his estranged girlfriend. After he killed Tatiana Tarasoff, her parents sued the University of California, alleging, in part, that the university was negligent in failing to warn a foreseeable victim. After several appeals, the California Supreme Court held that "when a therapist determines, or pursuant to the standards of his profession should determine, that his patient presents a serious danger of violence to another, he incurs an obligation to use reasonable care to protect the intended victim against such danger." The court found that a psychiatrist has a duty not only to warn but also to *protect* a known intended victim. In situations in which a patient threatens to harm an identified person, the psychiatrist should consider notifying the potential victim or the police or, if indicated, hospitalizing the patient.

2. Court decisions relating to the *Tarasoff* decision vary widely from state to state; some states have passed statutes that adopt a "*Tarasoff*" obligation to protect identified victims. In other states, appellate court decisions have also established this duty. Finally, many states have rejected this duty, and psychiatrists in those states cannot be sued for failing to protect a known intended victim. Because of the variability regarding this duty across jurisdictions, psychiatrists should be familiar with the law in the state in which they practice.

III   CRIMINAL ISSUES

The criminalization of mentally ill individuals has been an unintended side effect of deinstitutionalization, with more chronically mentally ill patients treated on an outpatient basis rather than in an inpatient setting. The Los Angeles County jail houses the largest number of persons with severe and persistent

---

TABLE 14–3   Criteria Used to Evaluate Patient Competency to Stand Trial

The patient understands the pending criminal charge(s) and potential penalties that conviction could bring.
The patient appreciates the roles of court personnel (lawyer, judge, prosecutor, jury, and witnesses).
The patient knows the potential pleas available and understands the process of plea bargaining.
The patient is able to control his or her behavior in the courtroom.
The patient appreciates the significance of evidence and witness testimony.
The patient is able to be appropriately self-protective.
The patient is able to describe a desired legal outcome.
The patient is able to communicate effectively with his or her lawyer.

---

mental illness in the United States. In adjudicating persons with mental illness, courts are faced with two issues: the mentally ill defendant's competency to stand trial and the defendant's criminal responsibility (i.e., legal sanity) at the time of the alleged offense.

A **Competency to stand trial (CST)**   CST is a criminal defendant's ability to understand court proceedings and assist an attorney in the preparation of a defense. In the 1960 U.S. Supreme Court landmark case *Dusky v. United States,* the court held that in order for a defendant to be considered competent to stand trial, he or she must have "sufficient present ability to consult with his [or her] attorney with a reasonable degree of rational understanding" and "a rational as well as factual understanding of the proceedings against him [or her]." Table 14–3 lists the trial abilities that are routinely assessed in a CST evaluation. If a criminal defendant is found incompetent to stand trial because of symptoms that are treatable with psychotropic medication, the U.S. Supreme Court has held that involuntary medication may be administered if the proposed treatment is medically appropriate, if there is reasonable probability that it would restore competence, and if it would further legitimate governmental interests.

B **Criminal responsibility or legal insanity**   Unlike CST, there is no constitutional basis for the insanity defense. Consequently, although all states must have procedures to ensure defendants' competency, the recognition of a defense of insanity is not required. Furthermore, each state must define the criteria to determine legal insanity. The insanity defense is rarely successful; fewer than 1% of felony prosecutions result in an insanity acquittal.

1. Determination of legal insanity requires that psychiatrists make a retrospective determination of a defendant's mental state at the time an alleged crime was committed. This can be difficult, especially if a long period has elapsed between the alleged crime and the time of the evaluation of criminal responsibility. It is most difficult when a defendant was acutely psychotic at the time of the crime but was subsequently treated and the psychotic symptoms have resolved before the evaluation. Consequently, in addition to a patient interview, evaluations concerning legal insanity require a review of police reports, defendant statements, witness and victim statements, the patient's psychiatric and medical records, and the defendant's functioning around the time of the alleged crime.

2. Psychiatrists who perform criminal responsibility evaluations should be familiar with the legal definition of insanity in their particular state. Most states use one of the following three standards of legal insanity.

    a. The **McNaughten standard,** named for an 1843 Scottish defendant, is the most widely used test of legal insanity in the United States. It requires that a person, as the result of mental disease or defect, failed to know the nature and quality of the criminal act he or she was committing or failed to know that the act he or she was committing was wrong.

    b. The **Model Penal Code,** also known as the **American Law Institute Rule,** states that a defendant should not be held responsible if a mental disease or defect impaired his or her capacity to appreciate the criminality of his or her conduct or to conform his or her conduct to the requirements of the law. It excludes illnesses that are manifested only by repeated criminal or antisocial conduct such as antisocial personality disorder or pedophilia.

    c. The **Durham rule,** the least restrictive of all insanity tests, merely requires that the crime is the product of a mental illness or defect.

IV CIVIL ISSUES

Civil courts settle legal disputes that do not involve violation of a criminal statute. In general, civil litigation involves a tort, or civil wrong, done by one party to another. **Intentional torts** are wrongdoings done with prior knowledge that damages may result. For example, a psychiatrist or other specialist who becomes involved in a sexual relationship with a patient may be held responsible for an intentional tort and ordered to pay punitive damages to the patient. **Unintentional torts** involve **negligence,** the concept that the act led to an unreasonable risk of causing harm to another, although the act may not have been intended to cause such harm.

(A) **Guardianship and conservatorship**   Whereas commitment laws are designed to protect patients from immediate harm to themselves or others, conservatorship and guardianship laws protect patients from financial loss and other less immediate harm that may result if their mental illness or defect impairs their judgment and ability to make decisions.

1. **Guardianship.** A guardian is a person designated by the court to manage the property and rights of another individual and to make decisions related to the physical well-being of that individual. A guardian may make decisions related to financial matters, living arrangements, and physical needs, including medical treatment. In some states, a guardian is called the **committee of the person,** reflecting the global decision making involved in the guardianship role.
   a. Patients who are declared globally incompetent and in need of a guardian may lose many civil rights, including the right to vote, the right to own a firearm, or the right to have a driver's license. Consequently, patients undergoing guardianship proceedings are granted rights of due process, including the right to representation by an attorney. A petitioner must show the court, usually by clear and convincing evidence, that individuals lack substantial ability to manage their property or provide for themselves or their dependents. Forensic psychiatrists may serve as experts to the court in these proceedings, describing specific patient impairments and the effect of impairments on patients' decision-making ability. The presence of psychosis, dementia, or other mental illness does not constitute incompetence per se, so a functional assessment must be performed.
   b. Traditionally, courts have appointed a guardian from the patient's family, usually with input from the patient. If a family member is not available, the court may appoint an attorney or other interested person to serve as guardian.

2. **Conservatorship.** A conservator, or limited guardian, is a person designated by the court to manage another person's financial affairs. Individuals in need of a conservator do not have to be declared globally incompetent. Therefore, they do not lose their basic civil rights. A conservator may pay bills, buy or sell property, and manage investments or other financial matters.

(B) **Testamentary capacity**   The simplest of all competencies, testamentary capacity is an individual's capacity to make a will. The law presumes that a person is of sound mind when a will is signed. An evaluation of testamentary capacity at the time the will is signed can prevent challenges to the will by family members after the death of the testator (i.e., person executing a will).

1. To have testamentary capacity, individuals must understand the nature and purpose of a will, their assets (legally, the extent of their bounty), their natural heirs, and their relationship to their heirs. In addition, their decision-making abilities must be free of delusion.

2. Only a small percentage of contested wills are overturned. Most successful challenges involve proof of **undue influence,** the manipulation or deception of the testator by others to gain the affections of the testator.

(C) **Workers' compensation and psychiatric disability**

1. **Workers' compensation.** Workers' compensation laws are designed to reimburse an employee for medical expenses and loss of income resulting from a work-related injury. These laws are also designed to prevent litigation for work-related injuries. In most states, this compensation can last for up to 1 year after the injury. Most states bar compensation for self-inflicted injury or injuries occurring at work if the worker was under the influence of alcohol or drugs. This has led

to increased drug screening by many companies. The three categories of claims for psychiatric injury can be described as follows:

    a. A **physical–mental claim** involves a physical injury that causes mental impairment. An example would be an employee who is unable to return to work after being physically injured in an industrial explosion and subsequently develops posttraumatic stress disorder (PTSD). If he or she is unable to return to work after the physical injury heals, a physical–mental claim may be filed.

    b. A **mental–physical claim** involves recurrent job stress that causes or aggravates a physical condition. For example, an automobile assembly technician who is required to work excessive overtime subsequently develops a bleeding gastric ulcer requiring hospitalization. Mental–physical claims can be difficult to prove because of the issue of causality.

    c. A **mental–mental claim** occurs if job stress leads to the development of a mental condition. For example, a policeman who witnesses the murder of a partner in the line of duty is unable to return to work because of depression that develops after this traumatic event.

2. Disability. The Social Security Administration (SSA) administers two disability programs, Social Security Disability Income (SSDI or Title II) and Social Security Income (SSI or Title XVI). As of 2010, more than 9 million disabled persons and their dependents receive some form of payment from the SSA, which has defined diagnostic categories of mental disorders for which disability payments may be awarded. In addition, functional disability must cause two or three of the following: restrictions in activities of daily living; difficulties with social functioning; deficiencies of concentration, persistence, or pace in the work environment; or repeated episodes of decompensation in the work setting, causing the worker to withdraw from work or experience a worsening of signs and symptoms of his or her mental impairment.

    a. SSDI provides cash benefits for disabled workers and their dependents if the worker has contributed substantially to the Federal Insurance Compensation Act (FICA).

    b. SSI provides minimal income for disabled individuals who have not made significant contributions to FICA.

D Psychiatric malpractice Psychiatrists are less likely to be sued for malpractice than their physician counterparts. The most common psychiatric malpractice claims involve, in order of decreasing frequency, incorrect treatment, suicide, improper diagnosis, and inadequate supervision of other mental health professionals.

1. Negligence. Most malpractice suits fall into the legal category of an unintentional tort. In malpractice actions, the plaintiff must prove the **"four Ds"** of negligence: **duty** on the part of the psychiatrist (a doctor–patient relationship existed), **dereliction** or breach of that duty (the treatment provided failed to reach a standard of care), **damages** suffered by the patient, and **direct causation** (if not for the action of the physician, the damages would not have occurred).

    a. Duty. The concept of duty requires the existence of a physician–patient relationship. Thus, a physician must have agreed to treat a patient.

        (1) After duty has been established, it can only be ended by a medically indicated discharge or by transferring a patient to the care of another physician.

        (2) Duty may be excused in certain emergency situations in which a doctor–patient relationship was not previously established. To protect physicians (and others) from liability if they provide treatment to unconscious patients at accident scenes in emergent life-and-death situations, some states have enacted "good Samaritan" laws.

    b. Dereliction. If it is established that the treatment given by the physician fell below an acceptable standard of care, then dereliction has occurred.

        (1) Most successful malpractice suits use an expert witness (i.e., a physician in the same specialty) to testify that the defendant failed to provide care that meets a minimal standard of the profession.

        (2) In cases of outrageous physician conduct, an expert may not be needed. Such cases are known as *res ipsa loquitur,* which is translated as "the thing speaks for itself." Physical assault of a patient by a psychiatrist is an example of such a case. In this situation, the burden of proof shifts to the psychiatrist in proving that he or she was not negligent. Most malpractice insurers do not cover damages resulting from these actions.

    c. **Damages.** Physicians cannot be held liable for inadequate patient care, even if the care was grossly negligent, unless the patient has suffered damages. An expert witness is frequently used to establish the extent of damages a patient has suffered. In recent years, juries have had an increasing tendency to award large amounts of money for pain and suffering, leading to large increases in malpractice premiums.

    d. **Direct causation.** When damages have occurred, the plaintiff must prove direct causation; that is, if not for the actions of the physician, the damages the patient suffered would not have occurred. This is the most complicated element of a malpractice claim and often requires proof of proximate cause. The foreseeability of the harm done to the patient becomes a central issue in direct causation. For example, failure to hospitalize a suicidal patient with a history of serious suicide attempts and a current suicidal plan might not represent direct causation if the patient commits suicide 2 years after leaving the care of the psychiatrist; however, it might be direct causation if the patient committed suicide within days of seeing the psychiatrist.

2. **Malpractice prevention**

    a. In almost all malpractice suits, great attention is paid to the medical record. For this reason, good prevention against a successful malpractice action requires the maintenance of a thorough medical record that clearly documents the psychiatrist's reasoning behind treatment decisions.

        (1) Progress notes should be legibly written, dated, and signed.

        (2) A suicide assessment should accompany any change in an inpatient's status, including addition and removal of suicide precautions or changes in observation levels.

        (3) The purpose of medications and their target symptoms should be documented.

    b. Progress notes should never be used to criticize the treatment of other clinicians, and nursing notes should be reviewed regularly by physicians. Psychiatrists who supervise other mental health professionals may be liable for their negligence as well under a legal concept known as *respondeat superior.*

    c. The best prevention against malpractice claims is the maintenance of a healthy therapeutic alliance with patients. Patients may initiate a lawsuit based on a perceived attitude by a psychiatrist rather than a specific action of the psychiatrist. Careful attention should be given to patients who express dissatisfaction regarding their treatment. Patients' complaints should be discussed thoroughly with the patient in a noncondescending manner. A sincerely expressed apology after a clinical mistake may go a long way in averting a lawsuit.

BIBLIOGRAPHY

Dusky v. U.S., 362 U.S. 402 (1960).

Grisso T, Applebaum PS: *Assessing Competence to Consent to Treatment.* New York, Oxford University Press, 1998.

Gutheil TG, Applebaum PS: *Clinical Handbook of Psychiatry and the Law,* 3rd ed. Philadelphia, Lippincott Williams & Wilkins, 2000.

Gutheil TG: *The Psychiatrist in Court.* Washington, DC, American Psychiatric Press inc., 1998.

Lake v. Cameron, 364 F.2d 657 (1966).

Rosner R (ed): *Principles and Practice of Forensic Psychiatry,* 2nd ed. London, Arnold, 2003.

Rosner R, Schwartz HI: *Geriatric Psychiatry and the Law.* New York, Plenum Press, 1987.

Sell V. U.S., 539 U.S. 166 (2003).

Simon RI, Gold LH: *Textbook of Forensic Psychiatry.* Washington, DC, American Psychiatric Publishing inc., 2004.

Tarasoff v. Regents, 17 Cal. 3d 425 (1976).

United States Department of Health and Human Services. HIPAA Administrative Simplification Statute and Rules. Available at:http://www.hhs.gov/ocr/privacy/hipaa/adminstrative. Accessed December 22, 2010.

Zinermon v. Burch, 494 U.S. 113 (1990).

Study Questions

Directions: *Each of the numbered items or incomplete statements in this section is followed by answers or by completions of the statement. Select the ONE lettered answer or completion that is BEST in each case.*

1. A 42-year-old woman has been treated for major depression with psychotic symptoms with medication and weekly individual psychotherapy for 1 year after a serious suicide attempt. Because of low energy, poor ability to concentrate, and psychomotor retardation, she has been unable to return to work. Her application for disability under her company's disability policy was denied, so she has hired an attorney and has filed a suit against the company. Her attorney contacts the treating psychiatrist, requesting an opinion about the degree of her impairment and whether she is disabled under the policy guidelines. Which of the following actions should the treating psychiatrist take?

- [A] Write a report to the attorney explaining the patient's impairments and degree of disability.
- [B] Send the patient's medical records to the attorney.
- [C] Call the patient and with her permission, the attorney, and suggest that they hire an independent psychiatrist to conduct a disability evaluation.
- [D] Call the attorney and ask for a copy of the disability policy.
- [E] Write a report to the attorney and company explaining only the patient's impairments.

2. Which of the following events is the most common cause of malpractice suits against psychiatrists?

- [A] Breach of confidentiality
- [B] Development of tardive dyskinesia
- [C] Incorrect diagnosis
- [D] Incorrect treatment
- [E] Patient suicide

3. A male psychiatrist enters a sexual relationship with a married, depressed woman whom he is treating. After the treatment relationship and the sexual relationship end, she sues the psychiatrist, alleging that her depressive symptoms have worsened because of guilty feelings about the sexual contact and breakup of her marriage. She also alleges difficulty in trusting her current physician. The judge rules that expert testimony is not needed to prove that the sexual contact violated a professional standard of care under which of the following legal concepts?

- [A] Direct causation
- [B] *Res ipsa loquitur*   "the thing speaks for itself"
- [C] *Respondeat superior*
- [D] Unintentional tort
- [E] Vicarious liability

4. Which of the following is an element in evaluation of competency to stand trial (CST)?

determination of criminal responsibility

- [A] The defendant has the ability to distinguish right from wrong.
- [B] The defendant has the ability to behave according to the requirements of the law.
- [C] The crime was a product of a mental illness.
- [D] The defendant can communicate effectively with a lawyer.
- [E] The defendant was delusional at the time of an alleged crime.

5. Which of the following psychiatric treatments requires that a psychiatrist obtain written informed consent from a patient?

- [A] Behavioral therapy
- [B] Group therapy
- [C] Supportive psychotherapy
- [D] Use of antidepressant medication — *does not cause tardive dyskinesia*
- [E] Use of a typical antipsychotic medication

6. A 36-year-old homeless man with a history of schizoaffective disorder is brought to the hospital. He is hallucinating, and his thinking is grossly disorganized. His hygiene is poor, and he appears malnourished. He does not behave violently in the emergency department, he denies suicidal or homicidal thoughts, and he refuses admission. When asked about his family, he replies they have been replaced by look-alike "doubles"; he reports that "the CIA is involved." An examining psychiatrist finds that the patient is grossly psychotic but not imminently dangerous. Which of the following statements about the patient is correct?

- A His condition meets commitment criteria under a police powers model. *— immediately dangerous*
- B His condition meets commitment criteria under a *parens patriae* model.
- C His condition meets commitment criteria under the *Dusky* standard. *— competency to stand trial*
- D His condition does not meet commitment criteria for involuntary hospitalization under any model.
- E He can be involuntarily hospitalized only if he threatens suicide or homicide.

7. An acutely psychotic woman with schizophrenia is voluntarily admitted to the hospital. After a history and physical examination are completed, the psychiatrist orders antipsychotic medication, which the patient promptly refuses. Which of the following steps should the psychiatrist take next?

- A Contact a family member to consent to medication.
- B Give the medication over the patient's objections because she is psychotic.
- C Consider the patient competent and convene an administrative panel to determine the need for involuntary medication.
- D Contact a judge to order involuntary medication.
- E Determine if the patient is competent to consent or refuse medication.

8. A 50-year-old nurse witnesses her coworker and friend being shot and seriously wounded by an agitated patient in the emergency department. She subsequently develops posttraumatic stress disorder (PTSD) and is unable to return to work for 1 month. She is in need of financial assistance. What type of claim should she file?

- A Workers' compensation: mental–mental type
- B Workers' compensation: mental–physical type
- C Workers' compensation: physical–mental type
- D Social Security Disability Income (SSDI)
- E Social Security Income (SSI)

9. Which of the following series are the elements of an unintentional tort in a malpractice case?

- A Duty, dereliction of duty, documentation failure, and damages
- B Duty, dereliction of duty, damages, and direct causation
- C Dereliction of duty, damages, direct causation, and documentation failure
- D Duty, damages, direct causation, and documentation failure
- E Purposeful action to harm the patient, damages, and direct causation

10. Which of the following is a recognized exception to the clinician's confidentiality obligation and does not require patient consent to release information?

- A Providing information to a patient's employer
- B Providing information to a patient's attorney
- C Providing information to a deceased patient's spouse
- D Providing information to a child protective services agency
- E Providing information to an insurance company

11. In *Tarasoff v. Regents of the University of California,* the California Supreme Court ruled that which of the following statements applies to psychiatrists?

- A They cannot be held liable for the malpractice actions of their employees.
- B They have a duty to warn known, intended victims of their patients.
- C They have a duty to protect known, intended victims of their patients.
- D They cannot be held liable for treatment rendered in an emergency.
- E They have no duty to third parties.

12. An 82-year-old woman is referred for a testamentary capacity evaluation by her lawyer. She is able to quantify her assets of $500,000 and identify her two surviving children as natural heirs. She has decided to leave her assets to a local charity to begin an educational trust fund for abused and neglected children. She is leaving some family heirlooms to her two children and has divided these items equally. When asked about her decision, she states that each of her children inherited $1,000,000 at the death of another family member (this has been confirmed by her attorney), and she would like to leave her assets to someone who really needs them. Although her psychiatric examination reveals mild memory impairment, there is no evidence that this has caused problems in her daily functioning. Which of the following statements about this woman is correct?

- A She has been unduly influenced.
- B She lacks testamentary capacity because she is neglecting her children in the division of her assets.
- C She lacks testamentary capacity because of memory impairment.
- D She is in need of a guardian.
- E She has testamentary capacity.

13. A legally appointed guardian is also known as which of the following?

- A A committee of the person
- B A conservator – assets
- C A curator
- D A petitioner
- E A testator

14. A conservator would be appointed to make which one of the following decisions?

- A Whether to sell shares of a declining stock owned by the person in need of a conservator
- B Whether to consent to a medical procedure
- C Whether to allow another family member to live with the person in need of a conservator
- D Whether to have the patient enter a nursing home
- E The specifics of the will of the person in need of a conservator

15. A psychiatrist serving as a fact witness might not be allowed to testify about which one of the following things?

- A The dates of psychiatric treatment of a patient
- B The criminal responsibility of a patient charged with a crime
- C The demeanor of a patient during a therapy session
- D The observed behavior of family members toward a patient
- E Comments the psychiatrist told another physician named in a malpractice suit

Answers and Explanations

1. The answer is C [*I A*]. It would be appropriate for the psychiatrist to send treatment records to the attorney or company but only after the patient has signed a release. The treating psychiatrist should avoid providing opinions about disability because a negative outcome for the patient (i.e., denial of disability in the litigation) could jeopardize the physician–patient relationship if the patient holds the psychiatrist responsible for the denial of disability. Such dual agency situations should be avoided.

2. The answer is D [*IV D*]. Improper treatment is the most common reason for lawsuits against psychiatrists, followed by suicide, misdiagnosis, and improper supervision of other mental health providers.

3. The answer is B [*IV D 1 b (2)*]. Expert testimony is not needed to establish dereliction of duty in a case of egregious misconduct by the psychiatrist, who, in this case, has a sexual relationship with a patient. The concept of *res ipsa loquitur* means that "the thing speaks for itself."

4. The answer is D [*III A, Table 14–3*]. The ability to communicate with legal counsel is one of the most important trial-related elements in an evaluation of competency to stand trial (CST). Distractors A, B, and C are standards used in determinations of criminal responsibility, depending in which state the crime occurred. The presence of delusions does not automatically impair CST unless it has a negative effect on a specific trial ability.

5. The answer is E [*II B*]. Patients should be provided information about all proposed treatments and should be afforded an opportunity to ask questions. Because neuroleptic medications carry the added risk of tardive dyskinesia, a potentially irreversible side effect, it is important to document the consent process in a written record. Traditional antidepressant indicators do not require written informed consent because they do not cause tardive dyskinesia.

6. The answer is B [*II A 2*]. The man could be involuntarily hospitalized in jurisdictions in which a *parens patriae* commitment model applies. This model allows involuntary hospitalization for patients whose mental illness is gravely disabling but who are not immediately dangerous to themselves or others, as long as hospitalization represents the least restrictive alternative. A police powers model would require that the patient is imminently dangerous to himself or others. The *Dusky* standard refers to competency to stand trial (CST), not involuntary hospitalization.

7. The answer is E [*II B 2*]. Before a substitute decision maker (family member or judge) is contacted, the patient should be assessed to determine if the patient is competent to give consent. A substitute decision maker should be used only if the patient is incompetent to make treatment decisions. Unless an emergent situation (assaultive or self-injurious patient) arises, medication cannot be given over the objections of a competent patient without administrative review (usually two or more psychiatrists). Disguising medication is unethical.

8. The answer is A [*IV C 1 c*]. This type of scenario would be a mental–mental claim under workers' compensation, in which a stressful work event led to psychiatric impairment. This patient would not be eligible for Social Security Disability Income (SSDI) or Social Security Income (SSI) until she has completed a workers' compensation claim and has been disabled for 1 year.

9. The answer is B [*IV D 1 a–d*]. The "four Ds" of a malpractice action are duty, dereliction of duty, damages, and direct causation. Although documentation is important in preventing malpractice claims, it is not a specific element of an unintentional tort.

10. The answer is D [*II C 1 a (3)*]. The exceptions to confidentiality are numerous. Most states have mandatory child abuse reporting laws. In addition, information can be released in emergent situations if physicians are acting in patients' best interest. Information can be released to physicians at a hospital that is accepting a transfer patient and to other professionals actively involved in the patient's treatment.

However, other releases require patient consent. Clinicians' obligation to maintain confidentiality continues even after patients are deceased.

11. The answer is C [*II D*]. *Tarasoff v. Regents of the University of California* states that psychiatrists have a duty to protect intended victims. This duty to protect might include warning potential victims, notifying the police, or hospitalizing a particular patient. Although some states have adopted the *Tarasoff* ruling, other states have specifically rejected it. Psychiatrists should be familiar with case law in their jurisdictions.

12. The answer is E [*IV B 1*]. This woman has testamentary capacity because she is aware of her natural heirs, the extent of her bounty (assets), and the nature and purpose of a will. There is neither evidence that this woman has been subject to undue influence nor evidence of a delusion. Memory impairment does not, by itself, preclude testamentary capacity. There is no requirement that patients leave their assets to their natural heirs; the patient is able to give a rational motive for her decision.

13. The answer is A [*IV A 1*]. In some jurisdictions, a guardian is called a "committee of the person," which is a reflection of a guardian's multiple decision-making capacities. A conservator does not make multiple decisions but merely controls a person's assets. A petitioner may file for the person to be declared incompetent and in need of a guardian, but the person may or may not be appointed by the court as the legal guardian.

14. The answer is A [*IV A 2*]. A conservator controls a person's financial affairs, including the management of investments. A conservator does not have the same global decision-making authority entrusted to a legal guardian. Decisions about living situations, including entering a nursing home and consenting to medical procedures, can be made by a guardian but not by a conservator.

15. The answer is B [*I B 1*]. In general, a fact witness may testify to person, place, dates, and events. A fact witness, even if the witness is a psychiatrist, may not render opinions regarding a legal issue unless specifically qualified by the court to do so. Testimony about criminal responsibility would require an expert witness, not a fact witness.

chapter 15

Impulse Control Disorders

NIOAKA N. CAMPBELL

Impulse control disorders are varying illnesses characterized by patients' failing to resist an impulse to perform an act that is harmful to themselves or others. Before the event the patient may experience tension or arousal. The *Diagnostic and Statistical Manual of Mental Disorders,* 4th edition, text revision (*DSM-IV-TR*) (1), lists several disorders in this category as **impulse control disorders not elsewhere classified.**

I INTERMITTENT EXPLOSIVE DISORDER

A Diagnostic criteria (1, 2)

1. **Several, discrete episodes of loss of behavioral control characterized by aggression toward persons or property** are the hallmark of this disorder. Commonly, the aggression assumes the form of a physical assault or the destruction of property.

2. **Precipitating events** or psychosocial stressors may be variable or absent and **are disproportionately insignificant** compared with the extent of the aggressive behavior.

3. **The aggressive episodes are not better accounted for** by other disorders/diagnostic categories and are not due to the direct effects of a substance or a general medical condition.

B Epidemiology The disorder is thought to be rare, but may be underreported. Intermittent explosive disorders are more common in men than in women, with some studies indicating a prevalence of 80%. Whereas men with these disorders are reportedly more likely seen in correctional facilities, women are more likely seen in mental health facilities. The mean age of onset is 18 years of age. Family histories reveal high rates of comorbid mood, anxiety, personality, eating, and substance use disorders (2).

C Etiology (2, 3)

1. **Psychodynamic etiologies** may include the outbursts as a mechanism of defense against possible **narcissistic** injury. Situations that directly or indirectly represent earlier deprivation or trauma may evoke the destructive hostility.

2. **Neurobiologic etiologies** are unclear, but some studies indicate a dysregulation in serotonin neurotransmission. In some patients, low levels of 5-hydroxyindoleacetic acid (5-HIAA) in the cerebrospinal fluid (CSF) were identified. There has also been an inferred correlation between elevated levels of testosterone in the CSF and aggression. Genetic studies have shown higher rates of explosive behavior in first-degree relatives.

3. The **differential diagnosis** must rule out all other psychological and neurobiologic etiologies that may cause aggression. The disorder may be differentiated from or comorbid with personality disorders (especially antisocial and borderline), psychotic disorders (schizophrenia), mood disorders (manic episodes), and disruptive behavior disorders (conduct and attention deficit hyperactivity disorder).

D Treatment is best aimed at a supportive alliance with combined treatment modalities.

1. **Combination treatment** of medication management and psychotherapy has the best, yet limited, success. Incarceration, institutionalization, seclusion, and restraint are measures that may control but not alter behaviors.

2. **Behavior modification** techniques have met with only modest success, as have conventional psychotherapies.

3. Various **medications** have also been used with some symptomatic benefit. Mood stabilizers (e.g., lithium), anticonvulsants (e.g., phenytoin, carbamazepine, valproic acid), β-blockers (e.g., propranolol), sedative-hypnotics, and selective serotonin reuptake inhibitors (SSRIs; e.g., fluoxetine, sertraline, paroxetine) have shown favorable responses in appropriately selected cases (2).

II KLEPTOMANIA

(A) **Diagnostic criteria** (1, 2)

1. Kleptomania is characterized by an **inability to resist multiple episodes of impulsive stealing in the presence of pertinent negatives.** Specifically, the stealing is not:
   a. For monetary value or to satisfy a personal need
   b. An expression of anger, retribution, or retaliation
   c. Symptomatic of an underlying psychotic disorder (e.g., in response to a hallucination or delusion)
   d. Accounted for by a conduct disorder, personality disorder, or mania

2. Individuals experience a **mounting sense of tension or anxiety before the stealing episode.**

3. **Pleasure,** then, is derived from easing this internal tension or anxiety after gratifying the irresistible impulse to steal, not from the object(s) stolen. This contrasts sharply with shoplifting, robbery, burglary, and other stealing behaviors in which the secondary gain derives from the object(s) stolen. In fact, it is common for the objects stolen in kleptomania to be hidden, stored, discarded, returned, or given away.

(B) **Epidemiology and etiology (2, 4)**   Kleptomania is believed to be rare but may be underreported. It is more common in females than in males, with an approximate ratio of 3:1. Many reported cases must be carefully evaluated in light of the secondary gain afforded by conscious attempts to avoid criminal prosecution (malingering). Onset is usually in the late teens to midtwenties. Because the disorder is rare, little is known of its epidemiology or its etiology. There is a high comorbidity with affective disorders and anxiety disorders in addition to other impulse control disorders.

1. **Organic etiologies** related to behavioral disinhibition remain poorly understood. Differences in serotonin metabolism have been proposed. Genetic studies have shown an increased association with first-degree relatives and obsessive-compulsive disorder (OCD) and affective disorders.

2. **Psychological etiologies** have been suggested, largely by psychoanalytic theorists who tend to view the behavior as an attempt to restore wishes, drives, and pleasures that were lost or at least frustrated during infancy and childhood. The symptoms tend to appear or worsen in times of increased stress. From a behavioral and cognitive standpoint, the behavior is self-reinforcing because of its habitual nature.

3. **Differential diagnoses** must rule out theft that may occur during other disorders such as psychotic illnesses or mania. Antisocial personality disorders, malingering, substance use disorders, and dementia may also include the characteristic of theft. Shoplifting is a common crime not attributable to a psychiatric disorder.

(C) **Treatment (2, 4)**   The literature is largely devoid of systematically controlled treatment studies and instead includes mostly single-case, anecdotal reports of either psychoanalytic or behavioral therapeutic modalities. Most patients avoid help until they are forced into treatment for legal reasons. SSRIs such as fluoxetine have shown effectiveness in some of these cases.

III PYROMANIA

(A) **Diagnostic criteria** (1, 2)

1. Pyromania is characterized by **multiple episodes of willful and intentional fire setting in the presence of pertinent negatives.** Specifically, the fire setting is not:

    a. For financial gain (e.g., insurance reimbursement)
    b. An act of sociopolitical insurrection
    c. One of a series of related criminal activities
    d. An act of vandalism or an expression of retaliation or revenge
    e. A response to a delusion or hallucination or impaired judgment
    f. Accounted for by an underlying conduct disorder, mania, or antisocial personality disorder

  2. Individuals experience a **mounting sense of tension or anxiety before the fire-setting episode,** which may sometimes be in the form of a building sexual tension and excitement (**pyrolagnia**).

  3. **Relief** of tension and anxiety or sexual pleasure is derived when the fire-setting impulse is gratified as well as during the aftermath of the fire setting.

B **Epidemiology** Pyromania is a rare disorder that accounts for only a fraction of all cases of fire setting. The disorder appears to be more common in males than in females, with a ratio of 8:1. Childhood onset is common, with more than 40% of those arrested for arson being under the age of 18. Individuals with pyromania appear to lack empathy of the physical destructiveness of their actions and consequences. Afflicted individuals maintain an **obsessional preoccupation with fire** in much the same way individuals with eating disorders maintain obsessional preoccupations with food. There is a high comorbidity with substance use disorders, affective disorders, personality disorders, and other impulse control disorders (2).

C **Etiology** Specific etiology tends to be obscured by the rarity of the disorder.

  1. An underlying **organic factor** is suggested by long-standing observations of high rates of fire setting in organically impaired populations. Serotonergic and adrenergic involvement has also been postulated as biologic factors.

  2. **Psychological theorists** have focused on the intrapsychic representation and meaning of fire. Such theories have emphasized issues related to sexuality, power, rage, and aggression as psychodynamic determinants, which may underlie this disorder.

  3. **Differential diagnoses** must rule out fire setting that may occur during other disorders such as psychotic illnesses, dementias, substance intoxication, or mania (2).

D **Treatment** The nature of the disorder is such that "treatment" most often occurs in penal institutions. No systematically controlled studies have been applied in this population. Fire setting in children is a serious issue. Treatment considerations would include requiring supervision and family therapy. There is no clearly defined role for pharmacotherapy in this disorder unless an underlying organic state is identified (2).

IV   PATHOLOGIC GAMBLING

A **Diagnostic criteria** (1, 2)

  1. Pathologic gambling is characterized by **chronic, progressive,** and **maladaptive gambling behavior,** as evidenced by five of the following:
    a. An obsessional, cognitive preoccupation with gambling
    b. Using increasing amounts of money over time to achieve excitement
    c. Repeated efforts to control, cut back, or stop gambling
    d. Irritability when attempting to stop gambling
    e. Gambling as a way of escaping problems or of improving mood
    f. After monetary loss, the patient returning the next day to "get even"
    g. Lying to family or others to conceal behavior
    h. Committing illegal acts to finance the gambling
    i. Impaired personal, social, educational, and occupational functioning as a consequence of the gambling
    j. Relying on others to provide money to relieve debt from gambling

  2. It is not better accounted for by a manic episode.

B **Epidemiology** Pathologic gambling is a relatively common disorder. Approximately 3% to 5% of the adult population can be classified as problem gamblers, with 1% meeting criteria for this disorder.

It is more common in men than in women; however, new modes of gambling have shown escalation in the poor, elderly, retirees, and women. The prevalence is more common in areas where gambling is legal (2, 5, 6).

C Etiology (2, 5, 6)

1. **Psychoanalytic theories** attempt to connect the behavior with various disturbances in psychosexual development (from the oral stage through latency) as well as with aggressive and libidinal drives. **Predisposing factors** may include extremes in parental discipline styles (either overly indulgent or overly rigid) and childhood exposure to parental gambling, parental substance abuse, or parental sociopathy.

2. **Behavioral theories** attempt to explain the behavior largely according to learning theory (i.e., that most pathologic gamblers are exposed to the behavior and ultimately "learn" through patterns of reinforcement).

3. **Biologic etiologies.** It has also been suggested that the behavior may be propagated through the activation of endogenous opioid systems or may be associated with serotonergic and noradrenergic receptor systems. Some studies show a possible dysregulation in the ventromedial prefrontal cortex–regulating process for decision making.

4. **Comorbidity.** Associations between pathologic gambling and both mood disorders and substance use disorders have been identified. Anxiety disorder, personality disorder, and attention deficit hyperactivity disorder associations have been described.

5. **Differential diagnosis** should include distinguishing this illness from social gambling that is seen in the majority of the population.

D **Treatment approaches** derive from the theoretic framework applied to explain the etiology. Both individual and group modalities have been applied (2, 5, 6).

1. The earliest **individual modalities** tended to be conventional psychodynamic approaches. Recently, **cognitive behavioral techniques,** including both aversive and desensitizing models, have been studied.

2. **Group modalities** have also played a more prominent role, particularly self-help groups such as Gamblers Anonymous, which have been structured consistently with a 12-step addictions model.

3. **Pharmacotherapy** efficacy has not yet been demonstrated in a significant role unless an underlying organic state has been identified. Early case reports have shown some improvement with antidepressants and mood stabilizers.

V TRICHOTILLOMANIA

A Diagnostic criteria (1, 2)

1. **Recurrent episodes of pulling out one's own hair in quantities sufficient to result in identifiable hair loss** are the hallmark of this disorder.

2. **Hair-pulling episodes are preceded by a sense of increasing internal tension and anxiety.**

3. When the impulse to pull has been gratified, the individual experiences a pleasurable sensation or at least relief from the internal perception of tension and anxiety. Of note is that hair pulling in this context does not typically induce pain.

4. It is not better accounted for by another mental illness or a general medical condition.

5. It causes clinically significant distress or impairment in social, occupational, or other important areas of functioning.

B Epidemiology (2)   The prevalence of the condition is unknown. The disorder usually begins in childhood and is believed to affect females more frequently than males, with a ratio as high as 9:1. Lifetime prevalence ranges from 0.6% to 3%. Trichotillomania must be distinguished from stroking, twirling, and fidgeting with hair, which may fall within a spectrum of normal behavior.

Scalp hair most commonly is involved; facial hair, eyebrows, eyelashes, truncal hair, limb hair, axillary hair, and pubic hair may also be involved. **Obsessional thoughts and other compulsive behaviors may be described.** In particular, specific rituals related to the disposition of the hair, including ingestion (**trichophagy**), may exist. Comorbidity with OCD and anxiety or depressive disorders is common, as well as eating disorders and varying personality disorders.

C Etiology **(2, 7)**   All etiologic theories are considered tentative and speculative at present.

1. One view holds that the behavior represents a form of **self-stimulation** in response to emotional deprivation. Significant disturbances in parent–child interactions are commonly described.

2. Other theorists emphasize the dimension of **self-mutilation** as a form of self-punishment in response to rejection, trauma, and loss.

3. Some features are consistent with a learned behavior, similar to the **habit disorders of childhood.** An association with OCD has been suggested.

4. Finally, it is possible that an underlying **organic substrate or substrates** may exist.

D Treatment   (2, 7)

1. **Psychodynamic and behavioral individual approaches have been described.** Psychodynamic approaches were more common historically, but recently behavioral interventions have been discussed more frequently. Desensitization, aversion, and habit reversal have all been described. Therapeutic efficacy of all individual modalities has been limited. Cognitive behavioral therapy has shown increasing promise.

2. **A variety of psychopharmacologic agents have been used.** Neuroleptics, anxiolytics, mood stabilizers, and antidepressants (clomipramine, fluoxetine) have met with only limited success. Some literature suggests that medications used to treat tic disorders may be of some benefit as well.

VI IMPULSE CONTROL DISORDER NOT OTHERWISE SPECIFIED

This is a diagnostic residual category within the *DSM-IV-TR* including disorders of impulse control that do not meet specific criteria for an impulse control disorder. Disorders in this category include compulsive buying, delicate self-cutting, repetitive self-mutilation, and compulsive sexual behavior (1, 2).

BIBLIOGRAPHY

1. American Psychiatric Association: *Diagnostic and Statistical Manual of Mental Disorders,* 4th ed., text revision. Washington, DC, American Psychiatric Association, 2000.
2. Greenberg HR: Impulse control disorders not elsewhere classified. In *Kaplan and Sadock's Comprehensive Textbook of Psychiatry,* 8th ed., vol. 1. Edited by Sadock BJ, Sadock VA. Philadelphia, Lippincott Williams & Wilkins, 2005, pp 2035–2054.
3. Felthouse AR, Bryant SG, Wingerter CB: The diagnosis of intermittent explosive disorder in violent men. *Bull Am Acad Psychiatry Law* 19:71, 1991.
4. Durst R, Katz G, Teitelbaum A, et al: Kleptomania: Diagnosis and treatment options. *CNS Drugs* 15: 185, 2001.
5. Petry NM, Stinson FS, Grant BF: Comorbidity of DSM-IV pathological gambling and other psychiatric disorders: Results from the National Epidemiologic Survey on Alcohol and Related Conditions. *J Clin Psychiatry* 66:564–574, 2005.
6. Potenza MN, Kosten TR, Rounsaville BJ: Pathological gambling. *JAMA* 286:141–144, 2001.
7. Christenson GA, Crow SJ: The characterization and treatment of trichotillomania. *J Clin Psychiatry* 57(Suppl):42, 1996.

Study Questions

Directions: *Each of the numbered items or incomplete statements in this section is followed by answers or by completions of the statement. Select the ONE lettered answer or completion that is BEST in each case.*

1. The motive for fire setting in pyromania is most strongly associated with which of the following?

- A Psychotic delusions
- B Secondary gain
- C Tension reduction
- D Terrorism
- E Vandalism

2. Which statement is most accurate with regard to the role of environmental precipitants in the aggressive outbursts in intermittent explosive disorder?

- A They are variably present and proportionate to the aggression expressed.
- B They are variably present and disproportionate to the aggression expressed.
- C They are invariably present and proportionate to the aggression expressed.
- D They are invariably present and disproportionate to the aggression expressed.
- E They are unrelated to the aggression expressed.

3. A 28-year-old woman steals a valuable pocket watch from a jewelry store. She is most likely to suffer from kleptomania if she:

- A Anonymously mails the watch back to the jewelry store
- B Gives the watch to her boyfriend for a birthday gift
- C Sells the watch to help pay her house payment that is in arrears
- D Sells the watch and deposits the money into savings
- E Displays the watch in a showcase along with other artifacts in her home

4. Which parental disorder would be most likely to contribute to the development of pathologic gambling in the parent's adolescent child?

- A Anxiety disorder
- B Attention deficit hyperactivity disorder
- C Bipolar disorder
- D Depressive disorder
- E Substance abuse

5. Which two impulse control disorders are more common in women than in men?

- A Trichotillomania and pyromania
- B Pyromania and intermittent explosive disorder
- C Intermittent explosive disorder and pathologic gambling
- D Pathologic gambling and kleptomania
- E Kleptomania and trichotillomania

QUESTIONS 6–9

For each disorder listed below, select the association most consistent with it.

- A Addiction
- B Factitious symptoms

C Irresistible urge
D Obsessive-compulsive symptoms
E Sexual excitation

6. Trichotillomania D

7. Pathologic gambling A

8. Pyromania E

9. Kleptomania C

Answers and Explanations

1. The answer is C [*III A 1–3*]. The motive for fire setting in individuals with pyromania is specifically not for secondary gain (e.g., to access insurance benefits), as an act of terrorism or political insurrection, or as an act of vandalism amid a constellation of delinquent behaviors. Neither is it in response to psychotic delusions or command auditory hallucinations. Rather, the motive for fire setting in individuals with pyromania is tension gratification and reduction, often of a sexual nature. Tension is relieved or sexual pleasure gratified only by indulging the impulse to set fires and its aftermath.

2. The answer is B [*I A, C*]. Multiple etiologies, including psychological and organic states, likely underpin this disorder. Environmental precipitants are only variably present, but when present, they are disproportionately minor compared with the extent of the aggressive behavioral outburst. Nonetheless, precipitants may not be identifiable with each explosive outburst. Regardless of the underlying etiology, exposure to violence and aggression likely contributes to the behavior. Elevated androgen levels have been implicated in some cases.

3. The answer is A [*II A 1–3*]. Kleptomania is believed to be an extremely rare disorder. It is qualitatively different from most forms of stealing in that secondary gain is not derived from the object stolen, but rather from gratifying the impulse to steal. Consequently, the objects stolen often are returned to their owner. Many "cases" may be false-positives secondary to malingering in an attempt to avoid criminal prosecution. There is no clearly defined treatment for the disorder; all treatments are relatively speculative at this point.

4. The answer is E [*IV C 1*]. Childhood exposure to parental gambling, substance abuse, and sociopathic or antisocial behavior have all been suggested as predisposing factors. Mood and anxiety disorders may occur along with pathologic gambling as comorbid conditions; they have not been linked vertically, however. The impulsivity of attention deficit hyperactivity disorder (ADHD) may contribute to susceptibility to this disorder; however, parental ADHD has not been shown to predispose children to the development of pathologic gambling.

5. The answer is E [*II B, V B*]. Most impulse control disorders occur more commonly in men than in women; however, kleptomania and trichotillomania appear to occur more commonly in women than in men.

6–9. The answers are 6-D [*V C 3*], **7-A** [*IV C 4*], **8-E** [*III A 2*], **and 9-C** [*II A 1–3*].

In addition to compulsive hair pulling, other obsessions or compulsions may be noted in trichotillomania. In addition, trichotillomania may be a symptom of an obsessive-compulsive disorder.

Pathologic gambling has much in common with the addictive disorders. Both involve continuation of the maladaptive behavior despite chronic, progressive, adverse consequences. Likewise, peer support groups that use a 12-step approach have been of benefit in both disorders.

Pyromania often is precipitated by sexual tension that builds before setting a fire and that is gratified sexually both by setting the fire and during the aftermath of the fire.

Kleptomania must be distinguished from other forms of stealing by the distinction that the stolen object does not bring secondary gain or gratification as it does in other forms of stealing. When stealing brings secondary gain by way of the value of the object stolen, the attempt to invoke an "irresistible urge" as in true kleptomania more likely represents malingering as a means of avoiding criminal prosecution.

Drug Appendix

Antidepressants*

	Starting Dose (mg)	Dose Range (mg)	Half-life (hours)
Tricyclic			
Amitriptyline (Elavil)	25 tid	50–300	15
Clomipramine (Anafranil)	25–100 qd	25–250	32
Desipramine (Norpramin)	25 tid	100–300	17
Doxepin (Sinequan)	25 tid	75–300	7
Imipramine (Tofranil)	25 tid	75–300	7.6
Nortriptyline (Aventyl, Pamelor)	25 tid	75–150	26
Protriptyline (Vivactil)	5 tid	15–60	78
Selective Serotonin Reuptake Inhibitors			
Citalopram (Celexa)	20	20–60	35
Escitalopram (Lexapro)	10	10–20	27–32
Fluoxetine (Prozac, Sarafem)	20	20–60	72
Fluvoxamine (Luvox)	50	50–300	15
Paroxetine (Paxil, Pexeva)	20	20–60	20
Sertraline (Zoloft)	50	50–200	26
Serotonin-norepinephrine Reuptake Inhibitors			
Desvenlafaxine (Pristiq)	50	50–400	10
Duloxetine (Cymbalta)	20 bid	40–60	12
Venlafaxine (Effexor)	100	300 (rarely to 375)	5
Serotonin Modulator			
Trazodone (Desyrel)	50	75–300	7
Norepinephrine-serotonin Modulator			
Mirtazapine (Remeron)	15	15–45	20
Dopamine-norepinephrine Reuptake Inhibitors			
Bupropion (Wellbutrin)	150	300	3–4
Monoamine Oxidase Inhibitors			
Irreversible			
Isocarboxazid (Marplan)	10 bid	20–60	Unknown
Phenelzine (Nardil)	10	30–60	2
Tranylcypromine (Parnate)	15	15–90	2

*Lower starting doses for elderly patients and individuals with anxiety disorders, especially panic disorders.
bid, twice a day; qd, every day; tid, three times a day.

Side Effects of Antidepressant Agents

Type of Agent	Sedation	Weight Gain	Sexual Dysfunction	Other
Tricyclic	Yes	Yes	Yes	Orthostasis, lethal overdose, anticholinergic
Selective serotonin reuptake inhibitors	No	No	Yes	Nausea, insomnia, headache
Serotonin-norepinephrine reuptake inhibitors	No	Rare	Rare	Nausea, insomnia, headache
Serotonin modulators	Yes	Rare	Rare	Trazodone may cause priapism
Norepinephrine-serotonin modulator	Yes	Yes	Rare	Anticholinergic, increased serum lipids
Dopamine-norepinephrine reuptake inhibitors	No	No	No	Seizures; same as Zyban
Monoamine oxidase inhibitors	Rare	Yes	Yes	Hypertension, many potentially lethal drug interactions, dietary restrictions

Mood Stabilizers

	Usual Daily Dose (mg)	Serum Plasma Level	Notes
Carbamazepine (Tegretol)	400–1,600	4–12 mg/ml	Liver function tests and CBC
Lamotrigine (Lamictal)	100–200	n/a	Liver function tests and CBC
Lithium	600–1,800	0.6–1.2 mEq/L	Renal and thyroid function tests and CBC
Topiramate (Topamax)	25–400	n/a	Liver function tests and CBC
Valproic acid (Depakote)	750–4,200	50–100 mg/ml	Liver function tests

CBC, complete blood cell count; n/a, not applicable.

Antipsychotic Medications

	Usual Oral Dose (mg/day)	Notes
Atypical		
Aripiprazole (Abilify)	10–30	Agitation, insomnia; IM and sol-tab available
Asenapine (Saphris)	10	
Clozapine (Clozaril)	300–600	Agranulocytosis risk
Iloperidone (Fanapt)	12–24	
Olanzapine (Zyprexa)	10–30	Sleepiness, weight gain; IM, depot, and sol-tab available
Paliperidone ER (Invega)	6–12	Depot available
Quetiapine (Seroquel)	200–800	Sleepiness, palpitations
Risperidone (Risperdal)	4–6	Cytochrome P_{450} effects; depot and sol-tab available
Ziprasidone (Geodon)	80–240	Sleepiness, agitation; IM available
Conventional		
Phenothiazines		
Chlorpromazine (Thorazine)	50–1,500	High side-effect profile
Piperidines		
Thioridazine (Mellaril)	50–800	Cardiac arrhythmia, retinopathy >800 mg
Piperazines		
Fluphenazine (Prolixin)	2–60	Depot available
Perphenazine (Trilafon)	16–64	
Trifluoperazine (Stelazine)	5–80	High side-effect profile
Thioxanthenes		
Thiothixene (Navane)	5–80	Monitor for pigmentary retinopathy; antemetic
Butyrophenones		
Haloperidol (Haldol)	2–60	Depot available
Dibenzoxapines		
Loxapine (Loxitane)	20–225	Similar to thiothixene: tardive dyskinesia
Molindone (Moban)	20–225	

IM, intramuscular.

Antiparkinsonian Medications

	Usual Dose (mg/day)
Amantadine (Symmetrel)	100–300
Benztropine (Cogentin)	1–8
Biperiden (Akineton)	2–6
Diphenhydramine (Benadryl)	25–200
Trihexyphenidyl (Artane)	2–10

Antianxiety Medications

	Starting Dose (mg)	Usual Dose (mg/day)	Approximate Dose Equivalent (mg)	Approximate Half-life
Benzodiazepines				
Alprazolam (Xanax)	0.25–1	1–4	0.5	12 hours
Chlordiazepoxide (Librium)	5–25	15–100	10	1–4 days
Clonazepam (Klonopin)	0.5–2	1–4	0.25	1–2 days
Clorazepate (Tranxene)	3.75–22.5	15–60	7.5	2–4 days
Diazepam (Valium)	2–10	4–40	5	2–4 days
Lorazepam (Ativan)	0.5–2	1–6	1	12 hours
Oxazepam (Serax)	10–30	30–120	15	12 hours
Miscellaneous				
Buspirone (BuSpar)	10–30	30–60	n/a	2–3 hours
Hydroxyzine (Atarax, Vistaril)	50–100	200–400	n/a	

Note: Selective serotonin reuptake inhibitors (SSRIs) and other antidepressant medications are indicated in the treatment of individuals with anxiety disorders:

Obsessive-compulsive disorder: Clomipramine, SSRIs.
Panic disorder: SSRIs, tricyclic antidepressants, alprazolam.
Generalized anxiety: Buspirone, SSRIs, benzodiazepines.
Stage fright: β-blockers.
Social phobia: SSRIs, monoamine oxidase inhibitors, buspirone.
n/a, not applicable.

Index

Note: Page number followed by t indicates table.

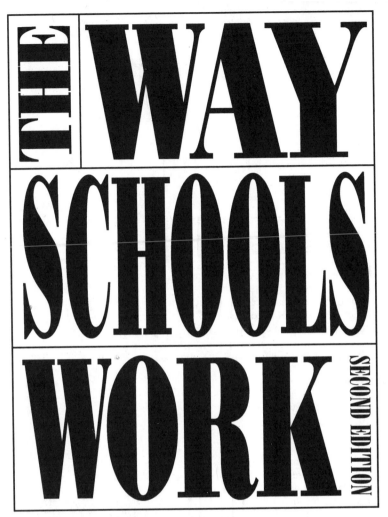

THE WAY SCHOOLS WORK

SECOND EDITION

A Sociological Analysis of Education

Kathleen Bennett deMarrais
University of Tennessee

Margaret D. LeCompte
University of Colorado, Boulder

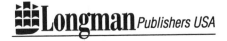

Longman *Publishers USA*

The Way Schools Work: A Sociological Analysis of Education, second edition

Longman, 10 Bank Street, White Plains, N.Y. 10606

Associated companies:
Longman Group Ltd., London
Longman Cheshire Pty., Melbourne
Longman Paul Pty., Auckland
Copp Clark Longman Ltd., Toronto

Acquisitions editor: Virginia L. Blanford
Production editor: Melanie M. McMahon
Cover design: Joseph DePinho, Pinho Graphic Design
Production supervisor: Richard C. Bretan

Library of Congress Cataloging-in-Publication Data

DeMarrais, Kathleen Bennett.
  The way schools work : a sociological analysis of education /
Kathleen Bennett deMarrais and Margaret D. LeCompte.—2nd ed.
      p. cm.
  Includes bibliographical references and index.
  ISBN 0-8013-1245-0
  1. Educational sociology—United States.   2. Education—Social
aspects—United States.   3. Education—Social aspects—United
States—History.   4. Educational sociology—History.   I. LeCompte,
Margaret Diane.   II. Title.
LC189.D36   1994
370.19'0973—dc20   94-21574
                                                      CIP

2 3 4 5 6 7 8 9 10-MA-98979695

We dedicate this book to four very special, talented women:
Rocklan McNeil
Elsita Leal
Amber Aguilera
Jennifer Walker

Contents

w/ Noguera on
Violence
+ Foucault
excerpt.
+ Klieband
Bureauc +
ed.

Five

v

Preface

We initially wrote this book in order to have a text that would provide our own students with a critical perspective on the sociology of schooling—particularly those students without a strong background in social theory. We wanted to explore different theoretical perspectives and challenge our students to think about the major sociocultural and political issues related to schooling. We also wanted our students to examine their own notions of schooling in light of these perspectives, particularly a critical, transformative perspective.

A special feature of this book is its strong historical bent both in the information presented and the way developments in theory have affected the way we look at and interpret the impact of schools. We have couched our discussion of contemporary schools within the context of their historical development because we believe the way schools are currently organized has been powerfully influenced by events and social policies of the past. Similarly, although our own interpretations and conclusions are informed by critical and feminist perspectives, they are, like the viewpoints of all social scientists, built upon the theoretical models and analyses of the past—especially functionalism and conflict theory. Because this text is an introduction to the way sociologists think about educational processes, we weave both classical and contemporary critical perspectives into each chapter. Each chapter usually begins with a descriptive, functional approach and concludes with a more recent critical analysis. It is easier to know where we currently are if we understand where we came from.

The chapters derive from subfields in sociology: social theory, the sociology of organizations, the sociology of work and professions, the sociology of knowledge, and the study of class, race, and gender.

Chapter 1 examines the theories that underlie how people conceptualize the purposes for which schools are organized, whose interests schools serve, and what should be taught. These theories are divided into three categories: (1) *transmission theories* of function and conflict, which argue that schools rather passively transmit the patterns of society unchanged from one generation to another; (2) *interpretivist theories,* which describe the workings of schooling through a microlevel analysis and build a bridge between transmission and transformation theories; and (3) *transformation theories,* which argue that through critique and human agency, people in schools can play a role in transforming society.

Chapter 2 examines schools as social organizations. First it presents a historical analysis of school organization especially as it has been shaped by concepts from business and industry. Then it examines both the internal organization and patterns of control within schools and districts, and the external matrix of local, state, and national agencies that impinge on their operation. It emphasizes both the apparent ambiguity of patterns of authority and the influence of political as opposed to pedagogical concerns.

Chapter 3 is a detailed discussion of a group often overlooked—the students. It examines the impact of societal change on the way children experience childhood and adolescence, the special ways children relate to and resist the influence of school, and the impact of peer groups and youth culture on schooling.

Chapter 4 examines teachers, administrators, counselors, and parents. It describes the greater control being given to administrators, at the expense of teachers, and it questions the extent to which teaching is really a profession. The chapter also examines gender bias in the work force and its impact on the power and prestige of teachers.

Chapter 5 is an analysis of the relationship between social class and education. It traces changes in thinking about the origins of social class hierarchy, as well as what has led to the acquisition of social power. It also examines the impact of social class on the structure of society as well as on the achievements of individuals, and it raises questions about the degree to which contemporary educational systems really are "fair," meritocratic, and egalitarian. This chapter sets the stage for similar analyses in regard to minority status and gender.

Chapter 6 examines the curriculum, what is taught both openly and covertly. It looks at the differences in power and prestige attributed to various kinds of knowledge, and it examines how curricular differentiation, or tracking and ability grouping, serves to sort children into niches roughly similar to those occupied by their parents.

Chapter 7 discusses the relationship between minority status and schooling. It examines the role of the federal government in providing equal opportunities for minority students. It also analyzes various sociological and anthropological explanations for the failure of minority students. This chapter concludes with a discussion of minority student responses in the form of assimilation, accommodation, and resistance.

Chapter 8 is an analysis of the relationship between gender and schooling, in both formal and informal curricula. In regard to the formal curriculum is a discussion of gender-identified subject matter, staffing of schools, and the portrayal of women. In regard to the informal curriculum is an examination of the hidden messages sent to females and males through class organization, instructional technology, and class interaction. Following a discussion of gender differences in academic performance and occupational outcomes, the chapter concludes with a discussion of feminism as related to schooling.

Chapter 9 presents an examination of how sociological analysis and critical insights might be used to develop alternatives to the current system of education. Here we examine the changing balance of power in schools and propose alternatives for school structures, pedagogical practices, and teacher education.

NEW TO THIS EDITION

This book is a major rewrite of the first edition. We have added many new discussions about current theories and debates in education, moved the key concepts section to an alphabetized glossary in the back of the book, and sprinkled activities throughout the text to involve students. Our goal was to write a book synthesizing the most current thinking in the field.

Throughout the book are inserted illustrative boxes containing stories from students, teachers, and administrators to help bring the sociological concepts to life. Some were contributed by students and teachers with whom we work, and some are from published sources. The stories represent the experiences of people positioned in a variety of social class, ethnic, and gendered locations to illustrate the complexity of the concepts we are exploring.

Chapter 1 has been completely reorganized and clarified in light of students' and colleagues' responses to the material. We have added a chart, "Social Theories at a Glance," to help crystalize the assumptions, key concepts, and major questions of each of these perspectives.

In Chapter 2 we include a discussion of reform and restructuring movements currently changing the shape and structure of schools.

In Chapter 7 we added a section explaining our use of labels for particular ethnic groups and we challenge European American students to explore their notions of ethnicity. We've provided a more elaborate discussion of race and ethnicity.

We significantly enlarged Chapter 8, adding sections on sexist language, sexual harassment, and sexual orientation. We included a discussion of psychological development based on recent work by Lyn Mikel Brown and Carol Gilligan. We also updated the vignettes at the beginning of the chapter so that Susan, whose story ended with her high school experiences, is now faced with differential treatment in her college and adult life. The chapter now concludes with a discussion of feminism and the major feminist theories: liberal, radical, socialist, poststructuralist, and black feminism or womanism.

Chapter 9 has been totally restructured around the theme of "changing the balance of power." It has examples of new transformative practices that are now evident in many progressive schools. We have added a discussion of the major transformative pedagogies and a chart that summarizes the focus of each perspective. In this discussion we examine democratic education, multicultural education, critical pedagogy, and feminist pedagogy—a discussion unique to this book. We have also added a discussion about current networks that are forming around transformation of school structures and practices.

Acknowledgements

We thank the many people who contributed to this book through their reviews at different stages in its development and through more informal discussions with us. We are extremely grateful to:

William Armaline, University of Toledo
Robert Barger, Eastern Illinois University
Phil Frances Carspecken, University of Houston
Rodney Clifton, University of Manitoba
Diane Cudahy, University of Tennessee, Knoxville
Donna Dehyle, University of Utah
Kathy Farber, Bowling Green University
Nancy Greenman, University of South Florida
Jim Harvey, University of South Australia
Lynn Hutchinson, Walsh University
Sally Oran, University of Tennessee, Knoxville
Joel Spring, State University of New York at New Paltz

This book is much better for their thoughtful comments and critical insights.

Our thanks to the Association for School, College & University Staffing, Inc. (ASCUS) for their permission to use salary and teacher demand tables from their 1993 Report: Teacher Supply and Demand in the United States. Our students are always interested in these data.

We thank the Honolulu County Committee on the Status of Women for permission to use their wonderfully helpful "Do's and Don'ts of Non-Sexist Language."

We thank Naomi Silverman, the editor of the first edition of this book, who began as our editor and became a close and valued friend.

We appreciate the work of Virginia Blanford, editor of the second edition of *The Ways Schools Work,* for her help and support throughout the process. Our thanks to Melanie McMahon, Chris Konnari, Ilene McGrath, and Louise Capuano at Longman who helped with the development of this edition.

We owe special thanks to our students as well as the collaborating teachers and administrators who contributed to the book through their stories and discussions. Their lively criticism has helped to make this second edition much clearer. In particular we thank Theresa Apodaca, Bonnie Cadotte, Caelin Creasey, Pilar Ferreira, Anna Gildersleeve, Lisa McCoy, Rocklan McNeil, Barbara Medina, Andrea O'Conor, Leanne Ross, Duren Thompson, Jennifer Walker, Robert Whittfield, and Tracy Wood.

Finally, we wish to thank Paul deMarrais and Sergiu Luca for their continuing and cherished support of our work.

chapter **1**

Theory and Its Influences on the Purposes of Schooling

INTRODUCTION

This book looks at schools and schooling from the perspective of the sociologist. Sociologists study the structure of society and the roles people play within it. Sociologists and psychologists think about schools and schooling differently in that psychologists tend to be interested in individuals while sociologists are interested in groups. Educational psychologists, then, are concerned with what goes on *inside* the minds of individual learners, while educational sociologists are interested in everything that happens *outside of* the minds of individual learners, including how learners interact with others and the characteristics of the settings in which they interact. Because most educational research has been done by psychologists, we believe that our sociological viewpoint will give a rather new perspective on schools.

Sociologists distinguish between *schooling* and *education*. The term **education** broadly refers to the process of learning over the span of one's entire life. Education begins at birth and continues in a wide variety of both formal and informal settings. Again, whereas psychologists study the psychological processes individuals undergo in learning and cognition, sociologists are more interested in the social or group aspects of learning.

Schooling is the learning that takes place in formal institutions whose specific function is the **socialization** of specific groups within society. Schooling is another name for socialization in schools, or the informal learning that groups of people, usually children, acquire about behavior in these schools. Sociologists who study schooling are interested in the characteristics of the people and institutions that make up educational systems, and particularly the dynamics of their interaction and operation.

As is the case with all social science disciplines, several different and competing theories exist within the sociology of education. While all sociologists share an interest in the same general phenomena, they use different theoretical lenses to interpret these phenomena. This chapter explores how sociologists with different theoretical perspectives explain the purposes of schooling. Keep in mind that these theories have evolved over time, growing from or in reaction to previous theories. They may share many concepts and methods. Some theories attempt to explain the way society works while others take these explanations, critique the current social order, and offer ways of working to transform the society. The principal questions addressed are the following:

What is the theory?

What are the purposes of schooling?

How does the theory relate to these purposes?

As you read this chapter, ask yourself which personal theories you use to explain the purposes of schooling.

The chapter begins with discussions of several key concepts, including the term *theory*, which will be used throughout the book. We then examine the various **theoretical frameworks** that have informed the sociology of education, showing how these frameworks alter interpretations of the purposes and impact of schooling. One of the primary theoretical issues addressed in the sociology of education is the process by which a society's ways of life, values, beliefs, and norms or standards for appropriate behavior are passed on from one generation to the next. Sociologists look at this process in two ways: as *social transmission* or as *social transformation*. In our discussion of transmission theories we explain **functionalism, structural functionalism,** and **conflict theory.**

Theories of transmission are concerned with description of the structural aspects of society (Parsons 1951, 1959; Weber 1947) and with how existing social structures facilitate the general functioning of society. For example, a sociologist might examine the social system within a school to understand how the values and behaviors of the society are transmitted and would find that American values such as neatness, efficient use of time, and obeying authority are emphasized in the daily routines of the classroom (LeCompte 1978b).

We then introduce **interpretive theories,** including *phenomenology, symbolic interactionism,* and *ethnomethodology*. These theories form a bridge to *theories of transformation*, which we discuss next. In the discussion of transformation theories we focus on **critical theories** and *feminist, postmodern,* and *poststructural* approaches. Transformation theories are less rigid than social transmission theories. Their central concern is the *transformation,* rather than reproduction, of the society (Burtonwood 1986). They also differ in how they view the role of individuals. While social transmission theories treat individuals as passive, transformation theories view individuals as having the capacity to become "empowered" (Ellsworth 1989). Rather than accepting the world as it is, they become agents for social action to improve their situation.

While many of these perspectives overlap, and many borrow heavily from each other, the primary difference between transmission and transformation theories lies in whether they concern *reproduction* or *production* of culture (Weiler 1988). Reproduction, or transmission, is concerned with how social structures are copied from generation to generation, regardless of external forces such as the activities or desires of groups or individuals. By contrast, theories of production, or transformation, give individuals' activities and desires an important role in the creation of culture. Theories of production describe the ways in which

> both individuals and classes assert their own experience and contest or resist the ideological and material forces imposed upon them in a variety of settings. Their analyses focus on the ways in which both teachers and students in schools produce meaning and culture through their own resistance and their own individual and collective consciousness. (Weiler 1988, p. 11)

WHAT IS THEORY?

In very simplistic terms, a **theory** is a world view, a way we organize and explain the world we live in. Theories are not necessarily impractical or complex. In fact, all human beings use theoretical thought every day.

> The informal explanations we use to guide our daily life as well as hunches we have about why things work as they do are *tacit* or lay theories. They derive from our own cultural background, academic training, life experiences, and individual personality traits. (LeCompte and Preissle 1993, p. 121)

We use theories about the weather to decide if we should take an umbrella to work, and "folk theories of success" (Ogbu 1987) to guide our career paths. Humans also have created theories to explain the operation of the natural universe, such as theories stating the relationship between energy and mass, or between moisture and the growth rates of plants. Similarly, we have developed theories to explain how the social world works, such as why job satisfaction and job performance are related and why people seem to develop conservative social attitudes as they grow older. We even develop theories about education, such as why higher occupational status usually is associated with higher levels of educational attainment, or why some ethnic minorities do poorly in school.

Social scientists generally use theoretical models or perspectives to organize their thought and inquiry. These models are "loosely interrelated sets of assumptions, concepts, and propositions that constitute a view of the world" (Goetz and LeCompte 1984, p. 37) or some significant part of it. Garbarino (1983) describes theory as a "statement of the principles presumably regulating observed processes, or one that accounts for causes or relationships between phenomena" (p. 5).

As we shall see, theory in both the natural and social sciences evolves because it is affected by historical and cultural developments. In general, theories change because we need more workable or accurate explanations for what we believe to be true. For example, science was guided for centuries by religious and philosophical theories that the sun revolved around the earth, and so all scientific inquiry was organized to support that belief. In time, however, as data amassed demonstrating that the earth revolved around the sun, support grew for a heliocentric view of our planetary system.

Social and cultural beliefs have similarly influenced theories about education. Throughout history people have observed that individuals who have higher levels of education tend to have higher social status, and a number of theories have been developed to explain this observation. At first they believed simply that the wealthy were smarter and capable of more education. Then, belief in the redemptory effect of education led people to believe that education would improve the human condition and help eliminate poverty, disease, and antisocial or immoral behavior. Schools, then, could make people better, if not actually wealthier. This belief justified the institution of schools for the poor, compensatory education programs, and a variety of social service practices. Later developments in social theory have changed our beliefs about the role and purpose of education. Now theorists believe that educational experiences, rather than leading to elimination of poverty and social differences, actually reinforce differences.

We all have acquired rather unscientific "pet theories" that we use to explain what goes on in the social world, including the schools. The poor performance of girls in mathematics is explained by a pet theory stating that math simply is more difficult for girls than for boys. A rationale for avoiding a Master's degree was the theory that school districts would not hire beginning teachers with a Master's degree because their salaries would be higher. Students who wanted to student teach only in a white, upper-middle-class district theorized that districts wouldn't hire teachers who had student-taught on an American Indian reservation or in the inner city.

Obviously some theories are more valid than others, but all of them help us to organize and understand our world. Many govern what we think about our educational experiences. At this point you might stop to consider some theories of your own. What theories do you use to answer the following questions?

Why are some students or some teachers more successful in school than others?

Why is teaching generally so little respected as a profession?

Why is the public so dissatisfied with the public schools today?

What leads some groups of students to be more successful in school than others?

We now begin a discussion of the three general categories of sociological theories that organize how sociologists think about schooling: social transmission theories, interpretive theories, and theories of transformation.

SOCIAL TRANSMISSION THEORIES

Functionalism

Functionalism, which has been the prevailing theoretical framework in the social sciences throughout the twentieth century, argues that society operates as does the human body: Like living organisms, all societies possess basic functions which they must carry out to survive.

For example, the human body is composed of many interdependent organs, each of which carries out a vital function. Every organ must be healthy and all must work together to maintain the health of the entire body. If any organ malfunctions, the entire body may die.

Similarly, societies, in order to survive, must carry out vital functions: reproduce themselves, recruit or produce new members, distribute goods and services, and allocate power. One of the most important functions is that of transmission. In the traditional functionalist view of social transmission, each elder generation passes on to each succeeding generation the rules, customs, and appropriate behaviors for operating in the society. They do so through the principal socializing institutions or transmitters of the culture, such as families, churches, and schools. By participating in these institutions, individuals accept their roles within the *social structure* of society. Functionalists identify not only the various functions within a society, but also the connections between the components of a societal system and the relations between different systems. For example, functionalists assert that if one socializing institution is not fulfilling its function, another will take over its role to maintain the equilibrium of the society. In today's society, functionalists would argue that as more families have both parents working, schools have taken over many of the functions formerly performed by the family.

Functional analysis has become an inescapable part of the training and worldview of all social scientists. Although they may not accept all the tenets of traditional functional social theory, all social scientists use its categories as basic analytic tools to describe social systems. However, functionalism has been criticized, both because it rejects conflict and change as viable and often valuable social processes, and because its proponents have asserted that it is the only approach that produces "objective," unbiased, or truly "scientific" findings. Functionalists may do this because their training has never presented alternative perspectives, and also because they are so steeped in the functional analysis approach that it appears to be the truth rather than merely one way of looking at the world. However, other theories are available, some of them variations of functionalism, and these may provide more adequate and/or critical explanations.

Structural Functionalism

An important variant of functionalism is **structural functionalism.** Based upon the assumption that human systems have an underlying but unobservable coherence based upon formal rules, signs, and arrangements, structuralists seek to understand human phenomena, such as systems of meaning, language, and culture, by identifying these underlying structures. Structuralists make inferences about underlying social structure based upon patterns observed in human life.

Central to structural functionalism is the conviction that social systems are like living bodies. Structures, like bodily organs, evolve to carry out vital functions in society, and they must maintain an equilibrium with each other in order for societal health to be maintained. Conflict, like an illness, is an aberration which the healthy system avoids and seeks to resolve as quickly as possible. Any change takes place only gradually in healthy systems, because it constitutes a disruption of normalcy. Revolutions and other forms of rapid change are signs of illness. Many structural functionalists came to believe that any social structure found in a system *must* have some function and probably serves some crucial need, even if that need is not immediately apparent. Some social scientists have used this argument to oppose change in general, especially in traditional societies, on the grounds that even practices that seem morally offensive, such as the cremation of Hindu widows upon the death of their spouses, must have utility within the given culture. They hold that to remove such structures might cause harm to the system and should, like surgery to the human body, be undertaken only with great care and in extreme circumstances. However, critics of functionalism contend that it ignores the notion—integral to conflict theories—that conflict and contradictions are inherent in a social system and, in fact, stimulate its adaptation to new conditions.

Functionalists view educational systems as one of the *structures* which carry out the *function* of transmission of attitudes, values, skills, and norms from one generation to another. Sociologists such as Robert Dreeben (1968), Emile Durkheim (1969), Robert Merton (1967), and Talcott Parsons (1951, 1959) have described this process. According to structural functionalists, educational systems perpetuate the "accepted" culture. The concept of "accepted culture" implies that there is a consensus on which values, attitudes, and behaviors should be transmitted. When conflict over values does occur, adjustments are made to regain consensus and keep the system balanced. For example, in mid-twentieth-century America, conflict arose over whether school curricula should portray America as a white-dominated society in which immigrants were expected to assimilate, or a multicultural society in which differences were celebrated. The past several decades have witnessed a variety of adaptations in curricula, a reflection of attempts to arrive at a new consensus.

Functionalism and the Purposes of Schooling. Functionalists believe that schooling serves to reinforce the existing social and political order. They assume there is consensus on the values and beliefs in society, especially on the allocation and use of power. Functionalism unquestioningly views the social system as benign and accepts existing class structures as appropriate. Because their perspective constitutes the current conventional wisdom about schools, the descriptions on the next few pages will seem quite familiar. We will soon examine other theories, however, and will see how interpretations of the purposes of schooling change when looked at through different theoretical lenses. Regardless of their particular orientation, though, theorists do not necessarily disagree with the functional description of how schools are organized; what they disagree on are the functions schools are said to have in society. They also differ in how they see the desired goals or purposes for schooling. The purposes attributed to schools fall into four general categories: intellectual, political, economic, and social. The following sections describe how these purposes are interpreted by functional theorists of education.

Divide your class into four or five groups. Have each group choose a different category of people to interview to determine what they consider to be the primary purposes of public schooling. Categories might include parents, students, teachers, administrators, community professionals, religious leaders, blue- and pink-collar workers, and others. Compare your findings in a class discussion.

Intellectual Purposes. The three primary intellectual purposes of schooling are the following:

1. Acquisition of cognitive skills (reading, mathematics, etc.)
2. Acquisition of substantive knowledge
3. Acquisition of inquiry skills (evaluation, synthesis, etc.)

If you were to ask a parent, student, or teacher why children attend school, the most common response would be "to learn." They would mean, to acquire the knowledge and skills enumerated above. In 1988 the U.S. Secretary of Education stated, "American parents want their schools to do one thing above all others: teach their children to read, write, and speak well" (E. W. Bennett 1988). Businesses and industry also view schools as institutions whose job it is to impart both cognitive skills and a body of substantive knowledge in the natural and social sciences. Recent outcry over high school students' lack of knowledge (E. W. Bennett 1988; Bloom 1987; Finn and Ravitch 1987; Hirsch 1987) has been over alleged inattention to this purpose of education. As will be discussed in Chapter 6, neoconservatives have begun a campaign to limit the function of schools to imparting skills and knowledge through a "core curriculum" that provides the same traditional liberal arts education to all students.

Political Purposes.   Schools also are viewed as places that must produce future citizens and workers. To that end, they serve four major political purposes:

1. To educate future citizens for appropriate participation in the given political order
2. To promote patriotism by teaching myths, history, and stories about the country, its leaders, and government
3. To promote the assimilation of immigrants
4. To ensure order, public civility, and conformity to laws

Functionalists believe that schooling facilitates knowledge about and integration into the political system. It is a means by which common social and political values are transmitted to young people and others, like immigrants, who initially may not share them. This goal has been one of the most important of modern public schooling (Carnegie Council on Adolescent Development 1989; Durkheim 1969; National Commission on Excellence in Education 1983; Spring 1988a).

Early American leaders believed that republican forms of government were required to educate citizens so they could participate wisely in the political system—vote, run for public office, and make informed decisions about government. Hence they believed publicly financed schools should be provided for all—at least all white males.

One of the earliest plans for free elementary education to both males and females was introduced to the Virginia legislature in 1779 by Thomas Jefferson. In his "Bill for the More General Diffusion of Knowledge" Jefferson proposed that public elementary schools be established in each county so that all children would receive three years of reading, writing, and computation. The most talented boys would then go on for free education in regional grammar schools. A final selection of the most talented boy from all the schools would then attend the College of William and Mary at public expense.

Jefferson's plan, unlike those in the New England and other colonies, envisioned an *articulated system* of schools from elementary school to college. An articulated system links requirements from each lower level to prerequisites in each higher one; students must master preceding levels before passing on to the next. Jefferson's plan sought to elevate a few males from the lower classes to the ranks of potential leaders. However, the plan did not explicitly teach citizenship. It emphasized a classical curriculum of Greek, Roman, English, and American history, rather than government or civics. Jefferson believed that literacy and a free press were sufficient for making wise political decisions.

Jefferson's plan provided no equal opportunities for women or minorities, and it was never enacted. However, it did formalize the idea that schools were critical to the development of leadership in a democracy. This type of thinking continues to inform the way many people view schools today.

Horace Mann, often called the father of American education, believed that schools not only should produce leaders but also should train citizens. Foreshadowing John Dewey and others, Mann felt that a national political consensus could be developed through the teaching of common values and beliefs in public schools. During Mann's tenure as Secretary of the Massachusetts Board of Education (1837–1848), political tension, mass immigration, and class conflict were causing great concern. Mann was active in school reform; as editor of the *Common School Journal,* he advocated the establishment of publicly supported elementary schools, open to children of all socioeconomic classes, to provide basic literacy and to instill social and political values for a unified American identity. Such a Common School would be the key to reforming society and creating a more stable union. His plan was supported by leaders of the dominant culture—industrialists, church leaders, and the business community—who felt that instilling respect for a common order would build a productive and complacent work force.

At the end of the nineteenth century the influx of immigrants from southern and eastern Europe prompted educators' efforts to assimilate newcomers. "Americanization" programs were established to teach language, customs, and laws. Especially after World War I, schools were used not only to Americanize immigrants but also to stimulate patriotism in all children. Reciting the Pledge of Allegiance and singing patriotic songs in school were viewed as training for later allegiance and service to the nation (Durkheim 1969; Spring 1988a). Participation in student government and competitive sports was encouraged in order to develop school spirit, which later would be transferred to the country.

Current curricular trends differ little from those described above. High schools require Civics and Economics, with special emphasis on the "free enterprise system"; children still learn political history and myths, and they still recite the Pledge of Allegiance; and political education and English as a Second Language (ESL) classes are required for recent immigrants.

Economic Purposes.   Schooling serves two major economic purposes:

1. To prepare students for later work roles
2. To select and train the labor force

Schools prepare students for the work force in part by teaching attitudes, technical skills, and social behavior appropriate to the work place, such as cooperation, conformity to authority, punctuality, gender-appropriate attitudes, neatness, task orientation, care of property, and allegiance to the team (Bossert 1979; Carroll 1975; Dreeben 1968; Jackson 1968; LeCompte 1978b). Schools also act as "sorting machines" (Spring 1976), categorizing students by academic ability and then pointing them toward appropriate career goals. In this way, schools create a meritocracy, a hierarchical social structure organized by ability, and they distribute individuals to fill the diverse roles required by a complex industrial work force. Such a meritocracy assumes that no major external impediments stand in the way of success for able, hard-working individuals (Young 1971).

Schools' **stratification** of students and creation of an ability-based hierarchical ranking serves to link occupational to social class differences in society. As the United States industrialized near the turn of the century, the concept of "human capital" and "manpower planning" came to dominate educational thinking (G. Becker 1964; Blaug 1970). The human capital school of thought, which originated in the late 1950s, calculates the rate of return from "investing" in schooling; it is measured by lifetime earnings minus the costs of education, including "opportunity costs," or the amount of money *not* earned while in school (Miles 1977; Schultz 1961). Humans are viewed as economic resources, and their laboring ability is likened to physical capital such as money, coal, steel, or electrical power. Just as physical capital can grow by being invested wisely, the value of human capital can be increased through higher educational levels.

Human capital theorists thus view young people as commodities in the labor market and view schools as the means of increasing the capacity of these resources by increasing their skill and knowledge. By supporting public education, industrialists invested in human resources just as they invested in physical capital and other kinds of resources. They also trained selected students for the work force. Industrial growth was believed to be intimately linked to a nation's ability to increase its supply of skilled human capital. School–business partnerships such as the "Adopt a School" program, whereby local businesses invest in schools, are a current example of the belief in human capital. This belief has been one of the strongest catalysts to the growth of educational systems in developing countries.

Social Purposes.   Schools serve three major social purposes:

1. To promote a sense of social and moral responsibility
2. To serve as sites for the solution or amelioration of social problems
3. To supplement the efforts of other institutions of socialization, such as the family and the church

In traditional societies the family, the churches, and the community transmitted social and moral values to youth for the maintenance of culture. As nations became more complex, children did not always follow the paths of their parents. More complex skills were needed for work, and schools were called upon more and more to assist in the training and socialization of children. Since the nineteenth century, schools have been viewed also as the primary institution for solution of social problems. In fact, in the 1890s the sociologist Edward Ross argued that the school had *replaced* the church and family as the primary instiller of social values, and he described education as an expensive alternative to the police (Ross 1901).

In the twentieth century, schools have been called upon to solve such problems as juvenile delinquency, poverty, child abuse, drug addiction, teenage pregnancy, sexually transmitted diseases, and highway safety. Social goals have become a very real and vital component of schooling.

Social services have been incorporated into schools on the grounds that well-fed, rested, and healthy children learn more readily and are less likely to drop out. They also are supported by the belief that children are more easily influenced in reform movements than are adults. Service programs also facilitate American egalitarian notions of equal opportunity and fair play.

This discussion of the purposes of schooling is a backdrop for exploring the various theoretical frameworks that have informed the sociology of education, particularly in the United States in the twentieth century. It is important to keep in mind that people interpret the purposes of schooling in accordance with specific theories about how schools relate to society. We have begun with the functionalist view, because it is the one with which people are most familiar. We now move to other views which, in our view, more closely correspond to the way schools and society actually are linked.

What do you think are the primary purposes of public schooling? How do these compare with the purposes of schooling discussed in this chapter?

Conflict Theory

Conflict theorists such as Karl Marx, Lewis Coser, Georg Simmel, and Ralf Dahrendorf believed that structural functional analysis, with its emphasis on social equilibrium and maintenance of existing patterns, is inadequate to explain the dynamism of social systems. They address questions not raised by structural functionalists, such as these:

1. What are the sources and the consequences of conflict in social systems?
2. How do conflicting groups organize and mobilize?
3. What are the sources of inequality in society?
4. How do societies change themselves?

Conflict theory, especially as developed by Marxists and neo-Marxists, states that the organization of a society is determined by its economic organization, and in particular by patterns of ownership of property. Inequality of property or of resource distribution, then, is the major source of conflict in societies. Insofar as schools are intimately linked to future economic opportunities, they too are institutions in which social conflict is played out.

Conflict theory has led to a rethinking of the relationship between schools, social class structure, and patterns of economic opportunity. Blau and Duncan (1967) first determined that the educational attainment of American males is a good predictor of their ultimate socioeconomic status. They further noted that the educational and socioeconomic status of sons tended to be the same as that of their fathers, indicating that status seemed to be inherited rather than transcended. Thus the system of class status seemed much more rigid than the egalitarian ideology of America purported. While interpretations differ as to whether it is the individual or the system that dictates one's ultimate destiny, the process of schooling clearly was linked to the structure of inequality as much as to opportunities, because of schooling's close ties to placement in the labor market. We now move to a discussion of reproduction as we examine the ways in which educational theorists explain how schools stratify—or rank-order—opportunity.

Reproduction Theory. The notion of reproduction represents the dark side of functional theories of transmission. Rather than viewing schooling as promoting democracy, social mobility, and equality, some theorists conceptualize schools as reproducing both the ideologies of the dominant social groups and the hierarchy of the class structure. In other words, schools serve as tools to keep wealth and power in the hands of the white middle- and upper-class groups.

According to these theorists (Boudon 1974; Bowles and Gintis 1976; Carnoy 1972; Carnoy and Levin 1985; Persell 1977), schools reproduce status in several ways. First, is the exclusive use of the formal language along with expectations for behavior of the dominant culture. This disadvantages the lower classes who do not speak the formal language, and also the middle and upper classes who engage in different behavior patterns (Bernstein 1977; Bourdieu and Passeron 1977).

Second, schools tend to magnify class differences by sorting individuals into occupational niches, not so much by their ability as by their social class origins. Thus children from middle- or upper-class families are thought to be more able and so are pushed toward professional or other desirable careers. Similarly, lower-class and minority children are viewed as less able and are placed in vocational curricula with lower job expectations. Children also are encouraged toward fulfillment of traditional gender roles.

Third, the status quo is reinforced by the fact that dominant groups control the major social and political institutions and they ensure that their power is never threatened. Giroux (1983a) summarizes this process of reproduction in schools:

> First, schools provided different classes and social groups with the knowledge and skills they needed to occupy their respective places in a labor force stratified by class, race and gender. Second, schools were seen as reproductive in the cultural sense, functioning in part to distribute and legitimate forms of knowledge, values, language and modes of style that constitute the dominant culture and its interests. Third, schools were viewed as part of a state apparatus that produced and legitimated the economic and ideological imperatives that underlie the state's political power. (1983a, p. 258)

Reproduction and the Purposes of Schooling.   The purposes seen by conflict theorists differ very little from those of functionalists. However, rather than accepting the status quo as natural, conflict theorists abhor the inequalities perpetuated by reproduction. Adherents to the concept of reproduction feel that public schooling operates so that the dominant class can maintain its place in a stratified society. Schools maintain class structure by preparing its members for stratified work roles, giving rewards for use of dominant language, and placing state regulation over most aspects of school life.

Three models of reproduction theory—economic reproduction, cultural reproduction, and hegemonic state reproduction—are used to explain how schools promote inequality and perpetuate class distinctions. Each model can be used both at the macrolevel, or schooling in the larger societal context, and at the microlevel, the more individual level of classroom and school practice. That is, some conflict theorists use large-scale quantitative analyses to study the relationship between reproduction and schooling, while others study interaction in small-scale settings such as classrooms to see how reproduction actually occurs.

Model #1: Economic Reproduction.   The economic reproductive model, which evolved from the work of Bowles and Gintis (1976), focuses on system blame, placing responsibility for social inequality on the schools. They link the failure of schools to reduce poverty and disadvantage to inequities in the economic structure of capitalist society (Carnoy 1972). This view, informed by traditional Marxism, states that power is in the hands of those who control wealth and capital and who maintain traditional class, ethnic, and gender inequalities. Stratification of work roles by race, class, and gender leave women, blacks, Latinos, American Indians, and other minorities at a disadvantage. The schools facilitate this stratification through their sorting and testing processes. Students are inculcated with skills, values, and attitudes considered appropriate for their later roles in the occupational hierarchy.

Correspondence refers to society's economic organization being mirrored in its institutions and vice versa. Thus if schools and churches resemble factories, this is so because the factory is the dominant form of economic organization in industrial society. Conversely, if schools are organized the way apprenticeships and workshops are, this is so because craftsmanship and skilled trades dominate the economic sectors. (See Chapter 2 for a discussion of correspondence between schools and factories.) Bowles and Gintis summarize the correspondence principle, which is central to their argument:

> The educational system helps integrate youth into the economic system, we believe, through a structural correspondence between its social relations and those of production. The structure of social relations in education not only inures the student to the discipline of the work place, but develops the types of personal demeanor, modes of self-presentation, self-image, and social class identification which are the crucial ingredients of job adequacy. (1976, p. 131)

Correspondence also refers to other aspects of societal organization being reflected in institutions such as schools. For example, schools tend to mirror the inequalities in society at large so that children learn, through both a hidden curriculum and an explicit curriculum, the skills and attitudes that will correspond to their later work roles. Jackson (1968) used the term **hidden curriculum** to describe implicit messages to convey "appropriate" values, beliefs, and behaviors to children. For example, by encouraging children to keep busy, complete their work neatly, come to school on time, wait quietly, and the like, schools teach behaviors needed in the labor market.

The hidden curriculum conveys different messages to children of different social class, ethnicity, and gender. Lower- and working-class children are socialized to accept authority, to be punctual, to wait, and to be compliant, while middle-class children learn to assume roles of responsibility, authoritative modes of self-presentation, and independent work habits. Teachers anticipate that middle-class children will need highly developed verbal skills but that lower-class children will not. Research in primary classrooms has confirmed that middle-class children are treated differently than are lower-class children. For example, during "sharing time," when children are encouraged to talk about themselves, teachers tend to give middle-class children feedback to enhance their self-presentation skills, while teachers of lower-class children tend to accept their students' presentation without correction or elaboration (Bernstein 1970; Labov 1972; Rist 1970).

Schools also reinforce gender differences. Studies show that males are called on more frequently, asked questions requiring higher-order thinking, given more criticism (both positive and negative), given more leadership responsibility, and generally provided with more teacher attention than are females (Sadker and Sadker 1985). The hidden message is that males are more capable and important than females. Researchers also have documented at the microlevel the connection between how social relationships in schools are organized and the implicit message about authority, work, and social roles and the values of the capitalist society (Borman 1987; Jackson 1968; LeCompte 1978b; Metz 1978).

In summary, the economic reproduction model provides insights into the relationships between social class, structural inequality in schooling, and reproduction of the social division of labor. It explains how initial class differences are reinforced by the structure of the school, so that students from lower-class backgrounds are relegated to lower-level jobs while middle- and upper-class students are rewarded with more desirable positions. However, this model has been criticized for its mechanistic, one-sided assumption that structure alone determines outcomes. Economic reproduction theory allows no room for individuals to act in behalf of their own destiny. It fails to explain **resistance** to authority, or the dynamics of relationships among students, teachers, and school staff. It is radically pessimistic, offering little hope for social change or alternative practices (Giroux 1983a, p. 266). This theory has also been criticized for omitting forms of domination based upon ethnicity or gender.

Model #2: Cultural Reproduction.   Cultural reproduction goes beyond transmission of the class structure alone. It examines how class-based differences are expressed in the political nature of curriculum content as well as in cultural and linguistic practices embedded in the formal curriculum. Bernstein's *Class, Codes and Control* (1977) analyzes these issues on both the macrolevel and microlevel. His studies, encompassing both the structures of and interactions in society, demonstrate that social inequalities begin in class-based differences in the family's linguistic codes, differences that are in turn reinforced by the schools.

According to Bernstein, the structure of society causes each class to develop a different family role system, each with its own mode of communication, which evolves as individuals participate in the shared assumptions and expectations of their class. Working-class life is organized around a family structure limited to traditional roles and positional authority based on age, class, and gender. It generates what Bernstein calls a "restricted" or "particularistic" code or meaning system, in which speakers use a shorthand communication, assuming that their intentions and meanings are understood by the listener. This code is described as "restricted" because its practitioners do not use an elaborate language system to make meanings explicit.

By contrast, the family structure of the middle-class is more open and flexible. It tends to rely on individual personality characteristics and personal relationships rather than on traditional, stereotypic roles. Because roles are negotiable, members of the middle class do not assume that meanings will be shared by listeners; hence they use what Bernstein calls an elaborated or universalistic language code to facilitate verbal communication. Differences between working-class and middle-class communication styles are illustrated by "How to Behave on a Bus" (see p. 16). Note the greater degree of directness and immediacy in the working-class dialogue. Working-class codes rely on the authority of the mother to obtain compliance, while the middle-class mother tries to obtain her child's compliance by means of rational dialogue.

Bernstein suggests that the elaborated or universalistic language patterns of the middle-class predominate in schools. Middle-class children are better able to participate in their own socialization processes because their language is similar to the language of schools. Since working-class students have less competence in the language of the school (or in Bernstein's words, have limited access to the elaborated codes of the socializing agencies), they often fail to understand exactly what is expected of them. They therefore respond inappropriately, perform more poorly, and reap fewer rewards for their efforts. Their poor academic performance leads them into preparation for vocational and blue-collar employment, whereas middle- and upper-class students are prepared for skilled and professional careers. In this way the class structure is maintained.

Pierre Bourdieu and Jean-Claude Passeron (1977) elaborated on Bernstein's notion of linguistic codes. Expanding on existing studies of class reproduction, they developed the concept of **cultural capital** to explain the function of schooling in the transmission of cultural and economic wealth. Cultural capital includes not merely language and social roles, but also the general cultural background, knowledge, and skills passed from one generation to the next. Cultural capital differs according to social class: Some has a higher "exchange rate" than others. High culture—that concerned with the arts, literature, and languages as well as communication skills, cooperative work patterns, creative endeavor, and what might be called "middle-class manners and behavior"—characterizes the middle and upper classes and is the most

---

How to Behave on a Bus

Working-Class Code:

MOTHER: "Hold onto the strap when the bus starts."
CHILD: "Why?"
MOTHER: "Because I said so!"
CHILD: "Why?"
MOTHER: "Sit down and do as you're told!"

Middle-Class Code:

MOTHER: "Hold onto the strap when the bus starts."
CHILD: "Why?"
MOTHER: "Because when the bus starts, you might fall down."
CHILD: "Why?"
MOTHER: "The bus jerks when it starts, and you might trip."
CHILD: "Why?"
MOTHER: "Sit down and do as you're told!"

---

highly valued. This type of cultural capital forms the basis of the overt and the hidden curriculum in schools.

Children go to school to add to their store of cultural capital, but working-class children find that their stock is undervalued. In fact, the capital they do have handicaps them. Since the schools embody the cultural capital of the middle and upper classes, children from lower social backgrounds who are not familiar with the codes will have more difficulty understanding the schooling process. The influence of cultural capital is especially pronounced in the first years of schooling, when their understanding and use of language is a major component in teachers' assessments of them. For example, students who respond in single words or short phrases rather than in complete statements will be perceived as less intellectually competent than their peers who speak standard English. They also will be judged less able if they do not make direct eye contact with teachers or if they use dialects such as Appalachian English, Black English (Labov 1972), American Indian English (Leap 1993; Spolsky and Irvine 1992), or the "village English" of Native Alaskan communities. These are the students who will be placed in reading groups for the "less capable" (K. P. Bennett 1986, 1991).

By contrast, students whose cultural and linguistic competence is congruent with school expectations will be considered academically superior. Schools reinforce the competencies already acquired by middle-class children, and since academic success tends to be associated with job success later on, this reinforcement in turn reinforces the existing class structure.

Model #3: Hegemonic State Reproduction.   A third model of reproduction is concerned with the complex role of governmental intervention in the educational system. The term **hegemony** refers to a social consensus created by dominant groups who control socializing institutions such as the media, schools, churches, and the political system; these institutions prevent alternative views from gaining an audience or establishing their legitimacy (McLaren 1989). The school is one of these agencies. Hegemony is created, at least in part, because schools reflect the ideologies advocated by the very state agencies that regulate the schooling process. For example, if state officials have mandated that sex education, AIDS education, drug education, driver education, or gun safety be taught in schools, districts must comply with those regulations.

Researchers in the hegemonic tradition argue that economic and cultural models of reproduction fail to consider how powerful the political intervention of the state is in enforcing policies that direct the reproductive functions of education. These researchers often refer to control by "the state," using "state" globally, without distinguishing among three kinds of "state" control in the United States—local, state, and national. Though these structures of power do not always coincide, Marxists would argue that all are products of a similar dominant culture and that the term "state" refers not to a political entity but to a general power structure. Giroux (1983a, 1983b) argues that hegemony is reflected not only in the formal curriculum, but also in school routines and social relationships and in the way knowledge is structured. The hegemonic model explains two functions which the state carries out in regard to schooling. The first involves the role of state and federal agencies in the actual production of knowledge taught in schools. The second involves state regulation of schools through certification requirements, length of compulsory schooling, and curriculum requirements.

THE ROLE OF THE STATE IN THE PRODUCTION OF KNOWLEDGE   At the national and state levels, government research reflects the interests of the party currently in power. According to hegemonic theorists, the state affects the production of knowledge by determining which types of research should be funded by the government. One of the earliest examples of federal involvement in educational research and the production of knowledge came in the 1950s following the Russian launching of Sputnik. Because federal officials believed that America was losing ground in the race to space, they encouraged talented students to study science and math. The National Science Foundation channeled funds into math and science curriculum-writing groups and, later, into summer institutes to train teachers in the use of new science and math materials. The National Defense Education Act also provided funds for college scholarships in science and mathematics, for new science and math equipment, and for purchase of curricular materials by local schools systems. Spring elaborates:

> . . . the National Institute of Education's main concern is the control of education by channeling of research interest into particular fields, which is ac-

complished by making available government funds for certain areas of research. The NIE, by designating priority areas for research, creates a potential situation wherein the production of knowledge about education is guided, by the means of attracting researchers into desired areas with offers of monetary support. (1985, p. 196)

The work of Anyon (1983, 1988), Apple (1979), Giroux (1983a, 1983b), Spring (1988b), and others illustrates the extent to which the production of knowledge is linked to the political sphere. A more detailed discussion of this process is presented in Chapter 6, where we examine the school curriculum.

THE ROLE OF THE STATE IN THE REGULATION OF EDUCATION   Political influence is evident in state control of teacher certification and assessment, compulsory education laws, curriculum mandates, and mandatory testing. The trend is toward more and more involvement by the states in the schooling process. For example, teachers in Tennessee, Texas, Georgia, and many other states are currently required to teach prescribed sets of "basic skills" on which the students regularly are examined for mastery by standardized tests. Where they are mandated, these basic skills constitute the major portion of the curriculum taught by elementary teachers.

The regulatory function also is performed by state-mandated exit examinations in reading, mathematics, and written composition, which are required for graduation from high school. Many states also require pre-service teachers to pass a National Teachers Examination for certification. Some states are considering ongoing competency testing to ensure that experienced teachers maintain their skills. As we shall describe in Chapters 2 and 4, many of these policies directly affect students, parents, teachers, and schools but are outside of their control (Giroux 1983a, 1983b; Spring 1985).

Hegemonic state reproduction theory, then, directs attention to the autonomy of national and state governments in exerting pressure on schooling. Its critics argue that while this theory attempts to explain macrolevel structural issues, it fails to consider the microlevel, or daily life in classrooms. It neglects the social relations among teachers, students, and school staff and how these interactions help them accept, accommodate to, or resist the role of the state in the classroom.

A Critique of Reproduction Models.   In summary, the three models for reproduction provide a structural view of the relationship between the work place and the schools, a view of the relationship between the dominant cultural and linguistic codes of the schools and those of the students, and an explanation of the effects of government on school policies and practices. In conflict theorists' view, the repressive economic, sociocultural, and political power of dominant groups reigns supreme and the system is to blame for students' failure to succeed and for the schools' failure to ameliorate social problems. In this view, the hegemonic power of the state leads the individuals to accept official explanations for their failure and therefore to place the blame on themselves.

Critics say that these theories are overly deterministic and one-sided. Some functional and conflict theorists have been criticized for their overreliance on quantitative research methods, for their unidimensional focus on social class and oppression based on ethnicity and gender (Clements and Eisenhart 1988; Delamont 1989; Ellsworth 1988), for the lack of empirical data in their analyses, and for their disregard of the power of individual human agency (Giroux 1983). Giroux explains that conflict theorists have "over-emphasized the idea of domination in their analysis and have failed to provide any major insights into how teachers, students and other human agents come together within specific historical and social contexts in order to both make and reproduce the conditions of their existence" (1983a, p. 259). Giroux argues that by avoiding a focus on human activity within social relationships, reproduction theorists offer little hope for change. While they have offered a different and often useful way of looking at schools as social and cultural transmitters, their view is a pessimistic one, giving no consideration to how individuals could interact to ameliorate or alter the constraints of the system.

Summary

Several themes emerge from our discussion of cultural transmission theories. Both functionalists and conflict theorists address the macro or structural aspects of schooling and its role in cultural transmission. The major differences between the two theories lie in their interpretation of cultural transmission. Functionalists believe in the existence of an underlying benign *consensus* on social beliefs and values and do not question its assumptions. Conflict theorists are critical of this assumption, arguing that social attitudes and values reflect the stratification in the society as a whole. They are concerned primarily with how schools serve the interests of dominant groups by replicating the existing social class structure and maintaining the division of labor necessary for a society stratified by class, ethnicity, and gender.

INTERPRETIVE THEORIES

Sociologists within the interpretive paradigm refer to themselves as phenomenologists, symbolic interactionists (Blumer 1969), or ethnomethodologists (Cicourel 1964; Garfinkel 1967). The common thread linking interpretivists is their focus on the *social construction of meaning* in social interactions. Interpretivists believe that human beings respond to each other and to their surroundings not so much on the basis of any objective or inherent meanings but on the basis of meanings assigned to people and settings by the people in them. Interaction and the assignment of meaning are affected by people's past experiences and beliefs, their current experiences in the given setting, and what they come to believe as interaction unfolds. This process is called the *social construction of meaning*. To interpretivists, reality is not fixed but is, at least insofar as it dictates human behavior and belief, negotiated in an immediate setting and depends upon the context. Such a fuzzy notion of reality might at first seem discomforting. However, consider how teenagers can be neat, helpful, well-behaved, and mature in *other people's* houses while remaining slovenly, slothful, irresponsible, and rude at home. Or how a perfectly well-disciplined class of students runs amok in the presence of a substitute. The construction of meaning is precisely why parents often transfer a child to a different school if the child has gained a reputation for being a troublemaker or a poor student. A chance to construct a new reality and new meanings often is all that is needed to transform a situation.

Interpretive Studies as a Major Shift in Research Methods

Interpretive researchers believe that the best way to understand human behavior is to examine real-world situations using qualitative or descriptive rather than experimental methods of inquiry. Interpretive approaches are a major departure from the quantitative studies which dominated the social sciences in the 1960s and 1970s, and the experimental studies which still dominate educational research. *Quantitative studies* use data from tests, surveys, or the census. These methods are indirect measures of actual behavior, since they ask people to recall what they did or to characterize their beliefs and actions in accordance with predetermined options designed by a researcher. *Experimental studies* try to place all elements of the research under the control of the researcher; anything the researcher cannot control is treated as bias or a threat to the integrity of the study. Neither quantitative nor experimental research is adequate for examining complex, uncontrollable, and multifaceted phenomena such as behavior in schools. By contrast, interpretivists rely heavily upon direct observation and open-ended interviewing in natural settings, frequently becoming participants; their major focus is on the details and nuances of interactions among people (Bogdan 1972; Erickson 1984; Glesne and Peshkin 1992; G. Jacobs 1970; LeCompte and Preissle 1993; Spradley 1980).

Interpretive inquiry has expanded tremendously since the late 1960s and early 1970s. It has grown beyond the discipline of sociology, and now researchers from a variety of disciplines are trying to understand the complex processes of schooling. Their studies are variously described as naturalistic, qualitative, descriptive, and ethnographic. Anthropologists of education, cognitive anthropologists, sociolinguists, and qualitative sociologists have begun to use the methods of interpretive inquiry. Their methods include long-term participant observation in classrooms, analyses of curricula, descriptions of methods and strategies used by educators, and extensive open-ended interviewing of those involved in schooling processes.

The three principal strands of inquiry that have influenced research in education are phenomenology, symbolic interactionism, and ethnomethodology. As we discuss them, note how each has influenced the others and contributed to an overall perspective in the social sciences.

Phenomenology

The key concern of phenomenologists is meaning. Phenomenologists study the social meaning of knowledge and what possessing various kinds of knowledge signifies. Phenomenologists such as Schutz (1972) and Berger and Luckmann (1967) viewed what we know, or reality, not as something given, but as constructed within the social interactions of individuals. This is so because people act upon their own definitions of reality *as if* they were fixed and true, not as if they were constructed and negotiable. Phenomenological researchers investigate these meanings that people construct in their personal interactions.

For example, researchers interested in the concept of a "good reader" can explore how meaning differs according to the actors and their social context. What a "good reader" is develops through interaction between teachers and students and varies from classroom to classroom. In Classroom A teachers may believe that being a good reader means being able to sound words out quickly and efficiently. In Classroom B the teacher may believe that being a good reader depends on how much of the text a child comprehends (K. P. Bennett 1986, 1991). A good reader from Classroom A would not necessarily be considered competent in Classroom B, because he or she might not conform to the meanings Teacher B assigns to good reading.

Symbolic Interactionism

Symbolic interactionists (Blumer 1969) link the construction of meaning to the roles that individuals and social structures play in creating meaning. While phenomenologists are concerned with *what* meanings are constructed, symbolic interactionists are concerned with *how* the meanings are made. To this end, they look closely at the processes of human interaction.

Symbolic interactionists state that people communicate meaning by using *symbols*—words, gestures, artifacts, signs, or concepts that stand for something else. Symbols are a shorthand and evoke a good deal more emotion or meaning than the actual object or concept. However, symbols can be confusing because they can have multiple meanings, which can differ from culture to culture, as the box on p. 22 indicates.

Symbolic interaction has introduced the individual into the study of social organization. Clearly, meaning is made by individuals. But society itself also is created by the meanings they make. As Blumer states:

> . . . social organization is a framework inside of which [individuals] develop their actions. Structural features, such as "culture," "social systems," "social stratification," or "social roles" set conditions for their action but do not determine their action. . . . Social organization enters into action only to the extent to which it shapes situations in which people act, and to the extent which it supplies fixed sets of symbols which people use in interpreting their situations. (1969, pp. 189–190)

Thus, unlike functionalists and conflict theorists, symbolic interactionists do not believe that people's actions and identities are dictated solely by their position in the social structure. Rather, what they do, who they are, and what they become are a product of what their past experiences have led them to expect is proper behavior. Personal identity incorporates all the things about them that give them a biological

Multiple Meanings in Symbols	
Symbol	***Meanings***
A wink	—A physical reaction to an itch
	—A sexual invitation
	—An indicator that something stated as true actually is false
The American flag	—A sacred emblem of national honor
	—Fabric with which to make a shirt
	—A mark of oppression
Not looking directly into someone's eyes	—Shyness
	—Respect
	—Evasive or shifty behavior
A red sports car	—Transportation
	—An indication of wealth and status
	—An adventuresome lifestyle

and social uniqueness. People may have multiple identities. To fully understand who they are and how they act, one must piece together their past and current history (Braroe 1975, p. 30). For example, hard-working college students may also be frazzled parents, diligent employees, members of an ethnic group, and lovers of classical or rap music. Each of these identities affects performance in school.

By expressing themselves in particular ways, people can attempt to control the responses of others to them, thereby influencing a definition of the situation to make it favorable to them (Braroe 1975, p. 27). Problems arise when people do not share a common definition of the situation. If they cannot arrive at a consensus on meaning, each may view the behavior of the other as inappropriate, hostile, or even evil. These disagreements in meaning—and the conflicts they create—often characterize events in schools.

Although symbolic interactionists may hold perspectives similar to those of functionalist or conflict theory, they do not explicitly address political issues. Apple describes this stance as follows:

> In the United States, England and France, it was argued that the questions most sociologists of education and curriculum researchers asked concealed the fact that assumptions about real relations of power were already embedded in their research models and the approaches from which they drew. As Young put it, sociologists were apt to "take" as their research problems those questions that were generated out of the existing administrative apparatus, rather than "make" them themselves. In curriculum studies, it was claimed that issues of efficiency and increasing meritocratic achievement

had almost totally depoliticized the field. Question of "technique" had replaced essential political and ethical issues of what we should teach and why. (1982, p. 16)

Ethnomethodology

Ethnomethodologists are more narrowly concerned with rules by which people order their social interaction and with the way these rules are communicated. Like structuralists, they search for the underlying "patterns for behavior" (Jacob 1987) which give coherence to social behavior. Ethnomethodologists believe that human beings work diligently at making their own activities make sense to others. However, this work is done unconsciously, and its products are taken for granted or go unnoticed by members of society. The leading proponent of ethnomethodology, Harold Garfinkel (1967), in a series of "experiments," explored the content of this work and the rules that govern it. For example, he sent his students home with instructions to act not as children of the household but as tenants or boarders. The surprise, resentment, and open hostility that ensued provided clues as to the unconscious rules that parents and other relatives believe govern the social roles of children.

Ethnomethodologists also study discourse, or conversation, since it is through conversing that people communicate to others their sense of the world. They are particularly concerned with how people "fill in the blanks" in discourse, making inferences about what is unsaid or about unfamiliar people and situations in order to maintain proper interaction (Abercrombie, Hill, and Turner 1984). Problems arise, of course, when the inferences made are incorrect. For example, many Cambodian parents were accused of child abuse when teachers noticed black smudges, like bruises, on the children's bodies. The smudges were, in fact, charcoal marks made during treatment Cambodians use to cure minor illnesses. Among the processes ethnomethodologists have studied in schools are classroom conversations, patterns of turn-taking and participation, and the asymmetries in speech exchange between teachers and students (Atkinson, Delamont, and Hammersley 1988).

How Interpretive Theorists View Schooling

Interpretive theory views schools as places where meaning is constructed through the social interaction of people within the setting. The interpretive approach to the schooling process gained prominence in the early 1970s when Michael F. D. Young in England announced the "new sociology of education," an approach whose key concerns were classroom interaction, utilization of the analytic categories and concepts used by educators themselves, and sociological studies of the curriculum (Young 1971). Questions to be explored in the new sociology of education included the social meaning of various kinds of knowledge, what its possession meant, and how it was distributed.

Interpretive inquiry was stimulated by various studies of reproduction, particularly the work of Bernstein (1977), who was interested in describing exactly how the process of cultural reproduction took place. According to Karabel and Halsey, Bernstein's arrival at the London Institute of Education in 1963 "played a crucial role in stimulating the emergence of a new approach focusing directly on the content of education and the internal operation of schools" (1977, p. 45). It sparked the development of phenomenological studies of schools.

An early example of the use of interpretive approaches is the work of Nell Keddie (1971), who worked with Michael Young at the London Institute of Education in the late 1960s and early 1970s. She explored what teachers know about their students and what they consider suitable knowledge for discussion and evaluation in the classroom. Keddie examined the organization of the curriculum, teacher–student interactions, and the terminology or categories into which educators divided their world. Careful use of observational techniques revealed that meanings constructed by educators resulted in differential treatment of pupils assigned to different ability categories. The teachers, while denying that student ability was associated with social class, suggested in concrete cases an intimate relationship between the social background and ability levels of their students. Thus the categories of meaning (for example, "poor children are poor learners") used by teachers led to tracking of students. When placed in tracks, poor learners use remedial books and receive less instructional time from teachers and more from aides than learners who are defined as more able (K. P. Bennett 1986). Differential treatment of students affects the internal structure of the school by creating a rigidly differentiated curriculum according to the perceived ability of students. Keddie's study further illustrated how this differentiation of curriculum impedes the academic achievement of lower-class students (see also Barr 1982; Page 1987).

The Contribution of Interpretive Approaches

You will recall that conflict theorists also discovered that students from different social classes received different types of schooling. However, conflict theorists looked at the macrosocietal level, using large-scale quantitative data, whereas interpretivists shifted the emphasis to microlevel qualitative analysis of interactions within schools and classrooms. They produced detailed descriptive analyses of these interactions, since they were concerned primarily with demonstrating that qualitative methods would provide "objective" descriptions of classroom processes. Many researchers who define themselves as symbolic interactionists, especially those in America, are careful to maintain this "objectivist" stance.

Interpretive theorists have been criticized for their single-minded focus on microlevel analyses to the exclusion of macrolevel linkages to social, political, and economic constraints—such as discrimination by class, ethnicity, and gender—described by critical and reproduction theorists. They also have been faulted because of alleged subjectivity of their research; critics asserted that interpretivists could not excise their own biases from their observations. However, interpretivists drew their research methods largely from the ethnographic literature of anthropology. They were trained to "bracket" or suspend their own beliefs and biases so as to describe classroom happenings from the point of view of the participants.

Summary

Interpretive theorists such as phenomenologist and symbolic interactionists study social meanings at the microlevel through qualitative or descriptive research methods. They are the precursors to theories of transformation in that they view the participants in their studies as engaged in the process of constructing culture through daily interactions.

SOCIAL TRANSFORMATION THEORIES

In this section we discuss sociological theories based on transformation, rather than transmission, of culture. It is important to remember, however, that these theories have evolved from those we have already discussed. Sociological thought builds upon, rejects, changes, and reformulates what has come before. Thus interpretive and critical theories of education draw upon functional and conflict theory. Unlike transmission theories, interpretive and critical theories are active, rather than passive. Participants engage in the social construction of their own reality, and both emphasize the need for microlevel studies. However, critical theorists go beyond simply exploring the agency of actors as they construct the meanings that structure their lives. Critical theorists focus on the construction of oppression and how individuals can emancipate themselves from it. In so doing, they forge a link between individual acts at the microlevel and social processes at the macrolevel, which the interpretivists fail to consider.

Critical Theory

Central to critical theory is a kind of negative but objective judgment which transcends simple fault-finding. It uncovers hidden assumptions that govern society—especially those about the legitimacy of power relationships—and it debunks or deconstructs their claim to authority (Abercrombie, Hill, and Turner 1984). Critical theory examines the current structure of society, in which dominant socioeconomic groups exploit and oppress subordinate groups. Critical theorists refer to active involvement by participants as *human agency* and believe that despite the influence of oppressive reproductive forces, hope for transformation of society is maintained because of the existence of agency.

Critical theory has its historical roots in a number of theoretical traditions. First, it combines both macro and micro analyses of social phenomena. It uses the analytic basis and many of the concepts of both functionalism and conflict theory. It shares with conflict theory a concern for social and economic inequality and a conviction that inequality is determined by the economic structure, especially the ownership of property. Like conflict theorists, critical theorists believe that inherent in social organizations are *contradictions,* which act as destabilizing agents to force change. Often contradictions can be found between social myths and beliefs and actual social behavior. For example, there is a contradiction between the American belief in equality and the simultaneous promotion of practices that create inequality of various groups. Critical theorists believe that contradictions are points of leverage within oppressive systems. As individuals learn to identify the contradictions that affect their lives, they also can become aware of the forces that oppress them. With growth in awareness, they can begin to transform their lives.

Critical theorists also borrow from symbolic interactionism and phenomenology. They believe that social reality is constructed and operates at multiple levels of meaning. However, they consider knowledge and understanding of meaning to be a source of inequality insofar as they are distributed unequally by race, class, gender, and other ascribed characteristics. Questions that critical theorists ask include the following:

What are the sources of inequality and oppression in society?

How do individuals experience life in social organizations?

How can individuals achieve autonomy in the face of societal oppression?

How are language and communication patterns used to oppress people?

How do people construct positive and negative identities?

Historical Roots of Critical Theory

Social theorists entered into World War I believing that however terrible the conflict might be, it was necessary to clean the slate of social, political, and economic evils. Once the war was over, they believed that the insights and methodological skills of social scientists could be used to create a new millennium. However, by the 1930s the rise of Nazism, the Great Depression, and the demise of the Weimar Republic made it apparent that World War I had not set the stage for Utopian developments. Neither war nor the new natural and social sciences had solved age-old problems, and the world was on the verge of another horrible war. The despair over these conditions destroyed a conviction that the sciences could solve human problems, a conviction that had persisted since eighteenth-century Enlightenment. Scientists were left believing that existing social science theory and methods were faulty and in need of radical critique or wholesale elimination.

Some of the principal critics of contemporary theory are discussed in the following sections. We provide only a brief glimpse at the works of these theorists and how their work has affected educational thought, but we encourage you to explore these works further on your own.

The Frankfurt School.   The Frankfurt School refers to a group of social theorists and philosophers who worked in Germany at the Institute for Social Research (1923–1950), which was connected to the University of Frankfurt. Max Horkheimer was the director of the Institute from 1931 until he retired in 1958. He coined the term "critical theory" to contrast what they were doing with the positivism of Descartes and Saint Simon (Tar 1985). Among the best-known of these theorists were Theodor Adorno, Herbert Marcuse, Erich Fromm, and Walter Benjamin. Members of the Frankfurt School, many of whom were Jewish, relocated the Institute to Columbia University in New York during World War II because of Nazi persecution, returning to Frankfurt in 1949. Its members' participation in American academic life, where they conducted a number of landmark empirical studies of race and prejudice, influenced generations of American scholars. Their critical perspectives are the foundation for critical theorists today.

Much like current work in critical theory, what emerged from their work was no single shared theory, but rather a perspective with several common elements. The analysis of the Frankfurt School was a critique of traditional or bourgeois perspectives, which had assumed that social phenomena could be understood through scientific methods of description, classification, generalization, and quantification. This traditional view, referred to as *positivism,* is patterned after that used in the natural sciences (Phillips 1987; Popper 1968). Knowledge gained by means of this type of research is presented as objective, value-free, and "scientific."

Frankfurt School theorists were critical of the positivistic model on the grounds that human phenomena could not be understood in the same way that physical phenomena could. Whereas positivistic research tends to ignore historical antecedents, critical theorists consider historical analysis central to understanding of social phenomena. The Frankfurt School members believed that neither social phenomena nor research methods—and even the decision to use specific methods—could be separated from their social and historical context. Both were embedded in social values and therefore could not be considered objective but rather were expressive of a particular theoretical or philosophical position. Critical theorists advocate recognition of this subjectivity through a process of self-criticism and self-reflection.

The Frankfurt School was critical of the economic determinism of Marxism because the latter ignored the influence of culture in the perpetuation of inequality and oppression. However, they shared a concern for injustice, oppression, and inequality and looked toward the radical transformation of social arrangements in order to increase human freedom.

Antonio Gramsci.   Gramsci was an Italian Marxist, both a theorist and an activist, who is best known for his *Selections from the Prison Notebooks,* which he wrote during eleven years of imprisonment for political activities during the 1930s, and which was translated into English in 1971. One of his most important contributions was his notion of the individual as an active rather than a passive agent, even in the face of extremely oppressive conditions. Gramsci was particularly concerned with the struggles of the working-class men and women in Italy and the ways in which dominant ideology of the state shapes individual consciousness. He used the term *hegemony* to describe the process by which the worldview of the dominant state maintains control through the socializing activity of institutions. (Recall our discussion of the hegemonic state reproduction model earlier in this chapter.) Gramsci believed that the state had the power to oppress but that individuals are active learners who produce knowledge and culture in their interactions within institutions. Gramsci argued that social change could occur only when revolutionary consensus—for which intellectuals provided a catalyst—was fully achieved among subordinate classes. However, once that occurred, alternative institutions could be created which would change the hegemony of the dominant groups. An example might be a group of female elementary teachers who resist the oppression of a male-dominated administrative structure by working together toward a structure in which they share in the governance of the school.

Jurgen Habermas and Michel Foucault.   Two other theorists who have contributed significantly to contemporary critical theory in education are Jurgen Habermas and Michel Foucault. Both are concerned with the relationship between knowledge and power. These theorists believed that knowledge is as important a social resource as land, money, or legal position. Those who control access to knowledge also control access to the power structure.

Habermas examined how restrictions on the flow of information contribute to inequality in society. He argued that valid knowledge derives only from open, free, and uninterrupted dialogue. Not even science is exempt from this dialogue. Habermas rejected the idea of an authoritative, neutral, apolitical science as well as the possibility of separating facts and values, since each is a product of social and historical context. Foucault also suggested that knowledge or truth is never free from the effects of history, power, and entrenched interests:

> Truth is a thing of this world: it is produced only by virtue of multiple forms of constraint. And it induces regular effects of power. Each society has its regime of truth, its "general politics" of truth: that is, the types of discourse which it accepts and makes function as true; the mechanisms and instances which enable one to distinguish true and false statements, the means by which each is sanctioned; the techniques and procedures accorded value in the acquisition of truth; the status of those who are charged with saying what counts as true. (1980, p. 131)

Paulo Freire.   Freire is a Brazilian educator whose work translates the notions of agency and power into strategies useful for educators. Freire has spent his life working with students and educators to challenge the constraints and inequities of traditional institutions. He draws on the radical "Catholicism of liberation" theology, which emphasizes the role of individuals in understanding and creating their own salvation, free from the mediation or definition of Church authority (Cleary 1985). Liberation theologians taught literacy skills to peasants by having teachers and students engage in dialogue over texts that were meaningful to them in their daily lives. Learning to read and talk about the conditions in which they lived gave peasants the courage to speak up against powerful agencies such as the government, the police, and the Church. Speaking up, in turn, led to efforts to transform their conditions of life.

One of Freire's central beliefs is that teachers must respect the culture of their students by providing opportunities for them to participate in their own learning. Teachers and students also must be self-reflective in discovering the ways in which state hegemony has structured their experiences. Freire views teachers and students as active agents in understanding, criticizing, resisting, and transforming schooling practices that serve to maintain a society that oppresses large groups of people.

Critical Theory in American Educational Thought

Since the 1970s a number of educational theorists have applied critical modes of thinking to issues of race, class, and gender in American education (Anderson, Apple, Aronowitz, Britzman, Fine, Giroux, Gitlin, Lather, McLaren, Tierney). In the pages that follow we discuss the thinking of Michael Apple and Henry Giroux, two of the earliest and most prolific American critical theorists of education. Their work has been stimulated in part by the inadequacy of both reproductionist approaches and interpretive theories to encompass the relationship between schooling and society. Apple and Giroux contend that reproductionist approaches examine only the macro-structural concerns of schools and that interpretive theories are limited to microlevel examinations of interpersonal interactions. Despite the fact that the methods used by interpretive researchers were a real breakthrough in our understanding of *how* educators and students interact to create social reality, they did not ask *why* these interactions proceeded as they did. Apple and Giroux used critical theory to unite the macro and micro approaches into one lens through which to view and understand the schooling process.

Critical Theory and the Function of Schooling

Critical theory assumes that schools are sites where power struggles between dominant and subordinate groups take place. A major theme of this work is an analysis of how schools are used to help dominant groups maintain their position of power, as well as how subordinate groups resist this domination. On the macrostructural level, critical theorists view schools as places where a class-based society is reproduced through the use of the economic, cultural, and hegemonic capital of the dominant social class. Giroux elaborates:

> Reproduction refers here to texts [language and communication patterns] and social practices whose messages, inscribed within specific historical settings and social contexts, function primarily to legitimate the interests of the dominant social order. I want to argue that these can be characterized as texts, as social practices *about* pedagogy, and refer primarily to categories of meaning constructed so as to legitimize and reproduce interests expressed in dominant ideologies. (1983b, p. 157)

Informed by conflict theorists, critical theorists contend that the power of dominant groups is reinforced within schools. By means of academic selection, socioeconomic stratification, and government regulation of curricular and pedagogical modes, dominant, white, male, and middle- or upper-class cultural standards are imposed on children.

Human Agency and the Production of Culture

On the microlevel, critical theorists view schools and classrooms as sites of cultural *production,* where people interact to construct meaning, much like those working from the interpretivist theories. Issues of power and control are worked out in classrooms by individuals. If those involved in the schooling process are able to resist the oppressive practices of schooling, and if critical consciousness can be developed by teachers, administrators, and students, schools can become sites of social change rather than of social reproduction.

The Influence of Critical Theory on Pedagogy

Critical educational theorists are deeply concerned with the art and practice of teaching. They argue that teachers must become "transformative intellectuals" and "critical pedagogues" in order to resist the oppression of the dominant ideology and to produce a liberating culture within schools. In other words, teachers must continue to be active, questioning learners. They must have knowledge as well as critical ability, so they can question not only their own practice but school structure as well. Students also must be taught to become active, critical, and engaged learners in an environment made stimulating. Critical theorists believe that their task is to uncover the ways in which dominant ideology is translated into practice in schools and the ways in which human agency mutes the impact of that ideology.

Critical Theory and the Purposes of Schooling

Critical theorists and reproduction theorists agree that the purpose of schooling is to serve the interests of the dominant classes. However, critical theorists point to a way out, emphasizing the power of individuals to structure their own destiny and to ameliorate the oppressive nature of the institutions in which they live. In many ways, the focus that critical theorists place on the liberating qualities of critical thinking resembles that of John Dewey and other educational philosophers who felt that an educated citizenry would facilitate the preservation of a democratic and egalitarian society. However, critical theorists have been faulted for failing to put their theory into practice. Much of their work consists of theoretical writing, much of it in obscure language unintelligible to the very teachers and students whom they hope to emancipate.

Imagine a group of teachers who were critical theorists. If they had the freedom to make any changes they wanted in their schools, what do you think they would do? What problems would they encounter and how could these be handled?

Critical Ethnography

We will now consider the research methods in the critical approach to understanding the process of schooling. The guiding concept is "collaboration," which means that these scholars attempt to work with the people being studied to help them achieve release from oppressive conditions, especially in the work place. In this stance, they resemble applied researchers everywhere; their research questions are guided by the interests of the clients rather than by notions of pure science or the interests of the researcher.

Researchers who call themselves critical ethnographers (cf. G. Anderson 1988; K. P. Bennett 1991; Gitlin 1989; LeCompte and McLaughlin 1994; Weiler 1988) approach schools from a critical perspective and also use qualitative research methods much like those used by interpretive researchers. They too draw on the ethnographic methods of anthropology and qualitative sociology, but they differ from interpretive researchers in their concerns and the questions they ask. Unlike interpretivists, who try to enter the field free from preconceived notions of what they will find there, so-called critical ethnographers *assume* and *explicitly state* that schools contain both empowered and disempowered groups of people. Many even advocate abandoning scholarly detachment for active confrontation with oppressive situations and individuals.

These researchers borrow from the **sociology of the curriculum** (discussed in Chapter 6) to explain how power is maintained through control of the flow of information, and how dominant groups use the curriculum, methods of instruction, and modes of evaluation to maintain their power. They also look at the way in which hegemonic state control at the macrolevel and the hidden curriculum at the microlevel serve to maintain social inequalities. Using the methods but not the detached perspectives of ethnography, they study the curriculum in an attempt to determine how hierarchically arranged bodies of knowledge (ability grouping and academic tracks) help stratify children to receive differential learning, marginalizing or disqualifying certain groups (including women, minorities, and members of lower socioeconomic classes) from positions of influence in society. Critical ethnographers study interaction to understand how dominant structures and practices are resisted by subordinate groups. By uncovering some of the ways in which school structures disempower groups, they hope to be able to propose transformative approaches to education.

Examine Table 1.1 to explore how functionalism, conflict theory, interpretivist theory, and critical theory explain students dropping out of school.

Other Social Transformation Theories

We have stressed throughout this chapter the fact that social theories change over time to reflect new ways of thinking and the impact of new information. The first challenge to accepted social science theories that is relevant here is conflict theory. The second challenge, begun in the 1950s, gave rise to the application of phenomenology and critical theory to educational and other issues. Called *post-positivism*, it attacked the notion that scientific knowledge, especially as exemplified in classical physics, chemistry, and mathematics, was the ideal toward which knowledge should strive, and the idea that scientists were infallible "paragons of intellectual virtue and fortitude, worthy of emulation by lesser mortals" (Phillips 1987, p. 17).

TABLE 1.1   Differential Theoretical Approaches to the Same Phenomenon: Dropping Out of School

Functionalism	1. What are the characteristics of the dropout population? 2. What role do dropouts, as a group, play in the social system of the school? 3. To what extent does dropping out serve to remove from schools those students for whom formal schooling is inappropriate or wasteful of public resources?
Conflict Theory	1. What are the social class origins of dropouts and at-risk students? 2. To what extent are disadvantaged students overrepresented among dropouts? 3. What structural sources of inequality lead to tension between students and teachers?
Interpretivist Theory	1. How do the patterns of interaction between teachers and students lead students to define themselves as failures?
Critical Theory	1. What patterns of resistance do students (and teachers) employ to resist the hegemony of the dominant order in schools? 2. What processes operate within the school to push students out?

Postpositivists believe that knowledge consists no longer of true statements, but rather of "statements that have been rigorously tested-and-thus-far-not-rejected" (Bredo 1989, p. 4). As a consequence, reality cannot be immutable and fixed. Scientific truth is neither verifiable nor completely falsifiable. It consists of whatever can, for the moment, be subjected to rigorous empirical testing, compared with the results of other tests, and warranted to be the most complete and accurate explanation yet obtained (Dewey 1929; Phillips 1987; Popper 1968).

Because postpositivism questioned the infallibility of scientific inquiry, it facilitated an attack on the capability of scientists to be objective. No longer could scientific inquiry be viewed as "value-free." Researchers began to realize that their own points of view inevitably shaped the direction and results of inquiry. Critical theorists have used this position to question the methods, theories, and interpretations of functionalists. Further, postpositivism helped to legitimate the use of nonexperimental, qualitative, and naturalistic research—the kind carried out in the real world by ethnographers, qualitative sociologists, and symbolic interactionists.

In the middle and late 1980s critical theory came under its own attack by social theorists such as postmodernists, poststructuralists, and feminists (Delamont 1989; Ellsworth 1989; Lather 1986). If postpositivism questioned the hegemony of science and rationality, *postmodernism* questioned not only the authority of traditional science, but the legitimacy of any authoritative standard or canon—whether it be in art, music, literature, science, or philosophy. *Poststructuralism* is a corollary of postmodernism; it attacks the assumption that societies are made coherent by underlying forms and structures, which it views as a form of authority. What poststructuralists object to is the notion that any fixed, nonnegotiable, ahistorical forms determine the structure of social life.

Postmodernism holds that dominant groups have controlled not only access to knowledge, but the standards of which knowledge is valuable and legitimate. Since it is Western European males that have been dominant, all art, music, science, philosophy, and social life have been governed by their standards. Only when the standards of other groups are equally powerful will the kind of free dialogue—and the valid knowledge—Habermas called for be possible.

While these approaches differ in their emphases and are as varied as the researchers who espouse them, they all draw on the analytic constructs of earlier functionalist and conflict approaches, as well as the postpositivists' attack on "hard science." They also, like interpretive theorists, accept the premise that reality is constructed of the sum of the realities of individuals interacting in any given setting. These approaches place great importance on presentation of the "multiple voices" (Geertz 1988, 1989) of all participants—especially less powerful participants such as women, members of minority groups, and students.

These critics of critical theory share a belief that it has merely substituted another form of hegemonic domination—that of the working class—for the elitism of traditional capitalists or bureaucrats. Because critical theorists have been concerned primarily with oppression of the working classes, and because their models are based upon analyses in Western European societies, critical theorists are, consciously or not, biased toward a working-class European perspective. Included in this perspective are patriarchal, male-dominated aesthetic values and social organization as well as individualistic, rather than collective, forms of human liberation. Critics of critical theory believe that models of resistance to oppression that are appropriate for working- and middle-class males of European descent may be inappropriate for non-European, non-working-class, and non-male individuals.

Perhaps most important, critical theory presents an oversimplified view of asymmetrical power relationships. Critical theorists assume that the end result of resistance, confrontation, and open dialogue will be some kind of consensus. However, they have made no systematic examination of the barriers unequal power relations create to the kind of expression and dialogue they advocate. "Critical educators have defined 'student voices' in terms of . . . being different from but not necessarily opposed to the voice(s) of the teacher or other students" (Ellsworth 1989, p. 7). However, especially in matters of cultural difference, matters of truth, and questions of who is entitled to receive privileges, consensus may be impossible to achieve. Further, the emancipation advocated by critical theorists is predicated upon Western and European notions of power and group relations. Imposing this view on people who are not part of that tradition is no less authoritarian, say the critics, than other kinds of oppression (Burtonwood 1986; Ellsworth 1989; LeCompte and Bennett 1992).

Table 1.2 presents a summary of the main concepts and questions addressed by the principal sociological theories discussed in this chapter.

In this chapter we examined functionalism, conflict theory, interpretive theory, and critical theory as they relate to schooling. Choose two of these theories to compare and contrast. Which theory most closely resembles the way in which you view the schooling process? Explain.

TABLE 1.2 Sociological Theories at a Glance

	Functionalism	Conflict Theory	Interpretive Theory	Critical Theory
Focus	Analysis of social and cultural systems with an emphasis on how order and equilibrium are maintained. Goal is to identify social system components and to describe how systems work with an emphasis on how order and equilibrium are maintained and transmitted.	Expansion of functionalism with an emphasis on conflict and change rather than order and maintenance. Goal is to arrive at a more realistic portrayal of social reality, one that includes an explanation of change, social disruption, and conflict.	Analysis of the constructed nature of social meaning and reality. Goal is to understand how people construct meanings.	Individual response to social, political, and economic oppression; inadequacy of current social theory to improve human condition. Goal is to unmask sources of oppression, to promote understanding of causes and consequences of oppression, and to encourage participation in liberation.

Assumptions			
1. All social systems are composed of identifiable and interconnected structures and institutions.	1. All social systems are composed of identifiable and interconnected structures.	1. Meaning is constructed through social interaction.	1. Analytic basis of functionalism and conflict theory as well as methods of interpretive theory are used.
2. Each social system, through its structures and institutions, must carry out certain functions to survive.	2. Economic organization, especially the ownership of property, determines the organization of the rest of society.	2. Individuals act on the basis of meanings they perceive.	2. However, conventional social theory is a bankrupt construction of ruling elites whose purpose is to perpetuate patterns of oppression in society.
3. Each component contributes to the overall health and order of the system.	3. While the basic categories and analysis of functionalism are accepted, traditional functionalism fails to explain the dynamism of social systems.	3. Meanings change in the course of interaction because of different perceptions held by the actors.	3. Humans are oppressed because power is hidden or disguised in language practices, communication patterns, and information flow defined and dominated by ruling elites.
4. Equilibrium is viewed as normal; disorder and conflict are viewed as pathological.	4. Inherent in social organizations are contradictions which cause their opposite—conflict is inherent.	4. Thus reality is not a prior given; it is based upon interpretations and it is constructed during interaction between and among individual actors.	4. Social life operates at multiple levels of meaning; knowledge and understanding of meaning are stratified and differentially distributed.
	5. Conflict and change are normal forces within social systems and contribute to their health and adaptation.	5. Reality is not fixed but changes according to the actors and the context.	

TABLE 1.2 (continued)

	Functionalism	Conflict Theory	Interpretive Theory	Critical Theory
Assumptions (continued)		6. Inequality of resource distribution is the major source of contradiction and hence conflict in society. 7. Conflict is manifested in bipolar opposition and is designed to resolve dualisms. 8. Conflict is dialectical; it creates new sets of opposing interests to resolve.		5. People are essentially unfree, inhabiting a world filled with contradictions and asymmetrical patterns of power and privilege.
Major Concepts	System, functions, goals, latent and manifest functions, adaptation, integration, institution and structure, norms, values, cultural rules, social equilibrium, and order.	The same concepts as in functionalism, plus others including legitimacy, consciousness, domination, coercion, subjugation, contradiction, dialectic, correspondence, ideology, strain, deviance, change, and adaptation.	Self, self-concept, mind, symbols, meaning, interaction, role, actor, role taking, role expectations, construction of reality, discourse, scripts, texts, communication.	Resistance, human agency, oppression, hegemony, domination, subordination, subjectivity, political economy, consciousness (false and true), stratification of power by race, social class and gender, ableness, sexual orientation, deconstruction.
Levels of Analysis	Macrolevel (groups, collectivities and their relationships—structural rather than individual level)	Macrolevel	Microlevel (individuals in interactions with others)	Macro and microlevels (integration of individual interaction with macrolevel social analysis). Meaning in interactions and texts.

Major Questions and Topics for Investigation	1. What categories organize the social world? 2. What structures and institutions constitute a given social system? 3. How are they interrelated? 4. How do they work to maintain order?	1. What are the causes and consequences of conflict in social systems? 2. How do conflicting groups organize and mobilize? 3. Where does power reside and how is it exercised? 4. What are the sources of societal inequality? 5. How do social systems transform themselves?	1. What meanings—both overt and covert—do humans attach to behavior patterns and objects in their world? 2. How do varying interpretations of meaning, expectations, and motivations affect human behavior? 3. How does the process of constructing meaning take place? 4. What symbols and rituals do humans create to structure their interactions?	1. What are the sources of inequality and oppression in society? 2. What is the experience of individuals within social organizations? 3. To what degree and how can humans achieve autonomy in the context of societal oppression? 4. How are research and oppression linked? 5. What patterns of language use, communication, and interaction do people use to oppress one another? 6. How are positive and negative meanings and identities constructed?
Critique	Too static: focuses on order maintenance that justifies the status quo; conflict and change come to be regarded as aberrations. There is some question whether there is consensus in society and whether the transmission of core values is based on a consensus model.	Does not define what constitutes conflict. Cannot resolve the question of order—how a society constantly in conflict can create order and stability.	Remains at microlevel; seeks no connections to determinants in external, social structural variables.	Lack of objectivity and neutrality in favor of stance of advocacy for the oppressed.

TABLE 1.2 *(continued)*

	Functionalism	Conflict Theory	Interpretive Theory	Critical Theory
Contributors	T. Parsons, C. Levi-Strauss, A. R. Radcliffe-Browne, B. Malinowski, R. Merton, E. Shils, E. Durkheim.	K. Marx, G. Simmel, R. Dahrendorf, L. Coser.	H. Blumer, G. H. Mead, R. Park, C. Cooley, R. Turner, E. Goffman, M. Kuhn, H. Garfinkel, A. Cicourel, H. Becker, J. Dewey.	T. Adorno, M. Horkheimer, H. Marcuse, H. Gadamer, M. Foucault, J. Habermas (In education: H. Giroux, M. Apple, P. Freire, M. Fine, L. Weis, P. Wexler, P. McLaren, J. Dewey, I. Illich).

SUMMARY

In this chapter we have tried to give some idea of how the theories that underlie social science thinking affect our beliefs about the purposes and operation of schools. The remaining chapters will discuss schools, their organization, participants, and purposes, using the language of sociologists. In some cases, we will first present perspectives that appear rather traditionally functionalist in their orientation. This is done because we feel that the earlier works established the foundations and developed the vocabulary for later analyses. Each chapter ends, however, with the critical analysis that is closer to our own thinking. As you read, consider how you, or other social theorists, might explain or interpret what is being presented.

chapter 2

The Social Organization of Schooling

INTRODUCTION

In Chapter 1, we presented the theoretical basis for a sociological analysis of schooling. In this chapter we present the organizational basis. We begin by describing the
internal organization of schools as they currently exist in most school systems, as well
as the many different groups that participate in the schooling process. As you read
this material, you may find yourself thinking, "Yes, but I know schools that aren't so
rigidly structured." We recognize there are schools today using less hierarchical organizations, alternatives to age-grading, and more developmentally appropriate curricula, particularly with current restructuring efforts. We hope you are fortunate

enough to be working in such a setting. However, we want you to consider traditional school organizations first, as a backdrop to later discussions on restructuring and alternatives. On the microlevel we describe the degree of influence of various participants at different positions within the organizational structure. We also present a descriptive and historical analysis of how school systems came to be organized as they are in the United States. This background will set the stage for a later examination of the impact of schools on society. Finally, we discuss recent efforts to change or "restructure" the organization of schools.

First we use a rather traditional analysis, describing school organization in terms of their functions and structures that carry these out. We then look more critically at how the structure of schools has changed in response to conflicts among various community constituencies whose interests should be served by the public schools. We have used the work of critical, or revisionist, historians because, like critical theorists in sociology, they question the validity of traditional interpretations of past events, asking in particular how these interpretations help to perpetuate cultural myths such as the belief that schools can eliminate poverty and promote equality and mobility. Among the themes we discuss are how business and industrial ideologies have affected the schools, the degree to which schools are pressured to serve economic, social, and political goals rather than intellectual or cognitive goals, and how school organization facilitates resistance to changes not congenial to dominant groups in the system or society.

THE INTERNAL ORGANIZATION OF SCHOOL DISTRICTS

Examining the actual structure of schools in an unbiased fashion is very difficult because both you, the readers, and we, the authors, have already spent most of our lives going to school. We are far too familiar with them to be objective! To facilitate the task, we use a device often employed by anthropologists—"making what is familiar strange" (Geertz 1973)—that is, treating something we know very well as if we had never seen it before.

Imagine that scientists from another planet—Mars, for example—have been sent to study the social institutions of Earthlings. Not knowing the language, they begin by describing the things they *see,* knowing that the physical setting of a social system often determines the behavior and attitudes of the people who live in it. They would probably use some Martian form of structural functional categories to organize their description.

The alien scientists would first be struck by the sheer size of the educational enterprise. They would note that school buildings are among the largest edifices in most communities, housing at least 250–300 people, except in the very smallest communities. From this they would infer that whatever happens in these buildings must be of great importance to the communities that support them, since so many resources are devoted to them. In fact, in many communities the educational system is the biggest industry, and the largest employer.

Differentiation as an Organizing Principle in Schools

During their first day of field work the aliens would note that everything in the school buildings is *differentiated*, or divided into clearly defined chunks or categories. Every chunk of space or time, every type of person, task, reward, or training, has a distinct function. The setting seems to abhor ambiguity, and where it exists, as in open-space classrooms, people try to impose a framework. From the clearly framed (Bernstein 1970) social and physical environment, the Martians infer that there are strict rules governing the use of such a place and the activities that can and cannot take place in its various sectors.

Differentiation of Space

Analysis of the use of space indicates that work predominates in schools and that teachers control and direct it. Work space for children is subdivided into two types: classrooms for academic work, and workshops and laboratories for vocational and other subjects that need to be taught but that require more equipment than books, papers, and audiovisual materials. It is clear from the predominance of classrooms over other kinds of work space that whoever runs the schools gives primary importance to book learning. A look inside the classrooms also verifies the existence of hierarchical authority relationships. Although desks and chairs may be moved around from time to time, the children usually face front toward the teacher, who is in charge. Although each school has some sort of recreational space or playground for the children, purely recreational activities, for both teachers and students, are not given high priority and are often preempted for other activities. Playgrounds become parking lots, and teachers' lounges become offices when space is tight.

Martian social scientists might have trouble classifying the large amount of space devoted to athletic fields and gymnasia, especially in schools for older children. Later analysis would confirm that these reflect cultural preferences for community entertainment. High school athletics are a major source of civic pride in many communities, especially in suburbs and smaller towns. The games are widely attended and well supported by local businesses and other sponsors. Schools are pivotal community organizations in other ways. Often the school auditorium or gymnasium is the only space in the community adequate for concerts, plays, and other cultural events. Rooms in the school are used for public meetings and by civic organizations. At every election the voting booths are located in the school's lobby, halls, or cafeteria.

Schools also contain service spaces that are used by both children and adults. These include assembly halls, a lunchroom (often these are combined and include a stage for various presentations), parking lots, and the nurse's office. Other spaces are presided over by adults for service to children, such as counseling and testing rooms, the cafeteria kitchen, the boiler room, and the maintenance shop. Still others, like lounges and bathrooms, are segregated, not only by gender but by age and status— one for adults and one for children.

The location of administrative spaces or offices reinforces the authority hierarchy noticed in the classroom. Visitors must locate them to obtain permission to be in the school, even if these offices are not located near the entryway of the building. Sometimes the offices are difficult to find. They may be located far from where visitors are allowed to park. Front doors may be locked, and imposing entryways make many schools seem forbidding. The Martian scientists note that this geographical arrangement helps control what goes on in the school and is often used to keep out people whom educators view as hostile.

Differentiation of Time

The alien scientists then make a key observation about the episodic nature of activity in schools: time is segmented and encapsulated; no activity lasts longer than approximately 50 minutes. Of that, a good portion is devoted to organizing the beginning and ending of activities (LeCompte 1974, 1978b, 1981). Use of the buildings is governed by bells or buzzers. Bells ring at regular intervals throughout the day, and in response people move from room to room and from activity to activity. To control the movement of children, they line up by gender and size under the watchful eyes of an adult. The early morning is a very busy period as hordes of children and adults arrive. In general, adults can enter the building any time, but children must wait for the buzzer and can leave only with permission. This process is more or less repeated in midafternoon. Although some people stay later to participate in after-school activities or projects, most children and many adults are gone within 15 minutes after the closing bell.

Differentiation of People

Following observations of the physical and temporal layout of the school, the Martians would begin to examine the differences among human inhabitants. In Chapter 3 we will discuss in detail the characteristics of student participants in schooling. Our purpose here is to analyze the structural differences between the way children and adults participate in the educational process. The Martian scientists interpret phenomena as these odd humans do, that is, they use human canons for distinction rather than Martian ones. They initially note that people in schools are differentiated by age, training, ability, and their purpose for being there. Only later do they begin to notice more subtle forms of differentiation and segregation by gender, ethnicity, and social class.

The anthropological "making things strange" means being careful not to take for granted the simplest and most obvious things. As we continue to use a Martian perspective to "make school strange," we have the aliens carefully document that students and other people in schools differ most obviously by age. Students are younger than teachers and staff. Age alone, rather than intellectual ability, determines when children enter school and at what grade level. Children are divided into classes or grade levels by date of birth. This is done for administrative convenience in processing the masses of people involved, but it creates many problems for instruction, because intellectual development and chronological age may be only vaguely related in some children.

A second and less obvious pattern of differentiation is that children are grouped by ability. Whereas the admission-by-age criterion reduces differences among children, ability grouping amplifies them (Dreeben 1968). In some ways this grouping permits school staff to overcome the instructional heterogeneity imposed by age-grading. As we shall see, however, ability grouping creates semipermanent cliques of differing social status and self-esteem, which often predict the occupational and social chances of their members (K. P. Bennett 1986, 1991; Eisenhart and Borko 1983; Powell, Farrar, and Cohen 1985).

Both children and teachers are differentiated by gender. Certain activities are designated only for girls, others for boys. Some activities, such as physical education, are not only differentiated by type, but segregated, so that the two sexes do not engage in the activities together. Some activities, such as teaching math and science, coaching football, and being an administrator, are more likely to be done by male than female staff members. The Martians also notice some differentiation of activities by ethnicity or race. Asians are concentrated in high-level academic courses but not in sports. African-American students are overrepresented in remedial, special education, and vocational classes; they also predominate on the football, basketball, and track teams, but not in golf, swimming, or tennis (see Chapter 7).

We will address these kinds of differentiation in later chapters, but they are important to note here as components of the organization of schools. The organization of instruction and the availability of subjects is predicated largely upon characteristics of the student population (Oakes 1985). Minority-dominated schools often provide fewer advanced courses and offer fewer electives. They are often more oriented to vocational training than schools whose students are expected to attend college. Teachers in these schools may complain that they have to teach many sections of remedial classes rather than advanced courses in their area of specialization. In addition, such schools often provide more support services and feel the need for ancillary staff such as security officers.

Differentiation by Employment

Adult participants in school are differentiated by the type of training they have received and whether or not they are paid for their work. The Martians notice that women teachers are more prevalent than men in all schools, especially those where younger students are housed. However, males outnumber females in administrative positions. Some of the adults work part-time; these include consultants and teachers who "float" among several schools teaching music, art, and physical education. Special services instructors, such as those who help disabled students or students with limited proficiency in English, often serve several schools because individual schools are unable to support a full-time employee in those fields. The marginal presence of these staff members means that what they do has little impact upon the day-to-day operation of the school. Their influence often wanes as soon as they are out of sight. There are also adults in schools who are not paid for their work; these include volunteers, parents, observers, and student-teachers.

In Chapter 4 we discuss in more detail the characteristics of adults who make up the work force in schools. Here we are only noting how children are distinguished from adult participants in schools: in the way they enter or are recruited to schools, in the rewards they hope to reap, in their training, and in the ancillary organizations that support their participation.

Differentiation in Recruitment

Perhaps the biggest difference between children and other participants in schools is how they enter or are recruited. Our alien social scientists observe that children come to school because they have to. Every child, regardless of his or her mental or physical condition, must attend some sort of school from approximately age 6 to age 16. Everybody else comes voluntarily—with the exception of parents, who come because their children must do so—either because they have a job there or because they have some special interest in education (Bidwell 1965; Nadel 1957).

Differentiation in Rewards

Because people come to school for different reasons, they expect different rewards. Children are somewhat short-changed in the immediate rewards category. The best they can hope for is a stimulating environment that is socially comfortable and intellectually challenging. Many teachers work hard to provide an environment that is intellectually rich, fun, and emotionally supportive. However, most teachers are severely constrained by the structures of time, organization, and governance already described. School staff try to reinforce the idea that learning is intrinsically worthwhile and that the payoff has substantial material value. They do so primarily by dispensing symbols—grades, gold stars, praise and awards, and eligibility for extracurricular activities. As Chapter 3 will show, not all students find these symbols intrinsically or extrinsically rewarding. Some students see little connection between their school experiences and their daily lives outside school. They cannot envision how what they do in school will result in economic rewards in the workplace.

Think back to your own experiences in elementary and high school. What were your rewards for participating in classes?

Staff members, on the other hand, not only garner immediate extrinsic rewards in the form of regular paychecks and long vacations, they may also reap the intrinsic rewards inherent in doing a job they have chosen, in working with children, in associating with professional colleagues, and in performing a task they deem necessary and socially useful. These rewards may pale, however, when working conditions grow difficult and inhibit opportunities for teachers to use their knowledge, skills, and talents (see Chapter 4).

Differentiation in Training

Children are grouped by ability in schools, but adults are grouped by the length and type of their training. Children are not specifically trained for the student role when they enter school; they are, in fact, there because they are deemed to be *in need of*

**Summary of the Criteria
for Differentiating People in School Settings**

Age
Gender
Social Class
Race/Ethnicity
Intellectual Abilities
Physical Abilities (or Disabilities)
Education/Training/Certification
Full-Time Work/Part-Time Work/Volunteer Work

---

training. On the other hand, professional staff such as teachers, administrators, and counselors have already undergone the rather lengthy training that gives them claim to expertise and to a certain degree of autonomy vis-à-vis students. Their training and subsequent experience lead them to feel that other adults—even parents of their students—have little competence in instructional or administrative practices. This feeling can create tension and sometimes hostility between school professionals and members of the outside community. Service personnel such as custodians, secretaries, and clerks also have some degree of training, but it is not specific to schools. Unlike the training of teachers, their training equips them for similar jobs in many kinds of organizations.

THE GEOGRAPHY OF CONTROL

Having established the organizing principles that humans use to differentiate events and occupants of schools, the aliens would next examine the impact of spatial arrangements on how people work in schools.

Spatial Decentralization

First they note that schools seem to come in two basic architectural types—multistory, rectangular brick buildings or sprawling campuses with many detached or semidetached buildings. Despite external variations, they possess remarkable similarities inside, resembling motels, with long strings of equal-size rooms placed on either side of long corridors, each room capable of accommodating approximately 30–40 children and an adult. The rooms are categorized according to the kind of tasks carried out in them: *work* and *recreational* spaces for children, and *administrative* and *service* spaces for adults.

Administrative space is typically arranged in clusters around a larger central waiting area. The aliens notice that architecture often follows cultural fads. Consequently, they make note of some exceptions to the motel-like construction of schools. For example, some of the buildings contain open space loosely divided by bookshelves. In most cases, however, this arrangement seems to be a vestige of the past, since temporary and semipermanent walls have appeared to redivide much of the space into more conventional arrangements.

They also notice that in most communities the school systems are geographically decentralized. Schools and central administrative headquarters are usually dispersed throughout the community, so communication from building to building or from one part of a particular campus to another takes some time, even with telephones and other communications systems to facilitate the process. The physical decentralization of school systems leads to structural looseness, or what many social scientists have called *loose coupling* (Bidwell 1965; Metz 1978; Weick 1976). We will leave our alien social scientists at this point since they have served their function to help us "make the familiar strange," and we will move on to explore this notion of loose coupling.

Loose Coupling and Its Impact on Control

Loose coupling refers to the fact that direct supervision and control are difficult in school systems. Both the geographic dispersion of supervisory staff and the "autonomy of the closed door" (Lortie 1969) contribute to loose coupling. In contrast to other types of organizations, such as factories, hospitals, and prisons, school supervisors cannot directly monitor teachers because they work in the privacy of their classrooms. Principals and their assistants cannot be in every classroom each day and may show up only once a year for mandatory evaluations. Similarly, central administrators do not usually visit each school building daily; in large school systems they may visit a particular school only once a year.

The motel-like configuration of most schools tends to isolate teachers both socially and professionally. Dispersion and closed doors affect the camaraderie of teachers. Departmental meetings are infrequent and devoted to business, so teachers may interact only with the staff members whose classrooms are across the hall and on either side of their own. In general, teachers spend most of the day in their own separate classrooms. They cannot leave their students unsupervised and have little free time to talk to each other. Elementary school teachers must often supervise students during lunch hour and before school. If breaks or planning periods are provided, they are devoted to lesson-planning rather than to developing solidarity with other teachers.

Loose Coupling and Teacher Autonomy

Although the isolation of teachers inhibits interaction, some researchers feel it helps teachers maintain a semblance of professional autonomy because it inhibits monitoring by administrators (Lortie 1969). On one hand, teachers may use the "autonomy of the closed door" to engage in innovative practices not approved of by their supervisors and colleagues. On the other, unmonitored teachers can avoid conforming to administrative dictates regarding even salutary innovation and remain traditional.

Although loose coupling does make the control of teachers more difficult, there are still indirect ways in which teachers are limited in their autonomy. For example, some states require a certain number of evaluations each year, sometimes unannounced. Thus teachers know that a supervisor can walk in at any time. In some such schools teachers develop an efficient grapevine so the evaluator's arrival is usually made known by the time his or her car key is removed from the ignition.

Another example of this indirect control is the heavy emphasis put on state-mandated proficiency tests for students. Teachers' autonomy is restricted by administrative pressure to prepare the children for these tests, and by the use of students' test scores to evaluate individual teachers' abilities.

DIRECT AND INDIRECT INFLUENCES ON DECISION MAKING

Perhaps the most incomprehensible aspect of American schooling is the ambiguity in patterns of control and decision making. The American educational system operates within a system of direct and indirect controls. The direct controls tend to operate at the local level, but as one moves farther from the home community, controls tend to be regulatory and indirect, consisting of guidelines and "strings" attached to funds beyond those raised locally. Functionalists view the support and concomitant control of nonlocal agencies as simply part of the system. Critical theorists, in contrast, believe that school systems are oppressive to the extent that local individuals are unable to determine their own destiny; hence they view the influence of state and national agencies, whether private or governmental, as evidence of further penetration into schools of the hegemony of dominant groups.

Indirect control also consists of the pressures deriving from a matrix of competing constituencies, all with a legitimate interest in what goes on in schools. Some, like school boards, superintendents' offices, and building-level administrators, are charged with the day-to-day governance of the system. Others, like local, state, and national governmental agencies and national accrediting associations, exercise regulatory and watchdog power. Still others, like parent groups, teachers' unions and other professional associations, youth organizations such as Scouts, and social service agencies, have an interest in the welfare of the adults and children who participate in school activities. More distantly related are community organizations such as churches, local employers, taxpayer organizations, cultural associations, political interest groups, and the media. While these organizations can attract a great deal of attention, they serve primarily as lobbies; they cannot regulate school activities directly. Who, then, does establish policies for and regulate the schools? We will begin with an examination of control at the local level, including the school board and the superintendency, and then will discuss how state and national interests influence local activities.

The School Board and the Superintendent

At one level, school districts are run by officials elected by the community. They establish overall policy, prepare and/or ratify the budget, approve curricular and instructional directions, and oversee the hiring of personnel. Although school boards represent the community and set educational policy, the real power at the local level generally rests with the professional chief administrator, or superintendent, whom the board hires. Superintendents are hired generally because they represent a particular educational philosophy or have a track record that appeals to the board. They are supported by professional staff, usually located in the central office.

The philosophy of school boards tends to reflect prevailing business ideology. Business and professional people dominate school boards, constituting more than three-fifths of the members nationally. Homemakers, usually middle- and upper-class wives of professionals, account for 7.2 percent, while skilled and unskilled workers account for 9.4 percent. Boards in larger cities and appointed boards tend to have an even larger proportion of business and professional members (Fantini 1975). In 1987 women made up 26.5 percent and African Americans 2.4 percent of the elected school officials in the country (Cull 1989).

Board members tend to be more fiscally conservative than their superintendents, but they are more open to change in other respects than the people who elected them. Many also tend to view election to the school board as a springboard to a further political career (Cull 1989). However, most board members lack expertise on educational issues. As old board members socialize new ones, the board becomes allied with the superintendent and dependent upon his or her expert knowledge. The role of the board often becomes one of legitimizing the actions of the superintendent to the community (Kerr 1973). However, we need to look at the community context in order to understand how specific boards interact with superintendents. For example, there have been boards that took a strong position on a school policy or practice, even removing superintendents whose philosophies differed from theirs.

The whims of school board decision making are limited, however, by state and national dictates regarding curricula, aid for special categories of children, and requirements for graduation and testing. Ties to local interests can create conflict with state and federal authorities. In recent years some districts have ended up in litigation because the actions of their school board violated the U.S. Constitution in regard to separation of church and state and equal protection of all citizens.

Attend a school board meeting. Find out about the background of the members. Notice the interactions in the meeting. Who speaks, who introduces new measures, and which positions do members take on different issues? What special-interest groups are in attendance? What role does the superintendent play? What types of actions are on the agenda? Who determined the agenda?

Limitations on the Power of the Superintendent

Although superintendents in large districts find it easier to maintain administrative independence than those in small districts, their actions are still somewhat limited. First, superintendents do not have absolute control over the ideological direction of education—that responsibility resides with the school board. However, since superintendents are appointed by the board, they often share educational philosophies.

Second, regardless of the size of the district, superintendents must maintain the support of the school board, as the story of Goose Pond Alternative School (recounted later in this chapter) illustrates. Much depends upon the political ability of a superintendent to maintain a consensus regarding policies he or she deems most important. Longevity in office depends partly upon the superintendents' ability to manipulate the flow of information to school board members so as to justify expenditures and either yield acceptable test scores or convince the board that academic progress is being made (Fantini, Gittell, and Magat 1974). Since priority is placed upon achieving consensus before matters are officially considered by the board, open board meetings often seem desultory at best (Kerr 1973).

Third, decisions are constrained also because they are not made in the same way as they are in business and industry. Major decisions are not made on a day-to-day basis. Many, like textbook and budget adoptions and curriculum changes, occur once a year or biennially.

Fourth, lines of control in school districts, even within the superintendent's office, are blurred by distinctions between *line* and *staff* areas of responsibility. Line and staff offices create separate hierarchies, each reports to the superintendent, but they are not accountable to each other. **Line offices** are the positions in an organization located in the vertical supervisory structure. People in lower-line offices report to and are supervised by those directly above them, who in turn report to and are supervised by those above them. These workers carry out the actual tasks for which the organization exists. In school districts, line offices are held by teachers, principals, assistant superintendents, and superintendents.

Staff offices occupy horizontal positions in the reporting structure responsible for tasks which are ancillary or consultative to the overall work of the organization. Counselors, secretaries, curriculum staff, and media specialists are examples of staff members in schools. Many staff offices are concerned with curriculum and instruction. They provide advisory assistance and monitoring to school-level personnel. They are responsible for developing curricula and providing staff development and training in the various subject areas as well as in specialized areas such as education for children who are handicapped or who do not speak adequate English. Lacking line authority, these offices can provide advice, develop materials, and train teachers but they cannot supervise or enforce the use of their products.

The offices responsible for vocational, gifted, remedial, alternative, and handicapped programs also may blur the lines of administrative control. While these offices may have staff functions, they also run programs. Some almost constitute districts-within-the-district, in that they often have responsibility for their own special schools, including hiring of teachers and administration of budgets.

Voluntary Organizations

A major source of pressure on school personnel comes from voluntary organizations whose members have an interest in the school but are not directly affiliated with it. They have power over schools as voters and as potential candidates for school board positions. In addition, they can petition the school board, appear at public meetings, and campaign for the support of their agenda. These groups include unions, parents, taxpayer coalitions, ideological "watchdog" groups who monitor the curriculum, and groups that pressure the schools to add or delete a variety of subject areas, including drug and sex education and school prayer. The activities of these groups are episodic, usually generated in reaction to some event. Because they can be unpredictable, these groups are most problematic for school systems. They often represent conservative special interests critical of what educators view as good innovative professional practice. Although school administrators circumvent them by following safe political policies, these groups can act as a strong deterrent to bold innovation and reform.

Teachers' Unions and Professional Organizations. The tension over whether teachers are workers or professionals with control over their work is echoed in arguments over status discrepancies: Should teachers be represented by professional associations or by unions? (See Chapter 4.) Here we will examine the origin of teacher efforts to act collectively and their impact upon control of schools. One faction of the educational profession—one that emphasizes the white-collar, professional nature of its work—has consistently pressed for an umbrella professional organization serving groups as disparate as classroom teachers, administrators, and college professors. The result, as we shall see, is not one big happy family, but a collection of warlike tribes who fail to further the interests of any of the participants. Another faction—this one conceptualizing the teacher–administrator relationship as one of management and labor—advocates *teachers' unions.* Teachers' unions have suffered identity problems because although their members are not blue-collar workers, the orientation of the organization, like that of steelworker and truck driver unions, is adversarial.

While teachers' unions have not generally wielded substantial power, their existence does serve as a check on excessive administrative use of power. Two watershed events, both in New York City, changed the pattern of relationships between unions and school managers. The first was the 1962 strike of the United Federation of Teachers (UFT), the largest teachers' local. It not only won raises for teachers, but kept the district from retaliating against those participating in the strike. The second was the Ocean-Hill-Brownsville strike in 1968, when an alliance of the UFT and the very conservative school administrators of the Council of Supervisory Associations fought off attempts to give control over hiring and firing of teachers to decentralized local school boards (Scimecca 1980).

Since these events, there is evidence that teacher militancy has initiated some important changes in patterns of control and power in education. While these changes are not universal, and their full effect is still unknown, they point the way to future shifts in the governance of education. First, the militancy of teachers' unions has tended to radicalize the National Education Association (NEA) and other more conservative organizations. Second, it has reduced the arbitrary decision-making power of school boards and administrators with regard to teachers. Third, it has made clearer the dichotomy between teachers' and administrators' interests. Fourth, it has greatly reduced the power of building-level principals. Because teachers can use their union representatives to negotiate directly with higher district officials, the principal can be circumvented (Scimecca 1980). Finally, because the teachers' unions have affiliation with national organizations, the growth in militancy may produce a more cosmopolitan outlook among teachers. It shifts teacher concerns from purely local problems and local solutions to state and national arenas (Brookover and Erickson 1975).

Invite a representative from your local teachers' association to speak to your class about the roles unions have played in the teaching profession. In preparation for this visit, develop a list of questions you would like this person to address.

Community Groups.   There are other adults in the community who may claim expertise in the field of education on the basis of special knowledge. Parents may claim expertise in children. Taxpayers may claim financial knowledge. Athletic boosters may claim knowledge of the sports programs. Consultants, textbook vendors, lobbyists, and special-interest groups such as churches and political parties may claim expertise in curricular materials and current issues. Businesspeople and local employers may claim expertise in vocational training.

At the local level, anything having to do with sexual behavior, religion, or finance can stimulate citizen protest. Groups might protest sex education classes, day-care programs for children of students, controversial books, tax increases, or school bond issues. These and many other issues pit school people against segments in the community and threaten school personnel control over educational matters. However, despite the energy of their involvement in schools, none of these groups is trained specifically for such a role in the educational enterprise. Unlike parents, they do not have an automatic and compelling voice in school operations, but they do represent the multiple constituencies whose interests penetrate the school.

Parent Groups.   The outsiders who do have a legitimate interest in the schools are the parents of the students. First of all, their activities can make a big difference in teachers' workload. Parents serve as volunteer aides, class parents, and librarians, provide transportation for field trips, sponsor extracurricular activities, and raise money for computers and other materials not provided by the budget.

Second, teachers, administrators, and researchers believe strongly that parent activity enhances pupil achievement. In Houston, schools where students had the highest achievement scores had five times as many parent volunteers as those with the lowest achievement (Tedford 1988). A strong correlation has been demonstrated between children's reading scores and whether or not their parents read stories to them (Boehnlein 1985). The War on Poverty of the 1960s and 1970s heavily stressed teaching parents how to help their children study. Further, success of the educational reform movement of the 1980s is believed to rest upon involving parents in their children's schooling.

However, the involvement of parents and other nonprofessionals is viewed with ambivalence by teachers and principals. They are truly comfortable only with volunteer efforts that they can control and that do not question their authority. They do not look favorably upon upstart student groups or underground community newspapers, unfavorable media publicity, or organized groups of reform-minded parents who are dissatisfied with their children's academic progress or the educational activities provided for them.

On one hand, parent groups can be perceived as a serious threat to the school because, as parents, they have legitimate access to school affairs. On the other hand, the tenure of a child in a school is relatively short, and if parents cannot be discouraged, co-opted, intimidated, ignored, or otherwise resisted, school personnel can always merely wait until the children move, drop out, or graduate. Stern (1987), for example, documented how public schools train African-American parents to accept unquestioningly the low evaluations given to their children, "cooling out" those who resist by locking the doors, canceling meetings, and retaliating against their children.

Identify community groups in your area that wish to influence education. What constituency do they represent? What changes would they like to see? What tactics and strategies do they use?

PATTERNS OF CONTROL BEYOND THE LOCAL LEVEL: THE PUBLIC SECTOR

State Jurisdiction

Each state has an educational agency whose organization parallels that at the local level. At the top is a chief officer or superintendent, a state board of education, and an executive branch or agency that carries out the activities of the department. State regulation specifies the scope of state support, establishes curriculum content and minimum time for each subject, sets minimum standards for student promotion and graduation, describes the rights and competencies of teachers, defines the characteristics of administrative structure, and creates rules for the physical safety of school inhabitants (Benson 1982; Wirt and Kirst 1974).

Examine your state's teacher certification requirements and compare them to your college's teacher preparation program. Examine the state curricular guidelines for students at the grade level or in the subject area of most interest to you.

Some state departments of education adopt curricular guidelines which teachers must follow, and many states approve a specific set of textbooks. State involvement in education was relatively limited until the mid-1960s. With concern for educational standards and accountability in the 1980s, we saw increased state involvement in the day-to-day workings in schools, particularly in regard to standardized testing and cur-

---

Attendance Policy

State law requires that all children between the ages of 7 and 17, both inclusive, be enrolled in day school. Excuses for absences for students in grades K‑8 must be made in writing or in person by a parent or guardian. High school policies for excusing student absences vary from school to school. Students with as many as five unexcused absences will be referred to the attendance and social services department. Students of high school age may lose their driver's license for excessive absences. Aside from the obvious need for students to be present in school on a regular basis, absenteeism decreases state monies available to local school systems.

SOURCE: This quote is from a 1994 policy document, county school district, Tennessee.

---

ricula. It has become common for states to work with test developers to create proficiency examinations that are administered statewide to students at designated grade levels. These proficiency tests have a tremendous impact on the way teachers handle the curriculum.

The passage in 1965 of Title V of the Elementary and Secondary Education Act, which provided federal funds to bolster the professional staffs of state education agencies, greatly increased state-level educational activity. It led, for example, to increased research, media, and consulting services to local school districts, and administration of federal funds for compensatory education. These activities had two effects. First, they increased the level of bureaucratization at the state level, and second, they permitted the federal educational policies to penetrate closer to the local level, thereby shifting the location of control in school systems. While national agencies still have little influence over day-to-day behavior in the classroom, districts that accept federal funds find that they are constrained to use them in specific ways and to carry out systematic evaluation of their actions.

The Role of the Federal Government

While the primary, day-to-day activities of educational systems are subject to governance no higher than the state level, regional and national agencies in both the public and private sector influence these systems by means of financial incentives, certification, court enforcement of constitutional and other national laws, and federally funded research.

Despite the fact that primary responsibility for education in America is reserved to the states, there has long been concern that extreme decentralization might lead to great inequalities in the educational services provided by individual states. In 1867 educators overcame their distrust of federal influence and established the first federal Department of Education. Its charge was limited to providing statistics and information about educational matters and promoting the establishment of an efficient educational system (Butts 1978).

Since that time, federal influence has grown, especially in the enforcement of equal opportunity provision. The courts have been used to ensure that these constitutional provisions were applied in local school districts. Although the power of the federal Office of Education has varied as it has gone through a number of title changes, this agency has provided financial aid to states and local districts for specific programs and has sponsored research on topics felt to be in the national interest. These have included vocational educational programs and the teaching of science, bilingual education, English as a foreign language, and foreign languages. Federal funds have also been provided for research on testing and assessment, desegregation effects, improvement in instruction in basic subject areas, and improvement in techniques for teaching the disadvantaged. In addition, the federal government has financed research and evaluation staff to ensure that funds are being used as intended. Since the 1960s each federally funded project has had a mandated evaluation component, even those carried out by local staff.

The federal government has provided scholarships and loans to special classes of individuals. These have included veterans of military service, under the Servicemen's Readjustment Act of 1944 (the "G.I. Bill"); those who study certain subjects such as foreign languages and science, under the National Defense Education Act; ethnic minority students, under War on Poverty legislation during the 1960s; and trainers of bilingual teachers, under Title VII of the Elementary and Secondary Education Act. Individual undergraduates have received Pell grants, while graduate study has been encouraged under the Smith-Mundt and Fulbright legislation, the National Science Foundation, and other scholarship and loan programs.

In addition, federal regulations protect the educational rights and welfare of certain groups of students, including the poor, the handicapped, and those with limited proficiency in English. Members of these populations have been provided with school nurses, lunches, certain medical examinations, clothing, remedial instruction, and other compensatory services. The national government has also enforced laws regarding discrimination on the basis of race, gender, religion, and national origin and has placed constraints on using schools for religious purposes. Because of affirmative action and laws outlawing discrimination in public agencies, schools in particular have come under close scrutiny by the Office of Civil Rights and the courts.

PATTERNS OF CONTROL BEYOND THE LOCAL LEVEL: THE PRIVATE SECTOR

Regional Accreditation Agencies

State monitoring of local graduation standards and instructional quality is reinforced by regional accrediting agencies. During the nineteenth century secondary school courses were so diverse that universities had no way of knowing what and how much their incoming students knew. They therefore established the practice of certifying the curricula of given schools and then accepting their students without entrance examinations. Eventually these certification practices were institutionalized, and the resulting agencies visited high schools to approve their curricula, certify their students, and "accredit" their programs. These agencies have made secondary school course offerings more uniform, at least for college-preparatory programs; it also has created an external watchdog function which reduces the autonomy of schools and districts.

Private Research Institutes and Philanthropic Foundations

While private institutions have far less money to dispense than does the federal government, they are far more accessible to local school districts. Operated by state, regional, and local corporations or funded by the legacies of philanthropists, they are often directed by charter to sponsor programs in the schools, especially to provide small grants for teachers. A few very large private research foundations, such as the Rockefeller, Ford, and Spencer Foundations, have a pervasive effect not only on the topics and methods of investigation, but also on the use of research data. In addition, recipients of awards from these agencies form an elite network of intellectual leaders whose judgment is sought on educational matters in both the public and private sectors (LeCompte 1972).

The influence of local businesses and industries is particularly powerful. School-business partnerships have been promoted heavily as ways to help minority youth enter the work force and reduce their dropout rate (see, for example, Hargroves 1987). Corporations also have loaned executives to school districts to teach specialty areas such as math, science, and computer technology. Vocational curricula in high schools often reflect the dominant industries in the community. The schools do initial training and students then are preferentially hired by local businesses.

THE SCHOOL AS A BUREAUCRACY

How did schools evolve into their current patterns of organization and control? School enterprises today are a great deal more complex than the one-time individual classroom and building. In fact, schools are large, formal, social organizations, similar to hospitals, corporations, and factories. These organizations are called **bureaucracies.** The term "bureaucracy" is neither an insult nor a reference to red tape and frustration, but rather, a term used by sociologists to describe large, complex, multilevel social organizations which are run by full-time professionals.

A Formal Definition

A convenient way to begin to understand bureaucracies is through functional theory as it was defined in Chapter 1. Functionalists define bureaucracies in terms of the tasks they perform and the organizational structures that carry them out. One characteristic of bureaucracy is that each task (function) the organization does has an individual, department, or group of people (structure) to carry it out. Imagine a typical organizational chart, in which the president occupies a box at the top, the lowest levels of workers are arrayed in horizontal rows of boxes at the bottom, and other tasks and departments occupy the space in between. Organizational charts specify the goals of the organization, what jobs are required to achieve them, and who shall carry them out. In effect, organizational charts provide a functional analysis of formal structure.

Bureaucracies embody a division of functions, much like that of an automobile assembly line, where each area of responsibility is clearly defined. Line tasks or offices—those that actually do the work of the organization—are arranged hierarchically, so that people lower in the organization are supervised by those higher up. Staff offices operate laterally. For example, design departments and quality control officials in the automobile industry advise line personnel but are not involved with the direct production of cars.

Obtain a copy of the school organization chart from the central office of your local school district. What do you think of this organization? How does it compare with the organizational chart shown in Figure 2.1? What organizational changes would you suggest to your local district?

According to Max Weber, the first theorist who completely delineated the characteristics of bureaucracy, workers in bureaucracies must be full-time workers, not volunteers or part-timers with divided loyalties. They must be rewarded according to their skill and training. Those with more training and responsibility are usually paid more and hold higher positions than those with less training and responsibility (Blau and Scott 1962; Dalton, Barnes, and Zaleznik 1968; Weber 1962). They may receive merit pay for objectively assessed exemplary performance.

Bureaucracies operate by means of rules which rationally and systematically establish *what* each person is expected to do—and often *how* they are to do it as well. These rules are the basis for systems of accountability and apply to all job-holders without favoritism. The rules can be found in job descriptions, by-laws, guidebooks, operating manuals, and handbooks of various kinds.

Clearly, a formal, functional definition of bureaucracy does not describe how most organizations really operate. Their sheer complexity makes it impossible to specify every action that might be undertaken. Individuals take on tasks that are not in their formal job description, bypass people or offices that are roadblocks, and bend the rules when necessary. Informal practices outside of the "normal channels" evolve to facilitate work (Blau 1955). These informal adaptations are necessary for organizations to function smoothly.

It is no accident that schools resemble other kinds of bureaucratic organizations in modern society. However, because institutions do not exist in isolation, the social context in which they have developed must be considered. Their history and physical arrangements, as well as the characteristics of their inhabitants, shape how people behave within organizations and how they feel about themselves and others. Bureaucratic organizations have assumed the shape they did because policy makers gave priority to order, uniformity, and efficiency (Katz 1971). Schools developed and

FIGURE 2.1

1994 ADMINISTRATIVE ORGANIZATION CHART
COUNTY SCHOOL DISTRICT*
528 SQUARE MILES
COUNTY POPULATION: 335,749

BOARD OF EDUCATION

SUPERINTENDENT OF SCHOOLS

ADMINISTRATIVE SERVICES DEPARTMENT
Assistant Superintendent for Administrative Services
Coordinator of Food Service
Coordinator of Transportation
Supervisor of Food Service
Specialist—Food Service
Supervisor of Transfers and Disciplinary Hearings
Supervisor of Student Information System
Supervisor of Athletics
Captain of School Security

BUSINESS AND PERSONNEL DEPARTMENTS
Assistant Superintendent for Business and Personnel
Specialist—Payroll Administrator
Specialist—Administrative Assistant to Assistant Superintendent
Specialist—Assistant Business Manager
Director of Personnel
Supervisor of Elementary Personnel and Evaluations
Supervisor of Middle School Personnel and Minority Recruiter
Supervisor of High School and Secretarial Personnel and Substitute Teachers
Supervisor of Data Processing for Payroll and Personnel
Director of Maintenance and Operations

CURRICULUM AND INSTRUCTION DEPARTMENT
Assistant Superintendent for Curriculum and Instruction
Director of Vocational Education
Coordinator of Research and Evaluation
Coordinator of Science
Coordinator of High Schools
Coordinator of Elementary Schools
    Supervisors (3)—Elementary Generalist
    Supervisor of Adult Home Economics
    Supervisor of Trade and Industrial and Technology Education

Supervisor of Social Studies

Supervisor of General Business, Office Education, Computer Labs and Vocational Improvement Program

Supervisor of Adult Basic Education

Supervisor of Language Arts (6–12)

Supervisor of Driver Education and In-School Suspension

Supervisor of Mathematics (K–8)

Supervisor of Mathematics (9–12)

Supervisor of Health Occupations, Home Economics, Marketing Education, and Cosmetology

Supervisor of Science

Supervisor of Physical Education and Health (K–8)

Supervisor of Physical Education and Health (9–12)

Supervisor of Gifted Education

Supervisor of Art

Supervisor of Music—Choral

Supervisor of Music—Instrumental

Supervisor of Adult Basic Education and Evening School

Supervisor of Computer Skills

Specialist—Alcohol and Other Drug Prevention Programs/Section 504

Specialist Foreign Language/ESL

Specialist—Computer Skills

Specialist—Teacher Center

PUPIL PERSONNEL SERVICES AND SUPPLEMENTARY SERVICES DEPARTMENTS

ASSISTANT SUPERINTENDENT FOR SUPPLEMENTARY STUDENT SERVICES

Director of Pupil Personnel Services

Supervisor of School Nurses

Administrative Assistant to Director of Pupil Personnel Services/Special Education Generalist

Supervisors of Resource and CDC Programs (2)

Supervisor of Psychological Services

Supervisor of Sensory Communications and Home/Hospital Services

Supervisor of Special Education

Supervisor of Consultative and Intervention Support Services

Supervisor of OT/PT

Supervisors of Chapter I Reading, Language Development, and Mathematics (2)

ADMINISTRATIVE ASSISTANTS

SUPERVISOR OF COMMUNICATIONS

SUPERVISOR OF BUSINESS PARTNERSHIPS

CHIEF NEGOTIATOR

* At the time this chart was constructed, the county district operated 88 schools: 55 elementary schools (building average enrollment of 451), 13 middle schools (building average enrollment of 892), 12 high schools (building average enrollment of 1,176), 1 center for dropouts, 2 vocational centers, 3 special education centers, and 2 early childhood development centers.

changed in response to these priorities in ways that paralleled the bureaucratization of large hospitals, governmental agencies, factories, and society in general.

Schools are a special kind of bureaucratic organization. While they share characteristics with other bureaucracies—such as the prisons, factories, and social service agencies with which they often are compared—other characteristics conspire to make them unique. In addition to the particular historical, cultural, and economic context in which they developed, they are differentiated in the type, specificity, and number of their goals. Schools also are unique in the ways people can participate in them, and in their multiple lines of power and control. In the sections that follow we will discuss the special characteristics of school organization, how they affect the people who work in them, and some of the political and social forces that were critical to the development of contemporary schools.

Think about the organization of the high school you attended. How was it organized? Who controlled the school? Who were the people in power positions? How did they maintain this power? Do you think this organization was effective? Why or why not?

Schools as Modified Bureaucratic Organizations

Schools, like many organizations, possess some, but not all, of the characteristics of bureaucracies. For example, while teachers and other school staff are in fact hired for their professional training and skill, and while they do have job descriptions that encompass most of their required duties, they generally are rewarded for longevity rather than for merit. In addition, their written job description may not include many of their required duties, such as grading papers after school and being involved in extracurricular student activities (see Chapter 4 for a detailed description of teachers' work).

Multiple Constituencies and Multiple Goals

Ideally, bureaucracies have clear and unambiguous goals, and their leaders possess fairly complete control over the means for realizing those goals. School bureaucracies clearly do not fit this model. Schools actually have many organizational goals—some ambiguous or diffuse, and others contradictory. For example, schools are expected to provide training suited to each individual child while adhering to instructional guidelines based on single texts, uniform procedures, and mandated mastery of specific content.

Schools have multiple goals because they have multiple constituencies and clienteles, each with their own agenda and each pushing their own goals. Added to this is the unique mix of national, state, and local financial control. Few educational systems in the world and few social service agencies in the United States are as subject to external pressures as are the public schools in America, where the electorate controls the purse strings. Most school districts depend upon revenue from local property taxes, much of which comes from people who have no school-aged children. Furthermore, school officials cannot operate independent of their community because it is usually the public that chooses the school board. In addition, by law, school board meetings must be open to the public, and community and parent groups can exert powerful pressure regarding the content of textbooks and other instructional materials, as well as teaching techniques and extracurricular activities.

Local control encourages diversity in schools but it also makes them an arena in often bitter conflicts over cultural values. Tension is produced when the ideologies of the community are at odds with those of the school staff or of government agencies. Often these tensions arise over the substance and delivery of curricula. As we will discuss in Chapter 6, religious fundamentalists fight with advocates of secular education, and back-to-the-basics advocates vie with developmentalists and humanists for control over the curriculum. As Apple (1993) and Brouillette (1993) have described, these conflicts become especially heated in times of budgetary shortages. Hard choices have to be made among disparate goals: Closing the alternative high school for pregnant teens is balanced against the firing of 30 special education teachers, which is weighed against the elimination of reading and math specialists or the dismantling of the swim team and the choir. If compromise cannot be reached, the various interests may end up in court. Conflicts over school goals have been generated over bilingual education (*Lau et al.* v. *Nichols et al.* 1974) and ethnic studies, prayer in school (*Engel* v. *Vitale* 1962; *Abington School District* v. *Schempp* 1963), racial integration (*Brown* v. *Board of Education* 1955), free speech for students (*Tinker* v. *Des Moines* 1969), and the teaching of creationism and secular humanism (*Smith* v. *School Commissioners* 1987).

The real mission of schooling becomes blurred under the onslaught of so many constituencies, each seeking control over some portion of school activities. In many districts the result of such conflict is goal displacement.

Goal Displacement

Goal displacement (Sills 1970) is a common malady in bureaucratic organizations. It occurs when procedural activities—the dos, don'ts, and how-tos of organizational life—become more important than the reasons for which the organization was created. Goal displacement occurs when the resources intended for a given task are diverted to another purpose, or when the survival of a procedure or a group achieves greater importance than the purpose for which it was originally created. We also see goal displacement when the means become ends in themselves, that is, when some practice that was adopted to help solve a problem begins to interfere with the organization's original goals.

Goal displacement can be found, for example, in the proliferation of programs for assessing students and teachers. These were initiated to ensure that teachers were teaching what was required and that students had mastered the subject matter. However, in many districts such tests now drive the curriculum, taking up almost as much school time as teaching, and becoming the focus of instructional content.

Another example can be found in teachers' organizations' protecting tenure;

they have been accused of maintaining teacher jobs at the expense of quality instruction. Teachers resist the firing of colleagues for incompetence because the firing of one might call into question the competence of others. Schools may continue to employ teachers who are incompetent, or who are racists, or who do not like children, or who have come to detest teaching—because there are so many legal and institutional obstacles to firing them (see Dworkin 1985b). In these cases, more energy is spent in avoiding change than in carrying out the original mission of the organization.

Schools are particularly vulnerable to goal displacement. Many of the issues we discuss at length later in this chapter are illustrations. In considering the social organization of schools and the extent to which they resemble other modern bureaucracies, you may find it helpful to think about who controls the schools in your community and the extent to which patterns of control affect what schools ultimately can and should do. You also may wish to examine how the original intentions of innovative educational practices come to be subverted.

What examples of goal displacement can you describe from your own experiences with school organizations?

HOW SCHOOLS BECAME BUREAUCRACIES

A bureaucracy as a social organization is a relatively modern phenomenon which developed along with a capitalistic economic system, political nation-states, industrialization, and demographic shifts to urbanization. Small organizations with limited purposes do not need many employees and can operate under informal and unwritten rules. However, as they begin to involve more people and carry out more activities, additional levels of management and coordination are created. Specialized individuals are hired for complex, technical tasks. The process by which organizations increase in size and complexity, add levels of hierarchy and professionalism, and begin systematically to subdivide tasks is called *bureaucratization*. Bureaucratization is not limited to schooling; it has penetrated virtually every modern social institution.

Origins of the Common Elementary School

Schools have not always been structured as bureaucracies. The "little red schoolhouse" frequently had no more than one classroom, a coat room, a shed for firewood or coal, and a field outside for recess. Even in urban areas, school buildings housing hundreds of students were generally one large room with a teacher and monitors to help with the instruction (Spring 1986). The schools' services were limited to book learning. In elementary school the teachers instructed children in the basic cognitive skills of reading, writing, and computation. While there were no classes in science or social studies as such, textbooks like Noah Webster's *Blue-Back Speller* and the *McGuffey's Readers* contained heavy doses of instruction in these subjects, as well as in literature, morals, and social values such as thrift, hard work, cleanliness, patience, abstinence, and correct social behavior. Because educators were concerned primarily with transmitting cognitive skills and cultural knowledge, the number of nonteaching staff required was minimal. Teachers swept their own classrooms and lit the fires to keep them warm.

In 1848 John Philbrick introduced the Quincy School in Massachusetts, a radical new design with three floors containing multiple classrooms and a large assembly hall on the top floor. Each classroom was designed for a teacher and 56 students. This design was a step toward bureaucratization of schooling because it differentiated teaching and administrative roles. Tyack quotes Philbrick's specifications for staffing of this school:

> Let the Principal or Superintendent have the general supervision and control
> of the whole, and let him have one male assistant or sub-principal, and ten
> female assistants, one for each room. (1974, p. 45)

Tyack refers to this type of organization, with a male administrator and female teachers, as a "pedagogical harem." The Quincy School, with its sex-role differences and hierarchical bureaucratic structures, became the model for urban schools in the United States in the late nineteenth and early twentieth centuries (Spring 1986).

By the 1880s "school-keeping" practices had changed dramatically. A relatively coherent system of elementary, or "common," schools had been established in every state, and what we call the "service sector" of education had expanded exponentially. Growth in the service sector was a critical factor in the bureaucratization of schools because it rapidly expanded the number of functions that schools were expected to carry out.

Establishment of Public Secondary Schools

In the early years of the Republic the demand for education was fueled primarily by an educated elite desirous of passing their status on to their children by means of college-oriented liberal arts instruction. Beginning in the 1830s the middle and upper classes began to advocate that publicly supported instruction in basic literacy and morality be provided for economically disadvantaged children. The implicit purpose of this instruction was social control—to ensure the continuance of a productive labor force and to forestall the civil unrest, drunkenness, and immoral behavior to which it was felt an illiterate and unindoctrinated working class would be prone (Boutwell 1859; Mann 1842; Resnick and Resnick 1985).

Many industrialists, civic leaders, and educators supported mass education, as did the business community, which saw little difference between running factories and keeping school. Compulsory attendance laws became common between 1880 and 1920. Labor unions applauded the removal of competitive and inexpensive youths from the labor market. With the passage of the Smith-Hughes Act in 1917, secondary schools added vocational and non-college preparatory, or "general education," streams to accommodate advocates of "democratization." The comprehensive, nonselective public high school became known as a "poor man's college" and provided all the education most people needed.

By the end of the nineteenth century the general structure of the American public educational system, both elementary and secondary, had been established. The public sector provided free or nearly free instruction from elementary school through land-grant colleges and universities, although it was clear that only a minority would avail themselves of postsecondary schooling (Katz 1971). Bureaucratization had gradually developed from the increasing size and complexity of the educational enterprise. Schools acquired principals; superintendents were hired to supervise groups of schools; and standards for hiring teachers, certifying the quality of schools, and graduating students were put into place.

During the first three decades of the twentieth century, the school structure continued to evolve as supporters of a powerful industrial ideology urged the shaping of schools along the lines of the most efficient American factories. The following sections draw heavily on the work of critical and revisionist historians such as Michael B. Katz, Joel Spring, Clarence Karier, Raymond E. Callahan, and Marvin Lazerson, who have questioned the conventional view that schools were established to support democratic and egalitarian ideals. While these ideals did motivate some supporters of public education, critical historians note how schools acted largely to reinforce existing patterns of social and economic inequality and benefit members of the dominant culture.

Addition of the Service Sector

The service sector began to develop in the late 1800s as civic leaders, educators, industrialists, and the churches targeted the elementary schools for the monumental task of upgrading the social and moral level of immigrant and working-class children. Between 1865 and 1900, 14 million immigrants were known to have entered the United States. Between 1876 and 1926 over 27 million immigrated, a number that exceeded the 1875 population by 50 percent. Whereas the original migrants were from England and Northern Europe, most of the newcomers during this later period were rural dwellers from central, southern, and eastern Europe whose languages, skills, habits, and ethnicity differed drastically from those of the established residents (Butts 1978, p. 229). Immigrants have continued to arrive at a rate of about one million per year (Callahan 1962). Since the 1970s, the greatest pressure for entrance to the United States has been from Latin Americans and Asians, especially from Southeast Asia.

It is difficult to imagine the fear that immigrants and the working class struck in the hearts of the affluent. Whether they were the Irish of the early nineteenth century, the southern and eastern Europeans later in the nineteenth century, or the Jews who came even later, unassimilated immigrants were viewed in America with the same suspicion as card-carrying Communists were during the "Red Scares" of the 1930s and 1950s, and as illegal aliens were in the 1980s and 1990s. They were portrayed as vicious, immoral, mentally deficient, lazy, unhygienic, and a threat to the social and moral fiber of the nation.

Part of the fear came from culture shock. The immigrants differed from established residents in language, religion, standard of living, and customs. Most important, they were—and still are—accused of taking jobs from the native-born. They also had little power and few influential advocates in government to oversee their interests (Higham 1969; The Massachusetts Teacher 1851). Established residents viewed education as a way to counteract the threat that immigrants posed to the social order. The type of education advocated was, however, a departure from prevailing practice. As the characteristics and needs of immigrants changed, pressures to provide appropriate education for them have also changed the schools.

Principal among the factors mandating social services to immigrants and the poor was growth of class conflict during the late 1800s. It was exacerbated by an almost rabid fear dominant groups had of immigrants and the lower classes. Concerns for law and order fueled the desire of policy makers to "Americanize" immigrant children as quickly as possible and to indoctrinate the working-class children with middle-class values (Higham 1969). Service programs were used to accelerate this process.

The service sector of schooling includes a wide variety of noninstructional activities such as medical inspections (1894), health and nutritional services (beginning in the early 1900s), rehabilitation for the handicapped (the 1920s), and school lunches (as an emergency measure during the Depression and made permanent in 1946). Legislation that was part of the War on Poverty in the 1960s added programs to reduce racial prejudice as well as a variety of support services, including dental care, clothing banks, free or low-cost breakfasts, after-school care, sex education and drug abuse advice, programs for pregnant girls, and mental and physical health counseling. Provision of these services has contributed substantially to the transformation of schools into large, complex, bureaucratic institutions.

Several themes provided impetus for the provision of social services. One was custodial and came from the belief that poor families were unable or unwilling to provide proper care for their children (Gumbert and Spring 1974). Another was the humanitarian acknowledgement that sick, hungry, and poorly clad children were too preoccupied with their physical needs to study. For families living in one-room apartments and amid grinding poverty, schools and settlement houses often were the only places where children could be fed, bathed, provided warm clothing, and given minimal medical care (Albjerg 1974; Butts and Cremin 1953; The Massachusetts Teacher 1851).

Schools as Custodians of Children

Over time, the school has become an all-purpose child-care institution whose services go far beyond training in the "three Rs." As the custodial functions of schools grew, teachers and administrators took on more responsibility for the health, well-being, and good behavior of young people—even in areas once considered the exclusive province of families and the private sector.

Some of these services, like drug, pregnancy, and prenatal counseling, day care, and driver education, are attempts to alleviate social problems, such as the many students who drop out because they become parents and the rising incidence of automobile-related fatalities. Other services, such as training in the performing arts, are designed to provide opportunities once available only to the wealthy. Still others, such as free lunches and medical exams, attest to our recognition that sick and hungry

The Fate of Goose Pond Alternative Jr./Sr. High School

Discussion of Goose Pond, the Cottonwood District's well-respected alternative school, occurred when there had just been a significant shift in the composition of the school board. Goose Pond had served seriously at-risk students since the 1970s. It was integral to the District's major stated goal: success for all students. Housed in an historic school building, it offered an individualized student-centered program with a 15:1 student teacher ratio. Though effective, Goose Pond was an expensive school to run, and its building was in need of repair. While previous school boards had supported the school, the agenda of the new school board was fiscally conservative. Noting the need for general financial retrenchment, board members questioned the amount of money to be spent on the Goose Pond facility. Stating that the district should not delude itself into believing it could heal all the world's ills, they targeted the school for closure. Dr. Roberts, the superintendent opposed the closing as openly as his status as a school employee would allow, knowing it was pivotally important that he maintain good relations with board members. They, however, rejected his argument that more funding should be assigned to help those most in need, arguing that social work should be left to social work agencies. According to their view, achieving the greatest good for the greatest number of students meant maintaining strong programs district-wide. In time of financial austerity, they felt, the district could not afford to keep open what they considered to be an inefficient school, despite a strong consensus among Cottonwood staff that the alternative school should remain open.

SOURCE: Brouillette 1993.

children cannot learn. Finally, some, such as classes and support services for the physically and emotionally handicapped, are congruent with the belief that all children—regardless of their motivation, aspirations, or limitations—are entitled to an appropriate, free education until age 21 or graduation from high school. Adding social service functions, with the accompanying resources and staff, has hastened bureaucratization. It also has added controversy, because the many constituencies who participate in and finance the schools seldom achieve a consensus as to whether these programs are legitimate school functions—as the controversy over Goose Pond Alternative School illustrates (see box).

A distinct feature of bureaucratization of schools in America was that, since there are no explicit constitutional provisions for schooling, states assumed responsibility for public education. Unlike in most other countries, where there is centralized national control, state and local boards oversee educational responsibilities. Placing school finance and governance under the control of local boards laid the groundwork for racial and economic inequality, because rich communities had more resources than poor ones. The public school system co-existed with independent private schools, whose numbers varied by region and which generally served special interests such as religious groups, those favoring alternative education, and the wealthy.

Urbanization, Consolidation, and Scientific Management

After World War II, global changes in the distribution of population, natural resources, trade, the labor market, and technology, as well as urbanization, industrialization, and changes in the labor force (Chafetz and Dworkin 1986) affected every facet of human existence and gave birth to modern society. In addition, during the past two centuries industrialization has caused the poor and landless to migrate to cities in every corner of the globe. Urbanization of the poor has increased the percentage of the economically disadvantaged (Chafetz and Dworkin 1986). It has also profoundly affected the locally controlled "little red schoolhouse."

The little red schoolhouse model was sufficient for relatively homogeneous small communities, but today more than 75 percent of the U.S. population lives in cities, where economic and ethnic diversity has exploded both the myth of the middle class and the myth of the melting pot. Concentration of the population into cities was accompanied by pressure for universal and compulsory education, in part because American cultural ideology promoted education as a means to improve one's social and economic condition. Education was no longer viewed as appropriate only for the affluent. It was needed both for nation building and for provision of the skills requisite for an industrial nation. However, pressures to expand educational opportunities often were conservative. While public education was, in fact, provided for children of the working classes and the poor, its content was different from the classical liberal arts training for the wealthy; it was more practical, oriented to civic training, and geared toward job preparation. Educational reform was equated with creating social and economic stability. It was a way to avoid taking more radical steps to solve problems such as urban poverty and social disorder (Katz 1971; LeCompte and Dworkin 1991).

THE SCIENTIFIC MANAGEMENT OF SCHOOLS

At the turn of the century America's cultural heroes were industrialists—Andrew Carnegie, John D. Rockefeller, J. P. Morgan, and others. Belief in the efficacy and virtue of big business and industry saturated American life. It was a logical extension of the "can-do" spirit of the legendary pioneers. Americans firmly believed that success—defined in terms of material acquisition—was the result of honesty and hard work. In keeping with another cultural myth—that America was an egalitarian, classless society (see Chapter 5 for further discussion of the "myth of the middle class")— they also believed that success had very little to do with social background or education. Since Americans tended to believe that businesspeople had made America great, they also believed that the best way to solve all problems was to subject them to good business practice. This notion meant that the value of any commodity, enterprise, or person was measured by marketability, the tangible contribution to sale value, or the ability of someone to get ahead.

The Rise of Taylorism

These ideas were embodied in a philosophy called "Scientific Management," whose chief exponent was an industrial engineer named Frederick W. Taylor. Taylor first came to prominence in 1910 when his theories of management were used as evidence in a widely publicized hearing before the Interstate Commerce Commission. The railroads had asked for an increase in freight rates to compensate them for higher wages granted to railroad workers. The government's lawyer, Louis Brandeis, argued in opposition that the railroads were being operated inefficiently and that if they introduced Taylor's new techniques of scientific management, they would be able to increase wages *and* also reduce costs. Taylor also suggested that his approach would result in more productivity from fewer workers. His ideas took the industrialized world by storm and were applied to everything from baking cakes and sewing trousers to carrying ingots of pig iron and getting students to study harder. Taylor's "scientific" operating principles included the following:

1. Management must be responsible for analyzing, planning, and controlling every detail of the manufacturing process.
2. Management must use scientific methods to identify the best methods for performing each aspect of every task carried out in the plant.
3. Each step in each task must be standardized, and tools must be developed that are appropriate both to the task and to the workers who are to carry it out.
4. Planning departments must be established to develop the science of each job, including the rules, laws, and formulae for its execution. These rules will replace judgments made by individual workers about how their work should be done.
5. Detailed records must be kept of every activity and transaction so that accountability can be established and traced.
6. Managers must carefully train workers in the exact execution of their tasks and must closely supervise them to make sure that they are following directions.
7. Assessment procedures must be established so that performance can be measured and exemplary performance can be rewarded.

Taylor's system which placed all power in the hands of managers and planners, introduced a rationale for meticulous observation, testing, and recordkeeping, and wrested from workers any control over the execution of their tasks. While it was criticized by individuals in industry and universities, the voices of protest were drowned out by the chorus of enthusiasm for a process that appeared to increase productivity while reducing costs. The outcry coincided exactly with a wave of dissatisfaction over the public schools (Callahan 1962).

Waste, Inefficiency, and "Laggards" in Our Schools

If businesspeople were the most capable individuals in America, then it stood to reason that they should be intimately involved in public institutions such as schools. The political reform movement of the early 1900s, generated from distrust of political machines, encouraged a shift away from political appointment of administrators. Council-manager forms of municipal government, in which an elected council hired a professional city manager, became popular because they were congruent with the desire for management by scientifically trained professionals rather than amateurs. School districts soon followed suit. Instead of hiring teachers to run the schools, they chose "professionals" — graduates from colleges of education that provided what purported to be professional training for school administrators. Communities elected to school boards businesspeople who evaluated school operation by the same criteria they used for factories. Educators became vulnerable to the same kinds of criticism as factory workers and managers: Why couldn't the product be manufactured more efficiently and at less cost?

Report after report alleged that educators were sadly lacking in both business acumen and accounting skills. Many could neither account for nor justify their expenditure of the taxpayers' money to the satisfaction of their boards and communities (Callahan 1962). Schools also were criticized for retaining large numbers of "laggards," or children who were over the normal age for their grade level. No one examined whether the so-called "retarded" children were immigrants with insufficient mastery of English for the work at their age level or whether they had been held back because they had failed courses. School efficiency came to be defined in terms of how fast children could be pushed through the grades: An "efficient" school had every child on grade level for his or her age, regardless of extenuating circumstances. Double-promotion or skipping grades was widely used as a cost-saving measure. Course offerings were judged by their cost per pupil and their utility in moving students right into jobs, notwithstanding any measure of intrinsic worth or external cost. School administrators also were criticized for the amount of time their buildings stood unused—in the summer, during holidays, and at night.

Solving such problems by application of businesslike practices accelerated the process of routinization, specialization, and bureaucratization. Pressured by taxpayers and school boards, superintendents had to go back to school to learn new methods. At universities, they became steeped in scientific management, a doctrine wholeheartedly embraced by education programs. With their degrees in hand, newly minted professional school administrators altered curricula, supervisory techniques, and instruction accordingly (Callahan 1962).

The Legacy of Scientific Management

Most of the changes introduced from 1915 to 1930, the heyday of the efficiency expert, were major departures from the tradition of "school-keeping." These changes became permanent and have welded the educational establishment ever closer to the image of corporate and bureaucratic America. Perhaps the most obvious change was the addition of a management stratum to the hierarchy. Teachers could no longer rise into administration without special training. While administrators still come through the ranks—most educational administration programs require three years of teaching—the requirement of a "professional" credential is here to stay. It is nearly impossible to be hired as a school administrator without certification from an approved graduate program.

Other changes were made in recordkeeping to codify attendance procedures, financial records, curricula, and time allocations for instruction. Many of the changes were needed to introduce system and rationalization into an enterprise that had become increasingly chaotic (Butts 1978). However, they also were harbingers of the paperwork avalanche which often overwhelms today's school staff.

The impact of Taylorism was also felt in equipment and design. Time-and-motion study experts developed tools suitable to both the job and the worker—for example, chairs that fit children's bodies and are an appropriate size, lighting that is adequate for reading, left-handed scissors, and big crayons which are easy for small children to hold. The efficiency bureaus established in some districts have evolved into departments of research, testing, and evaluation.

The efficiency movement also left more mixed blessings. One is the continued interest in split sessions and the year-round school as a solution to overcrowded buildings. More pervasive is the "platoon school" or "Gary Plan." The Gary Plan, named after the city in Indiana where the experiment was implemented, was based on the idea that schools would be more efficient if no room ever were empty. Space could be saved if one group—or platoon—of students were outside on the playground at all times so their classroom could be used by another group. Implementing such a plan required subdividing of the students, careful scheduling, and constant movement of people among the available rooms. It subordinated instruction to the dictates of a time clock, interrupting instruction regardless of student interest or the difficulty of the subject matter. Teachers could no longer decide how to allocate their instructional time, and students were ever more rigidly divided into batches by age rather than ability or intellectual interest. The Gary Plan lives on in the hallways of today's middle and high schools, as students move in batches every 50 minutes to a different classroom.

Taylor's human cost accounting survives in practices such as treating teachers as "FTEs" (full-time equivalents, or the number of workers multiplied by the number of hours worked each day), and demanding that course offerings justify their existence not on the merit of the material or the rigor of the course, but on the basis of per-unit cost calculated in "credit hour generation," or the number of students enrolled per course. Other accounting survivors include determining graduation requirements by counting "Carnegie units" (a specified number of hours taught in a given subject area), and the per-pupil-expenditure figures which appear before every school election.

The practices that probably have had the most impact upon the daily life of students and teachers include "Taylorizing" the curriculum into easily taught, measurable objectives, and the massive systems of testing students, teachers, and even administrators for academic competency and achievement. These practices, often instituted as part of educational reform measures, act systematically to **de-skill** teachers, removing from their control decisions over how and what to teach, as well as their prerogative to evaluate student progress. We discuss the impact of these practices in detail in Chapters 4 and 6.

The Impact of Scientific Management on Teacher Autonomy

Perhaps the most ominous legacy of scientific management is the authoritarianism built into Frederick Taylor's insistence on three principles: (1) granting managers absolute control over the definition, assignment, and assessment of tasks; (2) breaking down tasks into discrete, measurable subunits, and (3) requiring the complete and unthinking acquiescence of laborers in everything employers asked them to do. When applied to schools, these principles ultimately removed jurisdiction over instruction from teachers and changed the pattern of control and decision making in schools.

By the time Taylorism hit the schools in the 1920s, some shifts of control already had occurred. Many of the most important curricular decisions were being made outside the classroom. For example, accreditation agencies, school boards, administrators, and textbook committees decided what courses should be taught and which books would be used. All that remained to the teacher were how to teach the material and how to manage the children. Proponents of scientific management proposed that even these decisions be made centrally. On the grounds that teachers worked inefficiently at best, and could not be trusted to cover material adequately and objectively, curriculum and instruction were increasingly made "teacher proof."

"Professional educators"—usually university professors and administrators rather than classroom teachers—broke down instructional tasks into measurable "behavioral objectives" and then prescribed how they should be taught. While these practices organized and standardized instruction and facilitated assessment of results, they also prevented teachers from deciding what, in their professional judgment, was most valuable to teach and how to teach it. Teachers also no longer could rely exclusively on their own judgment for assessment of student ability. Children were grouped for instruction on the basis of external tests. Teachers were assigned textbooks which might or might not match the ability levels of their students. They were given scripted lessons which prescribed children's answers, and tests with which to assess student progress. Good instructional objectives were those accompanied by specified reading materials. Usually these also required a great deal of recordkeeping by the teacher—records that ostensibly were used to chart the children's progress but also could be used to monitor the teacher's conformity with the curriculum.

These reforms had the effect of enforcing progress. Teachers had to move their students through a certain number of curricular units per semester whether or not they felt the material had been covered adequately. Teachers could, of course, resist the imposition of lock-step curricula to some extent by relying on the autonomy of the closed door. They also could—and do—wait until the current wave of new ideas passes, a new superintendent is hired, or a new set of reforms are set in motion at the national level.

Management by Objectives in Cottonwood

Dr. Roberts explained that during the years prior to his arrival, "the district had received national recognition for the implementation of Outcomes-Based education and Computer-Managed instruction. It was also very centralized. Most major decisions and plans for implementation evolved directly from the central office administrators with little opportunity for input by those expected to implement the decision [the teachers]." And, as a curriculum specialist recounted: "We 'Benjamin-Bloomed' everything. I don't know whether you remember that era when objectives were the thing. We were all trained in writing objectives. In fact, I've had a number of courses from various universities on instructional objectives, goal setting, that sort of thing. So the district ended up, in every discipline, with an entire objective based curriculum. We wrote in that 86 percent of the teachers had to support an objective or it was revised or deleted. That became our curriculum."

SOURCE: Brouillette 1993.

As you continue through this chapter, ask yourself the following questions:
    How is your daily life in schools affected by practices grounded in scientific management?
    Can you identify features of your experiences that are governed by principles of efficiency rather than of good teaching and learning?

Schooling and the Hegemony of Corporate America

Schools now are criticized for mirroring corporate America and for too closely resembling factories. We need to remember, however, that the forces that led to bureaucratization were unleashed because people believed they led to highly desirable outcomes. The tenets of scientific management were introduced to the schools under the banner of the best-intentioned democratic reform. The alacrity with which scientific management was embraced illustrates just how powerful external control or "hegemonic domination" over education can be, as we discussed in Chapter 1.

    Because educators had so completely accepted the legitimacy of business ideology, no force was needed to induce them to adopt the structure, language, and practices of business. They did not foresee that scientific management had other, less desirable consequences. While the factory model was marketed on the basis of fostering efficiency, hard work, and entrepreneurship, it did not, in fact, train entrepreneurs. On the contrary, it fostered obedience rather than the risk-taking and nonconformity of industrial capitalism's early heroes. For this reason, the factory schools were most popular in the industrialized central cities, where the majority of the poor and working class lived, where financial shortages mandated money-saving practices, and where a hard-working, obedient labor force was needed by industry. There, schools that mirrored life in the factories flourished. In more affluent areas the rigidities and excesses of Taylorism were blunted, and the extras that were deemed wasteful by the efficiency experts, such as foreign languages, Greek, and smaller classes, survived to differentiate the education of the rich from that of the poor.

RESISTANCE TO SCIENTIFIC MANAGEMENT: RESTRUCTURING AND REFORM

Schools have continued to resemble factories, even those in campus-like structures. In fact, school reform legislation in the 1980s, which concentrated on entrance and graduation standards and the content and structure of instruction, accelerated the process. However, counterpressures are growing. Teachers, principals, parents, and others are exhibiting growing disenchantment with centralized control and their disenfranchisement in the educational enterprise. As early as the 1960s, decentralization movements constituted a critique of the increasing consolidation of schools for the sake of efficiency. In the sections that follow we will recount a brief history of efforts to reform the organization of schooling and instruction.

A Definition of Restructuring

In the 1980s a new buzzword, **restructuring,** emerged to describe any number of efforts to reform the schools. As an approach to educational change, it has been called the "garbage can" of school reform (Elmore and Associates 1990) because of its capacity to encompass almost any kind of change imaginable, or a "garage-like approach" to reform (Goldwasser 1994) because, like a garage, one can fit almost any kind of reform in it. Critical to our discussion, however, is that restructuring efforts constitute a rejection of the centralized governance and reductionist curricula advocated by descendants of Taylorism.

In general, restructuring involves one or more of the following:

1. Changes in the distribution of power between schools and their clients or in the governance structure within which schools operate
2. Changes in the occupational situation of educators, including conditions of entry and licensing of teachers and administrators
3. Changes in school structure, conditions of work, and decision-making processes within schools
4. Changes in the way teaching and learning occur or in the core technology of schooling (Elmore and Associates 1990)

Interview a school administrator who has been in your school district for a long time about the changes in organization over the past decade or more. What are some of these changes? What does this administrator think about the ways the bureaucracy has changed?

Decentralization: The Predecessor of Restructuring

The original idea for contemporary restructuring probably can be found in the decentralization movements to counteract extreme bureaucratic rigidity in large city school districts (Elmore 1990; Hess 1991; LeCompte and Dworkin 1991; Rogers 1968; Tyack 1990). The focus of decentralization is the structure of school district governance. It attempts first to dismantle nonresponsive, alienating, corrupt, top-heavy and expensive bureaucracies (LeCompte and Dworkin 1991). Decentralization was designed to make educational systems more responsive and accessible by reducing the size of the unit that people had to deal with daily and by locating administration in the community it controlled. Furthermore, it represented a reversal of the consolidation movement that had drastically decreased the number of districts over the previous 50 years (Tyack 1990).

Ocean-Hill-Brownsville in New York City (Rogers 1968) and the Woodlawn Experimental School District (LeCompte 1969) were efforts at this type of reform and paved the way for other large districts to decentralize and become more responsive to community diversity. Movements for decentralization were particularly attractive to community groups because they included a strong push for community, especially parent, involvement.

During the 1960s and 1970s this kind of decentralization was encouraged by federally funded projects which required "maximum feasible participation" (LeCompte 1972) in the form of citizen advisory boards, community liaison individuals, and the encouragement of Parent Teacher Organizations as a condition of funding. However, participation usually degenerated into tokenism or the continual recruiting of the same few members of the community who could be counted on not to rock the boat (Deyhle 1992; Reyes and Halcon 1988; Stern 1987). Further, increased community control, even as radical an approach as that documented by Hess (1991), has not proved a sufficient remedy for the unresponsiveness of "pathological bureaucracy" (Rogers 1968) or for low pupil achievement.

The "Excellence Movement": Standards for Students

Much of the current rhetoric surrounding restructuring can be construed as a reaction to the "excellence movement" of 1983–1986, which initially blamed poor student performance for the alleged demise of American educational quality. The excellence movement was given impetus by a large number of federal commissions and study groups whose charge was to examine the supposed fragile state of education in America. Their influence was typified by the report of the National Commission on Excellence in Education, *A Nation at Risk: The Imperative for Educational Reform*

Graduation Requirements

In order to receive a regular high school diploma, students must correctly answer at least 70% of the questions in each of the two sections—mathematics and language arts—of the Tennessee proficiency test, and shall have attained an approved record of attendance and conduct. In addition, verified handicapped students must have completed an individual educational program as confirmed by a multidisciplinary team. Regular students must complete 20 units of course work.

SOURCE: Quote from county school district publication, Tennessee.

(1983), and the Holmes Group's report, *Tomorrow's Teachers* (1986). *A Nation at Risk* described the failure of American education as a "rising tide of mediocrity that threatens our very future as a nation and a people."

The first wave of the excellence movement attempted to improve student performance by increasing the standards (see examples of increased graduation requirements in Table 2.1) to be met for promotion and graduation and by ensuring the competency of teachers to provide high-quality instruction. The mechanisms instituted in all 50 states included (1) increasing requirements for student graduation, (2) intensifying standardized testing, (3) establishing minimal competency standards

TABLE 2.1 Graduation Requirements[a]

Students Entering Ninth Grade in School Years:	1983–84 through 1990–91	1991–92 and 1992–93	1993–94	1994–95
English Language Arts	4	4	4	4
Mathematics	2	2	3	3[b]
Science	2	2	2	2
U.S. History	1	1	1	1
Economics	$\frac{1}{2}$	$\frac{1}{2}$	$\frac{1}{2}$	$\frac{1}{2}$
U.S. Government	$\frac{1}{2}$	$\frac{1}{2}$	$\frac{1}{2}$	$\frac{1}{2}$
Physical Education	1	1	1	1
Health Education	$\frac{1}{2}$	$\frac{1}{2}$	$\frac{1}{2}$	$\frac{1}{2}$
Free Electives	$8\frac{1}{2}$	7	7	7
Limited Electives	0	$1\frac{1}{2}$	$\frac{1}{2}$	$\frac{1}{2}$
TOTAL	20	20	20	20

[a]Graduation requirements taken from 1994 Tennessee county school district publication. Limited electives are to be chosen from among Mathematics, Science, World History, World Geography, Ancient History, Modern History, and European History.
[b]Beginning with the 1994–95 ninth-grade students, one of the three mathematics units must be earned in Algebra I, Math for Technology II, or the equivalent in an integrated mathematics curriculum incorporating standards of the National Council of Teachers of Mathematics.

for both teachers and students, and (4) tying teacher accountability to standardized test scores. With the "tide of mediocrity" decried by *A Nation at Risk* came metaphorical secondary waves of reform, one of which was restructuring.

Teacher Competence: "Excellence" for Teachers

Calls for improved student performance were soon seen to be empty without concomitant improvement in instruction. As a remedy, the second wave of excellence proposed a major revamp of training programs—including eliminating the baccalaureate degree in teaching and extending the program by a year—and a variety of methods for stimulating better teaching, including differentiated staffing, merit pay, and other incentives. Finally it was proposed that incompetent teachers simply be fired.

Beginning in the 1980s state departments of education became heavily involved in testing teachers' competency—so that those who failed even after remediation could be fired (see Shepard and Kreitzer 1987)—and in mandating the establishment of "career ladders" for teachers. Some of these proposals are a legacy from Taylorism and the 1930s efficiency experts, but they also are linked to the national educational reform movement of the 1980s. The establishment of state test development offices along with staff for assessment and enforcement, like the compensatory programs in the 1960s, increased the bureaucratization of state-level agencies and reduced local control over recruitment and promotion of staff and students.

"Excellence" reforms have been quite popular because they are relatively easy to institute. They avoid attacks on entrenched political interests because they do not radically alter basic structure, and they affect only those with the least power: teachers and students. They also have demonstrated little real impact on academic achievement or teacher performance (Malen and Hart 1987). Many of the proposed reforms, especially competency tests for in-service teachers and some of the schemes for accountability, have actually been detrimental. Competency testing in particular has done substantial damage to teacher morale (Dworkin 1985b; Shepard and Kreitzer 1987). Further, attempts to transform instruction by changing standards for teacher training are ineffective because schools cannot really be reformed with *new* teachers. New teachers represent only a fraction of the teaching staff. Reforms must be implemented with the existing teacher cadre, many of whom disagree with or do not understand what is being asked of them, while many more are burned out, entrapped, disinterested, isolated, or uncaring (LeCompte and Dworkin 1991).

Site-Based and Shared Decision Making

Building-level decentralization has been termed school-based or *site-based management.* Its purpose is to increase creativity and responsiveness to community needs (LeCompte and Dworkin 1991). Site-based management has now been appropriated wholesale by proponents of restructuring, though it began long before the term *restructuring* had the currency it now enjoys.

Site-based management devolves authority to a specific building principal, who is given far more control over the selection of curricula and instructional techniques, and sometimes over hiring and firing and budgetary matters. Depending upon how it is instituted, site-based management may or may not involve *shared decision making,* which gives additional power to other constituents in the school—teachers, parents, and students. It is this form of decentralization—or restructuring—that has been the primary locus of rhetoric surrounding empowerment. Because it includes lower participants (Merton 1967) (such as parents, teachers, students, noncertified staff, and local businesspeople) in decision making, and even gives them some areas of at least partial authority, it constitutes a shift of power away from higher participants (such as central office staff or middle management). Hence it "empowers" the lower participants.

However, site-based management is not a clearly defined term, nor is it without controversy. A number of studies have shown that teachers, administrators, and policy makers disagree over what should be managed at the site and by whom (Brouillette 1993; Goldwasser 1994; Hart 1990; LeCompte and Wiertelak 1992). For example, Dr. Roberts of Cottonwood School District clearly distinguished between site-based *management* and site-based *decision making* (see the box).

When major decisions remain the province of administrators, however, teachers retreat, as they did in the Pinnacle School District (LeCompte & Wiertelak, 1992). Site-based management also contributes to difficulty in overall district-wide planning, especially if principals take seriously a mandate to run their own schools as they think best. As Brouillette's (1993) careful ethnohistory of a site-based school district indicates, some principals use the latitude this gives them to initiate programs that subvert or counter the philosophy of the superintendent.

Interview a veteran teacher about changes in the school organization since she or he began teaching. What were some of these changes and what does this teacher think about them?

Dr. Roberts's Distinctions

Since my background reflected a participative approach to management, one of the things I began to do during my first year was to talk about decentralizing decisions that traditionally had been associated with the central office. . . . But site-based *management* is a misnomer. Site-based management [implies] that teachers, community members and others are going to be involved in managing the schools. This is not the case with our site-based decision making. The management of schools is an administrative function and people should understand from the very beginning that this movement is not intended to move the managerial functions from building principals and other administrators to staff and/or members of the community.

SOURCE: Brouillette 1993.

A Teacher's Retreat from Management

Site-based management just means teachers have to do what administrators should be doing. We have enough to do without having to run the school, too. What we have here in our district is "room-based management," not site-based management. I don't have any power to run the district, but that's OK. They just leave me alone. And I'm free to manage my own classroom the way I think is best.

SOURCE: LeCompte and Wiertelak 1992.

Changing Control of Teaching and Learning

A third kind of restructuring is *not* organizationally based but involves altering relationships of control in the content and delivery of instruction, so that the experience, knowledge, and participation of children are given more weight in the learning process. Some of the most active restructuring of this nature has come in language arts, especially in whole language programs. Many whole language advocates have appropriated the rhetoric of empowerment. Assuming that functional literacy empowers individuals by giving them "voice," they utilize a number of strategies to increase children's ability to make decisions about how they learn. One common strategy is to involve students in the choice of what they do, either by providing a cafeteria of learning centers or by letting them write stories on topics (or even in the language [Reyes and Laliberty 1992]) of their choosing.

Proponents suggest that by increasing skill levels in critical reading, writing, and inquiry skills, individuals develop a greater sense of self-awareness, which in turn leads to empowerment. This empowerment permits not only *recognition* of the forces that oppose disempowered or oppressed individuals, but also a *showdown* between individuals and the social structures that oppress them (Apple 1982; Ellsworth 1989; Freire 1970, 1985; Giroux 1983a, 1983b, 1988; Gitlin and Smyth 1989; McLaren 1989). Literacy then serves as a vehicle to social reform or revolution, depending upon the orientation of the writer (LeCompte and Bennett 1992).

Both critical theorists and curriculum theorists have drawn on the language, if not the procedures, used by liberation theorists such as Paulo Freire to justify their approach (LeCompte and Bennett 1990). However, much of the actual practice remains rooted in instructional practice and is not informed by social science theory. Often these pedagogical approaches promote methods that are most effective for middle-class children and do not take into account the special needs of other groups, thus rendering the techniques useless if not actually harmful (Delpit 1988; LeCompte and Bennett 1992; Richardson et al. 1989).

Find out what school reforms currently are being advocated in your community. Who is backing them? What problems are they meant to address? Do you think they will be effective?

The Juxtaposition of Restructuring and Empowerment

Considerable attention has been paid over the years to changes in the structure and content of the curriculum (Kaestle 1983; Kliebard 1986; Liston and Ziechner 1991; Tyack 1990), but the current calls for change explicitly link curricular and organizational changes with the concept of empowerment. In the forefront are some school–university collaborative projects initiated by critical theorists as a way to train teachers to be change agents, "critical pedagogues," and "transformative intellectuals" (Giroux 1988).

These new projects almost always, and we believe erroneously, link the terms *empowerment* and *restructuring.* The latter term refers to structural change in *systems* and implies a change in the locus of authority; the former refers to the psychological change in *individuals,* which presumably occurs as a consequence of structural change. The problem is that educators often are unclear as to which comes first, and how either is supposed to be generated. Lack of empowerment (that is, oppression), as described by critical theorists, is a consequence of unequal social relationships, and the presumed remedy uses a structural change model. As described by educators, however, increasing empowerment among lower participants requires a mental health model. With its focus on individuals, it is often vague or silent on structural change issues. As a consequence, it can be held accountable to charges of "blaming the victims" of oppression for not having empowered themselves.

It is an open question whether or not these programs will have a major effect on the power structure of schools. A major impediment seems to be that empowerment is based upon a model of participatory democracy, which seldom has proven long-lasting except in very small and homogeneous communities. And school districts and their constituencies, as we have noted in this chapter, are anything but small and homogeneous!

Two other factors mitigate against the success of entirely participative models such as those advocated by their two most active proponents, John Goodland and his I.D.E.A. model, and Theodore Sizer's Coalition for Essential Schools. The first, as Michael Apple (1993) suggests, is the general lack of cultural support for participatory decision making. Apple asserts that participatory democracy evolved in the small, homogeneous religious communities of New England and eventually became the town meetings still found in small communities in the region. However, the class and cultural patterns that facilitated this form of egalitarian decision making did not prevail throughout the United States. In no other part of the country did this secular form of governance succeed.

A second mitigating factor is the lack of support for shared decision making within the schools themselves. School practice has, for decades, emphasized a top-down form of management, whose justification is enshrined in standard business practice and embodied in scientific management. Furthermore, while "Small is beautiful" (Schumacher 1989) might have guided proponents of private schools, in the business of public education smallness has been expensive or impractical. Given these traditions, practices such as school-based management, which give principals and teachers primary control and empower communities to share in the overall direction of schooling, are unlikely to be viewed with open enthusiasm by the current educational administrations.

If you had the power to change the organization of schooling within a school district, how would you do it? Why?

SUMMARY

In this chapter, we have described the organization and control of school systems in America. Our goal has been to provide a context for the rest of the book, which describes the process of schooling and its impact upon participants. We hope that you have begun to understand that schools and educational programs are not neutral. In fact, they exist in a highly politically charged arena. Because schools have more contact with children than any other social institution (excluding the family), and because they are the single agency most amenable to public manipulation, the groups who control the schools have a profound impact on indoctrination and training of future generations. We believe that sociologist Max Weber is correct in stating that it is possible to tell a great deal about the power structure and patterns of social differentiation in a society if you can determine how the schools are organized, the content of instruction, and who benefits from attendance. In the chapters that follow we will explore these issues.

chapter 3

Youth Culture and the Student Peer Group

INTRODUCTION

Most sociology of education texts look at all aspects of schooling—curriculum, staff, hierarchy, buildings, unions, testing—except for the students for whom schools are intended. Notwithstanding, most studies of young people are carried out in schools, because that is where they are most accessible. Researchers seem to assume that schools are the only places children spend time. Perhaps this convenient fiction exists because schools are the aspect of the collective life of children most firmly controlled by adults.

Because researchers study children primarily in school, they have attributed far more prominence to school-related activities in children's lives than may be valid. Because we believe that the out-of-school events are at least as important as are those occurring in school, we will look closely at both types.

Until recently the voices of students simply have not been heard, even to describe what schools really mean to them. (See LeCompte & Preissle 1992 for a review of research on student perceptions of schooling.) As we shall see, how students actually feel about school often diverges widely from what educators would prefer. In fact, schools have lost a great deal of centrality in the attitudes and values of students. Furthermore, students' attitudes toward school are at least as important in shaping their educational experiences as how they are taught or how school is organized. An increasing number of children have become convinced that schools have little to offer them. In response they have become mentally, if not physically, absent from school more than they are present. For many, what goes on outside school is far more important. Teachers no longer can assume that their pupils share their views about the value of education. How long students stay in school, how committed they feel, and the quality of their performance often depend upon their social class, race, and gender as well as characteristics of the community, pressures from outside the school, and attributes of the school itself.

The term *student* refers to a social role and, unlike the term *child*, depends upon enrollment in an educational institution. Successfully enacting the role of "student" means mastering certain institutional requirements, whereas being a child does not. In this chapter we distinguish between children *as children* and children *as students*, in order to highlight the importance of out-of-school events to children and to their lives as students.

The first part of this chapter is devoted to the process of growing up and how it has changed. We define the terms **peer group, adolescence,** and **youth culture** and trace their development. We suggest that the cultural content of any given youth group is context-specific and that, while all young people face common developmental, economic, social, and cultural variables, how they respond depends on the circumstances in which they live.

It is clear that some special kind of energy exists between and among young people. In the minds of many social scientists this energy possesses enough force and longevity to generate a culture of its own. In modern society this culture conforms to its own internal norms, but it can be and usually is directed in opposition to the culture of parents, school, and adult institutions in general. On one hand, this opposition, however mild or intense, constitutes a way for young people to establish an identity separate from that of their elders. However, as a collective entity, the "student peer group" can be a major problem in schools for students themselves as well as for teachers and administrators.

Parents want their children to hang out with friends whose behavior and values are acceptable. Teachers are aware of the powerful influence friends have upon each other, and they separate children who habitually get into trouble when they work together. Social scientists cite studies demonstrating that one of the strongest predictors of a child's future is what his or her friends do. Police, probation officers, therapists, and social workers try to keep juvenile offenders away from the deleterious influence of their old friends.

In the next part of the chapter we look at how schools affect the lives of students and the impact of peer groups. We focus on young people's resistance to the inflexibility of their educational experiences, especially the social definitions and the standards imposed on them in school. Ours is a perspective most applicable to Western European culture and subordinate groups under its influence. Hence some of our assertions may not apply for some minority youth, such as Navajo teenagers. While these cultural biases should be kept in mind, the analysis provides a valuable perspective on the Western European definitions and cultural forms that dominate school life in the United States.

WHAT IS YOUTH CULTURE?

The two terms **peer group** and **youth culture** are often used interchangeably. However, they refer to quite different phenomena and have their origins in different social science disciplines. The term *peer group* comes from sociology and refers to a group of people who share special characteristics such as age, race, gender, or professional or social status. Peer groups are not synonymous with friendship groups, although friendship groups often consist of people who are peers.

Often the equality of peers is defined rather loosely. The phrase "a jury of one's peers" has generated many court battles over the degree to which the composition of a given jury really did equate with the social standing, race, gender, or ideology of the defendant. The same might be said of student peer groups. While they most commonly are defined as an age or grade-level cohort—a group of students who are the same age and in the same grade—that definition is too narrow. Many other factors, including differences in place of residence, social philosophy, dress, academic prowess, social status, race, religion, and interests, cross-cut similarities of age and grade level, so it probably is more accurate to speak of multiple peer groups rather than just one (Epstein and Karweit 1983). Leanne's story (see box on p. 86) reflects this multiplicity of peer groupings, as well as the widespread belief (discussed in Chapter 5) that we all are "middle class."

The term *youth culture* comes from anthropology and is a broader term than *peer group*. Anthropologists have defined *culture* variously as the way of life of a

---

Leanne's Story

This friend informed me that my family was the richest in _____ County. I figured if this was true, why did we always drink 2% milk? Plus, how come I never got one of those shirts with the alligators when I was in junior high? We never spent money. That's why I considered myself very middle class. So, on any given day, I am either middle class or upper middle class. In my mind, we had this ladder. There were a lot of people on the top, and even more on the bottom. I fit somewhere on the middle. Every day I moved up or down, or even stayed on the same rung. When I was in junior high, the thing I wanted most was to climb to the top of that ladder. That is where all of the "popular" people were. In junior high, I was not popular. I don't even think I was noticed. Now when I look back on it, I'll bet other kids felt the same way that I did. The social ladder: (1) popular kids, cheerleaders/jocks; (2) smart kids, nerds, but not a bad term; (3) me, I didn't really fit in any group; (4) druggers, head-bangers, really cool kids; (5) scuz, people who took vocational classes or woodshop. We wanted to fit in but didn't really. In high school my affections never laid with the popular kids. I did not fit in with them either, but they seemed to respect me. I was an artist and I dressed a little off-center, and I loved the group "Police." They were a big topic of discussion with these guys I liked who had a band. I also hung out at school with this guy who looked like John Belushi and wrote poetry. All of this was at school. I did not go anywhere after school with these people. I did not talk to them on the phone. Therefore, I wasn't really friends with them.

---

people (Linton 1945), what anthropologists have observed about the behavior of a group of people (Harris 1981), and everything having to do with human behavior and belief (Tylor 1958). In general, they agree that culture includes the entire body of attitudes, values, beliefs, and behavior patterns of a group of people (Spradley and McCurdy 1972). These include language, kinship patterns, rituals, economic and political structures, patterns of reproduction and child-rearing, life stages, arts and crafts, manufacturing, and technology (LeCompte and Preissle 1993).

Cultural development is profoundly affected by a people's physical environment. The environment strongly influences the possessions they make or buy, their family structure, religious beliefs, morals and sexuality, attitudes and behavior toward work and government, and patterns of dress, personal adornment, and recreation. The concept of culture also includes a historical dimension, because past activities of a group affect its current behavior, as do its beliefs about what will happen in the future.

Think back to your high school experiences. What were the student groups in your high school? Describe how these groups distinguished themselves from others. What did they call themselves? How did teachers and school administrators relate to each of these groups? Was there a relationship between social class background and peer group membership?

Can Youth Have a Culture?

Many scholars have argued that youth cannot have a culture, since individuals grow up and become non-youth; in the inevitable loss of their youth they lose the primary characteristic defining them as a part of the culture. Still other scholars argue that one can move into and out of cultures as one gains and loses the status that earns entry. For example, many professions, such as teaching, medicine, and the arts, and many institutions, such as prisons and religious organizations, develop sufficiently distinctive sets of attitudes, values, beliefs, and behavior patterns—even distinctive patterns of dress, personal adornment, and language—as to constitute cultures (Becker and Geer et al. 1961; Ebaugh 1977; Goffman 1959; Sykes 1958). In this view, individuals who cease to practice the given profession or who leave the institution are no longer a part of that culture, and in the same way youths grow up and leave the youth culture.

We do not feel that youth culture necessarily requires that individuals remain children, because youth culture can in fact be perpetuated as practices are passed from one generation of children to another. Bennett, Nelson, and Baker (1992), for example, describe the way succeeding generations of Yup'ik Eskimo girls learned cultural norms and folk tales through "storyknifing," a way of telling and illustrating stories by cutting pictures in soft sand or mud with a dull knife. Similarly, Lever (1976) discusses how gender differences in patterns of play teach children the social roles they will enact as adults.

We believe that *peer group* and *youth culture* are linked terms which must be used together. Youth culture is defined by those distinctive behavior patterns that children and adolescents develop, often in opposition to the power of adults and their institutions. These patterns differentiate young people first of all from adults, and then from other cliques and subgroups within their age cohort (for example, "punkers" are differentiated from "preppies" in American high schools). The peer group is the social entity that develops and practices youth culture. To the extent that the youthful peer group is defined by its relationship to school, we can speak of a student peer group. While peer group influence is important in the lower grades, it becomes more profoundly problematic for schools during adolescence, as Robert's story illustrates (see box on p. 88).

Developmental Factors in the Generation of Peer Groups

Conformity.   One of the characteristics of growing up is not wanting to be different from your friends. Children are fad followers. On one hand, they want to have the most up-to-date fashions, toys, and equipment. On the other hand, they don't want to be too different from their friends or to be caught liking or possessing something that others think is outrageous, outmoded, or stupid. Part of the herd instinct that afflicts young people involves role-modeling and trying on different identities exemplified by their friends or significant adult figures. Another part involves learning the norms and values of a group and trying to stay within them.

Robert's Story

Peer groups had a great deal of influence on me. I was a straight "A" student in elementary school. When I got to junior high, I became friends with a group of boys that wanted to be cool. Our leader was 16 and had a car in the seventh grade. My grades dropped somewhat to B's and C's. Looking back, I believe I did not want to be thought of as one of those "smart" kids. Most of the "smart" kids were from a higher class, or so I thought. I had no idea of going to college. When I got to high school, I began to run track and play football. My new peer group talked about going to college. My grades picked up somewhat, although I still did not want to be perceived as one of the brains. In my peer groups I was a follower, until I became more secure in athletics. However, by my junior year I was a leader in my group. Most of the guys wanted to do whatever I wanted to do.

It is important to note that the conformity of a young person is *internal* to the norms of his or her chosen peer group. Some kinds of youthful solidarity actually facilitate conformity to the norms of teachers and other adults, as was the case with the middle- and upper-class "earholes" described by Willis (1977). In other cases, such as Willis's working-class "lads" and Marotto's (1986) "Boulevard Brothers," peer group norms usually lead to the formation of groups that oppose the rules of adults.

Rebellion.   As much as most children abhor being different from others in their own clique, they find it equally distasteful to be similar to their parents. Rebellion against adult symbols of authority is an important component of growing up in modern urban societies, whether it consists of the cranky independence of a two-year-old or the outlandish dress and behavior of punk adolescents (Roman 1988). The rebellion of students of the 1980s may be seen in part as a conservative reaction to the radicalism of their parents in the 1960s, just as the worldwide student uprisings of the 1960s might be viewed as a reaction to the conservatism, alienation, and repression of the 1950s (Keniston 1968, 1971; Miles 1977).

The actual content and direction of student rebellion is hard to characterize, other than that it is in opposition to whatever strong adult presence, whether parental or institutional, is prominent in the lives of young people. Rebellion against authority may make these groups a mirror image of adult society: What is "bad" to adults becomes "good" to kids.

You hafta make a name for yourself, to be bad . . . [to] be with the "in" crowd. . . . It's just all part of growing up around here. . . . (McLeod 1987, p. 26)

He's the baddest, He shot a fucking cop. . . . That's the best thing you can do. . . . (McLeod 1987, p. 27)

Idealism. A third characteristic of young people that affects the formation of the student peer group in Western societies is idealism and a sense of immortality. We define *idealism* as a desire to transform the world and make it a better place. It is a

---

Jennie's Story

Especially during my high school years, I experienced a wide variety of peer groups at school. There were many different groups, and divisions were often based on one's interests. For example, one group was athletes and cheerleaders. Another was R.O.T.C. members. Yet another was made up of students in more advanced classes. There was a group of band members and one with drama students. There was another of those who were not focused on school and smoked, cut classes, and found themselves pregnant. Although there were some students who crossed lines and fit into several groups, they seemed to have a primary identity with one of the groups. I was probably most easily identified with the group of kids in more advanced classes. I was in the band during my freshman year and fit into that group until I quit. My sister was two years behind me in school. She was a cheerleader and that gave me a foot in the door to that crowd. I would have been called a "preppie" over a "punker" any day. I was influenced somewhat by the group in the sense of conformity. I was motivated to receive the high grades the others did, and to understand the information as they did. In most cases I was able successfully to conform. These were positive goals that I sought to achieve. I was influenced also by groups that made me appreciate where I was as an individual. I was thankful not to fit in with the crowd of pregnant girls, druggies, and dropouts, although they made up a good number of the student body. Because I grew up in a family that was intact and held high moral standards, I was somewhat of an exception to the norm, even within my peer group. The peer group that affected my life the most was the friends I had at my church. I felt that I fit in better with them than anyone at school. Another factor that influenced the peer group relations was socioeconomic status. Although this was not an absolute divider, there were obvious divisions within the student population. This factor caused me to realize that I was better off than many people I was closely associated with in the same school building. School peer groups were not a wonderful experience for me because I did not have an absolute place to fit in. I followed an "acceptance" response to surviving school and worked hard to make it a successful experience. Looking back on my high school years, I realized that I was not as bad off as it seemed at the time. I continue to be a well-adjusted person with a variety of friends in different peer groups.

tendency to simplify problems and look for unambiguous solutions. Doing so is a necessary stage in the development of a young person's personal philosophy (Belenky et al. 1986). While it allows them to be brave and capable of action on issues that adults, with their more sophisticated understanding of complexities, would sooner abandon, it also makes them prey to outrage and despair when solutions are delayed. Idealism also makes many young people indifferent to the dangers of practices such as truancy, drug use, reckless driving, and unprotected sex.

Their belief in invincibility, immortality, and high ideals permits young people to feel that they cannot be harmed by actions that would endanger most people. This confidence permits them to grow and to change in response to a changing culture by challenging existing definitions and ways of doing things. It also facilitates growth because it encourages risky behavior. In Western societies this attitude is important, because individuation and personal development are valued.

These characteristics of youth—conformity with peers, rebellion against adults, and youthful idealism—facilitate the growth of children away from their families into separate lives as mature adults. The desire for conformity leads to strong friendship groups of individuals who share (1) likes and dislikes, (2) attitudes toward work, family, school, and the opposite sex, (3) aspirations and expectations for the future, and (4) patterns of language, dress, and recreation. Cultural differences may cause variation in specific attitudes, but peer groups remain a major socializing force for young people in modern life. The relative indifference of young people to physical and emotional danger complicates their relationships with school, however, if the cultural patterns and attitudes of the peer group are antithetical or indifferent to behavior required for success in school.

Interview several high school students about the peer groups within their schools today. With the help of these students, make a chart to illustrate the status hierarchy of these peer groups. Which groups hold more power? How does this power get translated into privileges within the school and outside the school? How do these peer groups compare with the groups that existed when you were in high school?

Social and Historical Factors in the Development of Youth Culture

Certain structural characteristics of societies, such as age grades, clans, and schools with patterns of academic tracking, facilitate formation of youthful peer groups. In most cultures people identify throughout their lives as members of a generation or age grade. In some traditional cultures these groups have ritual significance and are recognized as one of the primary organizational structures in the society. Where each age grade performs specific tasks or functions integral to the support of the culture, as they do in certain East African and American Indian societies, the social structure of youthful groups does not promote opposition to the mainstream (Bernardi 1952, 1985; Bowers 1965; Evans-Pritchard 1940; M. Wilson 1963).

In contrast, in much of contemporary Western society youth groups oppose adult values and traditions. We believe that this has occurred because our system of schooling has changed the way young people grow up and caused them to develop and function with only limited contact with adult culture. In fact, in immigrant families adult–child relationships often are switched. Children become teachers to their parents, serve as interpreters, and act as intermediaries between the culture of origin and that of the new country (see, for example, Delgado-Gaitan 1988; Gibson 1988; Richardson et al. 1989; Sanjek 1992). Young people maintain stronger contacts with each other, the media, and their own youthful culture than they do with that of their families. In the pages which follow we will discuss how this situation has come about.

Socialization in Traditional Societies

Unlike animals, children are born without the knowledge or instincts to survive. Either by formal instruction or by watching others, they must be taught social, cognitive, and technical or mechanical skills. They also must learn the history and acquire the knowledge base of the people to whom they belong. This entire process is called **socialization.** In many pre-industrial, or traditional, cultures, where formal schooling is not the primary agency for socialization, children learn how to be adults initially by modeling the behavior of parents and family members. Later they may acquire more technical skills or sophisticated knowledge of the culture from indigenous specialists. Socialization takes place within and is controlled by the community and reflects its structure and values. Young people may "sow their wild oats," but they do not, as a *cohort* or a peer group, develop values and behavior patterns wildly at variance with those of their parents.

Puberty rites, whose purpose is to create a dramatic break in the developmental stream, signify a biological change from childhood to maturity, but there is no such clear distinction between youth and adult culture. Whatever culture young people have is a fairly close approximation of that of their parents. In these traditional cultures parents do not always tell children directly how to behave: It is assumed that they will learn by watching adults, and they do. Such education is not limited to learning how to herd sheep, make clothing, care for children, hunt seals, or farm. It also includes learning how to interact appropriately with others, participate in social life, and adhere to the moral precepts of the community. Only when children misbehave are they punished, and often then only indirectly, through the telling of stories or through gentle reminders (Basso 1984; Deyhle and LeCompte 1994).

Historically, children spent very little time in school. School learning was not necessary for most people, and only the very wealthy could afford the luxury of permitting male children to be out of the work force. Females, too, were needed at home, to help in child-rearing and household chores and to serve as adjuncts to the economic endeavors of women. For example, young Moslem girls in Africa, who are permitted to move freely in the community until puberty, facilitate the trading activities of their mothers, who are restricted by *purdah* to their family compounds (Schildkrout 1984).

To some extent these patterns still prevail. Until the twentieth century, American educators believed education to be wasted on girls. Even if they were intellectually capable of acquiring the necessary skills, jobs where they could use them were not open to females. Considerable doubt was cast not only upon the suitability of education for girls, but also on their ability to absorb it. As recently as the late 1880s the study of geography for girls was opposed because it might make them dissatisfied with their homes and inclined to travel (Curti 1971). Some educators—and even medical experts—believed math, science, and physical education to be so taxing as to cause mental and emotional deterioration and even damage to girls' reproductive organs (Fausto-Sterling 1985; Kaestle 1983). These beliefs—rather than patterns of discrimination or conflict between family responsibilities and careers in an era predating birth control and affirmative action—were used to explain why most of the few women who did become highly educated and had careers remained childless and unmarried. Women were relegated to the home, despite the fact that "careers" as sheltered-wife-and-mother-with-a-spouse-who-supported-her were always more myth than reality. Social beliefs ignored the fact that wars, the distant or intermittent employment of spouses, poverty, death, and abandonment left many women to a great extent responsible for taking care of themselves and raising families alone.

With the exception of a small elite whose male children did spend long years being educated, childhood for most remained a brief prelude to adult responsibilities (Aries 1962). In fact, until the 1920s, and then only in industrialized societies, adolescence for most young people, if it existed at all, was very short and included no more than a few years of schooling.

Adolescence as a Life Stage

Adolescence is a fairly recent phenomenon produced, as we shall see, primarily in modern industrialized societies. In traditional societies adolescence usually begins at the onset of puberty or the achievement of a certain age and is celebrated with special celebrations or rituals, such as a *bar* or *bat mitzvah* for 13-year-old Jewish children. It lasts only until marriage, the birth of the first child, or the point when the young person demonstrates economic self-sufficiency, mileposts that are achieved shortly after biological maturity. In these societies, youth are closely supervised by adults, and there are no great concentrations of young people. The period of youthful irresponsibility is short, and leisure time is limited or taken up by the need to work or to train for it, so young people have no opportunity to develop a distinctive cultural style separate from that of adults.

Adolescence as a Liminal State. Anthropologists (Gennep 1960; V. Turner 1969, 1974) define *liminal* points as social or developmental transitions—a period after leaving one clearly identified social status and before entering another. Liminal people exist in a state that is "ambiguous, neither here nor there, betwixt and between all fixed points of classification" (V. Turner 1974, p. 232). Initiates in fraternal orders exist in liminal states. So do brides on the day of their wedding before the actual ceremony; they are, in a sense, neither married nor single. Their in-between state is a state of **liminality.** We consider adolescence to be a liminal state because adolescents are neither children nor grown up.

Attitudes about liminal people are somewhat ambivalent. As novices, they are "structurally if not physically invisible in terms of [their] culture's standard definitions and classifications" (V. Turner 1974, p. 232). They are often thought to be in need of protection because they have not yet been socialized to know how to behave in their new role and they might do something that would harm them. They also pose a potential danger to others, because they do not as yet know the rules governing their new state in society and hence they could violate those rules with impunity. Therefore, in most cultures special precautions are taken to protect liminal people from actions that would endanger them or their future status, and other members of society must also be protected from their potentially asocial actions.

In traditional societies, rituals of passage from one social status to another generally include a period of liminality. During this period the initiates may be subject to avoidance taboos, be required to wear special adornments, be placed in a kind of protective custody, be isolated from other people, and made subject to special ceremonies or training. Turner suggests that this segregation emphasizes the equality and comradeship of people who are in a liminal state. It promotes development of group norms, cultural values, and a sense of community.

We believe that in Western societies, schools, especially high schools, act as the segregating and custodial institutions where the rite of passage from early childhood to adulthood takes place. Borman and Spring (1984, p. 238) suggest that adolescence in modern society is a period of transition in which adult status is incrementally achieved. During adolescence, youth occupy "multiple and conflicting statuses." They go to school full time . . . but they also work. They can drive a car and join the army, but they cannot vote or buy alcoholic beverages. They are biologically old enough to procreate but are considered too young by many parents to be told the "facts of life." Schools isolate adolescents in much the same way that formal rituals of passage do in traditional societies. In this way, they act as an incubator for youth culture.

Interview several high school teachers about the peer groups in their schools. Find out how they perceive the relationship of these peer groups to their academic performance in school. What kinds of student do they think are more able?

Schooling and Adolescence

Aries (1962) suggests that the recognition of adolescence as a life-stage is directly related to the lengthening of the mandatory period of schooling. In modern urban societies growing up is a more complex process than in traditional, usually rural, societies, and going to school is a more important part of a child's life. While recent growth in the "home schooling" movement (see Pitman 1987 for a description of home schooling and its supporters) and an increase in private school enrollment are evidence of groups that oppose publicly controlled learning, for the vast majority, childhood instruction takes place in public schools.

Further, the more technologically advanced a society is, the more years children spend in school. We believe that the number of years spent in school is associated with the development of strong peer relationships. As a consequence, the longer a society schools its children, the greater will be the tendency for them to develop a youth culture that is in opposition to adults, even where students change schools frequently. This is so because it is only in age-graded schools that so many people of the same age and sex are forced by law to remain in close proximity for so long.

Compulsory Schooling.   By the end of the nineteenth century universal primary school attendance had been mandated in most of the Western world. By the middle of the twentieth century serious efforts had been made to institutionalize primary schooling worldwide. The subsequent expansion of day-care, pre-school, secondary, and postsecondary school, especially in urbanized and industrialized countries, reflected a changing labor market, especially for women, as well as changing attitudes toward children and child-rearing. As the knowledge base deemed necessary for survival became more complex, and as custody of the young increasingly came to be supervised by the state, instruction was separated more and more from what parents can teach. Parents came to be viewed as incompetent to teach the cognitive and technical skills their children needed, and the family came to be viewed as an inappropriate place for this kind of instruction (Coleman and Hoffer 1987; Durkheim 1969). Children began to spend less time exclusively in their family, neighborhood, and close community and a correspondingly greater proportion of their developing years in institutions of formal instruction. With the institution of day care before and after school, students might be dropped off at 7:00 A.M. and not picked up until nearly twelve hours later. In many countries children of working parents often begin ''school'' in infancy and continue into university more than twenty years later.

Age Grade Segregation.   In school, young people are concentrated by age groups and segregated from contact with all adults but teachers and other school staff. Compulsory schooling isolates youth in a way which, as V. Turner (1969) suggests, facilitates the development of group solidarity. Idiosyncratic youth culture, especially one that is more or less in opposition to that of adults, developed hand in hand with the expansion of compulsory schooling and the concomitant creation of adolescence (Aries 1962). Schools gave students something to do in the long interval between childhood and adulthood and also provided a way for society to maintain custody over large groups of people deemed too old to be children and too young for the responsibilities of adulthood.

Separation of Biological from Social Maturity.   In contemporary Westernized and industrialized societies marriage or pairing off and the ability to support oneself do not coincide with or closely follow puberty. Instead, during the gap between biological and social maturity which constitutes adolescence, children are kept in a legally enforced state of liminality during which they are emotionally and socioeconomically dependent. Institutions, like schools, have substituted for the rituals of the traditional society, serving to protect liminal persons from themselves and society from them.

Protective Custody and Economic Dependence. Part of the custodial function of schools has been to protect adult laborers from the cheaper, and hence "unfair," competition of youthful workers. In the Third World young urban shoeshine boys, apprentices, "tour guides," beggars and car watchers, tiny rural shepherds, gardeners, and child-care providers perform critical economic functions for their families. However, in the industrialized West young people are denied substantial access to the labor market and often are paid lower wages than adults when they do work. They cannot support themselves well even if they want to. While Groce (1981) states that rural children differ from urban dwellers in that the former must perform many tasks of gardening, animal care, and housework, even they usually are not left to fend for themselves. Traditionally, children in the urban Western world bear few basic responsibilities. Upper- and middle-class children there enjoy a prolonged childhood enforced by economic dependence upon their families.

A second aspect to custody involves inhibiting sexual maturity and premature adulthood. Aries (1962) suggests that the prolonged period of immaturity common in Western society fostered ideas of childhood as a time of innocence, when children should be protected and given time for play and irresponsibility. This idea is associated with the romanticized Victorian notion that children—especially girls—are sexually naive, gentle, and nonviolent and that parents should preserve their innocence, closely supervise their passage through adolescence, and prohibit them from entering into early marriage. In Western societies children spend this stage of their lives segregated in schools and the military, where they acquire a protective veneer of intellectual, social, and vocational skills in preparation for the work force. Protective custody reinforces prohibitions against early marriage, parenthood, and exploitation in the work force, activities that are considered appropriate in traditional societies but an impediment to future economic well-being in modern ones.

In the first half of the twentieth century full-time employment was postponed until after high school. High school graduation came to symbolize the rite of passage into adulthood. However, decreasing economic opportunity and a glut of diplomas have substantially weakened the impact of high school graduation. This situation is changing, as we shall see. Global demographic and economic shifts have meant that many young people now must feed, clothe, and house themselves. Increasing poverty has transformed many children into *de facto* adults.

YOUTH CULTURE AND MODERN LIFE

Growing up is more complex than in the past for several reasons. As we have discussed, the lack of clear-cut rites of passage has blurred the distinction between childhood and adulthood. Second, increased crime as well as social, economic, and cultural pressures have made growing up riskier. Third, there are many obstacles along the way. Finally, even though adulthood takes longer to reach and involves more training than previously, it may no longer offer rewards commensurate with the effort. In the following sections we shall discuss how children have responded to this situation.

Material Culture

Patterns of Consumption.   Children in most of the Western world and in the urbanized portions of the non-Western world grow up in a world in which the monetary value of commodities is paramount. Children have become prime targets of advertising, because they have enough money to be consumers. For example, children in the United States 12 years old or younger spend more than $6 billion a year of their own money and influence more than $130 billion per year in household expenses (J. McNeil 1992). They are a market for fashionable clothes, up-to-date cars, electronic toys, and other consumer goods. The global village has spawned global patterns of consumption for children. Youngsters in Tokyo, Lagos, and Los Angeles look remarkably alike. Sometimes fads are adopted specifically because they represent a collective departure from the ways of parents. Fads sometimes go to school in the form of antisocial or antischool behavior, often constituting visible manifestations of an oppositional culture.

Youth Employment.   While children under the age of 18 in the United States still are legally regarded as minors, their relationship to the work world has changed. Most students from junior high through graduate school are employed. Prior to 1970 a full-time student from the middle class seldom had a substantial commitment to the work force. Working- and lower-class students often did, and still may have to work as teenagers to help support their families. Now many middle- and upper-class students become parents while still in school and must support their own children. Many more affluent students now work, not so much for basic necessities of life or even to save for college, but in order to buy clothes, cars, and other consumer goods their parents are unwilling or unable to provide (L. McNeil 1983; Powell, Farrar, and Cohen 1985). Regardless of their reason for working, more than 70 percent of 16-year-olds who are in school now work, and they are spending more time on the job. In 1970, 56 percent of the employed in-school male high school students worked more than 14 hours per week (Steinberg et al. 1982, p. 363). As a result, the centrality of school in their lives has been affected. Students now devote to working the time they used to spend on homework and extracurricular activities (Powell, Farrar, and Cohen 1985).

Jobs may provide an alternative source of self-esteem and gratification for students who do not do well academically or do not excel in athletics, school government, or other extracurricular activities. In fact, some studies have indicated that working a few hours a week may enhance performance in school. However, for the majority, jobs tend to interfere with school, especially when the immediate financial gratification supersedes the deferred gratification of success in school.

While students' jobs are not usually full-time, they may consume as many as 30 hours a week, often in the evening. However, schools still are structured for students who can devote all of their time to school-related activities. Teachers are faced with students who have little time out of class to read books, do projects, or work math problems. They might fall asleep in class because they worked late the night before or may refuse to let schoolwork interfere with their jobs. In response, teachers "dumb down" or reduce the amount and complexity of assignments, lower their aspirations for students, and teach less (McNeil 1985; Powell, Farrar, and Cohen 1985).

Technology.   Technological factors differ somewhat from other cultural factors in that they have habituated children to patterns of interaction, transmission of information, and communication radically different from those once common in schools. These advances have forced teachers and curriculum developers to change their expectations of what and how children will learn.

While television, video games, the telephone, calculators and computers, portable radios, and audio equipment are indeed cultural artifacts, their impact is more complex and powerful than the mere fact that some people have them and others do not. In fact, their presence has irrevocably altered human communication, and perhaps even perception and cognition. In the first place, these artifacts absorb a great deal—even the vast majority—of young people's leisure time. Teenagers on the telephone or with Walkmans glued to their ears, toddlers viewing the television set as their primary caregiver, and students who cannot do homework without the television or radio blaring—all are stereotypes that represent reality for a large percentage of children. The impact of these technological innovations is profound, controversial, and still being studied, but we wish to mention only a few.

First, these innovations eliminate face-to-face interaction. Telephone conversations lack the immediacy of visual, tactile, and olfactory contact, and answering machines are even further removed from communicants. In the classroom, computers and interactive video sometimes substitute for teachers, leaving children to work in isolation, each with his or her own keyboard.

Second, technological devices like calculators and video games shorten the period of attention needed to solve problems.

Third, they have most commonly been adapted for the simplest cognitive tasks. Instead of enhancing complex cognitive skills, computer-assisted instruction most often is used for simple memorization and recall. Simplifying knowledge to the presentation of single datum "factoids" and presenting them in the form of "sound bites" has penetrated many other aspects of life—entertainment, the media, and even religion. As a consequence, educators feel they must accommodate instruction to limited attention spans and simple solutions. No message or lesson can be longer or more complex than is considered manageable for the assumed attention span of a mesmerized child.

Fourth, use of technology further widens the gap between rich and poor. Schools in poor neighborhoods have fewer high-tech resources. Poor children cannot buy the computers that generate attractive term papers—and that many colleges require students to own.

Economics and Demography

Size and Urbanization.   Because children today must deal with people and distance on a scale far larger than any other generation, they face a paradox. As the external world becomes more familiar and intimate, their immediate surroundings become larger and more impersonal. On one hand, they live in a shrinking world where areas once remote and inaccessible now can be viewed nightly on television and visited by tourists. On the other hand, urbanization has made the once familiar strange. Most people now live in urban areas and in apartments rather than houses. Even the ostensibly bucolic suburbs have become urbanized. Families are renters rather than owners as the cost of homes prices most of them out of the market (Cohen and Rogers 1983).

As the supply of moderately priced rental housing decreases, many are faced with the specter of homelessness (Joint Center for Housing Studies 1988). The situation is so serious that the majority of homeless in the 1990s are families with children. The typical homeless person in New York City in early 1989 was a 4-year-old boy (*New York Times,* January 17, 1989). According to U.S. Department of Education estimates, 220,000 school-aged children are homeless and 65,000 of them do not attend school (Reed and Sautter 1990).

Adventure has become too perilous to be challenging. International travel is too familiar to be an adventure; adventure closer to home is too dangerous to be permitted. Parks are dangerous and there are few fields or open spaces where children can run and explore unsupervised. Even shopping malls have become centers of gang-related or criminal activity. The attendance zones of schools are so large that walking to school usually is impossible. Friends from the same school may live so far apart that it's difficult to visit each other. As a consequence, children either see only those children in their immediate neighborhood, or spend a lot of time driving or being driven to activities and friends' homes. Young people may be quite familiar with the customs of people on the other side of the globe but not know anybody on their block. Inner-city children may be even more isolated. In the housing projects, shelters for the homeless, and blighted neighborhoods where many urban children live, a visit to friends next door or even down the hall may lead to an encounter with drug-related violence.

Children may find it difficult to participate in any school-related activities before or after school, since most must come and go in accordance with a parent's schedule, timing of the bus route, or car pool. This constraint further reduces the capacity of the school to be of central importance to their lives and leaves them subject to the same social isolation afflicting urban adults. Under these conditions, the peer group's attitudes and behaviors are influenced primarily by street life and the media.

Poverty.   Even as school has lost its centrality, changes in families have made them less able to provide support and guidance. The increase in divorce and single parenthood means that the *normal childhood experience* will become life with one parent. The majority of children—59 percent of all children born in 1983, for example (O'Neill and Sepielli 1985, p. 3)—at some time in their lives will live in a single-parent home (Brown 1986). The percentage is even greater among many minority groups; 90 percent of African-American teenage mothers are unmarried.

More children than ever also are growing up in families that are very poor. In 1987, 25 percent of children under the age of 6 lived in families below the poverty line. One in six had no health insurance, and fewer and fewer were receiving public

---

Families in Poverty in the United States

* 23.3% of children aged 3 and under are poor.

* Nearly 22% of 3–5-year-olds are poor.

* Of children between the ages of 6 and 11, 19.9% or 4 million children are poor.

* Of children between the ages of 12 and 17, more than 16% live below the poverty line.

* Almost 50% of children living in a family headed by a person 25 or younger are poor.

* 56% of families headed by single African-American women are poor.

* Two-thirds of America's poor are white.

* Less than 9% of poor people live in the core cities of the United States; 17% of poor people live in rural communities and 28% live in suburban communities.

SOURCE: Reed and Sautter 1990.

---

assistance or food stamps (Children's Defense Fund 1988). Although at least 3 million children were eligible for Head Start in 1985, funds were available to enroll only 400,000 (Hodgkinson 1985). The rising incidence of divorce and unwed motherhood increased the number of children living below the poverty line, because female-headed homes are more likely to be poor. Of the children living in poverty in 1985, 50 percent lived in female-headed homes but only 12 percent in homes where a male was present. The situation is worse for minorities. Forty percent of all minority children live in impoverished homes, and the situation is worse in those headed by a female (Bayes 1988; O'Neill and Sepielli 1985).

Family Structure.   Even children in intact and "blended" nuclear families cannot rely upon the presence of a homebound parent, because maintenance of most households with children requires two incomes. What this means is that children are caught between the expectations of schools and the reality of their family life. Schools still operate as if most children have two heterosexual parents, one of whom is a full-time parent available for helping with homework, having parental consultations with teachers, making cookies, and other tasks. However, 51.9 percent of the mothers of children one year and younger are in the work force (G. Collins 1987). Up to 33 percent—over 4 million—of elementary school children are "latchkey" children (*Education Week* 1989; O'Neill and Sepielli 1985) who take care of themselves after school, get help with homework from a telephone hotline if available, and cope with overworked parents in the evening. They are expected to be emotionally mature and to demonstrate adult-like independence even in pre-school, because their parents have few economic or emotional reserves left after the pressures of daily survival (Woodhouse 1987).

Children are deluged with invitations to engage in illegal activities, use drugs and alcohol, and become sexually active. They find it easy to do so as drugs permeate all echelons of society. They see drug-related behavior where they work, on the streets, in their schools, and among their family members, and their parents often are too busy working to supervise them during their leisure time.

The Labor Market. The economic context of growing up in the latter part of the twentieth century for most young people, regardless of where they live, is one of frustrated aspirations and limited expectations. As the lower-paying service sector of the labor market grows, opportunities for lucrative positions shrink and there is less room at the top of the economic ladder (Bluestone and Bennett 1982). Young people must reduce their aspirations in accordance with the reality of the more humdrum, less lucrative jobs available (Littwin 1987). Competition for desirable professional positions is keen, feeding both a ferocious battle for those willing to join the fray, and hopelessness among those who deem the costs of competing to be too high. It also feeds racism and bigotry, as members of the dominant white culture feel unfairly disadvantaged by affirmative action programs. The lower-income white young men whom McLeod studied typify these feelings:

> [SHORTY:] "He got laid off because they hired all Puerto Ricans, blacks, and Portegis (Portuguese)."
>
> SMITTY: "All the fuckin' niggers are getting the jobs. Two of them motherfuckers got hired yesterday [at a construction site]; I didn't get shit. They probably don't even know how to hold a fuckin' shovel, either."
>
> FRANKIE: "Fuckin' right. That's why we're hanging here now with empty pockets. . . . hey, they're coming on our fucking land. . . . They don't like us, man, and I sure as hell don't like them."
>
> SHORTY: ". . . *Listen.* When they first moved in here [into the housing project], they were really cool and everything. We didn't bother them. But once more and more black families moved in, they said, 'Wow, we can overrun these people. We can overpower them.' That's what their attitude was." (1987, pp. 39–40)

Violence, Environmental Degradation, and Potential Annihilation. Today's children have immediate personal and global survival on their minds as well. In addition to the interpersonal violence they witness daily in the media, children see themselves or people they know being abused by parents. Their own parents abuse each other. Their schoolmates use drugs and carry guns and knives. Children worry about how to get through the school hallway or back home safely. Children living in urban communities worry about drive-by shootings in their neighborhood. Consider these statistics from the National School Boards Association's *Violence in the Schools:*

- Firearms are the leading cause of death of African-American males age 15–24 and the second leading cause of death for all teens in the United States.
- About 10 percent of youth (age 10–19) report that they have fired a gun at someone or have been shot at.
- One-fourth of all suspensions from school nationally were for violent incidents committed by elementary school students.
- Approximately 135,000 guns are brought into schools every day.
- One out of five weapons arrests in 1991 was a juvenile arrest; between 1987 and 1991 juvenile arrests for weapons violations increased by 62 percent.
- About 3 million crimes occur on or near school property each year. (National School Boards Association 1993, p. 3)

Schools and communities are actively working toward ways for making schools safer through a variety of programs, which involve protective as well as preventative measures. Protective measures include closed-circuit TV, gun-free school zones, drug-detecting dogs, establishment of "safe havens" for students, locker searches, metal detectors, phones in classrooms, search and seizure policies, and security personnel in schools. Preventative programs include conflict resolution and peer mediation training, multicultural sensitivity training, staff development, support groups, parent skill training, and home–school linkages (National School Boards Association 1993).

Growing up in the shadow of atomic, chemical, and biological war clouds, children wonder how growing up can be considered a viable proposition. The whole world might be blown up before they have any say in the matter. They know that activism in the 1960s neither solved the social and economic problems being protested, nor caused a revolution. James Gleick has suggested:

the explosion of the first atomic bomb stands . . . as the central moment in the history of our time, the threshold event of an age. . . . Its prelude was [a belief in] an irreversible mastery of science over nature; its sequel was violence and death on a horrible scale. (1989, p. 1)

These conditions spawn apathy and egocentrism among young people. All of them have made growing up in the past few decades a very difficult process, one requiring young people to set out upon virtually uncharted waters. One response has been simply to avoid growing up for as long as possible.

THE POSTPONED GENERATION

Joan Littwin (1987) suggests that middle-class young people in America have responded to the factors enumerated above by postponing adulthood. We feel that her phrase, the "postponed generation," fits more than just middle-class youth.

Being grown-up in Western culture means having economic self-sufficiency rather than biological maturity. Self-sufficiency means the ability to pay for one's own home, to support oneself, and to acquire and support a family. Until the late 1960s it more or less corresponded with completion of high school or military service—somewhere between 18 and 22 years—when individuals were old enough to work full-time and most could make a decent living. Increments of success were predicated upon obtaining skills that were not widely held by others or that were in demand. Schooling gave a competitive edge, whether or not it corresponded to increments of skill, because years of schooling served as a proxy for ability. Unfortunately, this is no longer always the case.

Inflation of Educational Credentials

As more and more people possessed the basic complement of schooling, the increment needed to stand out and be competitive increased. As more and more people need more and more education to compete for jobs, a real labor market dilemma arises: People are overeducated for the work they do. The level of schooling required to *obtain* many jobs is higher than the skill level needed to do the work. Littwin (1987) calls this disparity a "job gap," or the degree to which individuals must work at jobs that are below the level they expected to acquire, given their education and training. The job gap eliminates job slots to which the poorly educated or less skilled once aspired because more highly educated people who have revised their job expectations downward have filled those slots. Especially for graduates in the liberal arts, social sciences, and humanities—fields that historically held the most promise for creative individuals—interesting and desirable white-collar jobs are becoming increasingly scarce.

The job gap is aggravated by two factors. First, "our economy is very good at generating new jobs—but most of them are low-paying service jobs which require little education" (Hodgkinson 1985, p. 8). Since the number of young people who have done well in school exceeds the supply of entry-level jobs fitting their qualifications, many of the most talented young people must wait a long time to get any job, let alone one related to their chosen field (Borman 1987; Littwin 1987). In 1983 one out of every five college graduates worked in a job requiring no college education at all (O'Neill and Sepielli 1985).

The second factor exacerbating the job gap is current population trends. High birth rates between 1946 and 1964 produced the generation known as the "Baby Boomers" (see Figure 3.1). These individuals are now in their prime working years, increasing the number of people competing for jobs.

All of these factors prolong adolescence, or at least the period of time young people must wait before they can begin their life work. They also must adjust to a

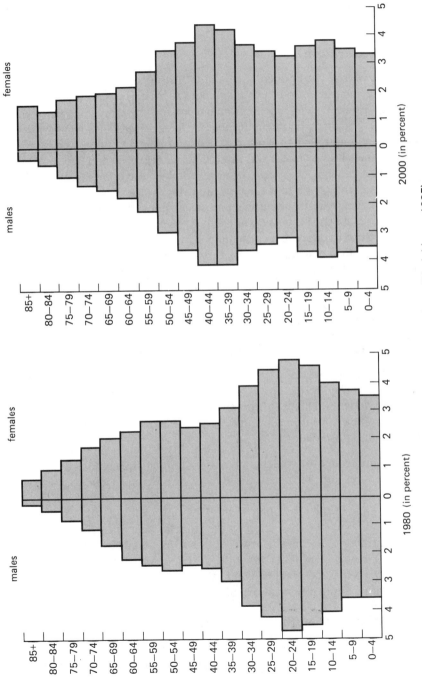

FIGURE 3.1 The Baby Boom Ages (Hodgkinson 1985)

lower standard of living than they expected, one perhaps lower than that of their parents, not only because of low-paying initial jobs (Borman 1987; Littwin 1987), but also because the jobs they ultimately get are less prestigious and lucrative than their aspirations indicated.

Postponed Maturation

The consequence is a "postponed generation." Its members start to grow up later than previous generations, and they take longer to attain economic independence. They may spend several years moving from one low-paying entry-level job to another (Borman 1987). They may be unemployable for long periods of time and have difficulty making a commitment to work that does not coincide with their aspirations. Both the academically successful and those who were less so and had lower aspirations suffer similar feelings of *ennui,* or boredom, because it is difficult for them to find gainful employment and to settle into family life.

Many also are unrealistic about what it takes to get and hold a job. Fine suggests that this is so because the schools do not provide them with information unless they are legally mandated to do so. As a consequence, students do not learn what it takes to get into college, join the military, or pass the GED. Fine's respondents, all dropouts, believed that "the GED is no sweat, a piece of cake . . . you can get jobs, they promise, after goin' to Sutton or ABI [trade schools and business colleges, most of which currently have dropout rates of close to 70 percent (Fine 1986; *New York Times,* June 28, 1989)] . . . in the Army I can get me a GED, skills, travel, benefits . . ." (Fine 1987, pp. 169–170). Hess et al. (1985), Powell, Farrar, and Cohen (1985), and others suggest that this situation is not unique to dropouts. An example:

> [To become a pediatrician] you have to go to community college for two years. Then you go to medical school for four years. After that you are an intern for two years. Then you are a regular nurse for two years. Then you do a residency, and after that you can be a doctor and start at $65,000 a year. (Firestone and Rosenblum 1988, p. 291)

Only the most motivated of students obtain realistic, adequate advice from school personnel (Cicourel and Kitsuse 1963; Powell, Farrar, and Cohen 1985; Sarason 1971).

A small decline in the job cohort in the 1990s may alleviate the situation somewhat, but there is evidence that although the Baby Boomers postponed having children for a while, their children will now create another population bulge. In addition, changes in the population will not affect the decline in professional jobs. The consequence for youth is that most will end up hitting a job ceiling at least for a while, and all will cope with extended periods of liminality.

Postponed Minority Youth

Most middle-class children eventually get back on track. However old they may be, they have a "safety net" of family connections and cultural knowledge which eventually helps most to work the system. Tobier (1984, quoted in Fine 1987) states that white high school dropouts living in affluent sections of New York are far more likely to be employed than African-American high school graduates from Harlem. The consequences of postponement for minority or disadvantaged youth are far more severe (see Table 3.1). They may never get started.

Many minority youth drop out of school, and many more graduate with minimal literacy skills. Even those who do graduate and are literate often find that no good jobs exist in their community (Wilson 1987). Deyhle (1991, 1992) found that high school graduation did not improve job opportunities for most reservation-dwelling Navajo youth, who ended up with the same low-paying menial jobs dropouts had. Minority youth in the inner city suffer from a flight of industry to the beltways and suburbs, and transportation networks often do not make it possible to travel easily to new work places, even if employers were willing to hire poorly trained adolescents. Some of the girls can become mothers, which is a culturally acceptable alternative (Deyhle and LeCompte 1994), but boys find themselves in a particularly desperate situation. In a society that values gainful employment above all other means of demonstrating self-worth, they find no jobs and nothing to do except drink and use drugs. Many die before the age of 30, often in ill-disguised forms of suicide such as substance abuse, fights, or motor vehicle accidents (see, for example, Conant 1988).

When they can find them, young minority men drift from one dead-end job to another. They often are unable to support themselves or a family except through illicit means—robbery, pimping for prostitutes, and the drug trade. These activities can land them in prison, if not in a morgue (McLaren 1989). The situation is worse on Indian reservations and in rural areas, especially where subsistence has been the traditional mode of life (Conant 1988; Deyhle 1988). These areas have no agricultural or industrial base and little hope for building one outside of the tourist industry, and most young people do not wish to follow traditional subsistence practices.

Although many middle-class youth postpone growing up by hanging out at home and working at make-do jobs they see as temporary, the poor, working-class, and minority youth may feel that they have no opportunity to grow up. Fine documents how minority youth know that "there ain't no jobs waitin' for me" (1986, p. 399). They pass their time hanging around street corners or other gathering places, talking, smoking, and drinking until they find some sort of work or get arrested (Marotto 1986). The hopelessness of their situation is illustrated by McLeod's description of the "Hallway Hangers'" reactions to a question about what they would be doing in twenty years:

STONEY: ". . . I could be dead tomorrow. Around here, you gotta take life day by day. . . ." (1987, p. 61)

FRANKIE: ". . . I live a day at a time. I'll probably be in the fucking pen. . . . I can work with my brother, but that's under the table. Besides, he's in [state prison] now." (Ibid.)

SLICK: "Most of the kids around here, they're not gonna be more than janitors. . . . I'd say the success rate of this place is, of these people . . . about twenty percent, maybe fifteen." (1987, p. 68)

TABLE 3.1 Civilian Labor Force—Employment Status, by Sex, Race, and Age: 1992[a]

Age and Race	Civilian Labor Force Total (1,000)	Percentage by Age Male	Percentage by Age Female	Male (1,000) Total	Male (1,000) Employed	Male (1,000) Unemployed	Female (1,000) Total	Female (1,000) Employed	Female (1,000) Unemployed	Percentage of Labor Force Male	Percentage of Labor Force Female	Percentage of Labor Force Male	Percentage of Labor Force Female
All Workers	126,982	100.0	100.0	69,184	63,805	5,380	57,798	53,793	4,005	92.2	93.1	7.8	6.9
16–19	6,751	5.1	5.5	3,547	2,786	761	3,204	2,613	591	78.5	81.6	21.5	18.5
20–24	13,703	10.5	11.2	7,242	6,357	884	6,461	5,799	662	87.8	89.8	12.2	10.2
25–34	35,103	28.0	27.2	19,355	17,847	1,508	15,748	14,594	1,154	92.2	92.7	7.8	7.3
White	108,526	100.0	100.0	59,830	55,709	4,121	48,696	45,770	2,926	93.1	94.0	6.9	6.0
16–19	5,744	5.0	5.6	3,019	2,464	555	2,726	2,297	429	81.6	84.3	18.4	15.7
20–24	11,539	10.2	11.2	6,097	5,462	634	5,442	4,993	450	89.6	91.7	10.4	8.3
25–34	29,538	27.6	26.8	16,510	15,364	1,146	13,029	12,222	807	93.1	93.8	6.9	6.2
Black	13,891	100.0	100.0	6,692	5,846	1,046	6,999	6,087	912	84.8	87.0	15.2	13.0
16–19	787	6.1	5.3	419	243	176	368	231	137	58.0	62.8	42.0	37.2
20–24	1,683	12.7	11.6	872	658	214	811	623	187	75.5	76.8	24.5	23.1
25–34	4,251	30.8	30.4	2,121	1,820	302	2,130	1,830	300	85.8	85.9	14.2	14.1
Hispanic	10,131	100.0	100.0	6,091	5,388	703	4,040	3,584	456	88.5	88.7	11.5	11.3
16–19	678	6.4	7.1	391	281	110	287	211	76	71.9	73.5	28.2	26.4
20–24	1,460	14.6	14.1	890	768	122	570	500	71	86.3	87.7	13.7	12.4
25–34	3,316	34.1	30.7	2,075	1,866	209	1,241	1,103	137	89.9	88.9	10.1	11.1

[a](For civilian noninstitutional population 16 years old and over. Annual averages of monthly figures. Based on Current Population Survey. We have omitted data on workers 35 years old and over.)

SOURCE: U.S. Bureau of Labor Statistics, *Employment and Earnings*, January 1992.

JINKS: "I think most of them, when and if a war comes, they're all gone. Everyone's going. But for jobs—odds and ends jobs. Here and there. No good high-class jobs." (Ibid.)

The problem is that even those young men who try to join the military as a last resort often find that they do not qualify academically. The result is a youth culture of hopelessness:

FRANKIE: "We were all brought up, all we seen is our older brothers and that gettin' into trouble and goin' to jail and all that shit. Y'know, seeing people—brothers and friends . . . dying right in front of your face. You seen all the drugs. . . . We grew up, it was all our older brothers doing this . . . the drugs, all the drinking. They fucking go; that group's gone. The next group came, our brothers that are twenty-something years old. They started doing crime. And when you're young, you look up to people. . . . And he's doing this, he's drinking, doing drugs, ripping off people. Y'know, he's making good fucking money; it looks like he's doing good. So bang. Now it's our turn. What we gonna do when all we seen is fuckin' drugs, alcohol, fighting, this and that, no one going to school?" (McLeod 1987, pp. 117–118)

The entire social system has become less and less responsive to the varied and sometimes desperate needs of young people. The opportunity structure also provides good jobs for only a few disadvantaged young people. The remainder are systematically pushed out of schools, which continue to hold out fraudulent promises of a good job in return for solid effort. For minority and poor children, equality of opportunity is a myth. Schools simply reinforce and widen the gap between rich and poor. Most, like Fine's dropouts, internalize the reasons given by the dominant culture for their failure, believing the system and its values to be legitimate and the failure to be their own.

THE LESSONS OF SCHOOLING

Going to school represents a sharp break from being at home. First, going to school introduces a new role: Children become students—one of the first institutional roles they acquire. Second, schools are structured differently from home (Dreeben 1968; Durkheim 1969). Functional theorists have suggested that families and schools are structured differently because they have different purposes and represent different values. They believe that the discontinuity schools create between the past and present experience of children is both necessary and proper. Citing the differentiation of function that modernization brings to social institutions, they argue that in complex industrialized societies no one institution such as the family can hope to impart all of the skills children need for adult life. Therefore, a division of labor evolves whereby the tasks of socializing the young can be divided. Each institution in which young people participate carries out the task for which its structure is most appropriate. The family, which is smaller, more intimate, and idiosyncratic, is responsible for the development of individual personality, close relationships, and specific moral values. The larger, more impersonal, diverse, and universalistic school is responsible for technical training, including cognitive skills, and for preparing children to be responsible citizens and workers. Coleman and Hoffer (1987) summarize the functional position, arguing that schools explicitly were an

> instrument that alienated the child from the family, an instrument that benefitted the child by bringing it into the mainstream of American society, but at a cost to the continuity and strength of the family. The cost was not great when a school served [an ethnically and religiously homogenous] local community, for then the culture of the local community pervaded the school and made it consistent with the functional community of adults whose children it served. The cost was great, however, for cultural minorities in [heterogenous communities]. (p. 140)

This cost, functionalists argue, is warranted in the face of community needs for order and consistency.

Critical theorists agree that there are differences between school and family life, but they argue that what schools actually do is to maintain the existing power structure and reproduce the system of social classes by mobilizing a work force stratified by class, race, and gender. They hold that schools do not train citizens to govern themselves and work in a meritocratic, egalitarian society. As one dropout put it:

> In school we learned Columbus Avenue stuff and *I* had to translate it into Harlem. They think livin' up here is unsafe and our lives are so bad. That we should want to move out and get away. That's what you're supposed to learn. (Fine 1987, p. 164)

In the pages that follow we will discuss the structural and organizational differences between school and family and will indicate how these differences help to prepare the ground for development of youth culture and its opposition to adults. We will also describe how children resist the power of teachers and school staff, as well as how educators have created institutions within the school to counteract their oppositional behavior. We will begin with a discussion of what children encounter when they enter elementary school and what it teaches them. Many scholars refer to this as the "hidden curriculum" (Jackson 1968), or the "tacit teaching to students of norms, values and dispositions that goes on simply by their living in and coping with the institutional expectations and routines of schools, day in and day out for a number of years" (Apple 1979, p. 14). After a discussion of elementary school, we will move to an analysis of high schools and their relationship to students.

Becoming a Student: Elementary School

Schools are not organized to coincide with the natural impulses of children, and they seldom involve a child's favorite activities. Because we are so familiar with them, we tend to forget that the way schools are organized is not inevitable but has evolved under the impact of social and political pressures.

We also forget that children are conscripts. Whereas staff are voluntary recruits because of their skills and professional credentials, children are involuntary recruits because of their age status as minors (Bidwell 1965; Nadel 1957). Nowhere else is such a large group of noncriminals forced to remain in an institution for so long, a fact that makes children's attitude about their participation diverge markedly from that of adults.

Crowds and Noise. The organization of schools is very different from that of the family. In the first place, schools are much bigger. Many people, on returning to their elementary school, are shocked to discover how small it was. But to children, the school building, no matter how tiny, still is much larger than their house or apartment.

Physical size is not the only difference. There also are many more people, and they are apportioned differently. A family in Western society usually contains no more than 3 to 7 members, but classrooms usually contain at least 28 to 30. The adult-to-child ratio changes as well. Families usually contain at least one adult for every two or three children, but in the classroom the ratio is closer to 30:1. This means that children in school receive significantly less adult attention than in the family (Dreeben 1968). In fact, schools are crowded, noisy places where adults are far outnumbered by children (Jackson 1968).

Coping with Diversity. Schools also are marked by considerably more heterogeneity than families. Most parents belong to the same racial, ethnic, socioeconomic, and religious group. In schools, however, children begin to learn about people who are quite different from themselves. Because elementary schools are tied to neighborhoods, the student body is usually more homogeneous than junior and senior high schools, but as children grow older, the schools they attend bring them into contact with more and more diversity and challenging social situations (Dreeben 1968). Homogeneity is becoming less possible in public schools as minority populations come to outnumber whites in the Western world. Desegregation programs also have made inroads into patterns of educational and residential racial segregation.

Even where the students form a homogeneous group, they may have very little in common with their teachers, ethnically, socially, or economically. They probably do not even live anywhere near each other, and they may be totally unfamiliar with the lives each leads outside of the classroom.

Losing Individuality and Being Categorized. While most adults recall the size differential between home and school, they probably do not remember how it felt to lose the sense of demographic uniqueness that the family provides. Unless a family has adopted children or has twins or triplets, it seldom contains more than one child of the same age and sex. Treatment of individual children in the family is predicated upon these age and sex categories. Behavior is deemed appropriate or inappropriate according to whether one is old enough to carry out an activity, young enough to justify specific actions, and of the correct gender to participate.

In school, however, children learn to be treated as members of social categories. First is age. Children are initially grouped exclusively by their birth date, and they discover that there are many boys and girls of the same age.

While language patterns, physical attractiveness, and general deportment do affect teachers' reactions to individual children, teachers make few allowances for special characteristics, and all the children are expected to conform to rather standardized patterns of behavior. In fact, it is treatment and grouping upon the basis of similarity of category, rather than upon individual differences, that constitute one of the hallmarks of life in school.

Separating Roles from Persons.   School is the place where children begin to learn the difference between parents and all other adults as well as to distinguish between social roles and the people who occupy them. They learn, for example, that the social role—its expectations and obligations—of teacher remains constant from year to year, even if the occupants change. They also learn that their teachers do not respond as their parents do and that staff are not present to nurture their individual idiosyncracies. Unlike parenting, teaching is a job, whose task it is to control children and to impart knowledge (Dreeben 1968). In fact, some researchers suggest that the differences between students and staff eventually diverge into "fighting groups" created from widely different interests in school and goals while there (Connell 1985; Waller 1932).

Learning to Achieve.   Another measure by which children are categorized is achievement. It is almost as powerful an influence on development as age, sex, and race (Dreeben 1968). This category begins to take shape before the child's arrival at school and remains almost immutable until school life ends, structuring the school experience and to a large extent determining the student's future occupational status. Children usually arrive at school already having taken "readiness" tests or with records of pre-school teachers and day-care workers. On the basis of these and sometimes additional tests, they are stratified for instruction according to their perceived ability to learn. The word "perceived" is an important one, because a child's ability is often subjectively defined and may have less to do with native intelligence than with behavior, ethnicity, and social class, as well as the teacher's affinity for the child and how a given school defines readiness (Eisenhart and Graue 1990; Graue 1994; Ortiz 1988; Richardson et al. 1989; Rist 1970, 1973; Rosenfeld 1971).

However they happen to be placed into ability groups, children are "tracked," "streamed," or "grouped" from the day they enter school. These groups are obvious to children, despite heroic efforts to disguise them. Tracks engender patterns of behavior and belief in children and play an important role in defining the kind of individual students believe themselves to be. An insidious characteristic of ability groups is that they construct failure. No matter how high the achievement of the lowest group is, children in it feel like "dummies," "retards," or "basics." Page (1987), for example, studied a "dream high school," where none of the students was disadvantaged, and even in this setting the lowest students—who might well have been the most advanced in an inner-city school—thought of themselves as "dregs" and a "circus," adopting the rebellious attitudes usually attributed to lower- and working-class students.

Ability groups are critical in the formation of student peer groups because they determine friendship groups. Study after study show that friendship groups form almost exclusively among students who study together and who share a common academic track record (K. P. Bennett 1986, 1991; Borko and Eisenhart 1986; Coleman 1961, 1965; Gamoran and Berends 1987; Gordon 1957). Students in the academic groups also tend to be the most popular students (Gamoran and Berends 1987, p. 427).

Evaluation and Gratification.   Schools and families also differ in the relative emphasis they place on different modes of evaluation (Dreeben 1968). Whereas families evaluate children on the basis of their individual personality, schools evaluate them primarily on how well they achieve in school. Impulse gratification is also handled differently. Parents are warned that, since young people are oriented to immediate rewards, they should not promise rewards that cannot be given or that must be delayed; schools, on the other hand, operate on the premise of deferred gratification. Teachers encourage children to believe that hard work now will yield tangible rewards in the future. Grades only symbolically represent the material rewards which will ultimately come. This promise is, of course, not particularly compelling to many teenagers, for whom the future is far away indeed.

Cognitive knowledge is not the only kind of knowledge children acquire in school. In elementary school children learn about the separation of student and teacher roles and something about appropriate sex-role behavior (Goetz 1981). They internalize the rules of the organization and construct their own definition not only of how to survive, but of how well they can be expected to do. They have some idea of the degree to which their efforts will pay off in grades, and they may have learned how to "make deals" with teachers as to how much they will be taught (Borko and Eisenhart 1986; Powell, Farrar, and Cohen 1985). Most of them have acquired some rudiments of the cognitive skills, and they have fairly well-formed personalities and sets of social relationships. By the time they reach high school, they are interested in other matters.

Becoming Pre-Adult: High School

The Opposite Sex.   In high school, students become deeply interested in working out their gender identity and relationships with the opposite sex. Especially for girls, sex complicates the development of attitudes and aspirations about work, careers, and their future. Weis (1988) and Holland and Eisenhart (1988) studied the "ideology of romance" (McRobbie 1978) which suffuses the lives of young women. Although Holland and Eisenhart (1988) studied college students, we feel that their analysis also applies to students in high school, who are only a year or two younger. Holland and Eisenhart stress the importance of the "world of peers" in the determining gender identity.

> [Students] spend most of their time around age mates, are constantly exposed to peer-organized activities, learn age-mate interpretations and evaluations of all aspects of . . . life . . . have most of their close, intimate relationships with age mates on campus, and learn ways to understand and evaluate themselves from those peers. (pp. 17–18)

Holland and Eisenhart (1988) suggest that the peer culture competes with schoolwork, derails some students, and affects even those who don't participate in it directly, because it creates a culture with which all students must cope. Whether they are identified as punks and badasses, greasers or jocks, preppies, nerds, or dropouts, young people cannot totally dismiss what the others say and feel about them, no matter how they try to distance themselves.

Most powerful of all pressures brought to bear on young people are those concerning traditional, gender-appropriate roles in romance, which have dampening effects on the self-image, aspirations, and efforts of young girls (Christian-Smith 1988; Brown and Gilligan 1992; Lesko 1988; Roman 1988b). We will talk more about self-esteem in young women in Chapter 8.

Getting Ahead.   Adolescents recognize that there are many areas of achievement. One is success in personal, social, and familial arenas. Another is demonstrated athletic prowess. A third is the status of conspicuous consumption. The fellow with the fancy clothes, expensive watch, and brand-new car smells of success, regardless of how these were acquired. A fourth, and the only one that schools are designed to facilitate, is success in academic and professional arenas.

Children go to elementary school to learn cognitive skills of reading, writing, and computation, and to high school to acquire both the knowledge base and the social skills and values that will fit them for various roles in the occupational structure. Their success in school is measured in terms of how well they do in these tasks, as measured by grades, teacher assessments, and standardized test scores.

Adolescents, however, know that the criteria for success in school are more diffuse and complex than just getting good grades. Two classic studies (Coleman 1961; Gordon 1957) demonstrated that grade point averages are of little importance in high school; extracurricular position or one's place in the juvenile social status system supersedes academic achievement. For boys the primary criterion was athletic prowess, followed by conformity to norms of in-school behavior, dating, dress, and recreation. For girls the highest positions went to the prom and yearbook queens. They gained this status by adhering to particular patterns of dress, giving service to the school, having a "good" personality and being friendly, being a leader in activities, and maintaining Puritan standards of morality. Grades still are relatively unimportant,

---

Amber's Dress Code

When I moved to College City from Denver, the kids all looked different from my old school. Like, they were all so . . . preppie! I like to look different . . . and I'm one of the only Hispanic kids. But the girls, they all had this thick straight blonde hair and little white tennies and tight jeans faded just right and white tee shirts and little gold chains. They all looked alike. I wear flannel shirts and baggy pants and boxers . . . [she laughs] . . . but under my pants! And I *don't* wear those little white tennies!

---

and although yesterday's teen queen wore bobby sox and pleated skirts whereas today's might "punk up" her hair, adherence to the prevailing adolescent dress code and standards for social behavior and recreation make all the difference in the status hierarchy (see box).

High grades alone are not sufficient to ensure a successful career in school even from the perspective of teachers, and conversely low grades will not always preclude students from feeling good about their life in school, being envied by their peers, and being defined as "successful" students. Many students consider social, personal, and familial achievement to be as important, if not more so, than academic achievement. They want very much to be accepted by their friends, and doing so means adopting the cultural values of their friends. If their friends do not value academic achievement, neither will they.

In point of fact, many can see little if any benefit, immediate or future, from the boring studies they slog through (McLaren 1980; McLeod 1987; Powell, Farrar, and Cohen 1985; Sizer 1984). Young people want to be in school, but less to study than because their friends are there. All they can do outside of school during the day is read, watch television, hang around on street corners and at shopping malls, and generally get into trouble. If their friends are anti-school, they may drop out, especially if they feel that conformity to school will alienate them from their peers. This circumstance is especially problematic for successful members of minority groups who are pressured to view conformity to school as selling out or "acting white" (Fordham and Ogbu 1986):

> People are afraid to show that they can speak grammatically correct English. When I do, my friends in my neighborhood will say, "you nerd!" or "Talk English!" or "Talk to us like we talk to you."
>
> I've been *per se* called an oreo because black as I am and bright, everybody thinks I'm too proper and talk white . . . and people tend to *tease* me.
> (Fordham and Ogbu, quoted in Erickson 1987)

An interesting reversal of acting white is the appropriation by rebellious *white* students of African-American hip-hop hairstyles and dress. Adoption of a stigmatized identity, or "acting black," led a number of white middle-school-aged girls to be spit upon and jeered at by their peers. Five dropped out, as did the few African-American students in their school (*New York Times* 1993).

Alienation from school is exacerbated when students respect very few of their teachers, because they feel either that teachers don't like or respect them or that they are incompetent to teach their subjects. Students form their opinions from the way teachers talk to them and treat them.

> Some teachers talk down to you like you're stupid when you ask questions. Some teachers embarrass you in front of the class. They make jokes about failed tests, poor grades, and things. (Firestone and Rosenblum 1988, p. 289)
>
> My teacher would put me on her knees in the corner and whip me with wet newspapers and the rest of the class would laugh. (Dixon, quoted by A. D. Greene 1989)
>
> The teacher laughed and said, "Well, here's a student who can't see how to get to class." [The speaker is a Navajo student whose name is Cantsee.] (Deyhle 1988)

Examples like these clearly indicate that the students' perceptions are sometimes correct.

The Extracurriculum

To channel the energy of young people and seduce them into school-related activities, educators have created an "extracurriculum" of sports, clubs, and entertaining activities to accompany the academic curriculum. These nonacademic functions of school help to contain the influence of the student peer group. They also fill the vacant time, which children are believed to have before and after school and on weekends, with activities sanctioned by the school. They reinforce academic standards because adequate academic performance and acceptable conduct are required for participation in these activities.

The extracurriculum also reinforces traditional gender roles. Activities for males emphasize what are considered appropriate male qualities of achievement, competitiveness, toughness, goal fulfillment in the face of pain and discomfort, and aggression. Girls' activities reinforce the fact that females are rewarded for having a pleasant, bubbly personality; neat, clean hair; a trim figure; and a calm, agreeable facade even under adverse circumstances, and for playing a supportive role to male activities (Eder and Parker 1987). Extracurricular activities also accustom students to the legitimacy of an unequal distribution of status and rewards in society, just as the academic curriculum does (Ibid., p. 205).

Visit a high school during its lunch period. What student groups can you identify? What distinguishes them from other peer groups? Discuss your findings in class.

Winners. The extracurriculum evokes a caricature of a white, middle-class American adolescent who does not have to work and whose life is filled with proms, sports, and cheerleading. Nevertheless, there are many students, of various social classes and ethnic groups, who "major" in the extracurriculum, finding the academic side of life too difficult or meaningless. They often are encouraged to do this by peers as well as by teachers and parents who believe that success in the extracurriculum is a boost to self-esteem. The importance of the extracurriculum to parents is highlighted by the practice of kindergarten "redshirting": Children who have the cognitive skills to begin school are held back a year so they will be more physically mature than their grade-level peers and can excel in sports (Eisenhart and Graue 1990).

The extracurriculum can even supplant academics: Athletes and other special students may be given undeserved passing grades to keep them eligible for outside-class activities. Controversy over this kind of pressure has led to the passing of "no-pass, no-play" legislation in many states, and to subsequent public outrage by coaches, alumni associations, students, beleaguered parents, and teachers on both sides of the issue.

What extracurricular activities did you participate in when you were in high school? Describe the students who participated with you in these activities by social class, gender, and race/ethnicity.

The dark side of extracurricular activities is the outgroups—the so-called wimps, nerds, losers, greasers, "badasses," punks, and delinquents—who cannot or will not participate. Until recently only the positive side of the caricature got attention. Studies conducted before the 1970s were concerned with suburban middle-class students or the white working class (Coleman 1961; Hollingshead 1949; Kahl 1953; Stinchcombe 1964). Parents and educators registered dismay at finding that the majority of students found academic work to have little intrinsic value and that, for most, the "gentleman's C" was the highest standard to which they aspired.

Yeah, if you're a straight A student, you get razzed. . . . (McLeod 1987)

[You have to] hang out at ____'s. Don't be too smart. Flirt with boys. Be cooperative on dates. (Coleman 1961, p. 371)

Losers. Middle- and working-class white parents in the 1950s and 1960s assumed that teenage hijinks and aversion to work would dissipate with maturity and that students would settle down and become productive members of the community. Nobody examined what became of the high school underclass—minorities, dropouts, the unpopular, and the poor. This disaffected and dropout population is now garnering a great deal of attention, since it is much larger than was previously believed. In most large cities it makes up nearly the majority of the population (Hess et al. 1985; LeCompte and Goebel 1987; Powell, Farrar, and Cohen 1985). It also is much louder and more manifestly violent in its opposition to school than the mild underachievement believed characteristic of the middle class. Further, its members do not eventually assimilate into a semblance of middle-class life. Rather, they remain a disaffected, underemployed and unemployed underclass as adults. This phenomenon raises some important questions:

- Why are students in general and resident minority groups in particular beginning to believe that going to school will not help them to succeed?
- Why do they sense that the American Dream does not apply to them?

To understand this, it is necessary to recognize that schools do not exist in isolation from the world community and that not all of the problems in schools can be resolved by classroom instruction. Rather, it is necessary to look beyond the confines of any given school and its community into the larger world society. As we have seen, the failure of the disadvantaged actually acts to preserve existing patterns of domination.

SURVIVING SCHOOL

In the preceding pages we have described what life is like for contemporary teenagers and how they spend their days. We have defined peer culture and explained how it developed. We also have discussed some of the societal issues that complicate the process of growing up. We have suggested that a critical aspect in the maturation of children is their long period of schooling, during which they learn from each other and establish collective ideas about the world and how to live in it. We also have suggested that adolescents find the ideas of their friends and the media a much more powerful influence than those of most adults.

However, young people differ according to sex, academic achievement, socioeconomic status, ethnicity, whether they live in large cities, suburbs, small towns, or rural areas, and by neighborhood. They also respond differently to school, both individually and in groups. While factors such as economic status and teenage parenthood contribute to the alienation of young people from school, the impact of these factors is heightened by the extent to which their friends are similarly alienated. Even very bright and highly motivated students with parents who help and even push them find it difficult to study when none of their friends does. Conversely, if students already are in trouble because of family divorce, pregnancy, low grades, difficulty in finding jobs, or knowledge of the shrinking opportunity structure, their potential for disaffection from school still depends upon how many of their friends are in similar trouble.

Valli (1983), who studied young women planning to become clerical and office workers, suggests that there are three possible forms of response to cultural institutions: acceptance, negotiation, and resistance. Which form a young person will choose in reaction to school depends upon how much hope this individual has for the future, and to what extent school will contribute to the realization of his or her aspirations.

Acceptance

Acceptance involves internalization of the school's promise that academic success and educational longevity will pay off. Students who accept this premise struggle to believe the American cultural myth of the linkage between education and occupational status (LeCompte 1987b; LeCompte and Dworkin 1991). Some work hard to maintain the status inherited from their family of origin, to take their putative place in the top echelons of society; others, like Horatio Alger, believe in the "rags to riches" story as they struggle to do better than their parents did.

Children who adopt this response generally come from any of several kinds of families. Most obvious are those from the middle class or the affluent Anglo and dominant culture, or immigrant families who, like many Southeast Asians, are well educated and once were wealthy but lost their status when they became refugees (Dworkin 1974). Most of these parents have themselves benefited from education and they push their children to do well. Even if they are not themselves educated, most know how to exert pressure on the school system when their children have problems, to negotiate to have their children placed in the best classes, and to help them with their homework. They also obtain tutoring, psychological counseling, and other kinds of help when it is deemed necessary (Ziegler, Hardwick, and McGreath 1989). Others who tend to do well in school are children of immigrants whose present situation, however bleak it may seem to native residents, is infinitely more promising than the opportunities they might have had in their former homes (Gibson 1987; Ogbu 1987; Suarez-Orozco 1987; Valverde 1987).

The "immigrant psychology" of hope (Ogbu 1987) helps to explain not only the hard work and academic success of refugee children from Southeast Asia, but also the fact that fewer children who were born in Mexico and then migrated to the United States seem to drop out of school than do Mexican-American children born in the United States (Valverde 1987). The issue is not limited to migration across national boundaries. McLeod (1987) points out that while both groups of high school young men whom he studied were from similarly impoverished and crime-prone backgrounds, the "Brothers," who were African American, experienced relatively greater academic success and expressed greater belief in the efficacy of school learning than did the "Hallway Hangers," who were white. McLeod suggests that the difference may be that the Brothers' families had moved fairly recently to the mostly white public housing project in which both groups lived, and they saw the project as an improvement over life in the ghetto. To the Hallway Hangers, whose families had lived there all their lives, the project symbolized the impossibility of escaping a dead-end existence.

Negotiation

Negotiators seek to make a deal. Negotiation is not wholehearted acceptance of the premises of schooling but rather a recognition that, while the payoffs for completing school may not be monumental, the consequences of not doing so are worse. The reasons for staying are unimportant. Students might be motivated simply by the wrath of their parents. The important point is that schooling has extrinsic rather than intrinsic value.

Negotiators try to complete their schooling with minimum effort. They may feel that most schoolwork is boring beyond belief (Eisenhart and Holland 1988, 1992; Powell, Farrar, and Cohen 1985; Sizer 1984), but they will work hard enough and conform sufficiently to the rules to ensure that they will obtain the necessary diploma or degree. Fuller's study (1980) of black Caribbean women students in England demonstrates how these students consciously or unconsciously negotiate an exchange of reasonable work for reasonable demands from their teachers. Negotiators may seek to minimize work by "scoping out" their teachers to find out what is expected and how to get around them. They may take less advanced courses which still meet graduation requirements. They may even make deals with teachers so they will be required to do minimal work and in exchange they will guarantee an orderly classroom without harassment.

While the most active and overt negotiators are older students, some researchers have described the process in elementary school. Borko and Eisenhart (1986) demonstrated how second graders in the lower reading groups induce teachers to simplify their lessons. When asked questions they thought were too hard, the children would respond either with difficulty or very slowly. Their teachers then assumed the work was too difficult and would subsequently "dumb down" their teaching, revising lessons to include less material. The students thus achieved their objective of making school less taxing. L. M. McNeil (1988a, 1988b, 1988c) has suggested that an unforeseen consequence of this interaction is, however, that students are progressively more handicapped in school. As they learn less, they fall further and further behind their classmates.

Although we have described it as such, much of the negotiation is not actually a consciously struck bargain, like a union contract. In fact, most students accept the inevitability of adult expectations and institutional constraints. The procedures for negotiating survival evolve as cultural knowledge within the student peer groups, which pass it on to each succeeding generation. Insofar as the rules for negotiation still require conformity to minimal academic standards, teachers may complain about the loss of student proficiency and energy but they do not define their students as engaging in active resistance.

Both accepters and negotiators cause little concern to school staff because their conformity gives the impression that they have bought into the premises of schooling. They follow most of the rules and are likely to graduate. Other students, however, do not wish to negotiate on the school's terms. We define these students as *resisters*.

Resistance: Its Definition, Purpose, and Types

Resisters are a problem for schools because they cause trouble and are likely to drop out. Resistance to institutional constraints is more than simple misbehavior. It is principled, conscious, and ideological nonconformity which has its basis in philosophical differences between the individual and the institution. It involves "withholding assent" (Erickson 1987, p. 237) from school authorities. Students who resist may disagree with the way they are treated on the basis of their gender, ethnicity, or social class; they may disagree with the academic track to which they are assigned; or they may disagree with the esteem in which any of these categories is held. They become resisters when their disagreement is actively expressed.

Resistance can serve to salvage the self-esteem or reputation of the individual engaging in it. In some cases, the acts of resistance do not entirely sabotage the careers of students.

Assertiveness. Schools consistently try to avoid, simplify, or deny the existence of resistance (L. M. McNeil 1988a, 1988b, 1988c; Page 1987; Powell, Farrar, and Cohen 1985). Some students, however, refuse to be silenced and demand the right to hold complex opinions or maintain contradictory consciousness (Gramsci 1971). Fine describes how Deirdre, a bright African-American senior, refused to accede to a teacher's demands that she decide whether the actions of Bernard Goetz, the New York City "subway vigilante" who shot four young men he thought were about to rob him, were right or wrong. From the supposedly silenced middle of the room, she declared:

> It's not that I have no opinions. I don't like Goetz shootin' up people who look like my brother, but I don't like feelin' unsafe in the projects or my neighborhood either. I got lots of opinions. I ain't being quiet 'cause I can't decide if he's right or wrong. I'm thinking. (1987, p. 164)

In another example, Rose (1988) was puzzled to find that African-American students in her college persisted in their use of Black English, even in written composition, despite the fact that they knew Standard English and realized that the practice would lower their grades. At first she thought it was a way to reinforce an African-American identity. The explanation the students gave, however, was that for their purposes, Standard English just did not sound right. Not using Black English was like not using inflection and punctuation. Standard English simply did not convey the meaning they wanted.

Hyperachievement: Beating Them at Their Own Game. A few students choose to repudiate the negative labels the school assigns to them. A dramatic example is that of Carrie Mae Dixon of Yates High School in Houston. An economically disadvantaged African American, she had been an orphan with no legal guardian since kindergarten. She was pregnant, unmarried, and the mother of a two-year-old. In third grade her teacher called her dumb for repeatedly getting in trouble in school. But she also was at the top of her class in every grade since the end of elementary school and graduated high school as valedictorian. She was accepted to university, awarded two scholarships for the fall, and now wanted to be a chemical engineer. The turning point was a classmate's insult. "After that, I decided I would show her who was dumb and who wasn't. . . . In tenth grade is when I found out what the valedictorian is. They explained to me that this is the person with the highest grade point average and I said, 'OK, that's what I want to be.' "

Plans for her valedictory address almost went awry when her principal decided that a pregnant valedictorian set a poor example for other students and so she could not participate in the graduation ceremony. It took national media attention to change the minds of the school officials (A. D. Greene 1989).

The kinds of resistance just described are used by students who are more or less successful in school. They may win peer approval or, like some of the students who "act white," not encounter so much adverse response from peers that they drop out. Other forms of resistance, however, lead to further alienation from school. Students may define the academic part of school as meaningless. Some may disavow schooling altogether, insofar as they not only do not identify with the academic part of school but also fail to find its extracurricular aspects alluring. These students choose alternative avenues for achieving status, some of them sanctioned or at least accepted by the establishment, others not.

There are a number of ways students express their alienation from and lack of engagement with school. Before discussing these, we need to note that most students engage in at least some of them at some point. These acts do not constitute resistance, however, unless they involve active, conscious, and principled opposition to a specific way in which the school has chosen to define a student.

Resistance may begin with simple nonconforming behavior and then be transformed into resistance by the negative responses of school staff. Student behavior will diverge further and further from what school staff find acceptable and bearable. Under these conditions, students who are dropout risks become "push-outs" — forced out of school by an establishment that will not or cannot accommodate them. As teachers, counselors, and administrators mobilize to neutralize, isolate, or otherwise eliminate the behavior (and often, the student engaging in it), students may find themselves in an ever less congenial environment — detention, suspension, remedial classes, and repeated confrontations with parents and school staff. They also may find that nobody cares to rescue them and stop the process.

Talk to a group of elementary school students and then to a group of high school students. Ask them what strategies they use to "get back" at teachers, what kinds of tricks they play on teachers, and how they get around assignments. Would you define any of these activities as types of resistance?

Boredom and Alienation: The Initial Phase of Resistance. Resistance usually begins when students stop studying or begin to engage in mild forms of smart-aleck behavior and vandalism. In an attempt to be considered more mature, they may begin to adopt what Stinchcombe (1964) calls symbolic adult behavior — use of drugs and alcohol, smoking, early dating and sex (Ekstrom et al. 1986). They get jobs, which make them feel good both because they involve some responsibility and because they provide funds to buy clothing, cars, and other goods with which to impress their friends. Girls may be happy to have a baby, despite feeling sorry because motherhood interferes with school and seeing friends (Deyhle and LeCompte 1994; A. D. Greene

1989; Sege 1989). Both jobs and babies can take so much time and energy that they seriously compromise a student's ability to cope with schoolwork.

Students who cannot get licit jobs or who find that they pay very little may engage in illicit ones—selling drugs, burglary, pimping, and prostitution. Alienated students often form gangs of similarly inclined peers and may go beyond simple vandalism and harassment to real terrorist tactics to intimidate both students and staff.

Tuning Out: Dropping Out in School.   The ultimate form of resistance is to stop coming to school. There are many ways to accomplish this. Some students start simply by sleeping in their classes. Those who have after-school jobs may doze as a logical response to lack of sleep. Others begin to cut classes. They don't leave the school building, they simply ditch the classes they find most distasteful. Selective class cutting is increasingly widespread. Hess and his colleagues (1985) have documented what they call a "culture of cutting," wherein students spend more time in the hallways and hiding places of the school than in class. These students are in-school dropouts, or "tune-outs." They are likely to be average middle-class students and those whom we have called the "negotiators." While they have not yet actually cut their ties with school, they are disaffected, and they receive little more instruction than students who actually have dropped out. They are, however, increasing in numbers, and they are at great risk of becoming dropouts.

Dropping Out: Giving Up on School.   Statistics on dropouts are notoriously unreliable. Even figures on the absolute number of students who fail to graduate are questionable. Some methods of analysis overestimate the dropout numbers, but most probably underestimate them significantly (LeCompte and Goebel 1987; Morrow 1986). However, since the 1960s at least 25 percent of any given age cohort in the United States failed to finish high school (McDill, Pallas, and Natriello 1985; Steinberg, Blinde, and Chan 1984). It probably also is correct that in most cities, and among what Ogbu (1978) has called "caste-like minorities"—African Americans, Latinos, American Indians—dropout rates exceed 40 percent and may be as high as 80 percent (Orum 1984).

It is even more difficult to determine *why* students drop out. Most dropouts do not appear at the school door to say goodbye. Like Carmen (see box on p. 122), they simply stop coming and eventually are placed in a "whereabouts unknown" category, then dropped from the records. Those who do announce their departure often lie about their plans. It is more socially acceptable to state that one has a job, is transferring to another school, or will join the military than to admit that one is simply giving up on school (Hammack 1986; LeCompte and Goebel 1987).

Most data on the reasons for dropping out consist of demographic correlations: Students, it is said, drop out because they are poor, are from minority or single-parent families, or are girls who have had babies. This descriptive data neither addresses the real motivations for leaving school, nor—because of its focus upon "victim characteristics" over which the school has little control—does it provide much assistance in remedying the problems. It is true that some young people must leave school in order to support their family or take care of siblings or their own children. However, the

---

Carmen's Story

By then I was hanging with a very rough crowd. My friends were into drugs, and soon I was doing the same. We shoplifted and stole everything we found that could be converted into cash. My parents were always on my case, and I ran away several times. I would come home only when I did not have any other place to crash. I would go to school while I was home, but my grades went down and I was not interested in school anymore.

Nobody in school ever took interest in helping me or learning about what had changed me. They only were interested in me going to school on a regular basis. I don't even remember talking to the school counselor. I think they gave up on me, and when I left I never looked back. I never even considered going back to school until I came here and at the Employment Office they told me about the program for farm workers.

SOURCE: Velasquez 1993, p. 91.

---

evidence suggests that the majority who leave school do so because of school-related factors. Many already were part of the culture of opposition to school, a culture that acts to exacerbate their difficulties by inducing them to violate norms of behavior or to engage in activities that interfere with schoolwork. For others who had serious personal problems, school requirements became the final straw.

In contemporary schools whose major task is the batch-processing and crowd control of huge numbers of children, little individual time and few resources exist for students with difficult problems, such as a need for child care or psychiatric care, or help for drug addiction or physical abuse. Many of these students with problems are defined as either intractable or just not the business of the school. For some, that indeed may be true. Schools cannot, for example, be expected to treat acting-out, psychotic students, or drug addicts.

Most students, however, do not fall into such extreme categories. They are bored. They hate school. The work is too difficult or too easy. Their degree won't amount to anything when they get out. The staff told them they were failures or unwanted. Teachers didn't care, were incompetent, or didn't understand. They were pregnant and embarrassed to "show." They couldn't find a baby-sitter. Their guardian was dying and they were needed for nursing care. They had no car and couldn't get across town to the dropout center. In all cases, the school was too inflexible to accommodate to their needs (Delgado-Gaitan 1988; Deyhle 1988; Fine 1986; Holley and Doss 1983; LeCompte 1985; Valverde 1987; Wehlage and Rutter 1986; Williams 1987). We believe that most students who drop out are those who were already at risk and were pushed out altogether by an unresponsive institution. It wasn't that they didn't learn how schools work—following the rules just didn't work for them.

SUMMARY

In this chapter we have discussed the formation of youth culture and the student peer group in the context of global patterns of consumption, technological change, the labor market, family structure, and cultural survival. It suggests that the advent of compulsory schooling and the prolongation of adolescence facilitate the development of oppositional youth culture. It also describes how curricular and extracurricular experiences socialize children for participation in a society stratified by achievement but biased by race, class, and gender. Finally, it suggests that students respond differentially to the realization that the rewards of schooling are mirrored in the rewards of society. Some accommodate to school and survive, others resist and drop out.

It is important for us to consider the experiences of students in schools within the broader cultural contexts. We cannot hold teachers and other school personnel responsible for finding solutions to all the serious problems facing youth today. Teachers can, and often do, provide meaningful environments for students, but they must compete with all of the societal forces—mass media, material consumption, violence, poverty, changing family structures—that are tremendous influences on the way young people construct meaning in their worlds.

chapter 4

The Labor Force in Education: Teachers, Counselors, Administrators, and Ancillary Staff

125

INTRODUCTION

In Chapter 3 we suggested that children go to school mostly to work at tasks set for them by adults. In this chapter we discuss the roles of teachers, counselors, administrators, and ancillary school staff, whose qualifications for being in schools rest upon specific professional training. These adults relate to the school differently from students because they *are* adults, because their participation is voluntary, and because they are paid and, at least in theory, can be fired for poor job performance. Students, on the other hand, "qualify" for attendance in schools simply by virtue of their age. Students, required by law to attend, are "involuntary recruits" who are not paid for the work they perform and cannot be fired for malfeasance (Nadel 1957).

We will limit our consideration of adults in schools to "educators," that is, professionals whose primary tasks are defined by their direct relationship to the teaching of children. Security personnel, maintenance engineers, dieticians, cooks, janitors, bookkeepers and clerks, personnel specialists, bus drivers, and gardeners also work in schools and are critical to their smooth operation. In many cases the relationships these workers form with educators and students are of profound importance to the teaching and learning process. For example, in his classic book, *The Sociology of Teaching* (1932), Willard Waller argues that janitors, all of whom at the time of his study were males, are among the most powerful people in schools and often serve as role models for male students. However, such staff members perform work such as

---

Anna's Story

I really enjoy working with the students. I love seeing the little "light bulb" go on in people's heads. Kids feel good when they "get it," and I enjoy conveying how much I love language.

Duren's Story

I love to teach. I get high on it. I love watching a kid "get it." I enjoy doing my job well. It changes, the people change, and the subject matter changes. If you're good, you'll never teach the same thing the same way twice. You can get summers off, you can get to know some wonderful people (students and parents), and you can continue to learn. You and the students can explore the world together.

---

preparing food, cleaning buildings, and hiring workers, tasks that can be performed in many kinds of institutions and that do not involve teaching children. The work of educators, however, is centered upon schools and school-like settings. While it may seem all too obvious, the practice of their profession also requires the presence of students—the too-often forgotten recipients of educators' labor.

How Do Sociologists View Educators?

Sociologists view teachers—and other educators—in the context of their work. This context includes how educators and the society at large define what they do. We will first discuss the definition of professions in general and consider whether or not teaching should be considered a profession. We will then examine the characteristics of educators, addressing the following issues:

1. How has the historical evolution of the profession affected its current development?
2. What are the demographic characteristics—such as age, sex, socioeconomic background, and race—of educators?
3. Is the profession stratified by race, class, gender, and other demographic characteristics?
4. What relationship exists between the demographic characteristics of teachers and the specific tasks to which various groups of educators are assigned?
5. Does this relationship affect the way educators carry out their tasks and how they feel about them?
6. What distinguishes educators as a group from people in other professions?

Finally, we will discuss teachers' work. Questions we will examine are the following:

1. What is the nature of educators' work?
2. How do the characteristics of their work affect how they behave and how they feel about their jobs?
3. What kinds of power and control do teachers have over their work?

4. Is power differentially distributed among various kinds of educators?
5. How does the relationship of educators compare with the labor market experience of other kinds of workers?

Throughout the chapter we will call attention to the tensions and ambiguities of power and status which constitute both the political and social context of those who work in schools.

ISSUES OF STATUS AND POWER: PROFESSIONAL ESTEEM AND PUBLIC DISREGARD

Education professionals have an image problem. Whether university-level or elementary school teachers, counselors or principals, coaches or superintendents, all educators feel there is a gap between the status they would like to enjoy in society and the power they actually wield. Neither social analysts, policy makers, the public, nor educators themselves can decide whether educational practitioners are scholarly professionals, like doctors and university professors, or members of the laboring work force, like clerks, salespeople, or skilled laborers. In part this is so because teachers' salaries are discrepant with what they "ought" to get, given the supposed value of the work they perform. It is clear that income does not necessarily correlate with social standing. For example, artists—writers, poets, musicians—may live at the poverty line despite the value of their creative contributions. The community services of teachers are considered so crucial that their right to withhold those services is often denied by laws forbidding them to strike. However, the public repeatedly demonstrates its unwillingness to pay for these services by establishing low salary scales and rejecting school tax levies and bond issues. Table 4.1 depicts teacher salaries compared with salaries in other occupations.

Even though they are considered to be professionals, public school teachers are ranked only slightly above electricians and musicians in indices of social status, and far below doctors, lawyers, dentists, college professors, and airline pilots. Their ranking in scales of occupational prestige has fallen steadily (Hodge, Siegel, and Rossi 1966, p. 325).

Teachers are ambivalent about their field. While they insist that their professional training, certification, and expertise justify community esteem, they often denigrate teacher education courses as the least rigorous part of their education (Lortie 1969, p. 24). Reflecting this ambivalence, there is widespread public belief that "anyone can teach."

One factor contributing to this ambivalence is that careers in teaching have different status levels for different groups. They are considered to be socially desirable for women and, until recent years, one of the highest attainable occupations for African Americans, Latinos, and American Indians. However, teaching is an entry-level position for white men if they move to administration, but a low-status dead end if they don't (Lortie 1969, p. 20).

Differential status also is based on age of students, subject matter, and gender.

TABLE 4.1 Average Starting Salaries of Public School Teachers Compared with Salaries in Private Industry, by Selected Position: 1975 to 1992[a]

Item and Position	1975	1980	1985	1986	1987	1988	1989	1990	1991	1992
SALARIES (dollars)										
Teachers[b]	8,233	10,764	15,460	16,500	17,500	19,400	NA	20,486	21,481	22,171
College graduates:										
Engineering	12,744	20,136	26,880	28,512	28,932	29,856	30,852	32,304	34,236	34,620
Accounting	11,880	15,720	20,628	21,216	22,512	25,140	25,908	27,408	27,924	28,404
Sales—marketing	10,344	15,936	20,616	20,688	20,232	23,484	27,768	27,828	26,580	26,532
Business administration	9,768	14,100	19,896	21,324	21,972	23,880	25,344	26,496	26,256	27,156
Liberal arts[c]	9,312	13,296	18,828	21,060	20,508	23,508	25,608	26,364	25,560	27,324
Chemistry	11,904	17,124	24,216	24,264	27,048	27,108	27,552	29,088	29,700	30,360
Mathematics—statistics	10,980	17,604	22,704	23,976	25,548	25,548	28,416	28,944	29,244	29,472
Economics—finance	10,212	14,472	20,964	22,284	21,984	23,928	25,812	26,712	26,424	27,708
Computer science	NA	17,712	24,156	26,172	26,280	26,904	28,608	29,100	30,924	30,888
INDEX (1975 = 100)										
Teachers[b]	100	131	187	200	213	236	NA	249	261	269
College graduates:										
Engineering	100	158	211	224	227	234	242	253	268	271
Accounting	100	132	174	179	189	212	218	230	235	239
Sales—marketing	100	154	199	200	196	227	268	269	257	256
Business administration	100	144	204	218	225	244	259	271	268	278
Liberal arts[c]	100	143	202	226	220	252	275	283	274	293
Chemistry	100	144	203	204	227	228	231	244	249	255
Mathematics—statistics	100	160	207	218	233	233	258	263	266	268
Economics—finance	100	142	205	218	215	234	252	261	258	271
Computer science[d]	NA	125	171	185	186	190	202	205	218	217

NA Not available.

[a]Except as noted, salaries represent what corporations plan to offer graduates graduating in the year shown with a Bachelor's degree. Based on a survey of approximately 200 companies.

[b]Estimate. Minimum mean salary. Source: National Education Association, Washington, DC, unpublished data.

[c]Excludes Chemistry, Mathematics, Economics, and Computer Science.

[d]Computer science index (1978 = 100).

SOURCE: Except as noted, Northwestern University Placement Center, Evanston, IL, *The Northwestern Lindquist-Endicott Report* (copyright).

Rocklan's Story

I care about children, all of them, and throughout my schooling I saw injustices occur to children because they were poor, who their families were, and these things always made me angry. I see teaching as a way to make a difference in the lives of children. I feel that I have been given many gifts and therefore I want to give something back. I have a love for knowledge and discovery and I want to share that with children.

The highest status is accorded to those who teach the oldest students. University professors are at the top of the status hierarchy, secondary school teachers and instructors in technical and vocational schools occupy the middle, followed by elementary school teachers, and day-care workers occupy the lowest ranks. Within these levels, teachers are differentiated by administrative rank, demographics, subject area, and the age and gender of the students. Supervisors and administrators rank higher than instructors. In general, women and minorities enjoy less status than men and dominant-culture individuals in the same position. Teachers of the "hard sciences" outrank philosophers, vocational educators, and English teachers. Teachers of graduate students and fifth graders outrank those who deal, respectively, with undergraduates and kindergartners. Those who teach women and minorities have less status than those who teach males and members of the dominant classes. Finally, differential status is accorded to specific philosophical outlooks. Since school bureaucracies are conservative and slow to change, change agents are stigmatized and the highest prestige is accorded to those who deviate least from the norm (Aronowitz and Giroux 1985).

These ambiguities and status differentials come from contradictions in the structural and historical evolution of the profession, the nature of teachers' work, patterns of control and status in the profession, the nature of career paths and the reward structure of education, and the age, racial, and gender characteristics of educators. We will discuss these from both a traditional functionalist perspective and the critical perspective which informs our own thinking.

CONTRADICTIONS IN THE STRUCTURE OF THE PROFESSION

Functionalists compare the structure and organization of teaching with those of other professions. They describe how differences in structure create gaps between the esteem in which teachers would like to be held by the public and their peers, and the low status they actually have. These gaps come from the nature and organization of tasks in teaching, how people are trained to execute them, and how much control teachers have over their performance.

Definition of a Profession: The Traditional View

Professions can be differentiated in terms of the complexity of tasks performed as well as the type, rigor, and duration of training and the nature of control, power, and autonomy in the profession. The relationship between the actual work done and the physical context in which it is performed also helps to differentiate professions. Max Weber first delineated the characteristics of the "ideal typical" professional, taking as his models occupations such as medicine, law, and the priesthood. Weber wrote that professionals shared the following characteristics: they were self-employed providers of services, they entered their profession because they were "called" to it out of some deep personal commitment, and their qualifications were based upon their possession of "expert" and esoteric knowledge. In addition, their knowledge base could be acquired by only a select few who underwent long and rigorous study. Their services dealt with serious, often life-or-death matters, and they were remunerated by fees from clients. Communication between professionals and their clients was legally privileged so that courts of law could not require its disclosure. Most important, entrance to these professions was controlled by professional peers, who set requirements for entry, training, and certification. Boards of peers also developed review processes to maintain standards and competence (Weber 1947).

Weber did not make value judgments about the relative merit of occupations; he simply provided a set of descriptors against which occupations could be compared. Today the profession that most closely approximates this standard is medicine. Education, on the other hand, deviates substantially from this model. Teachers are salaried and their communication with students is not legally protected. Other important deviations from the Weberian model include the nature of the knowledge base and the training required to attain it, the degree of control over entry to the profession, maintenance of standards, and the depth of commitment teachers, as a group, have to their calling (Etzioni 1969; Lortie 1969; Simpson and Simpson 1969).

Training.   One of the most obvious differences is in the training. Medicine, the priesthood, law, architecture, certified accounting, and other recognized professions require at least five years of training, including several years of rigorous study beyond college. Many also require a supervised apprenticeship or internship. In traditional teacher education programs, elementary and secondary school teachers typically spend only two undergraduate years in Liberal Arts courses. They then spend two years in pedagogical studies, where they learn how to teach the subjects they have just been taught. Only two years of content area instruction—equivalent to an Associate of Arts degree—and one and a half years of actual coursework in pedagogy are required. The remainder of the program is student teaching, which is experiential learning, located off-campus, and only lightly supervised by university personnel. In many colleges teacher training still resembles the normal school tradition, where teachers taught those just below their own academic attainment. One group of universities belonging to the Holmes Group (1986) now expects prospective teachers to complete a Bachelor's degree in Liberal Arts prior to a fifth-year Master's degree in teacher education.

The traditional knowledge base required for teaching, then, is not technical information requiring intellectually rigorous study, but rather experiential knowledge acquired primarily in apprenticeship or student teaching. Developing expertise involves adding to a "bag of tricks" rather than mastering complex levels of skill. Although the cumulative knowledge imparted to students is critical to one's functioning, no single piece constitutes a life-or-death matter.

It is illuminating to compare the "science" of education with the "science" of medicine. Both are applied fields that make use of information and techniques developed in the natural and social sciences (Ginsburg 1988), but one has high status and the other doesn't. The difference seems to be the seriousness with which medicine and other more traditional professions address the need for rigorous study prior to practice. Extensive advanced study in biology, chemistry, physics, and other background courses is required *before* the techniques of medical practice are learned. By contrast, the four years of teacher training are so crowded that there is little time, for example, for studies of the social and psychological anatomy of learning or the logical structure of mathematics and social studies. Students generally regard these courses as too theoretical, far less important than "how-to" methods for teaching discrete "factoids" (Morgenstern 1989) of reading, mathematics, and foreign languages.

National studies, including those by the National Commission on Excellence in Education (1983), the Rand Corporation (Darling-Hammond 1984), the Holmes Group (1986), and the Carnegie Task Force on Teaching as a Profession (1986), have questioned the quality of teacher training. Some have suggested requiring a fifth year of study in the "content areas" (The Holmes Group 1986). However, these suggestions, as well as others designed to make teacher education more rigorous, meet resistance both from university departments of curriculum and instruction, who see their control of teacher education eroded by course requirements outside their departments, and from students, who see that additional years of study produce no commensurate raise in pay.

Teacher education programs frequently are money-makers for their universities because they are cheap to operate. The per-student cost is less because the faculty generally are paid less than professors in other departments and because students do not use university facilities while student-teaching. Profits from education programs finance costlier programs, and universities are reluctant to reduce those profits by adding a year to the degree requirement.

Standards for graduation from teacher education are set by legislatures and are subject to the whim of fads and political pressures. For example, multicultural education courses, which were popular in the 1970s, virtually vanished in the 1980s. These are being reinstated in the 1990s with a renewed commitment to serving the needs of a diverse population.

Certification. Control of entry into the profession is another critical issue. In medicine and law, panels of doctors and lawyers set licensing standards. In contrast, it is market factors and legislative fiat that govern teacher certification. Furthermore, individual school districts can waive specific requirements if qualified personnel are not available. Teachers often are assigned to teach in their minor area of study, or in areas for which they have had no preparation at all. Certain subject areas, such as mathematics and science, bilingual education, and education for the handicapped, experience chronic shortages. Districts with shortages of certified bilingual or ESL teachers and large numbers of children who are not native speakers of English routinely hire English monolingual teachers on temporary certificates. These teachers are then paired, where possible, with bilingual aides or colleagues (LeCompte 1985). Where aides are used, they often provide the bulk of instruction to the poorest and most disadvantaged students (K. P. Bennett 1986, 1991; Ortiz 1988).

A national survey demonstrated how widespread these practices are. In some states the "percentages of high school classes taught by teachers who did not have a major, minor, or 20 quarter hours of preparation included Geography, 92%; Physics, 43%; Chemistry, 43%; Math, 36%; History, 32%; and English, 30%." Thus the areas most typically misassigned are in the core curriculum. Specialized offerings, such as fine arts and vocational education, are not so profoundly affected. The percentages in junior high schools and especially middle schools were even worse (Robinson and Pierce 1985). Table 4.2 presents data indicating that the shortage of qualified teachers will persist. Hospitals would never be permitted to hire a dermatologist to do brain surgery, no matter how severe the shortage of brain surgeons. However, such practices are routine in education.

Finally, a profession is considered a lifelong calling. However, as we shall indicate later in this chapter, teaching is treated as an interim career by family-oriented women, to be practiced at the convenience of marriage and child-rearing, and as an entry-level occupation for men and women who aspire to administrative jobs or other, more lucrative and less stressful careers. While many people do make teaching their life work, and while the rate of quitting decreases the longer a teacher remains in the profession, teachers on average have among the shortest career trajectories of all the professions. Individuals who actually begin teaching remain for an average of no more than about five years (Anderson and Mark 1977; Charters 1970; Mark and Anderson 1978).

Semiprofessions

Initial analyses of teaching equated it with the traditional "autonomous" professions. Functionalists next grouped teaching, along with nursing and social work, as a "semiprofession" (Etzioni 1969). Semiprofessions share some but not all of the characteristics of the classic professions. Like the traditional professions, they are white-collar occupations which provide services rather than produce goods. The training they require, however, is considerably less intellectually rigorous and time consuming. Their status is less legitimated. Their right to privileged communication is less well established, and their applicable body of knowledge is less esoteric.

The semiprofessions also have more supervision and societal control than the traditional professions. Practitioners are not typically self-employed; rather they are "bureaucratized," within formal service organizations. They receive salaries instead of client fees. They are "more" than clerks and secretaries, but "less" than doctors and lawyers (Etzioni 1969, pp. i–v).

TABLE 4.2 Relative Demand by Teaching Area and Year[a]

	1993	1992	1991	1990	1989	1976
Teaching Fields with Considerable Shortage (5.00–4.25)						
Special Education—Multiply Handicapped	4.40	4.47	4.42	4.39	4.14	—
Special Education—ED/BD	4.39	4.23	4.44	4.46	4.40	3.42
Special Education—LD	4.29	4.18	4.41	4.49	4.26	4.00
Speech Pathology/Audiology	4.28	4.37	4.53	4.41	4.25	3.63
Teaching Fields with Some Shortage (4.24–3.45)						
Special Education—Mentally Handicapped	4.22	4.33	4.47	4.48	4.29	2.87
Bilingual Education	4.18	4.15	4.15	4.35	4.45	—
Special Education—Deaf	4.17	4.41	4.21	4.34	4.12	—
Language—Other	4.04	3.53	3.67	3.41	—	—
Science—Physics	3.93	3.88	3.67	3.93	4.12	4.04
English as a Second Language	3.91	3.65	3.74	4.00	—	—
Science—Other	3.86	3.13	2.88	3.36	—	—
Special Education—Other	3.85	3.90	3.96	3.98	—	—
Special Education—Gifted	3.80	3.56	3.65	3.76	3.93	3.85
Science—Chemistry	3.79	3.68	3.84	3.62	4.01	3.72
Psychologist (School)	3.72	3.62	3.57	3.85	3.79	3.09
Language, Modern—Spanish	3.61	3.56	3.71	3.76	3.76	2.47
Teaching Fields with Balanced Supply and Demand (3.44–2.65)						
Library Science	3.43	3.61	3.53	3.76	3.60	—
Mathematics	3.43	3.53	3.58	3.91	3.83	3.86
Computer Science	3.41	3.25	3.36	3.84	3.75	—
Special Education—Reading	3.38	3.38	3.77	3.55	3.58	3.96
Counselor—Elementary	3.31	3.64	3.69	3.67	3.40	3.15
Science—Earth	3.24	3.14	3.33	3.15	3.55	3.44
Social Worker (School)	3.22	3.30	2.94	2.99	3.03	—
Data Processing	3.17	2.90	2.54	3.57	2.58	—
Counselor—Secondary	3.16	3.56	3.64	3.56	3.26	2.69
Science—Biology	3.16	3.08	3.04	3.17	3.35	2.97
Science—General	3.14	3.07	3.16	3.26	3.43	—
Language, Modern—French	3.13	3.13	3.24	3.22	3.51	2.15
Language, Modern—German	3.13	2.90	3.07	3.12	3.42	2.03
Technology—Industrial Arts	3.09	2.81	3.04	3.23	2.95	4.22
Agriculture	3.03	2.84	3.03	3.03	2.93	4.06
Music—Instrumental	2.91	3.09	3.27	3.23	3.20	3.03
Speech	2.88	2.85	2.72	2.78	2.95	2.46
Music—Vocal	2.81	2.95	3.10	3.12	3.00	3.00
Teaching Fields with Some Surplus (2.64–1.85)						
Home Economics	2.49	2.62	2.63	2.69	2.33	2.62
Journalism	2.46	2.64	2.59	2.66	2.76	2.86
English	2.44	2.94	3.05	3.28	2.97	2.05
Driver Education	2.42	2.31	2.82	2.57	2.71	2.44
Business	2.39	2.39	2.81	3.07	2.84	3.10
Art	2.25	2.11	2.21	1.96	2.24	2.14
Elementary—Intermediate	1.96	2.41	2.77	2.81	2.62	1.90
Health Education	1.89	1.90	2.17	2.02	2.03	2.27
Elementary—Primary	1.88	2.33	2.82	2.83	2.63	1.78
Teaching Fields with Considerable Surplus (1.84–1.00)						
Physical Education	1.61	1.70	1.85	1.72	1.78	1.74
Social Science	1.58	1.58	1.98	1.89	1.98	1.51

[a]Results for 1990 forward include Alaska/Hawaii; prior years are contiguous 48 states only.

5 = Considerable shortage; 4 = Some shortage; 3 = Balanced; 2 = Some surplus; 1 = Considerable surplus

SOURCE: From 1993 ASCUS (Association for School, College & University Staffing, Inc.) data supplied by survey respondents. In some instances, the averages are based upon limited input, and total reliability is not assured.

There is little agreement over standards for excellence in the semiprofessions. Both the establishment and enforcement of standards is affected by the needs of the employer bureaucracies. In addition, the knowledge base is applied and experiential rather than technical. While both professionals and semiprofessionals apply knowledge, semiprofessionals have less discretion over what they apply and how.

The authority of supervision over semiprofessionals is tenuous, since it is done by people who have had the same training, though more experience. This similarity in training is a source of tension and conflict. For example, school administrators all had to serve as teachers at one time, and teachers may question their dictates on the grounds that they do not have more training than the teachers. Another source of conflict is that teachers view administrators as management, not as colleagues or a respected reference group (Etzioni 1969, pp. v–xvi).

A Critical Note

Functionalists, in studying teachers' qualifications, compare teaching *up* to doctors, lawyers, and priests. Critical theorists, in contrast, focus on the character of teachers' work itself. They compare *down,* finding teachers to be more comparable to factory workers than to autonomous professionals. Both critical theorists and functionalists have examined the nature of control and power in the profession, including the fact that teaching is primarily a profession for women—a fact that they both use to explain many of the profession's unique characteristics. However, functionalists treat these asymmetrical patterns of control and power as understandable and unchangeable, while critical theorists view them as functions of the institutionalized patterns of oppression in modern capitalist society, conditions that perpetuate the weaknesses of the educational system—and that can and should be changed. We will next examine the themes of feminization, control, and work in teaching from both perspectives.

WHO BECOMES A TEACHER?

A Brief History of Women in Teaching

Teaching has not always been considered women's work. Until the middle of the nineteenth century most formal education, especially at the secondary level, was directed primarily at male students. For the most part, girls who were educated came from well-to-do families and were tutored in their homes. All teachers and administrators, whether of male or female students, were men.

Education Up to the Reformation. During the Hellenic and Roman eras, military leaders, town governments, and royal courts encouraged the establishment of public schools for the teaching of arts, rhetoric, music, literature, and grammar. With the fall of the Roman Empire, the thriving municipal schools for grammar and rhetoric also collapsed. By 400 A.D. literacy had survived only within the priesthood and among a very few aristocrats (Boyd 1966; Marrou 1956). Monastic orders preserved the remaining libraries, produced teachers, and copied books. The very few universities were governed by canon, or church law. Most professors were priests, and both teachers and students were treated as if they were members of the clergy. Some families of the nobility employed tutors and established schools for their own children and those of their entourage. These teachers often were priests who, like dancemasters and troubadours, were high-status servants.

The Protestant Reformation served as a catalyst for broader-based literacy. As the use of Latin as a *lingua franca* began to be replaced by the ancestors of modern European languages, songs and oral literature were developed in these, not ancient languages. By the time of Martin Luther, Latin was used only by priests and scholars. Literacy in Latin, however, was the key to the power of the Catholic Church hierarchy, since the Christian Bible was available at this time only in Latin and only priests were permitted to read and interpret it. One of the tenets of the Reformation was to reduce the power of priests by translating the Bible into the vernacular, making it accessible to all who could read.

The Reformation drew its power from the gradually strengthening middle and lower classes, groups that previously relied upon family socialization and apprenticeship to prepare young people for adulthood. Schooling for their children was deemed essential by Protestant churches and political leaders alike to inculcate in them the virtues of religion and the laws of society. As was pointed out in Chapter 2, because education then, as now, was viewed as a cure for social disorder, especially that allegedly fomented by the working classes, religious and civic leaders advocated the establishment of schools to indoctrinate the children of the poor. However, the existing educational system was designed only for an aristocracy and linked to university-level training for boys. It included tutoring in the traditional curriculum of Latin, Greek, grammar, rhetoric, and mathematics, followed by university training in law, medicine, or theology.

Towns and religious orders responded to the call for mass education by setting up primary schools which taught the rudiments of literacy, the catechism, and sometimes a little arithmetic. Thus was created a dual system of education: One strand was oriented to Latin, Greek, and the classics and led to university training for the rich; the other was conducted in vernacular languages and linked to vocational training for the poor (Resnick and Resnick 1985). Teachers for the former were required to have secondary school or university training, while those for the latter needed only to be literate. At best, they had some formal classes in pedagogy and had achieved one grade higher than the grade they taught.

The Entry of Women.   By the end of the 1600s, women were beginning to enter the teaching profession, although not in formal educational institutions. Dame schools, located in the women's homes, for neighborhood children, became a common way to learn the ABC's and the catechism. The English Poor Laws, enacted to ensure that poor children would not become public charges, encouraged apprenticeships. They also facilitated the education of orphans and girls from poor but respectable families, who learned to be governesses and tutors in the homes of well-to-do families, since, if unmarried, they would have no other respectable means of support.

Calvin E. Stowe Says Women Should Be Employed in the Elementary Schools, 1837

. . . Indeed, such is the state of things in this country, that we cannot expect to find male teachers for all our schools. The business of educating, especially young children, must fall, to a great extent on female teachers. There is not the same variety of tempting employment for females as for men, they can be supported cheaper, and the Creator has given [them] peculiar qualifications for the education of the young. Females, then, ought to be employed extensively in all our elementary schools, and they should be encouraged and aided in obtaining the qualifications necessary for this work. There is no country in the world where woman holds so high a rank, or exerts so great an influence, as here; wherefore, her responsibilities are the greater, and she is under obligations to render herself the more actively useful. I think our fair countrywomen, notwithstanding the exhortations of Harriet Martineau, Fanny Wright, and some other *ladies and gentlemen,* will never seek distinction in our public assemblies for public discussion, or in our halls of legislation; but in their appropriate work of educating the young, of forming the opening mind to all that is good and great, the more they distinguish themselves the better . . .

SOURCE: Knight and Hall, 1951, pp. 414–415.

Proponents of elementary school education, like Comenius and Froebel in Europe and Horace Mann in America, also encouraged the use of women as teachers of young children. Women were considered to be good influences on children. Their supposed motherly instincts, virtue, and less violent nature suited them for this work and served as a curb to the passionate, warlike nature of the young men they taught (Binder 1974, p. 124; Boyd 1966; Curti 1971). Perhaps more important, they were cheaper to hire than men (Boyd 1966; Curti 1971).

We need to remember that types of education were strictly differentiated by social class. The young children of the rich were taught at home and their education emphasized the classics, Latin and Greek. Older boys were taught by men at college preparatory academies and then were eligible to attend the university. If girls received any secondary training, it was primarily in the arts of homemaking and in those ornamental social skills deemed appropriate for upper-class women: French, fine needlework, music, dancing, and writing. Female teachers were restricted to teaching in their own homes, in the dame schools, or in those of the wealthy. Children of the poor received an education oriented to social control—sufficient literacy to understand the laws and contracts that governed their public life and labor and the doctrines of the Church.

The great influx of women into teaching began in the mid-nineteenth century through the Civil War period. The expansion of universal elementary schooling and the theretofore complete lack of schools for African Americans in the South, coupled with northerners' distrust of native southern teachers during Reconstruction, created a greater demand for teachers than could be filled by the available males. The "Yankee Schoolmarm" became a prototypical model for the female schoolteacher—single, dedicated, and often adventurous, willing to leave home and travel to hardship towns and frontier areas in search of the only jobs widely available for educated women (Kaufman 1984).

Teaching as Women's Work. The events of the nineteenth century shaped many of the patterns that characterize teaching today, the most important of which was the feminization of teaching. While the teaching profession entered the twentieth century with a work force dominated by women, men held virtually all of the administrative positions—a situation that prevails today.

From early times in America, teachers earned low wages. In areas dominated by subsistence farming they earned hardly more than common laborers. Only those lucky enough to teach in cities or in secondary-level academies attended by the wealthy could eke out a fairly comfortable living. A college graduate could make more money in almost any other profession. As a consequence, most male schoolmasters avoided making a career of teaching (Main 1966). The entry of women into teaching furthered the practice of paying teachers poorly; women were hired because they were expected to work for less than men.

Teaching was held in low esteem because, in an era that valued hard manual labor, teaching was defined as "easy." It did not require the full physical efforts of a man. Nor was it considered to be mentally taxing, since qualified teachers needed to attain only the level of education immediately higher than their students. Elementary teaching became a female-dominated field by choice (for women) and by default (for a very few men). By the mid 1880s training consisted of attendance at a high school or normal school (Lortie 1969). The persistent problem of high teacher turnover was institutionalized in the nineteenth century by the failure to pay men—or women—a living wage and by the requirement that women leave their job upon marriage (Lortie 1973, p. 488).

There is a long history of male resistance to higher education for women, or to giving university status to programs like normal schools which were designed for the training of women (Ginsburg 1988). Such resistance was justified on both gender and class bases. Higher education was considered unsuitable to the nature of women and a threat to male hegemony. Teacher education programs were denigrated for diminishing the status of universities with which they were associated (Ginsburg 1988) because they recruited both women and people from the lower socioeconomic classes, both groups of low status.

Critical theorists believe that recognizing the feminized nature of teaching is crucial to understanding the political, economic, and ideological modes of control in the profession. It is not the nature of the work itself that is problematic, but the fact that it is performed by subordinated, *female* workers whose position can best be understood through analyses of the labor process and patterns of class domination (Apple 1986).

During the early part of the twentieth century women poured into the teaching

---

Tracy's Story

Ever since the third grade I have wanted to be a teacher. Mrs. Salcido, my third-grade teacher, really turned me on to reading. She inspired me to make myself a better student. The effect she has had on my life is one that I hope to share with my students. Teaching is a very giving profession and I have always had the urge to help people. I feel that I really want to be able to see my success in reaching children in the classroom by seeing them graduate from high school and possibly go on to some form of higher education. If I can affect one student in the tremendous way Mrs. Salcido has affected me, it will be worth more than any salary given to me.

---

profession. First, as the barriers prohibiting their enrollment fell, an unprecedented number of middle- and upper-class women began to graduate from colleges and universities. For example, female enrollment in higher education rose from 29 percent of the total in 1948 to 51 percent in 1980 (O'Neill and Sepielli 1985, p. 27). In addition, government scholarships and preferential loan programs encouraged men and women to pursue careers in teaching.

Finally, even highly educated women in the 1950s and early 1960s found that sex discrimination in employment still precluded them from virtually all professional positions but teaching. Table 4.3 illustrates the male domination of school administration. The few women who do attain administrative rank do so by means of career paths markedly different from those of men (Grow 1981; Ortiz 1981).

Men usually go directly from teaching and coaching to line positions as assistant principals or principals in middle or high schools, and from there go to central administration. Women, by contrast, go from teaching to staff positions as curriculum coordinators or directors to line positions as elementary school principals, then to upper division schools, and finally to central administration. Sometimes they go directly from a staff position to central administration, but not often. Their career trajectory is usually slowed down by beginning in lower status staff and elementary school positions.

Not only are the type of tasks performed by educators rigidly differentiated by rank, but routes to these ranks as well as the incumbents themselves also are highly differentiated by gender. We will first examine demographic characteristics of the people who choose to become educators, then will consider the nature of their tasks and the structures in which these tasks are carried out.

Demographic Characteristics of Teachers

The most salient factor about teaching is its predominantly female work force. In 1983, the average teacher was a white, married woman in her mid-thirties with two children. She came from a middle- to upper-middle-class family, received her training

TABLE 4.3 Public School Employment by Occupation, Sex, and Race: 1982 and 1990[a]

Occupation	1982					1990				
	Total	Male	Female	White[b]	Black[b]	Total	Male	Female	White[b]	Black[b]
All occupations	3,082	1,063 (34%)	2,019 (66%)	2,498 (81%)	432 (14%)	3,181	914 (29%)	2,267 (71%)	2,502 (79%)	463 (16%)
Officials, administrators	41	31 (76%)	10 (24%)	36 (88%)	3 (7%)	43	28 (65%)	15 (35%)	37 (86%)	4 (9%)
Principals and assistant principals	90	72 (80%)	18 (20%)	76 (84%)	11 (12%)	90	56 (62%)	34 (38%)	70 (78%)	13 (14%)
Classroom teachers[c]	1,680	534 (32%)	1,146 (68%)	1,435 (85%)	186 (13%)	1,746	468 (27%)	1,278 (73%)	1,469 (84%)	192 (11%)
Elementary schools	798	129 (16%)	669 (84%)	667 (83%)	98 (12%)	875	128 (15%)	747 (85%)	722 (83%)	103 (12%)
Secondary schools	706	363 (51%)	343 (49%)	619 (88%)	67 (9%)	662	304 (46%)	358 (54%)	570 (86%)	66 (10%)
Other professional staff	235	91 (39%)	144 (61%)	193 (82%)	35 (15%)	227	58 (26%)	170 (75%)	187 (82%)	30 (13%)
Teachers' aides[d]	215	14 (7%)	200 (93%)	146 (68%)	45 (21%)	324	54 (17%)	270 (83%)	208 (64%)	69 (21%)
Clerical and secretarial staff	210	4 (2%)	206 (98%)	177 (84%)	19 (9%)	226	5 (2%)	221 (98%)	181 (80%)	24 (11%)
Service workers[e]	611	316 (51%)	295 (49%)	434 (71%)	132 (22%)	524	245 (47%)	279 (53%)	348 (66%)	129 (25%)

[a] In thousands. Covers full-time employment. 1982 excludes Hawaii, District of Columbia, and New Jersey. Based on sample survey of school districts with 250 or more students. 1990 based on sample survey of school district with 100 or more employees; see source for sampling variability.)
[b] Excludes individuals of Hispanic origin.
[c] Includes other classroom teachers, not shown separately.
[d] Includes technicians.
[e] Includes craftworkers and laborers.
SOURCE: U.S. Equal Opportunity Commission, Elementary-Secondary Staff Information (EEO-5), biennial.

at a public university, and was likely to teach in a suburban elementary school. She was not politically active and although she put in a slightly longer work week than the average blue-collar worker, she brought home a slightly smaller paycheck. She also was comfortable in her rather traditional gender role. She was older than her male counterparts by almost eight years, was somewhat less likely to have a Master's degree, and probably came from a family with somewhat higher socioeconomic status than the males (Feistritzer 1983; NEA 1963, 1972; D. Spencer 1986). Table 4.4 summarizes selected characteristics of public school teachers in 1990–1991.

Career Commitment: Teaching as a Second-Choice Job

Whether male or female, teachers are likely to have selected teaching as a second choice. The decision to teach is often made relatively late in college as students find that they lack the ability or financial and familial support to pursue a more desirable career (Holland and Eisenhart 1988; Pavalko 1970; Simpson and Simpson 1969). More college students transfer *into* education than out of it (Davis 1965).

Furthermore, most who enter teaching do not plan to make it their life work. One-third of those who are trained to teach never enter a classroom (Simpson and Simpson 1969). Sixty-five percent of beginning female teachers expect to leave within five years; 70 percent plan eventually to become homemakers. Although five out of six plan to return to teaching when their children are in school (Pavalko 1970), many do not. At any given time as many as 60 percent of those trained to be teachers are not in the classroom (Corwin 1965). In general, teacher turnover stands at about 17 percent of the cohort annually (Anderson and Mark 1977; Charters 1970; Mark and Anderson 1978). Increasing rates of divorce and single parenthood may have been changing this situation, however. By 1971 the number of female teachers with breaks in service had declined by 13 percent. In addition, attrition rates for both men and women tend to decline if they survive the first year or two of teaching (Charters 1970; Mark and Anderson 1978).

Commitment patterns for male teachers are similar, though for different reasons. Most men who enter teaching do not want to spend their lives as teachers; they plan to move into administration within five years. If they remain in the classroom, they express great unhappiness with their jobs by age 40 (Lortie 1973, p. 489). Another difference is in the percentage of male teachers with breaks in teaching service. Lortie found that the percentage increased by 6.6 percent, while the percentage of women who interrupted their teaching careers declined. These statistics indicate that men who remain in the profession try to leave it more often than women do, even given the female interruptions for child-rearing.

Intellect and Ideology

Although some studies indicate that those who enter education programs score higher on intelligence tests than the average college student (Pavalko 1970), many studies indicate that the standardized test scores and grade-point averages of teachers' college graduates are among the lowest of all college programs. This may be the case because the more able students drop out of teacher training. Pavalko (1971) indicates

TABLE 4.4 Public Elementary and Secondary School Teachers—Selected Characteristics: 1990–1991[a]

Characteristic	Unit	Age				Sex		Race/Ethnicity			Level of Control	
		Under 30	30–39	40–49	Over 50	Male	Female	White[b]	Black[b]	Hispanic	Elementary	Secondary
Total teachers[c]	1,000	312	732	1,003	514	720	1,842	2,216	212	87	1,298	1,264
Highest degree held:												
Bachelor's	Percent	84.1	56.4	43.8	41.6	44.7	54.7	51.5	50.8	61.0	56.7	46.9
Master's	Percent	14.4	39.1	48.8	49.9	47.0	40.1	42.7	42.1	32.9	38.7	45.5
Education specialist	Percent	1.2	3.4	5.9	5.9	5.3	4.3	4.5	5.0	4.3	4.1	5.2
Doctorate	Percent	—*	0.4	1.0	1.4	1.3	0.6	0.7	1.3	0.9	0.4	1.2
Full-time teaching experience:												
Less than 3 years	Percent	40.0	8.4	3.0	1.3	7.1	9.3	8.7	5.9	13.0	9.4	8.0
3–9 years	Percent	59.8	37.1	14.5	6.1	18.9	27.1	25.0	19.0	31.8	26.2	23.3
10–20 years	Percent	0.2	54.4	49.8	24.8	37.6	41.0	40.0	41.7	41.4	40.3	39.8
20 years or more	Percent	NA	0.1	32.7	67.8	36.5	22.5	26.4	33.6	13.8	24.1	28.9
Full-time teachers	1,000	283	650	925	481	666	1,273	2,015	199	81	1,170	1,169
Earned income (Dollars)		24,892	30,126	36,095	38,642	37,895	31,897	33,631	33,666	32,960	31,972	35,241
Salary (Dollars)		22,754	27,934	33,702	36,361	33,383	30,501	31,313	31,707	30,774	30,611	32,034
Supplemental contract during school year:												
Teachers receiving	1,000	121	231	313	122	353	434	701	49	25	238	549
Salary (Dollars)		1,675	2,045	1,914	2,088	2,663	1,357	1,977	1,664	1,709	1,172	2,276
Supplemental contract during summer:												
Teachers receiving	1,000	56	118	169	65	164	244	334	46	19	167	241
Salary (Dollars)		1,608	1,952	2,003	2,284	2,309	1,763	1,919	2,272	2,360	1,803	2,104
Teachers with nonschool employment:												
Teaching/tutoring	1,000	13	30	47	20	39	70	95	8	5	41	69
Education related	1,000	9	18	28	12	31	36	59	5	2	23	44
Not education related	1,000	32	63	91	42	130	99	203	16	5	52	147

[a]For school year. Based on survey and subject to sampling error; for details, see source. [b]Non-Hispanic. [c]Includes teachers with no degrees and associates degrees, not shown separately. *—represents or rounds to zero. NA = Not applicable.

SOURCE: U.S. National Center for Education Statistics, *Digest of Education Statistics*, 1993.

that of the women who did graduate and become teachers, those with higher measured intelligence were more likely to drop out of the profession. In any case, the appeal of teaching is not in its intellectual rigor. It appeals to the heart — to those who like working with people rather than ideas (Simpson and Simpson 1969) — or to those who have no more desirable alternative (see Dworkin 1986 and LeCompte and Dworkin 1991 for a discussion of teacher entrapment and "side-bets" which lure people out of the profession).

Teachers tend to be politically conservative: 16.9 percent describe themselves as conservative, while 43.6 percent describe themselves as tending to be conservative (NEA 1972). They also tend to be ambivalent about collective action in their behalf. In an early study, 21 percent felt that teachers should never strike and 64 percent believed that teachers should strike only in the most extreme cases, when all other means had failed (NEA 1970). More recently, when asked, "Do you believe public school teachers should ever strike?" only 10 percent said they believed teachers should be permitted the same right to strike as other employees (Ginsburg 1988).

Interview a leader of your local teachers' organization or union. What kind of organization is it? What has been the history of teacher organizations in your area? What obstacles have been overcome? How many teachers are active members?

Social Class Status

Data on the socioeconomic origins of teachers is mixed. Teaching traditionally has been thought of as an avenue for upward mobility. In 1911, 52 percent of teachers came from farm families and 26 percent had parents who were blue-collar workers, although the farm percentage has dropped steadily. By 1960 only 26.5 percent came from farm families and 30 percent from blue-collar families (Betz and Garland 1974). This change probably reflects a drop in the overall number of farm families and growth in the industrial sector, but it also reflects a substantial increase in the number of individuals from middle- and upper-middle-class backgrounds who chose to become teachers.

These figures, taken from Mason's (1961) often-quoted study, combined both rural and urban districts. They may somewhat underestimate the contribution of the urban middle class, since the impact of urban middle-class teachers is diluted by being combined with rural teachers. Rural teachers are fewer in number than urban middle-class teachers and teach in smaller districts. Consequently, they are less influential in education overall than the urban teachers with whom they were combined. Also, very importantly, the Mason figures are very old and reflect a time when there were more rural-origin teachers in the teaching labor force. As the country has urbanized, so has the teaching force, and the Mason figures don't reflect these changes (Hare 1988; Pavalko 1971). When figures from urban areas are examined, the contribution of the middle class to teaching is even higher, especially when figures for men and women are examined separately. The conventional wisdom that teaching is a career for those with blue-collar origins tends to be true for men as well as for the 5 percent of the teaching force that is Mexican American. However, white teachers, especially women, come disproportionately from professional, technical, managerial, and business backgrounds. Since the 1940s, African-American teachers increasingly have had similar backgrounds (Dworkin 1980). While women from upper-class backgrounds are overrepresented as new teachers, women from less-advantaged backgrounds are likely to continue teaching longer (Betz and Garland 1974). The reason may be that middle-class women have alternatives to teaching (Dworkin 1986). It also may be that women from the working classes, like men, see teaching as an avenue to higher status, or, as Maienza suggests, base their persistence in the job on the role model provided by their own working mothers (Grow 1981).

In any case, blue-collar children of both sexes seem to be encountering increasing difficulty in gaining access to teaching careers, perhaps because of both the rising cost of higher education and the curtailment of financial aid. Given the salary they can expect as teachers, few young people may want to burden themselves with the amount of debt a college education now requires. The consequences for the profession are that it will increasingly become a profession with white-collar and service-sector origins and that it will remain predominantly white and female.

Minority Teachers

While there are substantially fewer minority than white teachers, Gottlieb (1964) and Dworkin (1980) reported that turnover among minority teachers is much lower than for whites, perhaps because of their greater job satisfaction. Fewer desirable occupations were open to minorities, and these individuals are more likely to be upwardly mobile as teachers. While minority teachers were few and usually relegated to racially segregated schools prior to 1964, more African-American, Hispanic, and other minority teachers entered the profession during the period of educational expansion in the 1960s and early 1970s. Males, too, became teachers in increasing numbers to avoid being drafted. These changes, however, were temporary. When the draft was eliminated, the incentive for men to become teachers ended.

Curtailment of scholarships and other aid in the 1980s produced a drop in the number of minorities able to attend college at all, much less become teachers. Desegregation of school faculties in the 1970s and 1980s also contributed to the decrease in minority teachers. As segregated African-American schools were closed or consolidated with white schools, faculty slots were lost, and most commonly African-American teachers found that it was their jobs that were being eliminated or changed.

In addition, as discriminatory barriers in more prestigious fields eased, educated members of minority groups were no longer limited to teaching as the most prestigious occupation to which they could aspire. The result of all these factors is that the teaching force remains primarily white and middle class while school enrollments, especially in urban areas, become increasingly minority dominated (Hodgkinson 1985). More and more teachers are working with children whose background and ethnicity are radically different from their own. These conditions have important consequences for the amount of culture shock and stress teachers encounter on the job (Dworkin 1986; Dworkin, Haney, and Telschow 1988; LeCompte 1978a, 1985; LeCompte and Dworkin 1991).

What are the demographic characteristics of teachers and administrators in your local school district? How many males, females, and minority group members are represented in teaching and administration at each of the three levels: elementary, middle, and high school?

WHAT TEACHERS DO: CONTRADICTIONS IN THE NATURE OF TEACHERS' WORK

Teachers in the United States have inherited a "divided legacy." On one hand, education is believed to be essential to democratic citizenship, but on the other, it is housed in bureaucracies which subordinate individual learning to routine bestowing of degrees or "credentialing." Ironically, both notions are born of the same imperative. Democracy requires universal education, but the systems to provide it are so large that the complex, impersonal, and bureaucratic organizations required for their management are at cross-purposes with their educational goals (McNeil 1988a, p. 337).

Teaching also occupies a contradictory place in the occupational structure because it is neither an autonomous profession, like medicine, nor a bureaucratized occupation, like automotive assembly (Dreeben 1973, p. 453). Thus teachers are in what has been called a "contradictory class location" (Wright 1978). They are not blue-collar workers and cannot be expected to act like factory employees or clerks in large corporations. While many of them (especially men) have blue-collar origins, most do not adhere to working-class ideologies. At the same time, their status is not that of "real" professionals. The following sections will discuss the nature of these complexities and contradictions.

The Conditions of Labor

Contradictions in the status of teaching can be attributed, at least in part, to the type of work teachers do, the conditions under which they work, how their work is organized, and the differentiated sex ratio in the profession. We will begin with a functionalist analysis of the teaching profession, then examine what teachers do and what purposes these activities serve, and finally we will discuss how critical theorists conceptualize teachers and their work.

Classroom Conditions. Forty-five percent of the teachers in the United States teach in districts that have from 3,000 to 25,000 students. The average teacher works for a white male principal. Teachers' jobs require them to be in their classrooms 37 hours per week, and they perform 8 additional hours of uncompensated but required duty. They teach an average of 181 days each year, and most do so without help. Only 5.5 percent had their own teacher aides, while an additional 24.7 percent shared aides with one or more teachers (NEA 1972). These figures, compiled in the 1970s, have remained more or less unchanged, though mandated reforms such as portfolio assessment and increased recordkeeping for accountability have intensified (Apple

1992) workloads in the 1980s and 1990s. At least in reform-minded districts, then, the number of unpaid work hours has increased (Apple 1986, 1992; LeCompte and Dworkin 1991).

Teachers have little respite from their classrooms. Few have free periods, and the number who do has declined. Teachers have no coffee or bathroom breaks. A daily lunch break of less than 40 minutes, which has declined as much as 5 minutes since 1950, is often combined with supervisory duties in the cafeteria. Many teachers feel lucky to squeeze a 25-minute "child-free" lunch period.

Teachers also are badly outnumbered. While pupil–teacher ratios have been declining to some extent in the past decades, most classroom teachers face some 27 to 35 students every time they enter their rooms. Jackson (1968) states that nowhere except in schools are humans required to spend so much time so physically close to one another.

Classrooms have been described as "three-ring circuses" in which the competent teacher serves as ringmaster (Smith and Geoffrey 1968). The school day is characterized by high rates of interaction and frequent changes in activities—as often as every 5 seconds in an active classroom and every 18 seconds in a quiet one. Changes in who talks can occur more than 174 times each lesson, totaling 650 to 1,000 interchanges daily between teachers and students. Teachers themselves initiate as many as 80 interchanges per hour with students (Dreeben 1973, p. 464). Under some circumstances, the teacher can feel like a stand-up comedian with an audience full of hecklers. At best, the teacher ends the day with sensory overload.

Divide the class into three groups and assign students to interview elementary, middle, and high school teachers. Ask the teachers to describe what they do each day. How much time do they spend teaching? How much is devoted to nonteaching duties? What do they perceive to be the rewards of their profession? What factors are most disagreeable? How many plan to stay in the profession? In a class discussion, compare your findings.

Fragmentation.   Teaching is fragmented by everyday life in schools. The flow of instruction is regularly interrupted by announcements over the intercom, lunch count, children asking to leave the room, others coming in with notes or requests from other teachers, fire drills, assemblies, athletic activities, fights, and other contingencies. Sensory overload is exacerbated by such fragmentation. The physical design of classrooms seems highly conducive to frequent disruption, particularly in the lower grades. A teacher's primary task becomes to design learning activities sufficiently engrossing that pupils find them more attractive than outlawed alternatives (Jackson 1968, pp. 85–90). Teachers spend only about half the school day in actual instruction (Adams and Biddle 1970, pp. 41–45). Elementary school teachers may divide their time equally between instruction and classroom management (LeCompte 1978).

Teachers' work is fragmented also by the way the curriculum is organized, by bureaucratic time schedules, and by complications of school life which interrupt the flow of teaching. School knowledge is divided into subjects, the subjects into courses, the courses into chapters and units, and these in turn into sets of objectives (L. McNeil 1988a).

Despite recent calls for integrated and multidisciplinary curricula, most subjects are treated as if they have little if any relationship with each other. Reading in math has nothing to do with reading in social studies. In fact, there is fragmentation even within subject areas: Students study European history and art without ever considering relationships these subjects might have with each other or with history and art in America.

Teaching activities are divided into discrete time allotments, taught at specific times of the day. Teachers have little latitude to teach longer to make a point, to combine related content areas, or to omit unimportant things. Most important, the schedule allows teachers no time at all to meet with one another to plan joint activities. It is difficult to be carried away into a "grand sweep of history" or general theory of mathematics.

Isolation. Teachers, unlike virtually all other professionals, work in almost total isolation from other adults. In the motel-like structure of most schools, teachers get to see their colleagues only between classes or at lunchtime, periods when they often are engaged in supervisory tasks. If they have a free period, it is occupied with school tasks and shared by only a few of their colleagues. These conditions are obstacles to collegiality, sharing of ideas, or collective organization. What teachers know and feel about their job and about how well they are doing it is deepened through introspection over their experiences, rather than broadened through sharing of experiences and ideas with colleagues. In a sense, teachers are taught by their own students in that they are left very much on their own to determine what they are doing right or wrong (Lortie 1969, p. 469).

Control of Students. Knowing one's subject is not sufficient. Teaching is contingent upon the good will of students (Connell 1985). Teachers cannot just enter a classroom and begin to teach. They must first achieve a minimum level of order and attentiveness, as well as an agreement by the students to internalize what the teacher presents. The rules for this agreement constitute a "hidden curriculum." The hidden curriculum is as important to teachers as to students because competence in teaching is judged more by how orderly the classroom is than by how much students learn— perhaps because quiet is easier to assess than achievement.

School policies require that teachers be "fair." This means that they must exhibit affective neutrality around their students and judge them by uniform and universalistic standards. Students expect that their teachers will not play favorites. They also expect their teachers to keep order, explain things carefully, and not be boring (Nash 1976). These role expectations constitute an unwritten contract, violation of which precipitates student retaliation. Teachers maintain control only by balancing personal forcefulness with intimate teacher–pupil relationships. In order to accomplish this, teachers allocate rewards so as to establish their own power base while weakening the power of student peer affiliations to sabotage their activities (Bidwell 1965, p. 1011).

Lack of Tangible Results. Both the quality and quantity of what teachers do is difficult to assess. Connell succinctly describes this intangibility:

> Teaching is a labor process without an object. At best, it has an object so intangible—the minds of the kids, or their capacity to learn—that it cannot be specified in any but vague and metaphorical ways . . . [it] does not produce any *things,* nor, like other white collar work, does it produce visible and quantifiable effects—so many pensions paid, so many dollars turned over, so many patients cured. (1985, p. 70)

Because its product is elusive, teaching differs from both the factory work and the professional service sector to which it often is compared. Teachers can indeed count the number of their students who pass certain tests or courses, graduate from high school, or attain degrees. However, these measures are deceptive, because most teaching is cumulative and subjective. It is difficult to attribute to any one teacher the performance of any given individual or group of students.

Multidimensionality. While the work of teachers ostensibly is teaching, they do many other things as well. They develop instructional materials, coach athletic teams, and supervise extracurricular activities. Teachers serve on committees related to the academic and administrative operation of schools, engage in tutoring and counseling, and perform social work for students' families. They do police work in school corridors, lunchrooms, playgrounds, toilets, and buses.

The multidimensionality of teaching keeps the job from being boring, contributes to its appeal as a career, and is one of its intrinsic rewards. However, these activities are time-consuming; when they are added to time spent teaching in the classroom, preparing lessons, and grading homework and tests, teaching becomes much more than an eight-hour-a-day job.

Stress, Burnout, and Victimization

Teaching has grown more and more stressful over the years. We attribute this increase to several factors. First of all, schools have changed so much as a consequence of societal changes that they are almost unrecognizable as the institutions of twenty or thirty years ago. Consolidation has increased the size of schools and districts. Urbanization and growth in minority populations have increased student heterogeneity. Finally, the whole social, economic, and cultural context of schools has changed radically during the professional lifetime of most contemporary teachers (LeCompte and Dworkin 1991). This means that historical models of teachers' roles are no longer appropriate. While teachers have always counted discipline and crowd control among their primary professional concerns, the student body has changed to the point that there is little commonality upon which teachers can build adequate working conditions in the classroom. The result is the potential for unprecedented social and psychological job stress.

There are many sources for teacher stress. One source of stress is the discrepancy between what teachers expect to find when they enter the profession and what they actually encounter. Stress also develops when the rewards do not seem commensurate with the effort expended. Work **intensification**—the sense that nothing ever is

---

A Teacher's Angry Voice

It was just a difficult situation. I was not angry, just scared. I was angry at the school system as a whole, because it happened due to one of my students being beaten, thrown to the ground, and kicked by a bully in another fifth-grade class, on school time, in the lunchroom. Apparently, it was very vicious. My student was a small little guy, and the bully was horrible. He brags about having access to drugs and guns, etc. This is fifth grade, different classrooms. I got in there when it ended and took both of them to the principal's office. She handled it by suspending the bully for two days and read him the riot act about being a bully. I talked to my student. He didn't cry. He didn't want to be held. He was stiff. He said he was okay. When he came back into the classroom later he said he was fine. I thought it was all over. I was amazed at how well he took all of this. I should have done more, but I didn't. I thought, "Well, I guess that's okay."

About a week later, just before noon, I picked up a coat from his desk. It felt heavy. I just smiled. "What did you bring to school, ____?" I thought it was a video game or something. He looked a little stricken, and I could feel right through his coat that it was a gun. I have never owned one, but I could tell. I just told him to go outside with me. I got the coat and had him sit in the hall with me. I got ____'s assistant and had her watch my class. I took him down to the principal's office and had to wait for 20 minutes for her to show up. I held the gun, in the coat, next to me, not thinking about if it was loaded. It never dawned on me. I talked to him as we were going down the hall. He told me how he was going to get even with [bully], and he first considered killing him, then decided how he would just blow out both of his kneecaps, and was going to do it on the bus on the way home. He would get off at [bully's] stop and shoot him there. Then he was just going to walk home, and that [bully] deserved it. His older brother used to take care of his problems, and he didn't want to ask him any more. He was old enough to take care of them on his own. In fact, one of his older brothers had been killed a year earlier, and so he was going to handle it himself. He never cried, he was very frank and open about it. I felt awful. If we had intervened more somewhere along the line, and really thought about how he'd been put down and recognized that something like this might have happened. I was just shocked and shaken.

A Teacher's Angry Voice

Well, we [teachers] would eat together, but kind of like in shifts, and since I was doing third grade then, I overlapped with second grade and fourth grade. It was such a small school, I think we all ate together—second, third, and fourth. It reached the point where I couldn't stand to eat with them anymore because they were racist, and the jokes and things that they would say—I had a hard time keeping my mouth shut. I knew that I was already in a precarious position there and just had to get through the year. If I became embroiled and said what I really wanted to say, it would become even more difficult.

I try not to be too outspoken, especially in the South. I've had a lot of teachers tell me, "Well, you aren't from the South. That's why you are willing to speak out and not sit back and let things happen." But I felt that I sat back a lot more than I am inclined to, and I don't think I got messed with nearly as bad as the other two teachers did. They didn't say anything; they kind of hunkered down and closed their door. . . . The people [in Seattle] are very outspoken and not willing to sit down for anything. Down here, it's kind of like, "Do what you will with me. It's okay. I'm here to be walked on." I found it very interesting. I have often had teachers say to me that they are just shocked that I would not accept some things.

subtracted from your job description—and **de-skilling,** the limiting of teacher autonomy through mandated curricula and policies developed at administrative levels, contribute to this kind of stress. Work overload and de-skilling lead to alienation.

Faced with stressful situations, teachers may develop a sense of inadequacy to carry out assigned tasks. What teachers conceive of as "add-ons" aggravate this sense of inadequacy. In today's context of school reform and restructuring, teachers are called upon to change their pedagogical practices. They may come to view innovation as something to be added to what they already must do. In large part, this interpretation is accurate, however, it impedes reform. Teachers finding it difficult to substitute a new strategy or task for an old one, simply do both. They define each innovation as potential work overload, therefore they can become particularly resistant to new ideas.

Burnout is a common name for a sociological concept called **alienation.** Alienation is a sense that life has become meaningless, that one is powerless to make the changes necessary to restore meaning to one's life and work. One can neither understand nor control one's destiny because the rules that once made life predictable are no longer effective. One is *personally isolated* and without allies to improve the situation, *personally estranged* from the kind of person one thought oneself to be, and *culturally isolated* from the community and context of which one is a part (Dworkin 1985b, p. 7; LeCompte and Dworkin 1991; Needle et al. 1980; Seeman 1959, 1967,

1975). All of these conditions characterize the working situation of an increasing number of teachers. The result often is that teachers "wear out" or "burn out" (Dworkin 1986).

Teachers burn out for a variety of reasons. Some burnout occurs as a consequence of the sensory overload described earlier. Teachers usually cannot take a restorative sabbatical from their jobs. Isolation also increases the likelihood of burnout in two ways. First, as we have indicated, the physical layout and scheduling constraints of schools give teachers few opportunities to blow off steam with other teachers. Second, because teachers tend to find most of their friends among other teachers, they get less input from people with other viewpoints (Ginsburg 1979). Expectations also play a role. People are attracted to teaching because they perceive teachers as catalysts for student learning. When they find that they are unable to make children learn—whether because of institutional or time pressures, student misbehavior, or interpersonal conflicts—they become subject to stress and burnout (Needle et al. 1980).

In addition, many teachers feel unsafe at work. Every year 12 percent of teachers report that they have been robbed at school. Twelve percent also say that they avoid confronting students because they are afraid of them. One percent per month are physically attacked at school. In a 1993 survey on school violence 60 percent of responding urban districts reported student assaults on teachers. Twenty-eight percent of all responding districts (urban, suburban, and rural) reported student versus teacher violence (National School Boards Association 1993). In another study 72 percent of the teachers felt concern about the vandalism and destruction of property in school (Phillips and Lee 1980). The majority of reported violence takes place in secondary schools, but elementary teachers are not immune.

While many reports have minimized the amount of actual danger in schools, perhaps more important is the dismaying feeling that "you might be next." Seventy-five percent of teachers knew someone who had been verbally abused, and 35 percent knew someone who had been physically attacked (National School Boards Association 1993). The installation of metal detectors in middle and high schools in both urban and suburban school districts, the use of police guards and drug-sniffing dogs in large urban districts, and the rising indices of drug use and crime among pre-teens give these feelings of victimization and vulnerability additional credence. The result is a widespread disaffection with the profession.

In a major study of teachers, nearly one-third indicated that they felt their work to be meaningless and that they felt powerless to do anything about it (Dworkin 1986). These feelings were most common among those in the demographic majority—female, white, middle class, under 30 years old, and with less than five years of experience. Elementary teachers were more likely to feel stressed than secondary teachers. Significantly, feelings of discrimination, victimization, and burnout were more likely to occur when teachers were "racially isolated," that is, in a school where the predominant race of the student body was different from their own (Dworkin 1986). As we have indicated, demographic change in the coming decades will likely aggravate the cultural estrangement engendered by racial isolation (Hodgkinson 1985) and consequently increase culture shock among teachers.

THE REWARD STRUCTURE OF TEACHING

Teaching traditionally has produced few extrinsic rewards for excellent performance. Most of its benefits are intangible, coming from classroom activity and interaction with children. Standardized salary schedules preclude bonuses or merit raises. (See Table 4.5 for the current average teachers' salaries by region.) Teaching also has a "flat" career trajectory. Teachers cannot be promoted for good teaching except by moving into administration, which means leaving the classroom. The only tangible rewards administrators can give to teachers concern working conditions: a desirable classroom, assignment to gifted students, a free period, permission to teach a specialty course, or time off to go to a conference.

Merit Pay

Many districts have tried a merit pay plan and discarded it. The major complaint about it is that the criteria for establishing merit are vague, subjective, and too prone to administrative manipulation. Teachers may not trust their administrators to be fair. Teacher organizations also reject the concept of merit pay, because it has taken them years to achieve equal pay for teachers across disciplines and grade levels.

Career Ladders

As a consequence of the reform movements of the late 1980s, many states have mandated "Career Ladder" programs, which attempt to eliminate the flat trajectory of the profession. These create levels in teaching based upon seniority, advanced preparation, and excellence in performance. Career ladders are a variation of merit pay but they attempt to avoid subjectivity by making the steps for acquiring merit very explicit. Systematization of career ladder steps has been criticized, however, for turning teaching performance into a rigidly prescribed and routinized activity. Current research indicates that career ladder programs have not fundamentally changed teachers' work roles, responsibilities, and reward structures. In fact, existing distinctions in rank among teachers became the basis for levels in the career ladder, with the result that those who had always been favored continued to be (Malen and Hart 1987).

Critical Area Pay

Incentive systems of a different kind have also been initiated. "Critical area pay" has been instituted to encourage certification in areas with few teachers, such as math, science, and bilingual education. Another form of critical area pay is given to teachers willing to work in inner-city schools or in neighborhoods with high crime rates. Critical area pay adds substantially to the remuneration of some teachers but does not enhance the profession overall. As Dworkin (1986) indicates, teachers feel that increases in pay are inadequate compensation for adverse working conditions.

TABLE 4.5 Estimated Average Annual Salaries of Total Instructional Staff and of Classroom Teachers, 1993–94

Region and State 1	Average Salary of Instructional Staff 2	1993–94 Average Salary of Classroom Teachers — Elementary School 3	Secondary School 4	Current $ 5	All Teachers — % Increase Over 1992–93 6	Purchasing Power In 1984 $ 7
50 STATES AND D.C.	$37,701	$35,258	$36,765	$35,958	2.7	$25,098
NEW ENGLAND	44,751	40,809	40,351	40,583	3.2	28,320
CONNECTICUT	51,100	48,900	51,000	49,500	2.4	34,548
MAINE	32,049	30,483	32,140	30,996	2.5	21,630
MASSACHUSETTS	47,774*	39,370*	39,370*	39,370*	3.0*	27,474*
NEW HAMPSHIRE	38,599	36,402	36,346	36,372	7.2	25,382
RHODE ISLAND	39,992	39,212	39,318	39,261	3.5	27,898
VERMONT	35,503*	36,043*	36,043*	36,043*	3.5*	25,152*
MIDEAST	46,132	43,845	46,031	44,853	4.9	31,300
DELAWARE	39,031	36,853	38,111	37,469	3.5	26,147
DIST. OF COLUMBIA	39,257	41,936	48,534	42,543	9.9	29,688
MARYLAND	41,755	39,101	41,067	39,937	3.1	27,870
NEW JERSEY	47,635	44,199	47,283	45,308	6.2	31,618
NEW YORK	47,800	45,800	47,800	46,800	4.0	32,689
PENNSYLVANIA	44,698	42,890	44,515	43,688	6.0	30,487
SOUTHEAST	31,642	30,055	30,858	30,364	2.6	21,189
ALABAMA	30,015	28,705	28,705	28,705	6.5	20,031
ARKANSAS	29,038	27,092	28,626	27,873	1.6	19,451
FLORIDA	33,423	32,020	32,020	32,020	2.7	22,345
GEORGIA	32,128	30,456	30,456	30,456	1.3	21,253
KENTUCKY	32,834	30,881	33,228	31,582	1.5	22,039
LOUISIANA	30,560	28,508*	28,508*	28,508*	3.2*	19,894*
MISSISSIPPI	26,162	24,816	25,744	25,235	3.6	17,610
NORTH CAROLINA	30,895	29,602	29,804	29,680	1.2	20,712

TABLE 4.5 *(continued)*

| | | 1993–94 Average Salary of Classroom Teachers | | | All Teachers | |
| | Average Salary of Instructional Staff | Elementary School | Secondary School | Current $ | % Increase Over 1992–93 | Purchasing Power In 1984 $ |
Region and State 1	2	3	4	5	6	7
SOUTH CAROLINA	30,730	29,690	31,230	30,190	3.3	21,068
TENNESSEE	31,173	29,520	31,380	30,037	3.7	20,961
VIRGINIA	33,928*	31,996*	34,794*	33,128*	2.5*	23,118*
WEST VIRGINIA	31,656	30,241	30,972	30,549	0.8	21,318
GREAT LAKES	40,277	37,775	39,775	38,746	2.6	27,088
ILLINOIS	42,335	39,042	45,789	40,989	6.1	28,604
INDIANA	37,331*	36,155*	36,372*	36,255*	3.4*	25,300*
MICHIGAN	46,392*	42,500*	42,500*	42,500*	-2.5*	29,658*
OHIO	36,000	34,500	35,900	35,700	3.5	24,913
WISCONSIN	37,543*	34,865	37,171	36,644	2.0	25,572
PLAINS	32,991	31,221	32,757	31,818	3.0	22,204
IOWA	31,880	29,714	31,684	30,760	2.1	21,465
KANSAS	35,640	34,178	34,178	34,178	4.0	23,851
MINNESOTA	37,309	35,566	37,761	36,146	3.0	25,224
MISSOURI	31,386	29,465	31,079	30,227	2.9	21,094
NEBRASKA	31,595*	29,564	29,564	29,564	2.8	20,681
NORTH DAKOTA	26,359	25,539	25,452	25,508	1.2	17,800
SOUTH DAKOTA	24,977	25,098	24,993	25,199	3.7	17,585
SOUTHWEST	31,446	29,534	30,563	30,036	2.1	20,960
ARIZONA	39,794*	31,680*	31,680*	31,680*	1.0*	22,107*
NEW MEXICO	28,383*	27,072*	27,989*	27,922	5.2	19,485
OKLAHOMA	27,730	26,086	27,571	26,749	3.2	18,666
TEXAS	31,046	29,912	31,136	30,519	2.0	21,297

					%	
ROCKY MOUNTAINS	31,650	29,946	31,226	30,581	1.7	21,341
COLORADO	34,911*	33,236*	34,439*	33,826	0.8	28,605
IDAHO	28,994*	27,593*	28,084*	27,803*	2.9*	19,402*
MONTANA	29,358	28,024	28,535	28,210	2.1	19,686
UTAH	29,068	27,235	28,630	28,056	3.0	19,579
WYOMING	31,200	30,250	30,370	30,310	0.8	21,151
FAR WEST	42,078	33,020	40,109	39,095	0.6	27,282
ALASKA	46,649*	46,581*	46,581*	46,581*	1.2*	32,506*
CALIFORNIA	44,210*	38,628*	42,436*	40,289*	0.6*	28,115*
HAWAII	37,671	36,564	36,564	36,564	0.3	25,516
NEVADA	35,603	33,355	34,799	33,955	-0.5	23,595
OREGON	38,500	36,500	38,120	37,150	3.5	25,911
WASHINGTON	37,468	35,478	36,417	35,860	0.3	25,024

*Data estimated by NEA.
SOURCE: National Education Association Research, 1994. 1993–1994 Estimates of School Statistics. Washington, D.C.: NEA. Reprinted with Permission.

DE-SKILLING, ROUTINIZATION, AND THE ENFORCEMENT OF BUREAUCRATIC CONTROL

Teachers control only certain aspects of their classrooms. Lortie says that teachers' decision making is characterized by "variable zoning" (1969, pp. 13–15), meaning that they have "hard" jurisdiction in areas where their judgments will not be questioned and "soft" jurisdiction in other areas. Lortie and other functionalists suggest that the privacy of the closed classroom door ensures that instructional decisions can be "hard" ones for teachers, though they have less discretion over recordkeeping and other administrative matters. This area of "hard" decisions, teachers' area of discretion or autonomy, is one that strengthens their sense of professionalism. However, to the extent that teachers have discretion or empowerment in classrooms, "that which is most central and unique to schools—instruction—is least controlled by specific and literally enforced rules and regulations" (Lortie 1969, p. 14) and also is least under surveillance by the administration.

As schools have become increasingly bureaucratized, critical researchers have noticed erosion in the "harder" areas of teacher discretion. Apple describes the degree to which decision making about curriculum and instructional matters has passed out of the hands of teachers, leaving as their exclusive province only the control of behavior in their classroom (Apple 1982, 1988). He calls this phenomenon "de-skilling." It accompanies "teacher-proof" technological innovation in the delivery of instruction—computer-assisted instruction and other pre-programmed forms of teaching—as well as behaviorally based curricula with pre-specified teaching programs and lessons "bits." De-skilling strips from teachers the ability to make decisions about what and how to teach, the ability to utilize their training and expertise. De-skilling most often affects work typically performed by women—secretaries, clerks, and nurses in addition to teachers. Of particular note is that de-skilling is often associated with intensification of the teacher's workload.

Cuban suggests that teachers directly influence only five areas of classroom decision making, all related to the groupings and spatial arrangements:

1. Arrangement of classroom space
2. The ratio of teacher-to-student talk
3. Whether most instruction occurs individually, in small groups, or with the entire class
4. Whether or not learning or interest centers are used by students as a normal part of the school day
5. The degree of movement students are permitted without asking the teacher (1984, p. 5)

These are all basically management concerns and deal with matters other than the content of instruction. Decisions about curricula and content are made by local and state educational agencies, which mandate the subjects to be taught and the time to be allocated to each. State textbook committees also generally provide a list of ap-

---

A Teacher's Angry Voice

I can remember one [experience of anger in school]. It happened just before the end of school, and the reason I took it so hard was because I was tired. I had been through a lot all year, and we had all of the children in our school outside in the heat of the afternoon watching. The city police brought their dogs and they brought samples of drugs. They were showing how the dogs would hunt out the drugs. At other schools, they bring in clowns; at (name of school), they bring in dogs and drugs, right? That angered me in the beginning.

---

proved textbooks. Individual school districts may use teacher committees to help choose books from the list, but individual teachers may not select alternatives. Even teachers' choice of supplementary books may be restricted by community watchdog committees and district regulations.

The use of standardized subject-area criteria and normative testing also excludes teachers from decision making about curricula. In response to calls for improved standards, accountability programs have been instituted in almost every state. Much reform in the 1900s is, in fact, driven by assessment. To the extent that school districts gear course content toward externally developed tests, teachers lose control of daily classroom instruction. This is especially true when promotion, retention, and graduation of students is tied to performance on the tests.

Loss of control over content is a serious matter, because it prevents teachers from using skills they developed in their area of specialization. However, de-skilling can take even more insidious forms. Teachers may even lose control over *how* they teach. "Teacher-proof" curricula come not only with instructional objectives, but with lesson plans, mandated readings and exercises, pre- and post-tests, and supplementary activities. Such curricula routinize and bureaucratize the teaching process, hedging it with rules and regulations and making it difficult for teachers to improvise, create, or follow up on what they think is important.

L. McNeil's (1988c) case study comparing the attitudes and behavior of teachers before and after institution of educational reform programs amply documents the effect that de-skilling has upon enthusiastic and dedicated teachers. She describes how, in the name of improving student performance, the content of courses in one large school district was "taken apart, sequenced, numbered, and sub-numbered," not by teachers but by central-office test producers in a manner "perhaps unwittingly modelled on the activity analysis which efficiency experts used for pacing activities on an assembly line." Their purpose was to create measurable objectives for each component of the curriculum, then develop tests that assessed student mastery. Ultimately, uniformity of instruction and assessment of students was to be ensured for each student in the district. The result was to transform the tasks of the teacher into a set of "generic behaviors."

McNeil states that these curriculum reforms generated an immense amount of new work for teachers. Not only were they required to teach what they perceived to be much more material (the value of some of which they questioned), but both the instructional management systems and the preoccupation with administrating and grading tests generated a massive volume of paperwork. Teachers felt they had become little more than assembly-line workers or clerks, whose job was merely to organize, disseminate, and process predeveloped tasks.

Many of the teachers in McNeil's study engaged in principled resistance to this bureaucratic control. Some left teaching. Faced with an overwhelming volume of content to cover, some gave up on good teaching. They eliminated written composition altogether. Teachers engaged in omission of controversial issues, and compression or "defensive simplification" of complex topics. They taught students simply to recognize concepts rather than to understand them, and they presented outlines and lists to be memorized rather than analyzing and synthesizing the material. While these strategies undoubtedly made instruction less onerous, they also made teachers feel unprofessional and made them less credible in the eyes of students. Teachers neither answered serious questions from students nor seemed to have any demonstrated expertise (L. McNeil 1988b).

Reskilling and Alienation

The educational reforms of the 1980s not only increased teachers' workload but also changed the content and focus of tasks. While being "de-skilled" as they lost control over instructional matters, they were "reskilled" to manage complex technological and behavioral systems for students. Many responded, at least initially, with enthusiasm and competence. Apple (1986) attributes this reaction to the fact that they *were* learning new skills, even though these skills were clerical and out of their areas of competence. The process of learning new things, as well as the fact that they were in fact working long, hard hours, made teachers feel as though they were doing a good job. Because most teachers also believed that American education is in need of reform, they also believed they were participating in exciting educational innovation. They felt that they, in conjunction with external reformers—district administrators and state agencies—were defining the problem and working toward a mutually satisfactory way to solve it. Their efforts might have been illusory, however, because as the examples in Chapter 3 from Cottonwood School District indicate, the ultimate effect of centralized curriculum management is to remove control from teachers.

McNeil, by contrast, found meaning to be constructed in a different way. Teachers in the school she studied already had been defined by themselves and the district as excellent teachers in an exemplary magnet school. They interpreted the district's imposition of a reform program as an indication that they were no longer considered experts, and they resented the loss of status and control. We feel that the situation McNeil describes is more common. However, Dworkin's research (1985b, 1986) on teacher burnout indicates that principals and other administrators can lessen alienation in these circumstances. Regardless of the level of stress they encounter, teachers who view their principals as supportive are less likely to resist activities or experience burnout.

More recent innovations in education are centered on teacher empowerment and shared leadership. Whole language, the reading and language curriculum based on the natural language of students, and integrated curricular approaches place teachers at the center of decision making in their own classrooms. Democratic leadership or shared school governance movements encourage teachers to work with administrators regarding school policies and programs. We will talk more about these alternative and innovative approaches in Chapter 9.

Brainstorm with your colleagues a list of the satisfiers and dissatisfiers of teaching. Discuss both the difficulties and rewards of a career in teaching.

ADMINISTRATORS AND ANCILLARY STAFF

Having outlined the general conditions under which teachers work, we now move to a discussion of the work of administrators and ancillary staff. Initial experience as a teacher is the common denominator for all professional-level staff in public schools.

Administrators

Virtually all school administrators, whether they supervise teachers, counselors, bus drivers, evaluators, or recordkeepers, are required to have teacher certification. Entrance to administration programs in universities, which is required for most public school administrators as well as faculty in colleges of education, typically requires at least three years of teaching in elementary or secondary schools. This requirement guarantees a certain uniformity of outlook in the educational profession. It also ensures that a large proportion of professional staff will be drawn from the same pool of recruits.

Administrators do not constitute a representative sample of teachers, however. While they resemble teachers in social status, political views, and religious affiliation, administrators differ radically by gender. For example, 93 percent of U.S. high school principals in the mid-1970s were male (Boocock 1980). While searching for respondents for a survey of female U.S. school superintendents, Frasher et al. (Grow 1981) were able to locate only 131. Of the 82 who responded to the survey, over 70 percent served in school districts with an enrollment of fewer than 3,000 students. Although more women are moving into school administration, they continue to be underrepresented in these leadership positions. For example, in 1990, 38 percent of the principalships and assistant principalships were held by women (U.S. Equal Employment Opportunity Commission 1990). In 1990, 33.7 percent of all local school board members were women. In 1991, only nine of the fifty chief state school officers were women (American Association of University Women 1992).

Male and Female Career Patterns.   In addition to the dramatic difference in numbers, male and female school administrators appear to follow different career patterns once they move from the classroom. While there have been few comparative studies of male and female administrators, Maienza's study (Grow 1981) indicated that men who enter administration appear to have decided to do so early in their careers. Male administrators typically taught for a little more than six years, started and completed graduate school in their thirties, and had about eight years of administrative experience, usually as a secondary school principal or in an upper-level central office post, before attaining their first superintendency.

By contrast, females did not decide to become an administrator until after finishing the Master's degree. They entered and completed graduate school in their forties or fifties and attained their first superintendency after almost thirteen years of lower-level administrative experience. Only five years of the delay in career advancement seem attributable to breaks for child-rearing. (In fact, while most male administrators are married, women, especially at the superintendent level, tend to be single—either widowed, divorced, or never married [Good 1981].) Women's careers lead through lower-level central office positions to elementary principalships, not from secondary principalships and upper-level central office positions to the superintendency (Gaertner 1978). As Ortiz puts it:

> Men are more likely than women to occupy those positions with greater potential for power and opportunity as well as those at the upper levels of the hierarchy. Male mobility tends to be vertical through a series of line positions entailing the administration of adults. . . . Women tend to move through positions involving instruction and interaction with children from which vertical movement is rare. (1981, p. 81)

Minorities. Ortiz also points out that members of minority groups tend to be limited either to instructional duties or to supervision of other minorities. Because they are viewed as specialists in minority problems, as principals they tend to be assigned to schools defined as "problems" because of their large minority enrollments. Reyes and Halcon (1988) call this "type-casting" and the "Brown-on-Brown" taboo. They suggest that the very fact that minorities are considered experts in the problems of their own people disqualifies them as experts on the problems of others. They are regarded primarily as crisis managers rather than administrators capable of handling the broad range of responsibilities required in higher positions (Ortiz 1981). This perception limits the appointment of minorities to "one per pot" (Reyes and Halcon 1988) and reduces their chances for promotion.

Counselors and Ancillary Staff

Like teachers and administrators, counselors also must first be certified as teachers. Like administrators, counselors are not a representative sample of the teaching population. They tend to be older, male, and white. While we tend to think of schools primarily in terms of the activities of teachers, both the number of counselors and other ancillary staff in schools and their importance in educational functioning have grown dramatically in the past decades. In 1980 there were over 32,000 counselors in the United States (Boocock 1980). Their presence "bears witness to at least two things. There are problems in the school, and the usual personnel cannot, or have not been able to, resolve them" (Sarason 1971, p. 127). They are an indication of the growth in what in Chapter 2 we called the "service sector" in education.

Counselors often are counted as instructional personnel, so their numbers tend to deflate statistics on pupil:teacher ratios. However, counselors do not teach, and their career paths are different from that of teachers. They generally acquire a Bachelor's degree in teaching and experience in the classroom, followed by a Master's degree or doctorate, usually in guidance and counseling or school psychology. The relationship of counselors to overall administrative control in schools is more ambiguous than that of teachers, as is their status. While they have more education than most teachers, they do not acquire it in instructional areas. They have substantial power over students (Cicourel and Kitsuse 1963; Sarason 1971) but they are peripheral to the predominantly instructional life of the school.

The Contradictory Role of Counselors. Feelings of discrepancy between role expectations and actual accomplishments probably are greater for counselors than for any other school professionals. Originally, counseling was designed for academic purposes only. Counselors were placed in secondary schools as curricular offerings differentiated into more than one academic stream. They were responsible for the clerical function of ensuring that students were placed in appropriate classes and fulfilled the necessary requirements for graduation. They also helped students find and apply to appropriate colleges and universities. However, today both their training and the expectations parents, students, administrators, and the public have of them have broadened considerably.

As educators became aware of the importance to cognitive learning of social, emotional, and psychological factors, counselors were expected to engage in "social work," attempting to solve the psychological problems that kept students from learning. Their graduate training came to reflect a more clinical or therapeutic orientation. Counselors were customarily assigned 200 to 300 students in a given grade level. Now, student-to-counselor ratios of 420:1 and 350:1 are commonplace. Powell, Farrar, and Cohen (1985, p. 49) report that administrators in a school with a 200:1 ratio felt that their situation approached the national "ideal."

Even with a 200:1 ratio, the burden for seeking help falls primarily on students, who may not even know that they need advice. Even when students do get an appointment with a counselor, their average visit is less than ten minutes. Often the counselor has not had time to review student records before seeing them. Paper work is overwhelming. Though counselors are charged with seeing that eligible children receive appropriate special-needs programs and that the multiple standardized test scores are recorded, many students do not get placed in programs appropriate to their capabilities and minority children fail to get the encouragement and guidance they need to stay in school and aspire to college. Fully 75 percent of counselors' time can be consumed with these clerical duties, leaving little for the therapeutic interactions which they prefer and are trained to do. The result is that only those students with serious problems, aggressive parents, personal persistence, serious discrepancies in their records, or visibly flamboyant misbehavior will receive attention. Even many normally achieving students reach their senior year without realizing that they have serious deficits in their transcripts which will prevent them from graduating.

Functionalists view the activities of counselors as part of the status allocation function in society. That is, counselors help the school to function as a mechanism for social differentiation, sorting students by perceived abilities into academic, vocational, or remedial curricula commensurate with what is believed to be their occupational role (Cicourel and Kitsuse 1963). While the decisions are supposed to be made on objective grounds, from indisputable data such as test scores, Cicourel and Kitsuse demonstrated how other, more subjective measures played a role in student placement. These include counselor judgments of student social class and whether or not the student was perceived to be popular, a good athlete, a trouble-maker, or an underachiever. These judgments are critical, because they can conclusively bar students deemed unable to perform—for whatever reason—from the courses of study that they want or that would help them achieve their potential.

More problematic is that the increasing power of counselors over a student's academic—and occupational—destiny is not distributed equitably. Students whom counselors see most are those who need it least: those with a high level of academic achievement and extracurricular participation, who are from the middle and upper classes and have seldom been in trouble (Armor 1969). Shultz and Erickson (1982) describe how this process takes place, suggesting that the differentiation is facilitated by language patterns. Counselors can avoid spending much time with students by manipulating them to ask certain questions and to give answers that fail to elicit the needed help. Fine (1987) calls this a "policy of enforced silencing" (p. 167) and discusses how information about the consequences of dropping out is systematically withheld from students. We submit that enforced silencing also precludes disadvantaged students and women from getting adequate information about courses to take, job requirements, and ways to get into colleges and other forms of higher education. We will talk in more detail about the relationship of social class, race, and gender to academic differentiation in Chapters 5, 7, and 8, where the impact of variable treatment of students by teachers, administrators, and counselors will become apparent.

THE NATURE OF ADMINISTRATIVE WORK IN SCHOOLS

The daily routine of school administrators is almost as multidimensional as that of teachers. As we have indicated, school administrators are recruited from the ranks of teachers. Promotion is based upon further examination or experience as a school administrator, a practice that closes off the system to outsiders and non-school administrators (Fantini, Gittell, and Magat 1974). Historically, administrators served as instructional leaders. Some still return occasionally to the classroom, and many districts require that they do. Labor in the schools, however, has been increasingly subdivided both functionally and temporally. The resulting bureaucratization has created a rather wide split between instructional and administrative duties (Bidwell 1965). Those at the bottom of the chain of command—teachers and principals—find it difficult to make daily decisions without constantly looking upward for approval, but those in the central office are so removed from building-level activities that actions constantly are delayed or postponed. Sometimes this delay is deliberate as bureaucrats use the structure to avoid making decisions they would rather avoid (Rogers 1968). Distance leads to distrust. Central office staff believe that building-level personnel, especially teachers, are too close to the action to maintain objectivity and flexibility while teachers and principals see the central office staff as being in an ivory tower far from the firing line (Rogers 1968).

A number of researchers have described the daily activities of typical school administrators (Cuban 1984; Borman and Spring 1984; Wolcott 1973). Because of the great diversity of schools as well as recent changes in how administrators are expected to do their work, we shall outline the categories of responsibility for school-based and central office administrators. In so doing, we will illustrate the tensions and ambiguities inherent in these roles.

Loose Coupling and Variable Zoning

The gradual change from instructional to administrative responsibility has created contradictions between the role of educational managers and what Lortie (1975) called "zoning" in their areas of legitimate authority. On one hand, because they have been teachers, administrators claim special understanding of teachers and instructional problems. On the other hand, they are viewed by teachers as management, not labor, and as lacking expertise in the teachers' own subject areas. Teachers readily accept principals' authority as legitimate only in noninstructional matters. These include financial matters, parent relations, and contacts with agencies outside the school (Becker 1953).

This division produces constant tension in matters of control and supervision, aggravated by the loose structure or "coupling" of schools (see Chapter 2). Because of the closed classroom door and scattering of buildings and personnel, top administrators have little day-to-day contact with teachers, and therefore limited capacity for direct daily supervision (Bidwell 1965; Dreeben 1973, p. 452).

Principals also have limited power over hiring and firing of teachers. They must choose from among those screened by central office staff and sometimes must take teachers transferred from other schools. They can fire teachers only in the most extreme circumstances. In most cases, undesirable teachers can be transferred to another school only if a willing recipient can be found.

While schools resemble bureaucracies to some degree, the decision-making routine of top administrators differs substantially from that of chief executive officers in corporations. In the first place, decision making in schools is scheduled and routinized. Budgets are established annually or biennially, and the remainder of the fiscal cycle consists of administering decisions that were made long before. Hiring is done at the beginning of the school year. In the second place, school officials have little control over fund raising, other than lobbying for tax increases or state or corporate beneficence. How much revenue schools receive is in the hands of taxpayers.

Some researchers have attributed to this routinization the relative lack of crises and emergencies in school decision making. However, it is our belief that neither the periodic nature of fiscal and personnel decisions nor the absence of crises over sales, marketing, and procurement mean that schools operate peacefully, especially in urban areas. The crises that occur are of a different nature and require different, largely human relations skills.

Maintenance of Fiscal and Professional Standards

One area of potential crisis for school administrators is fiduciary; school leaders, as public officials, are caretakers of public funds. They also are responsible both to governmental agencies and their public constituencies for maintenance of appropriate standards, both professional and personal, of school staff. These are the touchiest areas for school people. Instructional mismanagement is not dramatic and takes a long time to be noticed, but fiscal mismanagement or behavioral impropriety creates the kind of scandal that topples superintendents and causes principals to be fired.

Quality Control versus Autonomy

At the same time that their managerial and fiscal functions have expanded, school administrators are experiencing pressure from policy makers to exercise more supervision over instruction. Responsibility for quality control, coordination, and monitoring to ensure uniform competence among high school graduates falls to administrators, from building-level principals to the central office. However, the structural looseness of schools and the long period of time over which cohorts of students are trained provide many opportunities for exercise of autonomy in teaching. Administrators are therefore pressed to institute rationalization and routinization of instruction and assessment (Bidwell 1965, pp. 976–977), thereby further bureaucratizing schools and removing control from teachers.

A number of reforms, including restructuring and site-based management, have encouraged administrators to exercise more control over instruction. Their increased control has had two effects. First, administrators, like teachers, experience work overload and burnout. Many feel that they cannot adequately supervise instruction and also carry out all their administrative duties. Second, serious monitoring of instruction contributes to de-skilling. It is resented by teachers, who see their "hard" area of jurisdiction over instruction eroded. Principals are caught in the middle, like factory supervisors who must enforce reform upon an unenthusiastic work force (Borman and Spring 1984).

Business Managers.   Schools also have experimented with dividing the duties of the principal. Principals would become "instructional leaders" or "headmasters" who supervise teachers and help implement the curriculum. A specialist trained in business administration rather than education would handle the business aspects of schooling, especially those dealing with finances. While this plan is congruent with the efficiency movement described in Chapter 2, it has had a mixed reception. Principals are uneasy about the loss of control over budgetary matters, especially if the business manager reported directly to the central office. Teachers worry about more direct supervision by principals. We can expect to see more of these innovations in the future, but their impact upon overall school governance still is unknown.

A further issue is the impact of such division of duties on the principal's role and authority. While these proposals seem a sensible way to lighten the load for building-level supervisors, it also promises to subject them to the same de-skilling and loss of control that afflict teachers.

Relationships with the School Board and Community

Public relations is among the most important functions of school administrators. Principals must establish relationships with the parent-teacher organization and cope with those parents whose children are problems. Blumberg (1985, p. xiii) suggests that conflict is the most appropriate orientation for understanding the nature of a superintendent's work. Superintendents must maintain the uneasy balance between advice and control with their lay school boards. This task is made more difficult by the fact that, until recently, school boards exercised direct managerial control over district activities. Boards have been reluctant to relinquish this power, and since they can fire superintendents who dissatisfy them, one of the primary responsibilities of superintendents is to maintain good board relationships. Doing this can be difficult where racial and economic divisions produce disagreement over educational goals and procedures.

Principals and superintendents develop a range of strategies to maintain consensus and to prevent community conflicts from interfering with school operation. These strategies include lobbying board members on important issues in advance of meetings and/or peppering them with so much information before meetings that they cannot assimilate it all and must rely upon the judgment of the superintendent. Superintendents may hide important policy issues in meeting agendas laden with personnel, budget, and other diversionary topics. A cardinal rule is to see that open conflict never erupts in public meetings. As a result, many decisions are made first in executive sessions (Fantini, Gittell, and Magat 1974; Kerr 1973; McGivney and Haught 1972).

SUMMARY

In this chapter, we have outlined the contradictory nature of the teaching profession. We have suggested, with the functionalists, that the work of educators really does not equate with that of the traditional professions. We also have traced the development of forces that are removing teachers and building-level personnel from the center of control.

The patterns of control and training that prevail in teaching make it difficult for teachers to acquire the pay and prestige they desire. The fact that teacher work has come to be defined as female work acts to reduce its status.

Control of standards also is an issue. How teaching is carried out and who is permitted to teach is more a function of external political, ideological, and economic pressures than of concerns over expertise and technical skill. Teaching is work deemed critical to the operation of society, but often for reasons irrelevant to pedagogy. While critical theorists have argued that teachers must transform the conditions of their work, we suggest that the proportion of teachers actually trying to do so is minuscule. Teacher militancy at the collective level seems limited. A hopeful sign, however, is the fact that teachers engaged in union activity are more concerned with increasing their autonomy and control over curriculum and with respect to administrators than they are with bargaining over wages (Falk, Grimes, and Lord 1982).

The crisis in urban education of the late 1980s and 1990s (Kozol 1991) bodes well for the possibility of change. We share the caution articulated by Michael Apple (1993), who believes that while there is much about public schools in the United States that needs reform, attacks alleging that *all* public schooling is defective are dangerous. Public schooling, whatever its flaws, is a democratizing institution, which provides considerable opportunity for the underclass to achieve upward mobility. An all-out assault on the public schools provides ammunition for a conservative political movement whose agenda is privatization of schooling and subsequent sequestering of privilege for the more advantaged members of society. We challenge readers to examine each critique and each accolade leveled at the schools for its immediate as well as its long-term consequences for education in the United States.

chapter **5**

Social Class and Its Relationship to Education

Chapter Overview

INTRODUCTION

WHAT IS SOCIAL CLASS?
   The Historical Perspective: A Hierarchy of Class and Virtue
   The Genetic Perspective: A Hierarchy of Intellect
   The Sociological Perspective: A Hierarchy of Wealth

THEORETICAL BEGINNINGS: MARX, WEBER, AND BOURDIEU
   The Contributions of Karl Marx
   The Contributions of Max Weber
   The Contributions of Pierre Bourdieu

SOCIAL INEQUALITY AND THE STRUCTURE OF SOCIETY
   Social Mobility
   Caste and Class
   Occupational Attainment

THE MECHANISM OF CLASS BIAS IN EDUCATION
   Test Scores
   Ability Grouping
   Structural Inequalities in Funding
   The Social Construction of Identity

SUMMARY

INTRODUCTION

In the previous chapters, we have discussed the characteristics of schools and the people who participate in them. We now turn to an examination of the impact schools have on children. This chapter begins with a discussion of social class, for several reasons. First, the variable social class constitutes perhaps the single most powerful source of inequality in society. Second, social class was one of the first factors, besides intelligence, examined by modern sociologists as a possible source of the differences in achievement. Explicating the relationship between social class and education has been one of the most important contributions sociologists have made to our understanding of education.

Notions of social class are so inextricably linked to our thinking about ethnicity, race, and gender that it is difficult to discuss them separately. This is especially true in the United States, where we tend to ignore social class origins, placing more emphasis on race and ethnicity. Most people in this country see themselves as middle class. In Europe and Australia people tend to differentiate social class positions more clearly. The experiences of women, people of color, and people from impoverished and working classes have long been neglected in the literature. Nevertheless, it is important to consider all aspects of a person's experience. We have attempted to disentangle them in this chapter as well as Chapters 7 and 8, to clarify their individual impact and to show the complexity of the interrelationship among education, class, ethnicity, and gender.

The first section of the chapter discusses the history of the concept of class and some of the most important thinkers who have contributed to its development. Next we look at the way social class and education interact to stratify society into a class structure. Finally, we examine some of the mechanisms in systems of education that lead both to reproduction of the existing class structure and social class bias in what purports to be a meritocracy based upon achievement.

WHAT IS SOCIAL CLASS?

Before we can talk meaningfully about the relationship between social class and education, we must understand what the term *social class* means and how it has become a key concept in how we think about our world. A *class* of things is a category—a number of things grouped together because they share common characteristics. Social scientists define social classes as groups of people who share certain characteristics of prestige, patterns of taste and language, income, occupational status (though not necessarily the same jobs), educational level, aspirations, behavior, and beliefs. Social classes are **stratified,** arranged in a pyramid-shaped hierarchy according to members' wealth, power, and prestige. *Wealth* refers to the control of material resources or economic clout, *power* refers to authority in the political realm, and *prestige* refers to the control of ideological resources or cultural influence. One's place in society depends upon the amount of superiority he or she has in all of these realms.

Throughout history, thinkers have had different opinions as to why certain kinds of people have occupied high positions in the hierarchy and others have occupied the bottom levels. As we shall explain, the social scientific view based upon socioeconomic status is a relatively new way of thinking about class.

To which social class do you think your family of origin belonged? What social class do you think you belong to now? What evidence do you use for giving yourself a particular social class assignment?

The Historical Perspective: A Hierarchy of Class and Virtue

what does it mean when a T says of a S: "He come from a good family"

People confuse a hierarchy of social class with a hierarchy of moral virtue and intelligence. Historically, this confusion has had a profound impact upon social and educational policy. It comes from the fact that the concept of social class is a very old one, predating by centuries the social science disciplines of sociology, economics, political science, and anthropology, which use it as an analytic concept.

The historical perspective is based upon notions of aristocracy. Until very recent times philosophers, religious leaders, and politicians, as well as the general population, believed that class status was determined by how valued, wise, and virtuous a person was. These ideas were reinforced by the concept of the "divine right" of kings to rule. People from the highest social classes were considered, merely because of their birth rank, to be the brightest and most virtuous, and therefore the most capable of ruling. For example, it was believed that kings and queens were anointed by God and ruled with God's permission, and they were held up as behavioral exemplars. The American Puritans too felt that wealth and prestige in this life were indications of God's favor and a guarantee of salvation in the hereafter. High levels of wealth and prestige, as well as of educational attainment, were seen as resulting from hard work, great spirituality, or moral superiority rather than, as was more often the case, from family inheritance.

In reality, many gentlemen were not very gentle, nor were all kings kingly, nor all ladies ladylike. Characteristics that were attributed to a superior intellect and morality often simply were functions of superior wealth. It was a great deal easier to be clean, kind, gentle, well educated, cultured, and generous if one were fortunate enough to be born into an affluent family. The illiteracy, social deviance, crime, moral depravity, lack of hygiene, brutish behavior, and general lack of culture common among the lower classes were believed to be innate or hereditary tendencies rather than a function of environmental influences.

This kind of thinking had a powerful influence on popular thinking. It argued against both social welfare programs and attempts to include the poor in decision making in their own behalf since they were not thought to be capable of such elevated behavior. Social Darwinists even argued that social policies to help the poor would be harmful, since they would only encourage the reproduction of people who were mentally or morally defective and would waste resources that could better be used for more deserving populations (Spencer 1851, 1898; Sumner 1883). The only rational response was to learn to live with poverty, rescuing those few "deserving poor" whose values could be shaped to resemble those of the middle and upper classes. This kind of thinking still exists today and impedes serious attempts to eliminate poverty and oppression.

Because class status was considered to be hereditary, few philosophers or social theorists considered that the association between affluence and virtue, leadership ability, literacy, and the like might be circular. However, their beliefs did not hinder attempts to use the schools as a means of social control. Educators developed curricula designed to teach obedience to the law, temperance, sexual restraint, good hygiene, thrift, and punctuality—all values acceptable to the upper and middle classes. In fact, some of the earliest educational sociologists felt that schools were the only appropriate place to learn civic virtues. As was explained in Chapter 3, Durkheim believed that as societies modernized, parents no longer could prepare their children adequately for adult life. Families had to specialize in what they could do best—developing the individual personality—while to the schools fell the task of nation building, that is, developing citizens capable of adhering to the laws of the land and carrying out their responsibilities to the state.

Durkheim developed his ideas in a 1901 treatise called *Moral Education* (1969), which was based upon a series of lectures he delivered to pre-service teachers. His ideas of moral education are echoed in contemporary theories of poverty which describe the incompetence of poor families to raise and educate their children. Courses in citizenship, health and hygiene, free enterprise, and other virtues are still popular, representing an effort to use the schools to create a consensus on acceptable ways of relating to the political order.

The Genetic Perspective: A Hierarchy of Intellect

Traditionally, then, social class was associated with morality. A modern variation has been to equate it with intelligence, as measured on so-called intelligence tests. People observed that the poor usually were badly educated, and they assumed that poor people and minorities had low educational attainment because they lacked intelligence. This conventional wisdom, coupled with the racism of the nineteenth and early twentieth centuries, led to a considerable volume of "scientific" research supporting a causal relationship between intelligence and social class. Studies of brain size and shape, or "craniometry," "proved" that women, lower-class people, African Americans, and other minorities had inferior brains with less cranial capacity than or different construction from those of Europeans. The connection between class and intelligence was bolstered by the advent of IQ testing, since lower classes and minorities scored lower on these tests.

Samuel George Morton, for example, attempted to show that Asians, Africans, and Native Americans were intellectually inferior to Northern Europeans because their brains were smaller. His research method was to weigh the amount of birdshot poured into the cranial cavities of skulls from various ethnic groups. Unfortunately, whenever he obtained results counter to his claims, he manipulated the data. The results of these studies have since been shown to be based upon misinterpretation or fraud (Gould 1981). Gould feels that Morton intended no fraud, however: "All I can discern is an *a priori* conviction about racial ranking so powerful that it directed his tabulations along preestablished lines" (1981, p. 69). The work of others, however, was not so innocent.

Sir Cyril Burt (1883–1971) was one of the most influential educational psychologists of his time. He was a pioneer in testing and mental measurement, and from the beginning of his career believed that intelligence was an innate and immutable characteristic. Nature, not nurture, determined one's destiny. Furthermore, people were poor because they—and their parents—were less intelligent. The observed differences in achievement between social classes were the consequence of hereditary intelligence. Not until after his death did investigators determine that the vast majority of Burt's research was based upon data flawed by inadmissible carelessness, fakery, omission, and outright fraud (Gould 1981, p. 235).

Despite the flimsiness of their work, these researchers have left a powerful legacy. As late as the 1970s Arthur Jensen (1969), William Schockley, and Richard Hernstein (1973) could publish articles in respectable scholarly journals advocating educational and social policies based upon the premise that the intellect of minorities, especially African Americans, was genetically inferior to that of whites. *+ how of course The Bell Curve – Hernstein again: C. Murray*

The Sociological Perspective: A Hierarchy of Wealth

As sociologists, we reject the notion that class status and virtue are synonymous or that class is a function of innate intelligence. We also reject attempts to teach children to accept the status quo as the only legitimate alternative to social chaos. While we do believe that class status and associated behaviors and attitudes are, to some degree, inherited, this heritability consists not so much in genetic factors as in the fact that a child's environment has a profound effect upon his or her development. Furthermore, because our work is informed by critical theory, rather than treating class status and its attendant inequalities as a given, we view class identity as "constructed"— that is, we believe it develops through interaction with other people over time. A child *becomes* an upper-class prep school graduate with medical school aspirations, or a lower-class teenage mother about to drop out of school, not because they were born into a particular kind of family but because their background set up expectations for their behavior and also influenced how others would react to them. The net of mutual expectations is not totally inescapable, but it does, to a large degree, affect the direction of individual development.

Examine your family's genealogy. Were there changes in social class status over the generations? To what do you attribute these changes?

Sociological Definitions of Class, Status, and Power. When sociologists look at the inequalities that rank-order groups, they distinguish among class, status, and power. *Power* refers to the ability to realize one's will, even if others resist. Weber suggests that power legitimated by others constitutes *authority,* while power not legitimated is *coercion* or force. The term *status* refers to a state of being or position. In sociology it connotes the distribution of prestige (Gerth and Mills 1953) based upon what people have—including material goods, where they live, who their family and friends are, the extent and type of their education and training, and their occupation. Status is associated with culture. Status groups

> subjectively . . . distinguish themselves from [one another] in terms of categories of *moral evaluation* such as "honor," "taste," "breeding," "respectability," "propriety," "cultivation," "good fellows," "plain folks," etc. Thus the exclusion of persons who lack the in-group culture is felt to be normatively legitimated. (Collins 1977, p. 125)

Sociologists believe that status and power are a function of *social class.* They define class as groups of people who share similar economic life chances because they have similar opportunities in the labor market. For Weberians, class is positional, a function of one's occupation, income, and to some extent educational level. For Marxists, class is relational, a function of one's interaction with others in the processes of production. Specifically, one's class is determined by the amount of political and cultural power as well as the extent to which one both owns the means to one's own livelihood and can hire or control the labor of others.

Some sociologists divide the social hierarchy into six classes: upper-upper, lower-upper, upper-middle, lower-middle, upper-lower (or working class), and lower-lower (Bensman and Vidich 1971). Marxists divide it into three strata, according to the kind of work their members do and how much control they have over their own labor. At the bottom are the *proletariat,* workers, or manual laborers, who own no part of the places in which they work, whose tasks are completely controlled by their supervisors, and who have to sell their labor to others. The *ruling classes* consist of two groups: (1) *capitalists,* who own their means of production, do not sell their own labor, and do purchase the labor of others; and (2) *petty bourgeoisie,* who own their means of production, do not sell their labor, and also do not purchase that of others (Wright and Perrone 1977). Capitalists, who include landed aristocrats, benefit from the "surplus capital," or profits generated by workers. In this formulation, teachers are considered to be workers, because they neither supervise labor nor own their means of making a living (Wright and Perrone 1977).

Marx wrote at a time when land ownership as a source of power was diminishing. His description of society better fits an eighteenth-century factory and industrial pattern than it does today's technologically oriented economy, where managers and professionals replace traditional capitalist owners, and manual labor and heavy industry have lost importance to service sectors in an "information" society. However, his ideas about social organization and the origins of power, inequality, and conflict are still powerful. Table 5.1 summarizes and to some degree updates Marx's ideas of social class structure.

Regardless of their orientation, sociologists agree that people with the most wealth, power, and prestige are at the apex of the social class pyramid and are influen-

TABLE 5.1. Expanded Marxist Criteria for Class

	Criteria for Class Position			
	Ownership of the Means of Production	Purchase of the Labor Power of Others	Control of the Labor Power of Others	Sale of One's Own Labor Power
Capitalists	Yes	Yes	Yes	No
Managers	No	No	Yes	Yes
Workers	No	No	No	Yes
Petty Bourgeoisie	Yes	No	No	No

SOURCE: E.O. Wright and L. Perrone, "Marxist Class Categories and Income Inequality," *American Sociological Review 42* (1977), p. 34.

tial in controlling policies and practices that maintain their position. While power comes from various sources—the political structure, business, the media, and the military (Domhoff 1967; Mills 1956)—these sources tend to overlap. The degree of overlap, as well as the means of exercising control, often are not obvious to the majority of the population.

The Material Conditions of Life. Peter McLaren uses a Marxist definition of *class:* the "economic, social and political relationships that govern life in a given social order." He states that inequality in society is based upon the concept of *surplus labor* and the unequal access people have to it. Surplus labor is the work done beyond what is necessary for the workers' survival, and the subsequent profits that others earn from their efforts. According to Marxist or critical analysis, surplus labor is the genesis of social class variation. Social class relations "are those associated with surplus labor [or profit], who produces it, and who is a recipient of it" (McLaren 1989, p. 171). The amount of surplus labor is a measure of the degree of exploitation in a capitalist society, because it represents the extent to which those who profit from it are not those who produced it.

The critical perspective that informs this book stresses that social classes originate in the material, and specifically the economic conditions of life. These are at the center of human activity. They involve using the forces of production—or levels of technology, land, labor, capital, and available energy—and the social relations of production—or how human effort is organized—for productive activity (Persell 1977).

Membership in a social class is determined by the way people relate to the economic and material conditions of life, how much of them they control, and how much they are beneficiaries of the productive efforts. Those individuals who control more of or who benefit more from the economic order are those at the top of the pyramid. Those who control less and benefit less are toward the bottom. Because stratification patterns are patterns of social and cultural domination and subordination, it may be more accurate to use the term *structure of dominance* (Weber 1947, p. 426) than the common sociological term *social stratification* when referring to economic and social hierarchies. Those who control more and benefit more also have more power or more capacity to dominate others.

Social classes, or the structure of power and domination, are differentiated by the prestige and status ascribed to them within the hierarchy as well as by the actual power they wield. Members of a social class do not need to know one another, although they usually choose their friends and associates from their own class. Nor need they be aware that they are a member of a class to belong to one. Some theorists would argue that class cannot exist without class consciousness—people have to know that they belong to it for a social class to exist. Others argue that one purpose of educational ideology is to keep people from being aware of their class position so that they remain satisfied with the status quo. Critical theorists believe that as people become conscious of their class membership, they begin to develop opposition to the oppressive practices that have masked class differences and preserved the status quo. One of these practices is to foster social beliefs that deny the existence of oppression and inequality. *Do such practices actually exist? What is one example?*

The Mythical Middle Class: Control through Ideology.   Ideologies are "way[s] of viewing the world . . . that we tend to accept as natural and common-sense." They provide the categories, concepts, and images through which people interpret their world and shape their behavior (McLaren 1989, p. 176) and, in doing so, they are instruments of **hegemony**, a kind of domination without the use of force.

Hegemonic domination operates through "social forms and structures produced in specific sites such as churches, the state, schools, mass media, the political system, and the family" (McLaren 1989, p. 173). There is no need to institute more stringent means of social control—such as exclusionary laws, imprisonment, and torture—when there is general agreement that the status quo is legitimate, even if not personally satisfactory.

Class consciousness is very low in America because our cultural ideology describes us as an egalitarian society. Americans generally refuse to assign each other to a hierarchical social ranking. Traditionally, most describe themselves as "middle class," regardless of their actual income, occupation, or education (Persell 1977). You might ask your friends or classmates to identify the social class that most accurately describes their own background to see if our argument fits them.

The consensus that everyone is "middle class" is one way in which actual class differences are hidden in the United States. Hegemonic domination is facilitated by this "myth of the middle class," because this social ideology maintains the domination of the existing class system. The common belief that any differences are only a matter of degree is a convenient fiction that allows us to ignore extremes of wealth and poverty. It is facilitated by the low visibility of the rich in America, who are segregated in private neighborhoods, schools, social clubs, and occupational circles (Persell 1977, p. 31) and the equal invisibility of the poor. Until recently, it cost middle- and upper-class Americans very little effort to avoid an encounter with homelessness or abject poverty. However, during the 1980s and 1990s the myth of a relatively "classless" society has been exploded by the growth and visibility of the poor, especially the underclass of the inner cities (Wilson 1987). That the poor do not revolt against their condition is a function of the power of ideology. Members of the underclass have internalized what schools have taught them: that people are rewarded for hard work. Even if they do not believe that they live in an egalitarian society, they tend to feel that they, not the system, are responsible for their plight. Either they weren't lucky enough, didn't have the ability, or just didn't work hard enough.

i.e. they to buy the ideology

That is why schools play such an important role in maintaining existing patterns of domination. They perpetuate a middle-class ideology which states that status and social mobility in American society are based upon merit, earned competitively, and facilitated by schooling. These attitudes achieve legitimacy because some individuals actually do benefit from the system. However, those for whom the system pays off most are those who already were advantaged—white middle- and upper-class males (Rosenfeld 1980; Wright and Perrone 1977).

Think back to your experiences in elementary and secondary schooling. Were you aware that children came from different social classes? How? How did differences in social class status affect children's school experiences? Give specific examples from your own experiences.

THEORETICAL BEGINNINGS: MARX, WEBER, AND BOURDIEU

Both Karl Marx and Max Weber were concerned with the relationship between class and education, though from different vantage points. Both felt that educational systems were a reflection of the societies in which they were embedded. They differed as to what they felt was the basis of that society. For Marx, the structure of society and of domination and subordination was based upon the economy, or the production and distribution of goods and services. Weber, however, felt that domination was based upon more than economics. Critical to his analyses were politics and government, or the organization of power and authority, and their relationship to educational systems in a variety of societies, industrialized and others. Bourdieu rejected the Marxist emphasis on the economy as the only basis for class structure; he added the correlate of power, which comes from acquiring specialized forms of social and cultural knowledge. In the following sections we explore these notions more fully.

The Contributions of Karl Marx

Marx never treated education extensively. He considered that educational systems, like systems of esthetics and religion, were simply a part of the societal superstructure which came from and corresponded to the economic base of society.

Class Analysis. Marx made explicit the relationship between social class and economic power and demonstrated how it creates a hierarchy of classes within a society. His analysis was so powerful that social scientists have been "Marxists" ever since, at least insofar as class and stratification have been critical to their analysis of social structure. Marxist analysis initially focused on class and caste at the structural level; it did not examine either the relationship of education to class or the functioning of schools as organizations. Later Marxist theorists did posit a relationship, stating that the educational system provided a legitimizing function for capitalist systems (Bowles and Gintis 1976; Scimecca 1980). Schools acted to defuse class antagonisms, as we shall explain later, because they indoctrinated students to accept the belief that the position they attain is the best they can achieve (Scimecca 1980, pp. 9-10). In this way, the school system was critical in reproducing the social class structure from one generation to another. This position has been adopted by critical theorists as well.

Marxists and neo-Marxists also believe that there is a tight causal link between and across subsystems, so that changes in one subsystem directly lead to changes in the others. The supposed existence of such links can be applied to education to bolster the argument that education is closely linked to generations of economic inequality. While most people who wish to use the schools to solve social problems are reformers rather than Marxist revolutionaries, using an education-economy link to eliminate poverty and other social ills has had powerful appeal to educators, policy makers, and social scientists. Especially with regard to education, however, current research has shown the links to be indirect and weaker than reformers would hope (LeCompte and Dworkin 1991). We will talk more about this later in this chapter.

Dialectical Analysis. Perhaps most important to Marx's approach is the use of *dialectical analysis.* This is a method by which all assumptions are assumed to contain their own contradictions or opposites. Propositions believed to be true are analyzed as if they were false. For example, dialectical analysis would permit us to question the truism, "All men are created equal," asking what was meant by the terms *men, created,* and *equal.* We then would determine if all men—or women—were equal and under what circumstances, if any.

Dialectical analysis provided a framework by which the legitimacy of all conventional assumptions about the relationship between wealth and power could be questioned, including assumptions that made moral virtue the basis of social class hierarchy. Dialectical analysis also made it possible to identify sources of inequality, exploitation, and oppression and helped to forge an understanding that wealth was not necessarily a sign of superior effort or morality. On the contrary, Marxists looked at possession of great wealth in a bourgeois society as a sign of ill-gotten gains, attainable only through the exploitation of others.

Critical theorists have used the concept of dialectical analysis to raise questions such as the following:

- Why is it that working-class children get working-class jobs while the children of doctors and other professionals become professionals?
- Could it really be true that the reason 40 to 70 percent of minority children in many major cities drop out of school is that they lack sufficient intelligence or ambition to graduate?

- Do the rewards of the educational system really go to those with the most intellectual merit?
- Why is it that schools in poor urban neighborhoods or rural communities are desperately underfunded, while neighboring suburban schools offer a wide variety of programs to children in clean, safe, and well-equipped schools?
- What are the consequences of educational reform? Will it really improve the achievement of minorities and the poor?

Alienation. Another major contribution of Marx has been a socioeconomic rather than a psychological definition of *alienation.* The sociological approach to alienation has contributed greatly to our understanding of why teachers burn out and students lose interest in schoolwork (Dworkin 1985b, 1986; LeCompte and Dworkin, 1991). Marx felt that workers could find meaning only in work that they directly controlled and in places whose ownership they shared. They were "alienated" to the extent that they had no control over what they did and how it was done.

However Utopian that notion may sound in a world of multinational corporations, accelerating buyouts, and consolidation of companies, alienation remains a powerful concept to explain industrial sabotage, teacher burnout, and other forms of occupational disaffection. To Marx, alienation simply meant that one's work place is so far removed from those who actually control the work, and so far removed from those who use the products, that the daily activities become meaningless. To cope with this boredom and meaninglessness, people may engage in self-sabotage in the form of shoddy work or rudeness, or may even destroy equipment, products, and materials.

Marx's concept of alienation is reflected in critical theorists' concept of de-skilling and its impact on teacher morale. Chapter 4 examines the impact of de-skilling through works by Apple (1986), Dworkin (1986), and LeCompte and Dworkin (1991).

The Contributions of Max Weber

Unlike Marx, Weber discussed education at length. He was especially interested in the curriculum and the types of students. He felt that each society created educational systems uniquely suited to indigenous systems of power and authority. These systems were used to select and train the leaders of the society. An analysis of schools' characteristics and populations would reveal who got into school and how, and an examination of what was taught would reveal what kinds of information were deemed important for different groups in the society.

Education and the Structure of Authority. Weber distinguished among three kinds of authority: traditional, charismatic, and rational-legal. They were found in different kinds of societies but were not predicated entirely upon the existence of a particular economic structure. Each type of authority required a different leadership style: Traditional societies produced kings; charismatic authority was that of the hero or guru; rational-legal forms required bureaucrats and civil servants. Each leadership type mandated differences in modes of training and education for elites (Persell 1977; Weber 1947, pp. 426–434). Weber used three case studies to identify the different systems: the Mandarin Chinese (traditional), Christianity (charismatic), and the industrial civil service of late nineteenth-century Europe (rational-legal).

A key contribution of Weber was his understanding of (1) the degree to which the educational system could facilitate the succession of elites through merit and rationally assessed competence, rather than through inheritance or some other nonrational means of selection; and (2) whether or not the curriculum could be standardized and graded. Only rational-legal forms of authority with their emphasis on competence and expertise required such standardization. If authority were based on charisma, leadership could not be taught; it was based upon "discipleship," and one could only wait for leadership capabilities to be awakened and demonstrated in some sort of trials or magical rites. And traditional kings were not trained; they ruled, competent or not, by virtue of "divine right" and their ability to survive attempts to remove them from the throne.

Merit and Achievement.   Weber understood that societies based upon meritocracy (Young 1971) could recruit able individuals for positions of wealth and power regardless of their initial social standing. Where achieved merit was the basis for rewards, it was possible to use educational systems to facilitate social mobility and exchange of ruling groups. Even within these societies, however, those who benefited most from the educational system were those who already were somewhat advantaged.

The Contributions of Pierre Bourdieu

Having determined the basis for the establishment of social classes, sociologists then turned to an examination of the dynamics and impact of class structure. Among the questions they asked were the following:

- What characteristics distinguish people in various classes?
- Can people move from one class to another, especially to a higher class?
- What rigidities stand in the way of movement from one class to another?

In Chapter 1 we discussed class differences in language and communication patterns. But class differences are based upon differences more profound than language and communication alone. To understand fully what differentiates people in one social class from those in another, we must examine the concept of cultural capital.

Distinctions between Class and Culture.   The terms *class* and *culture* are often confused. For sociologists, class is a position in the hierarchy or status. Culture is the way people express that status, or "the particular ways in which a social group lives out and makes sense of its given circumstances and conditions of life" (McLaren 1989,

---

Javier's Story: Former Migrant/Current ESL Teacher

School was someplace where I didn't have to go. It was a memory born in Del-icias, Texas, and since we had left El Paso. [It was] an activity that only hap-pened now and then. School was a world of children's games, more gringos than I ever seen, and spanking by someone called the principal, who punished children for things they said. . . . School was the place where I was ridiculed for my clothes, my way of reasoning, and for my neck, my elbows, my hair, and my hands, which were cleaned by my mother and judged by the school.

School was Mrs. Peters, who enjoyed so much to march the kids from the migrant camp out to the water fountain in the hall, hand us a bar of soap, and then bring out the whole class to watch as she ordered us to wash our necks. "Look, don't you know how to wash your neck? It is filthy." It amazed me that Mrs. Peters could assume that there was plentiful water for bathing; my view of the world was that water for this purpose was limited everywhere, not just as it was at the camp. She led me out to the water fountain and gave me a small piece of soap. As I stood there scrubbing, she went into the classroom and brought out some kids to stare at me. Her voice echoes in my ears: "His mother must live like a pig . . . pig . . . pig."

SOURCE: Velasquez 1993, pp. 106–107.

---

p. 171). Culture includes the distinctive language, ideologies, behavior patterns, atti-tudes and values, artifacts, dress, and shared historical experiences of a group of peo-ple. Javier's story (see box) illustrates how culture and class work together to shape social perceptions.

Cultural Capital. Taken together, all of these cultural patterns constitute *cultural capital* of a group—the ways of talking and acting, moving, dressing, socializing, tastes, likes and dislikes, competencies, and forms of knowledge that distinguish one group from another (Bourdieu 1977). Cultural capital is a resource, and just like natu-ral resources, not all forms of it are valued equally. The social value of cultural capital is a function of the prestige of the group that possesses it; or conversely, the prestige of individuals depends upon how much of what kind of cultural capital they own. In Chapter 1 we discussed cultural reproduction, explaining how children in school are evaluated on how closely their cultural capital mirrors that of the dominant society, the latter reflected in the requirements for success in white middle-class schooling. Those who do not meet the school's standards for whatever reason—dialect, commu-nication style, manners—may be perceived as being less capable than those who do.

Cultural capital is an important concept to critical theorists, because it is made up of factors to which people react in social interaction and which shape the con-struction of social beliefs and social realities. Insofar as members of subordinate groups refuse to conform to the norms or to value the cultural capital of dominant groups, differences in people's cultural capital can provide a starting point for the development of resistance and oppositional culture.

SOCIAL INEQUALITY AND THE STRUCTURE OF SOCIETY

Marxian and Weberian analysis laid the foundation for our understanding of the complex relationships between schools and societies, both at the macrolevel of societal organization and at the microlevel of the organization of teaching and learning. Educational sociologists have been concerned at the macrolevel in the following areas: (1) social mobility, (2) relationships between classes, (3) academic achievement and educational attainment, (4) social stratification and patterns of inequality, and (5) the occupational structure. Until the 1970s, sociologists were concerned primarily with effects: how "inputs" to education—such as parents' education, occupation, and income, and certain attitudes such as college and occupational expectations—affected "outputs" of education—such as test scores, high school completion, college entrance, and occupational attainment. What went on *inside* the schools was of little concern (Hargreaves and Woods 1984; LeCompte 1978b, 1981).

Since 1970 greater attention has been paid to the microlevel of schooling, that is, what actually happens in schools to create the inequalities school attendance seems to produce. We will discuss processes at the microlevel later in this chapter and in Chapters 6, 7, and 8.

Social Mobility

Social mobility refers to the movement of individuals and groups up or down from the social class of their birth to others. Mobility takes place through intermarriage or by acquisition of the cultural capital associated with the new status.

Up the Social Ladder. In a meritocratic society, education has been the key to upward mobility. It takes place in two stages. First, one must acquire at least some of the characteristics of the upper class, most important of which is a level of education that will provide competence in higher-status jobs and give a luster to social and intellectual interaction. Second, one must learn the social graces and habits of behavior of the class to which one aspires. Practicing for status is called *anticipatory socialization* (Srinivas 1965). It is reflected in the desire of parents to send their children to the "right" schools.

Americans tend to conceive only of upward mobility, and they encourage their children to get as much schooling as possible so that they can do better than their parents. Poverty in the lower classes has been attributed to an absence of the ambition or necessary ability to acquire an adequate education. However, upward mobility can exist only where there is room for expansion on the socioeconomic ladder. Room at the top is created when those at the top stratum are removed or decreased in number, either by lower birth rates among the elite, social upheaval, or geographic relocation of those hoping to move upward—in the past, for example, by moving to the colonies or out on the frontier—or by the creation of new economic opportunities, such as the computer industry. It has been possible for generations of Americans to ignore the possibility of downward mobility, both because the economy offered a wide range of opportunity and because social status has been heavily based not upon cultural standing, which had to be inherited, but upon economic wealth, which could be earned. The United States was blessed with expanding economic and geographic frontiers which provided opportunity for some people to escape their original destinies. The prestigious cultural goods associated with upper-class life could, in large part, be purchased once wealth had been acquired.

This model is, however, deceptive, because it is based upon a limited number of "deviant cases." Strategies that worked for a few who did "make it" were applied indiscriminately to everyone. Hence the Horatio Alger stories, in which a poor boy's hard work and diligent study won him wealth and the hand of the factory owner's daughter, became the model to which the general population aspired. The Alger stories contributed to hegemonic myths which held that if you didn't get rich and inherit the factory, you just hadn't worked hard enough.

Down the Social Ladder. The fact is, however, that not everyone can move up. Most societies are fairly stable and there usually are as many individuals moving down as are moving up. Where room at the top constricts, the net mobility downward may exceed movement up, no matter how much education people can acquire. This phenomenon appears to be occurring in the United States, as the society decapitalizes, industry moves to developing countries, and high-paying jobs in the industrial and professional sectors are reduced in number or replaced by lower-paying, less-skilled jobs in the service sector (Bluestone and Bennett 1982).

This situation is a real problem for the United States for several reasons. First, it devalues education, exploding the myth of the payoff for hard work in school. It creates educational inflation as increased educational attainment in the face of fewer appropriate jobs makes diplomas less valuable than before. College degrees are now required for jobs that once needed only high school diplomas. The prospect of downward mobility weighs particularly heavily on middle-class and poor students, for whom education represented their only hope to maintain status or escape proletarianization, or a descent into the working class (Miles 1977).

It also affects patterns of reward and control in school. Teachers no longer can promise their students that if they work hard to learn and if they respect the teacher, they will be rewarded with a good job. Finally, the anticipation of downward mobility can lead to student alienation and unrest as the promised "good life" seems further and further out of reach to an increasingly large group of young people (Keniston 1971; Miles 1977).

Caste and Class

Up to now we have been talking only about social *class*. Membership in a social class is not fixed, even though in many societies movement from one class to another is limited and often takes place only through marriage. However, where *castes,* rather than classes, structure a society, movement may be existent.

Membership in a caste is rigidly hereditary and is defined by occupational status. Caste members inherit the occupations of their fathers and are forbidden by law and social custom from engaging in any other profession unless it has the same assigned social status. Social interaction between castes is limited and intermarriage is forbidden. Often caste differences are highlighted by differences in dress, patterns of food consumption, ethnicity, language, and religion. Low-status castes often are stigmatized; anything associated with a low-status caste is considered polluting to a member of a higher caste. As a consequence, people from different castes cannot eat together or live in the same neighborhood.

Caste-based societies provide little opportunity for individual mobility. Using the case of India, Srinivas (1965) and Rudolph and Rudolph (1967) describe *group* mobility; certain low-caste groups have begun to raise the status of their group by becoming educated, changing their occupation, becoming vegetarians, and adopting the religious observances of Brahmins. The Rudolphs' research indicates that an increase in education is not sufficient. These groups had to change their *cultural capital* as well.

Castelike Minorities. Castes usually have not been thought to exist in the United States. However, Ogbu (1978, 1983, 1987) points out that the status of native-born, stigmatized minorities, such as Mexican Americans, American Indians, and African Americans, is "castelike." We might also argue that Appalachians could be included in this listing. Ogbu believes that the systematic patterns of discrimination these groups have experienced over many generations have transformed them into a virtually hereditary underclass of impoverished people. They do poorly in school as a group, regardless of the special programs set up for them, and are able to obtain only those jobs at the lowest end of the labor market. They share a fatalistic perspective: Since no amount of work will lead to a better job, why try?

Ogbu also makes the important point that the disabilities under which castelike minorities labor are contextual rather than inherent. When members of these groups escape to a society that does not discriminate against them, they can be as successful as any other migrant group. As Gibson's work with Punjabi students in California demonstrates, they often can do this without forswearing many aspects of their traditional culture (Gibson 1988).

In Chapter 7 we will further discuss minorities, education, and inequality and will also provide an update of Ogbu's perspectives on minority status and failure. Some scholars have criticized Ogbu's analysis for its overly simplistic and deterministic view of the impact of labor market structure (Erickson 1987). Others argue that his analysis fails to account for the fact that minority children often conform to, rather than behave antagonistically toward, the authority structure and norms of the school (D'Amato 1987). His discussion, however, points out that schools are among the primary locations where the process of social differentiation takes place. Children who start out there with ostensibly equal capabilities end up sorted into groups whose achievement is markedly different. Furthermore, these differences in achievement are explained, in large part, by differences in social class (or castelike status). Regardless of their ethnicity, poor students tend to study with poor students and rich students tend to study with other rich students. The remainder of this chapter will discuss how this process occurs and what its consequences are.

Occupational Attainment

Functional theorists in the sociology of education felt that educational systems played three roles in the larger society. First, they attributed to schools the functions of socialization for citizenship and social control (Durkheim 1969). Second, they believed that schools were sites for the meritocratic selection and training of leadership cadres (Weber 1947). Finally, they believed schools were where individuals were meritocratically selected and trained for specific occupational roles.

The last function is accomplished by means of two mechanisms: (1) the differentiated curriculum, which prepares students either for vocational careers or for higher education and professional training, and (2) the system of grading and ability grouping, by which students are placed into curricula appropriate to their ability and interests and to their ultimate career. In the United States sociologists and educators preferred to believe that status was based upon achievement. To do so, they had to demonstrate that social status was not inherited. Therefore, education, not family background, would have to be the most important predictor of educational and occupational attainment.

The Blau and Duncan Model. Blau and Duncan's (1967) landmark study of young men examined the relationship between family background variables, including father's occupation and education, and the level of education and occupation attained by their sons. Blau and Duncan tried to develop a model to predict mathematically how much education contributed to individual occupational attainment. Their model had a profound impact upon the way social scientists thought about the relationships among education, occupation, and socioeconomic status. They did find that the impact of all educational factors combined—including mother's and father's education, the individual's educational aspirations and actual years of education completed, and the individual's motivation as measured by grades and standardized test scores—was the single largest contributor to one's life chances.

However, there were some significant limitations to their work. First, they looked only at white males. More important, the correlations were not overwhelming, indicating that education contributed only about 30 percent of the total predictive power to the model. Other sociologists then attempted to improve the predictive power of the model by adding other factors. Perhaps best known of these attempts was the work of Sewell, Haller, and their associates.

The Status Attainment Model. The so-called "Wisconsin Model" (Sewell, Haller, and Portes 1969, 1970; Sewell, Haller, and Ohlendorf 1970; Sewell and Shah 1967; Jencks, Crouse, and Mueser 1983) asked the following questions:

1. What are the relative effects of family background and schooling on subsequent attainments?
2. What is the role of academic ability in the attainment process?
3. How do aspirations and motivations determine attainment and what is the role of family and school in providing support for aspirations? Do

> social psychological variables merely transmit the effects of family back-
> ground and/or ability or do they have an impact of their own? (Campbell
> 1983, p. 47)

These sociologists suggested that attitudinal factors in family background and aspira-
tional variables were important links between ascribed (or family background) status,
educational attainment, and ultimate occupation. In other words, family influence
was not just passive. Families transmitted to children an active desire toward certain
occupational goals and an expectation of reaching these goals. They also examined
the influence of "significant others"—teachers and parents. Some sociologists even
interviewed children and their parents to trace the impact of parents' aspirations for
their children (Kahl 1953).

However, these studies did not explain why families from different social classes
produced children with different goals, nor did they examine the constraints on occupational attainment imposed by both market conditions—supply and demand for
given services—and by patterns of discrimination—both legal and customary (Persell
1977).

The Rosenfeld Model: Race and Gender Bias. As was mentioned earlier, Blau
and Duncan's model looked only at whites, failed to examine the impact of mothers
on sons, and did not discuss daughters at all. R. Rosenfeld (1980) replicated both Blau
and Duncan's work and the status attainment models for women and African Americans. As she suspected, the model was not nearly as good a predictor for women or
for African Americans as it was for white men. In the early stages—the first six years
after completing school—white men and women receive about the same wage and
status returns on their investment in education. However, after six years the picture
changes dramatically.

> At their potential, white men receive greater returns to their human capital
> [education and training] than white women. They receive higher returns in
> terms of both status and wages to their years of formal schooling, get greater
> returns in terms of status to their white collar training, suffer less of a status
> disadvantage from having some formal preparation for a blue collar job, and
> receive considerably greater wage returns from both kinds of training. (R.
> Rosenfeld 1980, p. 604)

Only nonwhite males do worse than white women.

The most important factors in ultimate occupational attainment for women are
related not to education but to the labor market. They include previous work experience, the types of jobs available, and the degree of discrimination encountered.

The Contributions of Occupational Attainment Researchers. Despite their
limitations, the work of these investigators clarified several important ways that the
meritocratic model did not work as predicted. Blau and Duncan and the status attainment researchers found that the impact of education on achievement could not be
explained without one's taking social background into account. This was so because

the most powerful predictor of educational level obtained was found to be the social class background of parents, as measured by their income level, occupation, and education.

Their work also called into question the American view of meritocracy, which assumed that intelligence or ability was equally distributed throughout the population, not skewed by social class. If a meritocracy really existed in America, researchers would have found that each social class was represented in the various ability groups in proportion to the percentage in the population. For example, if 10 percent of students were recipients of public assistance, then 10 percent in each of the ability groups in the school—remedial, vocational, and college prep—should be students from welfare families. The same should be true of the representation of wealthy children. However, what researchers found was that children from higher socioeconomic status families were greatly overrepresented in classes for high-achieving students as well as in college preparatory schools, higher education, and professional jobs. Similarly, there was a significantly higher percentage of lower-class students in the remedial, vocational, and non-college preparatory classes than their percentage in the school population.

This measure of over- and underrepresentation meant that something was impeding the smooth operation of meritocracy. It became an indicator of inequality and class bias. Rosenfeld confirmed that the same indices of over- and underrepresentation among women and minorities meant meritocratic criteria also did not apply to them.

The Marxist Model: Class and Income Inequality.   Very few studies of the causes of social inequality have used Marxist categories of analysis. However, one important study (Wright and Perrone 1977) does examine three classes—workers, managers, and employers—to see what impact social class, in Marxian terms rather than in education, occupation, and family background, has on economic inequality. This study demonstrated that the class model is more powerful than status attainment models in predicting where a person will end up in the class hierarchy. Class matters more than education, and even overrides the effects of education.

Even with high levels of education, working-class children will not achieve as much prestige as children from the upper classes. This is so because working-class children, handicapped by their background, cannot translate their education into as much occupational prestige and economic success as can upper- and middle-class children with the same education or less. Studies like these provided a catalyst for identifying the mechanisms by which biases against the poor and working class impeded their performance.

THE MECHANISM OF CLASS BIAS IN EDUCATION

Discussions of the relationship between class and educational achievement are almost inextricably meshed with discussions of race, since castelike minority status, poverty, and low rates of educational achievement are highly correlated. However, we will argue that while patterns of discrimination create castelike conditions for some people and certainly systematically disadvantage women, nevertheless social class or patterns of economic domination and subordination create far more important distinctions among people. Hence, rich people, of whatever race, religion, or gender, are far more similar to one another than they are to poor people of their own race, religion, or gender. These differences are created, supported, and enhanced by participation in educational institutions.

Test Scores

Initial studies of social class impact used student test scores on standardized tests as a data base. This research was quantitative in that it looked at test scores as output measures and tried to predict them by looking at a variety of independent measures, such as sex, type of curriculum, mother's education, father's education, income, and race. All of these studies indicated that test scores are stratified by social class, ethnicity notwithstanding.

Ability Grouping

Test scores, however, proved to be insufficient to explain why differential learning according to social class existed, because they could not uncover the processes by which children were differentially treated. In the 1970s a strong interest in microlevel observation of classroom interaction developed. This work began to demonstrate how profoundly social class affects the placement of children in ability groups, because it showed the extent to which teachers grouped students on the basis of their *perceptions* of how able students are, rather than entirely on the basis of assessed competence. These perceptions are based on daily interactions with others and negotiations with teachers and are complicated by children's gender and cultural identities. Because lower-class children often lack the cultural capital congruent with school life, they are judged to be less able. Teachers classified children who were clean, were quiet, and acted respectfully as brighter. Teachers also tended to favor children who shared their own values, regardless of the student's measured ability. Sometimes teachers were notably poor judges of actual ability. They also had difficulty giving failing grades to students they liked. Unfortunately, since most teachers either were born into or have acquired the cultural capital, habits, and aspirations of the middle class, they now find many students in their classrooms who do not share their values (Brophy and Good 1970; Delgado-Gaitan 1987; Heath 1983; Ortiz 1988; Rist 1973; G. Rosenfeld 1971; Spindler 1987).

It is fair to say that teacher *perceptions* of a student's ability are a far more accurate predictor of a child's group placement than is measured intelligence or even standardized test scores (Cicourel and Kitsuse 1963). While all teachers take into account a child's past record—often too seriously—they may disregard evidence they disagree with, citing their own professional diagnosis skills as authoritative (Richardson et al. 1989).

As we will point out in Chapter 6, tracking or ability grouping acts to differentiate students further because it profoundly affects the amount and type of learning made available. Tracking affects the kind of control teachers exercise over their pupils. The treatment students receive in school also reflects the kind of cultural capital they bring to school.

Teachers interact far more with high-track students, for whom they hold higher expectations. These students are praised more when they are correct and criticized less when they are wrong than are students for whom teachers have low expectations (Allington 1983; Brophy and Good 1970; Grant and Rothenberg 1986). They are far more likely than lower-track students to be given autonomy in doing their school work, are more often expected to work independently, have better opportunities to engage in higher-order thinking skills, and are given access to innovative programs such as computer programming. They will be punished less for infractions of the rules, and will be given more chances and greater encouragement if they do poorly, if only because teachers fear the adverse reaction of middle- and upper-class parents.

By contrast, teachers of lower-class students employ custodial forms of behavior management. While much money and effort may be poured into special programs to enhance achievement, the programs often are remedial and simply repeat previous material. Where computers are used, they are used simply for drill-and-practice. Less capable students in the lower tracks get fewer hours of actual instruction and less rigorous coursework. "Pull-out" programs of special tutoring actually diminish the time spent in regular instruction (K. P. Bennett 1991; Delgado-Gaitan 1988). Teachers of the poor do not expect their students to do well and, assuming that they will fail, interact with them less, give them less encouragement, and worry less about the dropouts. These findings have been confirmed in studies of classroom interaction (Borko and Eisenhart 1986; Rist 1970); in interview studies with low-achieving students (Fine 1986; McLeod 1987; Valverde 1987; Williams 1987; Willis 1977); and in analyses of curriculum distribution and content (Anyon 1990; K. P. Bennett 1991).

All of these findings are complicated by race, but one can find the same patterns of neglect and custodialism in schools serving poor white students as are found for poor African-American and Latino students.

Structural Inequalities in Funding

Social class backgrounds of students are often replicated in the schools they attend. In his powerful book *Savage Inequalities* (1991), Jonathan Kozol carefully documents the inequalities in how schools are financed. The formula for school funding is based on local property taxes so local districts support and govern their own schools. According to the "foundational programs" introduced in the 1920s, supplemental state funds were provided to help equalize funding in poorer districts, with these state funds being based on attendance. In addition, federal funds are provided for federally mandated programs such as special or bilingual education programs. On the average, school districts in the United States rely on local property tax for 40 to 45 percent, the state for 40 to 45 percent, and the federal government for 7 to 10 percent of their funds. Wealthier districts are able to provide better facilities and more programs. They are able to offer higher salaries to attract better teachers and administrators.

Dissatisfaction with these methods of financing schools began in the 1960s in a class-action suit filed in 1968 by Demetrio Rodriquez and other parents in San Antonio. The families lived in the city's Edgewood District, which was primarily poor and 96 percent nonwhite. Despite one of the highest tax rates in the area, the district could raise only $231 per pupil, even with state supplements. Another section of the city was able to raise $412 per pupil with a lower tax rate, plus state and federal funding. In 1971 a federal district court in San Antonio ruled that Texas was in violation of the equal protection clause of the U.S. Constitution because the equalizing effects from the state aid "do not benefit the poorest districts" (Kozol 1991, p. 214). This decision was later overturned by the U.S. Supreme Court on the basis that education as a right is not explicitly protected by the U.S. Constitution and "the Equal Protection Clause does not require absolute equality" (Kozol quoting Justice Lewis Powell, 1991, p. 215).

Observe two primary school classrooms, one in a poor urban area and one in a middle-class suburb. Pay particular attention to factors that help to identify children according to social class backgrounds. Can you distinguish between differences attributable to class and those that are a consequence of minority status? Observe the children in both classroom and playground situations. From your observations, what role do you think social class plays in the school experience of the children? Compare the two settings. What do you think of the school experiences provided to each group of children?

It is state constitutions rather than the U.S. Constitution that refer specifically to public education, usually saying that the state will provide common public schooling for all its children. Lawsuits filed in the 1980s in states such as New Jersey, Kentucky, and Tennessee have attacked the funding formulas used for schooling on the basis that inequalities in these states are in violation of their constitutions. The disparity in school funding from poor to wealthy districts acts to reproduce social class because it results in inequitable education for children already stratified by their family's social class. Even *within* districts, funding disparities exist. For example, in his analysis of school funding in Chicago, Hess (1991) found that the schools with the poorest students actually received less per capita funding for instruction than schools with the wealthiest students.

The Social Construction of Identity

Some very early studies pointed to the ways social class was inherited. In his study of "Elmtown," Hollingshead (1949) suggested that children who grew up on the "wrong side of the tracks" remained there, as did *their* children. In the late 1970s critical analysts began to look even more closely at classroom interaction in an attempt to explain the processes by which social class is replicated. They used the methods of symbolic interactionists (see Chapter 1), an approach holding that people do not simply react automatically and unconsciously to any "stimulus or pressure they are subjected to, but they make sense of these pressures in terms of frameworks of meaning they have built up through their lives" (Hargreaves and Woods 1984, p. 2). The symbolic interactionists have discovered what these frameworks of meanings are, how to get people to talk about them, and how they reciprocally affect behavior and beliefs as people engage in social interaction. They have explained the *reflexive,* reciprocal nature of human behavior as people "work at" constructing reality around them.

H. S. Becker (1953), for example, described teachers' notions of the "ideal" student and showed how teachers treated pupils in accordance with how closely they approximated that ideal. Poorer, more disadvantaged students were far from the ideal. For them, teachers lowered standards for performance, spent more time in discipline and less in instruction, and taught more slowly. (See also Firestone and Rosenblum 1988; Page 1987; Powell, Farrar, and Cohen 1985.) As a consequence, the students became even more academically disadvantaged as the school year progressed. Other researchers have demonstrated how students treated in this manner pay less attention in class (Eder 1982), come to define themselves as "poor students" or "slow learners" or simply as "not college material," and adjust their performance standards and aspirations accordingly (McLeod 1987; McLaren 1986; Page 1987; Willis 1977). Erickson (1987, p. 336) has described this occurrence as "school failure," a reflexive process by which "schools 'work at' failing their students and students 'work at' failing to achieve in school . . . [school failure, in this sense, is] something the school does as well as what the student does." Elsi's story (see box on p. 90) describes how one bright student was turned into a failure in this way.

Interview a teacher. What is the teacher's social class background? What is the social class background of her or his students? Does this teacher believe that social class background plays a role in students' schooling experiences? In what way? Write a personal reaction to this interview.

Resistance. Schools do not fail all students with whom they are mismatched, and some students actively "withhold assent" (Erickson 1987) to educators' attempts to "cool them out" of the system. Early work by critical theorists blamed teachers for the failure of students, focusing on how their labeling of students destroyed students' self-esteem and stunted their intellectual growth. Data elicited from students bolstered the attack on teachers, detailing conflict and hostility among pupils, teachers, and other staff.

More recent studies have examined the patterns of mutual interaction between the inhabitants of schools. Researchers have begun to describe how people "work at" school, how both teachers and students come with preconceived notions and definitions with which they mutually construct the reality of their life in school. While much of the empirical research in this area has looked at negative effects—how negative self-concepts for both teachers and students are constructed and how they both resist being defined in ways detrimental to a positive self-image (see the discussion in Chap-

Elsi's Story: From Gifted Third Grader to High School Dropout

Elsi's mother, Maria, came from Guatemala when she was 15 to work as a maid for a wealthy family in the Southwest. She separated from Elsi's father, a Mexican American, shortly after Elsi was born. Life has been hard since. "Sometimes that lady, she just calls me the day before and says, 'I don't need you today, Maria.' And for her, it's OK, but I have to find somebody else's house to clean. That's why I want Elsi to stay in school. She can get her education and have a better life."

Elsi did very well in school, and in third grade she was tested and accepted for the SIGHTS (Supplemental Instruction for Gifted and High-Achieving and Talented Students) program at her school. SIGHTS provided pull-out instruction in science, art, and other enrichment areas three times a week. Elsi blossomed in the program. "I love SIGHTS," said Elsi. "I want to be a scientist and SIGHTS is the only place I get to study science." At the end of the year SIGHTS was eliminated in favor of a "school-within-a-school" gifted program which, though a full-day program, could accommodate only one-third as many students as SIGHTS had. The school held a lottery to fill its places and Elsi wasn't chosen. Back in a regular classroom, she was crushed, and her grades fell. "I really miss science. That's what I really liked to do. Maybe I'm just stupid." By fifth grade Elsi had given up, and by eighth grade she had failed English, Math, and General Science. Worried that Elsi was hanging out with a "bad crowd" and distraught over her grades, Maria tried unsuccessfully to transfer her to a parochial school nearby. After interviewing Elsi and Maria, the principal of the nearly all-white, middle-class school declared that Elsi "just wouldn't fit in" and that Maria "just wouldn't feel comfortable" in the support activities required of all parents. In tenth grade Elsi dropped out of school to help her mother clean houses.

ters 3 and 4)—a number of ethnographic researchers have begun to explore ways in which "working at" school can be turned from a negative to a positive process.

One perspective which focuses on ameliorating the impact of cultural as well as class differences is typified by Erickson (1984, 1987) and scholars from the Kamehameha Early Education Program in Hawaii and the Center for Cross Cultural Studies at the University of Fairbanks, Alaska (Au 1979, 1980; Au and Jordan 1981; Barnhardt 1982; Jordan 1984, 1985; Moll and Diaz 1987). These researchers identified aspects of the child's natal culture which could be utilized in classrooms to help students bridge the mismatch between home and school culture.

Empowerment.   Another approach which concentrates more on a social class perspective is a recent branch of "critical pedagogy" (McLaren 1989, p. 162) which views the mutual construction of meaning as an opportunity for manipulating interaction in school. It advocates using schools to promote empowerment of subordinated and marginalized groups within society, especially teachers, minorities, the poor, and women.

These researchers believe that schools can be used to help people become conscious of the forces that oppress them and learn strategies to overcome them, thereby becoming "empowered." They emphasize the importance of researcher collaboration with teachers as a means to raise the consciousness of teachers and students. Their efforts so far have been limited more or less to individual schools and classrooms. Translated into a curricular philosophy, this work involves believing

> in conceptions of learning as something that happens to an individual as an internal and subjective action, as a process of inquiry and discovery; knowledge as something that can only be personally acquired and not given; as truths in each of us rather than as fixed and finite truths "out there"; of development as personal growth, as the transformation of powers already present; of classrooms as communities of learners helping each other . . . for the enhancement of all. (Ashcroft 1987, p. 155)

As Chapter 9 points out, this perspective also is limited. While it develops awareness of patterns of hegemonic domination, its efforts are constrained by its focus on microlevel and psychological processes rather than larger political and structural correlates of oppression (LeCompte and Bennett deMarrais 1992).

SUMMARY

In this chapter we have demonstrated how our ideas of social class have changed over time, and how even scientific explanations of why people are rich or poor were affected by social and cultural traditions. Social class status is inextricably linked to educational achievement and occupational attainment. The work of sociologists, however, has exploded some of the beliefs of educators. We now know that what appears to be intellectual merit may actually be the product of special treatment in the schools, given because of one's social class status. Similarly, what appears to be a student's lack of ability may be a product of teacher perceptions, based on the student's lower-class status, plus the student's response to negative assessments by the school system.

The process by which students fail—or achieve—in school is composed of a complex set of factors. It is insufficient to say:

> Kids are lazy—or poorly prepared.
> Teachers are incompetent—or hate kids.
> Parents don't care—or don't know how to help their kids.

All of these explanations may contain some truth. But the reality of inequality in education is a mixture of many things, all of which are played out reflexively in the arena of schools and classrooms.

In the chapters that follow we will look more closely at how the curriculum widens the differences between students of different social classes. We also will discuss the impact of race and gender on educational achievement.

chapter **6**

What Is Taught in Schools: Curriculum and the Stratification of Knowledge

INTRODUCTION

Think back to your own experiences of schooling. What subjects were you taught in elementary and secondary school? How were the subjects taught? How were students grouped for instruction? How did your teachers organize this instruction? How did they choose what to teach? How did you interact with your teachers in different classes? How was your learning evaluated or assessed? What kinds of learning activities did you engage in? You might consider these questions about your own schooling as you read this chapter on curriculum and the stratification of knowledge.

We begin this chapter with a consideration of traditional notions of curriculum theory which have dominated how educators viewed what is taught in schools. We then consider **curriculum** from a critical sociological perspective, using concepts from the **sociology of knowledge,** a subdiscipline of sociology which is broadly concerned with notions of what counts for "knowledge" in a society (Berger and Luckmann 1967). Critical theorists believe that dominant groups in society define legitimate knowledge. Since curriculum represents the knowledge taught in school, the **sociology of curriculum** is concerned specifically with school knowledge and relationships among the curriculum, schools, and dominant groups in society (Giroux 1988). In this chapter we contrast the sociological view of curriculum with that of traditional educational curriculum theorists.

We then provide a discussion of formal and hidden curricula and the stratification of curricula for different groups of students. In so doing, we will address the following questions:

1. What is curriculum?
2. What types of curricula are used in American schooling?
3. What knowledge is included in these curricula?
4. What values and attitudes are taught through the curriculum?
5. How does the curriculum change over time in response to sociocultural needs and political interests?
6. Who determines what is taught in schools in the 1990s?

WHAT IS CURRICULUM?

A curriculum, usually thought of as a course of study or a plan for what is to be taught in an educational institution, is composed of information concerning what is to be taught, to whom, when, and how. Consideration of the curriculum must include its purpose, content, method, organization, and evaluation (J. McNeil 1985).

A simpler but more comprehensive way to think about curriculum is that it is *what happens to students in school.* More than the formal content of lessons taught, it is also the method of presentation, the way in which students are grouped in classes, the manner in which time and tasks are organized, and the interaction within classrooms. The term *curriculum* refers to the total school experience provided to students, whether planned or unplanned by educators. By conceptualizing the curriculum this broadly, we are able to include its intended as well as unintended outcomes.

Traditional Curriculum Theory

Traditional curriculum theory comes from psychology and subject area studies in pedagogy rather than from sociology. Traditional curriculum theorists assume that the body of knowledge to be taught is a given, objective and free from biases. The assumptions about traditional curriculum theory are summarized by Giroux:

> (a) Theory in the curriculum field should operate in the interest of lawlike propositions that are empirically testable; (b) the natural sciences provide the "proper" model of explanation for the concepts and techniques of curriculum theory, design, and evaluation; (c) knowledge should be objective and capable of being investigated and described in a neutral fashion; and (d) statements of value are to be separated from "facts" and "modes of inquiry" that can and ought to be objective. (1988, p. 13)

Traditional curriculum theorists are concerned with determining the best ways to impart a given body of knowledge to people. Rather than focusing on what knowledge is to be taught, they emphasize how a given body of facts, concepts, and understandings can be transferred effectively and efficiently directly from teachers to learners. Colleges of education have curriculum specialists who train pre-service teachers and graduate students in the "science" of curriculum design. The history of traditional curriculum theory is a history of the application of rational, scientific principles to the management of "objective" bodies of knowledge. Models for the development of curriculum are produced by these specialists. They view knowledge as something to be managed by state departments of education, school boards, administrators, and teachers and to be given to students, usually in the form of prepackaged designs, kits, formulas, approaches, materials, and/or lists of skills and objectives. Educators categorize and manage knowledge, and students are required to master it.

Sociologists of knowledge, the "new" sociologists of curriculum (Giroux 1988; Liston and Zeichner 1991), and **reconceptualist** curriculum theorists (Pinar 1989; Shaker and Kridel 1989) challenge these assumptions made by the traditional curriculum theorists. The central questions for critical theorists of curriculum is not *how* to manage knowledge, but what kinds of knowledge are included in the curriculum and whose interests are served.

Sociology of Knowledge and Sociology of Curriculum

The term *sociology of knowledge* was first used by the German philosopher Max Scheler in the 1920s (Berger and Luckmann 1967). The sociology of knowledge is concerned with definitions of knowledge, particularly with how knowledge is constructed through the social interactions of individuals. In their classic book *The Social Construction of Reality: A Treatise in the Sociology of Knowledge*, Berger and Luckmann state:

Common sense "knowledge" rather than "ideas" must be the central focus for the sociology of knowledge. It is precisely this knowledge that constitutes the fabric of meanings without which no society could exist. The sociology of knowledge, therefore, must concern itself with the social construction of reality. (1967, p. 15)

Implicit in the sociology of knowledge is the fact that humans construct and modify knowledge within their social interactions. Knowledge is not an "objective" body of facts but is constructed by humans and therefore is value-laden.

Critical sociologists assume that knowledge is power and that different types of knowledge are provided or withheld according to one's place in the social structure of society. They ask questions about whose knowledge is in the curriculum and whose knowledge is omitted. As we will illustrate later in this and subsequent chapters, certain kinds of knowledge are provided to or withheld from certain groups of people on the basis of gender, race, ethnicity, and social class status. Those in power can use their influence to advocate inclusion of certain types of knowledge in the schooling process.

Rather than a conspiracy by one group over another, the transmission of a particular curriculum occurs as a result of a complicated system of historical and cultural beliefs, hegemonic ideologies, pressure groups, and textbook markets. For example, in the 1980s and 1990s tensions arose among policy makers, educators, and the popular media as groups worked to replace the traditional Western liberal arts curriculum in colleges and universities, which were centered largely on the experiences of white males, with a multicultural curriculum more representative of the experiences of women and people of color. These efforts were countered by a conservative backlash (Apple 1993) whose "official knowledge" is composed of a "core" curriculum based on what is purported to be the best that Western civilization offers (E. W. Bennett 1988; Bloom 1987; Hirsch 1987). Two central concerns in the sociology of knowledge, then, are: (1) what knowledge is valued? and (2) how do certain types of knowledge become reality in the everyday lives of individuals within the society through social interaction in schools?

Research on the *sociology of curriculum* began in the early 1970s. Berger and Luckmann's definition of the sociology of knowledge provided a theoretical framework for subsequent studies of the knowledge taught in schools. School knowledge became the focus of studies known as the *sociology of the curriculum,* or sometimes the *new sociology of education* (Giroux 1988). Michael F. D. Young (1971) announced a marked shift in the sociology of education when he proclaimed the emergence of a "new sociology of education" at the Institute of Education in London. His edited volume, *Knowledge and Control: New Directions for the Sociology of Education,* was instrumental in promoting the sociological study of the school curriculum, and with its publication, the "importance of [this] area of sociological study came to be widely recognized" (Whitty 1985, p. 13).

The sociology of the curriculum examines how different types of knowledge are provided for different groups of students, or how curriculum is organized and stratified. It views curriculum within the social context of schools and as a reflection of interest groups within the broader society. For example, in examining the curriculum, sociologists ask:

1. How do schools group children for instruction?
2. How much and what kinds of knowledge are presented by the teachers in these groups?
3. How do teacher–student interactions differ from one level group to another?
4. How are different people in society represented in school texts?
5. Are there differences in the amount of information and types of content provided in the curriculum according to the ethnicity, social class, and gender categories of students?

Sociological research on knowledge and curriculum has added much to our understanding about how schools work. We have learned that in addition to the formally stated, explicit curriculum, there is an implicit, or **hidden curriculum** that imparts beliefs and values to students. The following sections will explore both the formal and hidden curriculum of schools.

Ideological Interests in the Formal and Hidden Curricula

A central concern of critical theorists is uncovering the ideological interests embedded in both formal and hidden school curricula. Giroux explains that there are two kinds of **ideology:**

> Theoretical ideologies refer to the beliefs and values embedded in the categories that teachers and students use to shape and interpret the pedagogical process, while practical ideologies refer to the messages and norms embedded in classroom social relations and practices. (1983b, p. 67)

The former addresses explicit curricula; the latter is concerned with hidden or implicit curricula.

In order for us to understand the various and competing ideologies inherent in schooling in the 1990s, we need to look at the formal curriculum as it developed throughout the twentieth century. In the next sections we will look at what is taught in schools from the perspective of both formal and hidden curricula. The following questions asked by critical theorists guide our discussion:

1. What counts as curriculum knowledge?
2. How is such knowledge produced?
3. How is such knowledge transmitted in the classroom?
4. What kinds of classroom social relationships serve to parallel and reproduce the values and norms embodied in the accepted social relations of other dominant social sites?

5. Who has access to legitimate forms of knowledge?
6. Whose interests does this knowledge serve?
7. How are social and political contradictions and tensions mediated through acceptable forms of classroom knowledge and social relationships?
8. What compromises are made among dominant and subordinate interest groups in the selection of a curriculum that represents the official knowledge to be taught in schools? (Apple 1993, p. 68)
9. How do prevailing methods of evaluation legitimize existing forms of knowledge? (Giroux 1983b, pp. 17–18)

WHAT IS TAUGHT: THE FORMAL CURRICULUM

The debate about what knowledge should be included in the curricula of American public schools is as old as public schools themselves. Since schools are highly political institutions, the content and form of instruction depend in large part upon which socioeconomic interests wield power in society. Since different groups disagree both over the relative value to be accorded to different kinds of knowledge and over the appropriateness of various kinds of knowledge for different groups of people, there *never* has been a consensus over which body of knowledge was appropriate for all the children in all the schools.

Today many interest groups compete to influence what knowledge is transmitted in schools and how this transmission takes place. Spring's (1988a) discussion of the textbook publishing industry provides an excellent examination of the conflicting interest groups and their effects on educational policy and practice. He describes how the particular textbooks chosen determine what curricula will dominate in a school system, since textbooks often serve as the curriculum. These choices are powerfully influenced by negotiations among the textbook publishing industry, state and federal educational policy makers, special-interest groups (teachers' unions, associations of school administrators, parent-teacher associations, religious organizations, etc.), and corporations. All of these interest groups differ radically in their beliefs about the purpose of schooling, its role in transmitting ideas and values, and which ideas and values should be taught. Publishers, interested primarily in making a profit by capturing a large share of the lucrative textbook market, take seriously the challenges of special-interest groups. Anything in the texts that may offend particular groups can eliminate their books from a state's textbook adoption lists. Therefore they produce inoffensive books lacking both controversial material and varying perspectives on issues. Although these textbooks present what appears to be "objective" knowledge, they actually contain selective information considered "safe" by the publishers. Educators are not warned that, as critical consumers of texts, it is crucial for them to determine whose knowledge and perspectives are represented and whose are omitted.

During the 1980s and 1990s conservative religious groups targeted textbooks for careful scrutiny regarding content they believed to contradict the teachings of the

Hawkins County Textbook Controversy

Vicki Frost, spokesperson for the parents, explained her view of the way the Holt Basic Reading Program portrayed traditional gender roles:

I see . . . the *terrible* dominance of role elimination and pro-feminism without any balance for traditional. I mean, every fairy tale was turned into a modern-day women's liberation movement in the story. And there was not one traditional fairy tale where they had the princess bein' rescued. But they made a point in the teacher's manuals to say . . . "We're bringin' you a modern-day fairy tale. And we're gonna contrast it in the teacher's manual to the old traditional one." And the old traditional fairy tale makes the princess look like she's frail and weak. But the modern-day princess is strong, not particularly pretty. She's clever. And she always saves the king or the kingdom or kills the dragon. And . . . you just think, "well, what's a fairy tale?" But it's what's behind . . . the moral or the lesson taught. And when you have that constantly fed, that at the end of seven years, . . . when you hear they have to write about "What do you think about the ERA?" . . . And when you've been given just one point of the issue, how will they respond? You know, that's the concern . . . the greatest concern's there's no balance. No balance whatsoever.

SOURCE: Dellinger 1991, p. 130.

Bible. For example, in a series of events from 1983 to 1988 known as the Hawkins County textbook controversy, a group of fundamentalist Christian parents in Hawkins County, Tennessee, challenged the content of the 1983 Holt Basic Reading Series (*Mozert* v. *Hawkins County Public Schools*). The parents, under the leadership of Vicki Frost, claimed that the reading program adopted by the county schools taught values that violated their personal religious views. They opposed, for example, teachings about evolution, magic, other religions, pacifism, rebellion against authority, situational ethics, promotion of human autonomy (as opposed to the primacy of Christ), feminism (see quote from Vicki Frost in the box), and one-world government. In December 1986 U.S. District Court Judge Hull decided in favor of the plaintiffs, awarding them approximately $50,000 in compensatory damages and stating that their children could attend school without attending reading classes where the Holt readers were used. In August 1987 the Sixth Circuit Court of Appeals reversed this decision, and in February 1988 the U.S. Supreme Court denied further appeal. This particular controversy illustrates the seriousness with which the content of textbooks is scrutinized by special-interest groups. It is easy to see the impact such a case might have on the textbook publishing industry—or on school districts faced with the need to maintain multiple sets of textbooks to satisfy multiple-interest groups.

Despite the lack of consensus about what should be taught in schools and how it should be delivered, identifiable trends in curricular knowledge appear throughout the history of American schooling. Kliebard (1986) has described these trends in *The Struggle for the American Curriculum: 1893–1958*. He illustrates how the formal curriculum has always been the result of conflicting ways of interpreting the goals of schooling (discussed in Chapter 1). Kliebard argues that four major types of curricula have dominated twentieth-century schooling: humanist, social efficiency, developmental, and social meliorist.

The Humanist Curriculum

The humanist curriculum is the model for the so-called "traditional liberal arts" program. Humanists view schools as the "guardians of ancient tradition tied to the power of reason and the finest elements of [Anglo] Western heritage" (Kliebard 1986, p. 27). They believe that the purpose of schooling is to develop the intellect by transmitting a core of the finest elements of this heritage to all members of society. This position was argued in 1983 by Charles W. Eliot, president of Harvard University and chairman of the National Education Association's Committee of Ten. The committee's report emphasized a K–12 curriculum that would increase students' reasoning power through traditional academic subjects (foreign languages, mathematics, literature, sciences, history, and the arts), which would be offered to all students whether or not they intended to go to college. The Committee of Ten believed that being taught a common core of subjects in the best possible ways was the best way to prepare all students for life (Kliebard 1986).

This same humanist viewpoint is embodied in E. D. Hirsch's *Cultural Literacy: What Every American Should Know* (1987) and was promoted in 1988 by former Secretary of Education William Bennett in his pamphlet, "James Madison High School: A Curriculum for American Students" and in his guidelines for "James Madison Elementary School" (1988). Bennett's curriculum proposals are designed for "mastery of a common core of worthwhile knowledge, important skills, and sound ideals" (E. W. Bennett 1988, p. 7). His plan prescribes a curriculum of seven core academic subjects. The core for high school includes four years of English; three years each of social studies, mathematics, and science; two years each of foreign language and physical education/health; and one year of fine arts (music history and art history). Bennett's plan for grades K–8 proposes a similar curriculum consisting of English, history, geography, civics, mathematics, science, foreign language, and fine arts. The curriculum ignores the literature of non-European cultures and includes twentieth-century American art and music only "if necessary."

While this assemblage of subject areas seems appropriate, what is problematic in a multicultural and multiethnic society is that it would, in traditional humanist style, emphasize only an Anglo-American cultural heritage. Such an emphasis reflects functionalist assumptions that a consensus on what should be taught in schools does exist and that the purpose of schooling is to transmit this knowledge from one generation to the next.

The Social Efficiency Curriculum

Among the most profound influences upon pedagogy has been social efficiency theory. As Chapter 2 described, social efficiency theory was developed from principles of scientific management, a movement based upon studies of organizations and industrial psychology. Social efficiency theorists believe that schools should facilitate the smooth functioning of the nation's economy by sorting citizens into job slots according to their abilities. Advocates of social efficiency believe that applying techniques of industry to the management of schools will make them efficient, smooth-running machines for transforming students into workers well equipped for a well-run economy. In Chapter 2 we examined the political context by which educators came to link schooling with work-force training and social engineering, as well as how scientific management affected the scheduling of the school day and the use of school buildings. Here we will examine the form and content of a "scientifically engineered" curriculum.

Rather than advocating the development of a core curriculum for all students as humanists do, the social efficiency curriculum prescribes different programs of study according to differences in students' abilities as measured by standardized testing. Programs of study usually include a college preparatory program, composed of the same academic core advocated by the humanists—literature, social science, natural science, mathematics, and foreign languages—and separate programs for students whom educators consider to lack the ability or interest to master the academic curriculum. These students, who are not "college material," are placed in vocational, commercial, and general courses that will prepare them for jobs not requiring a college education. Many of these courses have the same names as academic subjects in the college preparatory program, but they are presented less rigorously and at a lower conceptual level.

The tenets of the efficiency movement also affected how knowledge was conceptualized and evaluated and how learning tasks were organized. Cognitive skills and substantive knowledge were broken down into component parts, and learning was organized around the mastery of sets of behavioral objectives based upon those components. For example, in reading, curriculum specialists organized phonetic skills into lists according to perceived level of difficulty. Beginning consonant sounds were to be taught before short and long vowel sounds, which were to be taught before vowel diphthongs. These lists of skills were then written into behavioral objectives which teachers checked off as children mastered the skills. Study of more advanced skills was predicated upon mastery of earlier ones. In primary grades and remedial classes in particular, these practices persist. The teaching of phonics has played a significant role in the reading curriculum. However, this system disadvantages children who do not respond well to such an intensive phonetic skills approach to reading.

Elimination of "waste" also became a critical concern in the social efficiency curriculum. Students were to be moved through school as quickly as possible, and to that end, the degree to which children could be kept "on-task" became a measure of effective teaching. "Waste" also was defined as spending time on the teaching of "unnecessary" subjects. Necessary or useful knowledge was defined as that which could be used immediately in a job setting; hence subjects like Latin, history, and foreign languages were viewed with suspicion. In his article "Elimination of Waste in Education" (1912), John Franklin Bobbitt argued that students should be scientifically measured to predict their future role in society so that they could be taught only what they would later need to fulfill this role. A differentiated curriculum would solve the problem of "waste," since knowledge and skills that would not be used would not be taught.

Gender, too, played a role in curriculum planning. Since males and females would fulfill different social and vocational roles, student instruction should be tailored to gender-based adult roles. The training suggested for females generally was limited to general literacy and homemaking skills. (See Chapter 8 for more detail on the gendered curriculum.)

Development of the differentiated curriculum relied upon "scientific" and "objective" methods of testing, assessment, and measurement. In the 1920s and 1930s I.Q. testing came to be viewed as an accurate, scientific measurement by which children's native capacities could be determined. Educators considered it to be an effective way to determine how to place students in school programs appropriate both to their abilities and to their anticipated occupation (Kliebard 1986, p. 109).

By the mid-1960s testing had become a major part of the school curriculum. Continued routine use of standardized testing and curricular tracking provide evidence that the influence of the social efficiency experts is alive and well in American schools. Currently all 50 states have laws mandating state-regulated testing (D. Brown 1990). Increasingly these tests represent high stakes as rewards and sanctions for schools are being based on students' performance on state-mandated tests. The tests are used to provide evidence of school, program, and teacher effectiveness. They are used to justify accreditation of school districts and certification of students for completion of specific grades (Brown 1990).

In Tennessee, for example, teachers in second through tenth grades must administer the state-mandated Tennessee Comprehensive Assessment Program or "T-CAP." A Tennessee teacher describes the role these tests play in her teaching:

> When I came up to fifth grade, I really didn't know everything that would be covered in the fifth grade, so one of the teachers said, "Well, this skill will be on the achievement test, and you'll find this on the achievement test, and you'll find this on the test." And I know to teach my children survival skills that I had to teach those. Let's just face it, that's just the way it is. You know, I tell them, "This may be on the achievement test and this is something that I really want to stick." (Brown 1990, pp. 102–103).

Tennessee Comprehensive Assessment Program scores are released to the media, and scores of schools across the state are compared in local newspapers. One teacher described how these comparisons profoundly affect what is taught:

One of the neighboring county's scores were higher than ours last year, so there were problems here. Our principal came back from a principals' meeting and said, "Your test scores *will* come up. We will do a better job in this or this area." And he said, "I want you to pay attention especially in reading and math."

The National Center for Fair and Open Testing, operated by a consumer group which refers to itself as "Fair Test," estimates that American elementary and high school students take more than 100 million standardized tests yearly. Approximately 44 million of these tests are intelligence and admissions tests. The rest are measurements of achievement and basic skills (Fiske 1988). American educators and public officials continue to believe that standardized testing is an accurate method for monitoring students as they move through schools. In the elementary schools tests are used to place children in reading ability groups, special education classes, and gifted and talented programs. In high schools students are tested to determine their placement in either the general, college preparatory, or vocational curricular track. A later section entitled "Stratification of the Curriculum" presents a complete discussion of testing and tracking.

The Developmentalist Curriculum

The developmental curriculum comes from clinical and developmental psychology and is the only one of Kliebard's curricula that is "student-centered." Its focus is the individual learner rather than the needs of society or the importance of a particular body of knowledge. It also is concerned with helping people understand knowledge both experientially, that is, in the context of the real world, and intellectually, abstracted from the real world (Reisler and Friedman 1978). Developmentalists believe that curriculum should be designed to meet the needs of individual students throughout their stages of intellectual, social, and emotional development. Central concerns are the motivation, interests, and developmental stages of students. Students should be taught when they are intellectually and emotionally ready to learn rather than in accordance with their chronological age. Learning also should be structured so that children enjoy what they are doing while learning.

The developmentalists mandated a radically different role for teachers. They were to be partners with children in the learning enterprise rather than bosses. Some metaphors used for teachers provide clues to this shift in pedagogy. Teachers are described as advisors, supporters, observers, learners, facilitators, and senior partners (Silberman 1973). Experiential education, the open concept school building, the open classroom, middle-school philosophies, and cooperative and collaborative decision making and instruction all are legacies from the developmentalists.

Because of his emphasis on child-centered activities, John Dewey is one of the theorists most often associated with this type of curriculum. Both A. S. Neil's school, Summerhill, established in the 1920s, and the alternative or "free schools" of the 1960s were based upon these ideas. Spring (1989) notes that of Kliebard's four types of curriculum, the developmentalist has been the least influential on American public school curricula, even though colleges of education rely heavily on theories from developmentalists such as Rousseau, Dewey, and Piaget in the training of pre-service teachers. One sees little evidence of this approach in the daily activities of public schooling.

Despite its limited impact on public schooling overall, developmentalism survives in private and alternative schools and increasingly surfaces in special programs in the public sector. A contemporary example of a developmentalist curriculum is the "whole language" approach to the teaching of reading and writing skills in elementary schools. Drawing on their own language experience, children learn to read by telling and writing their own stories rather than relying on basal reading textbooks. The whole language philosophy includes the notion of an "integrated curriculum" in which language arts, math, social studies, sciences, fine arts, and other subjects are taught together through thematically organized units. For example, a teacher and students exploring a unit on zoo animals could integrate geography, children's literature, art projects, language skills, and knowledge from the sciences and social sciences to explore this topic. In recent years the whole language curriculum has gained greater support from teachers and administrators because it uses the developmental stages of children rather than standardized measures of ability to guide instruction. Current research in alternative forms of assessment, particularly portfolio assessment, has contributed to administrators' acceptance of this approach.

Another example of the developmentalist curriculum is in the work of the National Association for the Education of Young Children (NAEYC), summarized in the publication, "Developmentally Appropriate Practice in Early Childhood Programs Service Children from Birth Through Age 8" (1987). This work contrasts a developmentally appropriate curriculum to the traditional curriculum in primary schools. Other concerns about the inappropriateness of the traditional curriculum recently have surfaced among advocates of middle schools (Carnegie Council of Adolescent Development 1989; Connors and Irvin, 1989; Wiles and Bondi 1981; Williamson and Johnson 1991).

In the 1990s developmentalists in curriculum planning and implementation have achieved clear and strong—albeit minority—voices in public schools and colleges of education. American education is still far from using developmental curricula as the primary approach to teaching/learning processes in schooling.

The Social Meliorist Curriculum

Second to the efficiency movement in its impact on American education is social meliorism. Its tenets constitute a counterpoint to the tenets of social efficiency. According to social meliorists, schools should facilitate social change by producing students who will fight inequities and oppression and make the world a better place. The social meliorist curriculum came to the forefront of educational reform during the early 1930s as a reaction to scientific management, although it already had a long history among philosophers in Europe and America from Martin Luther and John Locke to Horace Mann and John Dewey. While Dewey provided inspiration to the

---

Components of Appropriate and Inappropriate Practice for 4- and 5-Year-Old Children—Curriculum Goals

Inappropriate Practice:
Experiences are narrowly focused on the child's intellectual development without recognition that all areas of a child's development are interrelated.

Children are evaluated only against a predetermined measure, such as a standardized group norm or adult standard of behavior. All are expected to perform the same tasks and achieve the same narrowly defined, easily measured skills.

Appropriate Practice:
Experiences are provided that meet children's needs and stimulate learning in all developmental areas—physical, social, emotional, and intellectual.

Each child is viewed as a unique person with an individual pattern and timing of growth and development. The curriculum and adults' interaction are responsive to individual differences in ability and interests. Different levels of ability, development, and learning styles are expected, accepted, and used to design appropriate activities.

Interactions and activities are designed to develop children's self-esteem and positive feelings toward learning.

SOURCE: Bredekamp 1986, p. 54.

---

developmentalists, he also was a strong believer that schools and teachers should serve as agents of social reform.

Among educators, George Counts and Harold Rugg are perhaps the best-known advocates of this position. As early as the 1920s Counts had advocated that educators act as agents of social change. The Great Depression, however, gave impetus to his stance. In his book *Dare the School Build a New Social Order?* (1932), Counts encouraged teachers to organize in order to bring about social justice and reform through the educational process. Like John Dewey and others, he viewed the public school curriculum as a tool for correcting social and economic injustices.

Rugg's social studies curriculum in American History was first published in 1929 and was very popular throughout the 1930s. However, an indication of how subversive social meliorism can seem to vested interests is that this program, which addressed issues of racism, class conflict, and the struggles of oppressed people, was forced off the market in the 1940s by conservative political action groups (Spring 1988a). In some towns Rugg's materials were even burned.

Currently the educators most closely allied with the kind of social meliorist curriculum presented by Kliebard are those known as feminist or critical theorists and pedagogues (cf. Apple 1986; Britzman 1991; Ellsworth 1989; Giroux 1983a, 1983b, 1988; Gitlin and Smyth 1989; McLaren 1989; Weiler 1988). The core concern of both feminist and critical theorists is an examination of patterns of subordination and domination in society: Who has access to power and why? As a consequence, stimulating the struggle against oppression based on gender, race, ethnicity, and social class is an essential element in such a curriculum.

At the center of the social meliorist curriculum is the notion of conflict and struggle. Students are provided with different perspectives on events and are encouraged to engage in critical examinations rather than merely reading texts and accepting the viewpoint of the author. A variety of texts are used to analyze all sides of an issue. For example, in a social studies discussion of the nineteenth-century "Western expansion" of white settlers into Indian lands, texts could include original documents, oral histories, diaries, novels, and treaties as well as talks by Native Americans. The term "Western expansion" could be deconstructed to determine whose interests are served by this label, and alternatives, including "Western colonization" or "conquest of indigenous peoples," could be chosen to describe the point of view of American Indians. Social meliorists believe that active student engagement through project-centered instruction is crucial to developing meaningful dialogue, critical thinking, and various perspectives of historical events. The underlying assumption of critical and feminist theorists is that by actively grappling with issues of struggle, domination, and oppression in the curriculum, students will work toward building a more democratic society.

The Formal Curriculum in Schools Today

The influence of all four of these curricula is likely to be visible in public schools, but social efficiency theorists have had the strongest influence. Their emphasis has been on efficiency, testing and measurement, and differentiated curricula. Administrators are still taught to be scientific managers of their schools. Public schools in the United States today continue to organize knowledge into discrete subjects to be taught in 50-minute blocks of time. Secondary school teachers still are subject matter specialists who work alone in isolated rooms with little time to develop different pedagogical strategies or to discuss professional issues with colleagues. Even at the elementary and middle-school level, departmentalized teaching, with children moving to different teachers' rooms for various subjects, is common.

Team teaching, project-based learning, flexible scheduling, whole language instruction, constructivist approaches to mathematics, integrated curricula, and cooperative approaches to schooling are currently in use by innovative teachers and administrators but are not the norm. Schools continue to base the stratified curriculum on standardized assessments of academic ability, rather than creating a curriculum based on research on child and adolescent development, the effects of ability grouping and tracking, or differences between school culture and the community cultures of children. Individual teachers or groups of teachers may be guided by social meliorist or developmentalist theories, but at the institutional level there is little systematic evidence of social meliorism or developmentalism in the standard curricula of public schools.

WHAT IS TAUGHT: THE HIDDEN CURRICULUM

The term **hidden curriculum** was first used by Edgar Z. Friedenberg in a conference in the late 1960s. This term called attention to the fact that students learn more in school than is included in their formal instruction. Giroux defines the hidden curriculum as "those unstated norms, values, and beliefs embedded in and transmitted to students through the underlying rules that structure the routines and social relationships in school and classroom life" (Giroux 1983b, p. 47). The hidden curriculum consists of the implicit messages given to students about differential power and social evaluation as they learn how to work in schools, what kinds of knowledge exist, which kinds are valued by whom, and how students are valued in their own right. These messages are learned informally and are sometimes, but not always, unintentional outcomes of the formal structure and curriculum of schooling. Giroux further suggests that in addition to information about the social relationships in school life, the hidden curriculum conveys messages both through the "form and content of school knowledge" and through the "silences," or what is left out.

For example, over the course of the school year a typical American high school history class would include very little formal curricular content that addressed the history of women and/or people of color. There would, however, be much text and discussion devoted to the white male military history of the United States. These omissions and inclusions give students a clear but implicit message about what knowledge society considers to be valuable and what is not.

Further, the hidden curriculum can be observed in social interaction. For example, traditional sex roles are reinforced by the way the teachers assign classroom tasks. Girls may be asked to clean up the room while boys may be asked to carry books or other heavy items out of the classroom. Middle-class children may be challenged by teachers to "try harder" while poor or working-class children are urged to "do the best they can." Girls may be discouraged from enrolling in advanced math and science classes, or teased when they enroll in them anyway (Holland and Eisenhart 1990).

While most writers have viewed the hidden curriculum primarily as the unintended outcome of the schooling process (McLaren 1989), we think it is important to understand that the hidden curriculum is often intended and considered desirable by school personnel. In fact, children can flunk out of school more readily by failing to behave in accordance with the hidden curriculum than they can by doing poor academic work. Teachers reward a hard-working slow student but penalize a high-achieving troublemaker or nonconformist.

The purpose of the hidden curriculum is to produce specific outcomes for later life, particularly to prepare students to accept as legitimate specific patterns of social behavior, positions in the social class structure, attitudes toward gender roles, and occupational placement. Functionalists and some interpretive theorists who view these behaviors, attitudes, and values as necessary for participation in society consider the hidden curriculum to be a necessary part of schooling. On the other hand, reproduction and critical theorists are more likely to examine the hidden curriculum for the extent to which it reinforces gender, social class, and minority group inequalities.

The Hidden Curriculum and Work Roles

Jackson (1968) argued that the hidden curriculum prepares students for the world of work by emphasizing such skills as learning to wait, accepting authority, coping with evaluation, and adhering to the demands of institutional conformity:

> Yet the habits of obedience and docility engendered in the classroom have a high pay-off value in other settings. So far as their power structure is concerned, classrooms are not too dissimilar from factories or offices, those ubiquitous organizations in which so much of our adult life is spent. Thus, school might really be called a preparation for life, but not in the usual sense in which educators employ that slogan. Power may be abused in school as elsewhere, but its existence is a fact of life to which we must adapt. The process of adaptation begins during the first few years of life but it is significantly accelerated, for most of us, on the day we enter kindergarten. (1968, p. 3)

LeCompte (1978b) has argued that these attitudes and values are embodied in a core of activities which teachers require of students as minimal behavior standards in the belief that without these behaviors, learning cannot take place. In the typical classroom today we see students sitting quietly at individual desks placed in straight rows or tidy clusters, with the teacher's desk in the front of the room. Students are expected to work individually from textbooks or worksheets without talking to each other. They are supposed to raise their hands to answer or ask questions and wait to be called on by the teacher. In striving to achieve these ideals, teachers provide hidden messages whose intent is to prepare the students for appropriate behavior in later work roles. The model of work embodied in these messages resembles the hierarchical working of a factory or other large-scale industrial enterprise, and it may be appropriate for some kinds of occupations. However, when it persists throughout pre-baccalaureate training, it is archaic, because it is incongruent with the working conditions and training required in most high-status and professional jobs, where employees are organized into teams, which work creatively and cooperatively with each other. Even today the factory model still predominates for most students; only high-status children systematically receive training whose hidden curriculum prepares them for professional work (Anyon 1990).

The organizational structure of schools teaches children that the social world of adults is hierarchical. Even in so-called restructured and site-based schools, administrators still manage teachers, teachers manage children, and children manage their assigned tasks. Teachers determine what children do in school, when, and how. Children learn that school knowledge comes from the teacher and from the textbook and that teachers evaluate how much they have learned by their performance on tests and classroom assignments. The evaluation process is external and performed by someone in a higher position. Anyon explains that daily life in this type of organizational structure provides practical ideological support for unequal distributions of power in society. . . . [T]he present unequal organization of authority in classrooms and schools not only indicates unequal power in society, but may reify and legitimate this in consciousness, thus fostering the impression that unequal power is natural, logical, or merely "in the order of things" and inevitable. (1988, pp. 178–179)

Children quickly discover that learning takes place individually and in quiet settings. It is "good" classroom behavior to sit quietly and "do your own work." "Keep your eyes on your own paper" helps to reinforce this message. Even cooperative groups most often mean those who sit still, not those who collaborate. Working together is discouraged except in groups organized by teachers. Even in classrooms where cooperative learning activities are stressed, children learn that there is a particular time period set aside by the teacher in which to engage in cooperation with peers. In such an individualistic school culture, it is not surprising that cooperative groups often become internally competitive, in a way that, as Deering's study of a middle-school classroom documents, derails the whole process.

CINDY: We got everything in!

KENNY: Yeah! You shoulda seen! We made Aaron do his work instead of fooling around. We kept telling him to work!

CINDY: Every time he'd goof around we'd call the teacher over and we'd get him in trouble! So he actually behaved himself for once! (1992, p. 141)

Schools require that students be punctual, clean, and neat, make efficient use of their time, take care of their equipment, work individually, and learn how to wait if they need something. Absenteeism is frowned upon and generally noted on evaluations. Classroom interaction conveys the message that there are different roles and expectations according to social class, race/ethnicity, and gender (for more detail see Chapters 5, 7, 8, and 9). Students who exhibit appropriate behavior in response to these school expectations are rewarded and displayed as role models to others. These rewards are both at the school and district level in the formal presentations at assembly programs and at the classroom level through teachers' evaluative comments. For example, here are several typical comments made by teachers:

- "I like the way Mary is waiting."
- "I like the way you wrote your name so neatly on the top of the page, Sally. Could you try to do that next time, John?"
- "You are really working hard on that math sheet, Sam."

The Hidden Curriculum and Perceptions of Knowledge

The organization of schools implies that both the structure of knowledge and social relationships are hierarchical. Knowledge is organized according to its perceived difficulty and its social value. Students who are expected to learn quickly are given lessons containing information that is more complex, higher on the cognitive scale, and more culturally valuable than are children who are deemed less able. Working-class children are less often placed in classes of higher mathematics and foreign languages and more often placed in vocational and industrial training than are middle-class children (Oakes 1985). The effect is to prepare the latter for college and professional careers, and the former for life in factories and blue-collar jobs of less status.

Despite the close interrelationship of many academic subjects, knowledge often is broken up into discrete courses, compartmentalized, and given to students as pieces of knowledge to be assimilated within certain periods or time slots. For example, students may have 30 minutes for reading, 30 minutes for language arts, and 15 minutes for handwriting. They are taught art divorced from history and mathematics devoid of science.

As a result, children fail to become seekers of information. They learn that knowledge comes from an external source such as the teacher or the selected textbook for the course, that there is usually one way to learn a skill, and that skills are taught by specialists. For example, in many classrooms reading is synonymous with phonics. A good reader comes to be perceived by other children as one who can "sound out words," not necessarily one who understands what the sounds mean. Deyhle, for example, describes how Navajo students who can't read nevertheless "act reading" during a silent reading period (1992). They turn pages and look attentive, even when their books are upside down or covering a well-disguised comic book.

Students learn that information is structured around multiple choice and true-false answers. They become uncomfortable with ambiguity—responses are either right or wrong rather than involving complex and often contradictory perspectives. The tasks assigned and the types of questions asked in classrooms reinforce this notion. Knowledge is seldom presented as complex, ambiguous, or something to be questioned; rather it is presented as "objective" fact. This approach is reinforced by standardized testing programs, which may drive the curriculum. Students are seldom encouraged to think that "knowledge" might be subjective, based on a particular historical context or social setting.

The Hidden Curriculum, Perceptions of Competency, and Self-Concept

Children who master the messages in the hidden curriculum, as Amber has (see box), learn how to "do school" successfully. Those who have difficulty understanding the instruction of the hidden curriculum, for whatever reason, often are perceived by teachers as less than competent students. In a study of reading in a first-grade classroom, K. P. Bennett (1986) discovered a hidden curriculum for measuring reading performance, one that had little to do with how well students understood what they read. Instead it addressed issues of *performance* in reading, including learning to (1) use the correct reading posture by sitting straight, still, and quietly; (2) watch and listen to the teacher when she spoke; (3) use a paper "marker" to keep the place in the book; and (4) demonstrate "comprehension" of the reading material by restating *verbatim* what was read in answer to questions the teacher took directly from the

Amber's Story

I came to this school from the city. We went on this choir trip back to Denver, and I, like I knew all the places and where the "jects" [housing projects] were and what they were called and the College City kids just like, wow! How do you know all that? I'm Hispanic. And the teachers, they were afraid I was going to bring my friends from Denver to visit the school and they said I couldn't. My best friend came from Denver, like me. We just hang out together. And the teachers are always watching us. We were out in the school yard under a tree and just talking, and the assistant principal came up and said we had to be smoking! He even smelled our breath . . . and we were just talkin'! I dress different, too [see "Amber's Dress Code" in Chapter 3]. I got good grades in my old school, but here it's a lot more advanced. It's hard and I had to study pretty hard. At first the teachers were always on my case. I hugged a boyfriend in the library and I had to go see the assistant principal. They were always watching me. The other kids could do things and nobody would notice. Then they tried to put me in a different class [a lower ability track]. I *know* how to write for school work, but when I talk, I just talk like I do, and the teachers listen and think I don't know anything. They were always watching me. But now I think they know me better and they're more used to me. I don't have so much trouble now.

text. Children who could exhibit these skills consistently were considered "good readers" and were put in the top reading groups. Those who had difficulty meeting these behavioral expectations or who refused to conform were considered to be less competent readers and placed in lower-ability groups, often without reference to standardized test scores which indicated that the placements were inappropriate. "She can't keep her place" or "He doesn't listen" or "She won't sit still in reading group" was enough to label a child a poor reader. Research by Eder and Felmlee (1984) and Grant and Rothenberg (1986) support these findings. How many adults could conform to such standards? One need only watch the behavior of adult teachers in faculty meetings to question whether adults can be as quiet, sit as still, and listen as well as children are expected to do.

Social standing in the peer group also is affected by academic placement. Children tend to choose for friends classmates who are in the same ability group or track as their own, so the social organization of schools comes to reflect the academic organization (Borko and Eisenhart 1986). This grouping has a profound effect upon self-concept. Children internalize the teachers' evaluations of them as well as their standing in the social organization of the classroom. Since they see the teacher as the authority figure and expert, they blame themselves for their lack of ability and low status. Anyon argues that the individualistic focus and evaluation structure of schools teach children that they are responsible for their own failures and academic shortcomings. Schools teach students that the reason for failure lies in their own "lack of motivation, low ability, disadvantage or inattention." Schools foster "blaming the victim" by shifting the terms of failure to the student rather than to the "failure of the institution to meet the student's needs by providing successful pedagogy" (Anyon 1988, p. 179).

Observe a classroom of your choice. Take extensive notes on what is happening there, trying to write down verbatim as much classroom dialogue as possible. What activities are the students and teacher engaged in? Analyze your observations according to the notion of a hidden curriculum. What are the implicit messages given to students in this classroom?

STRATIFICATION OF THE CURRICULUM

When sociologists talk about social stratification, they are referring to the hierarchy in society in which people are arranged according to how much they have of goods valued in that society. For example, in American culture, wealth, power, and prestige are highly valued. People who have more of these things are considered to be more valuable and therefore occupy the upper levels in the hierarchy. Both the formal and the hidden curriculum are similarly stratified. Today's schools are organized so that children are assigned to curricula according to the location and resources of the school, the age of the children, the number of children per classroom and—most important—the school's expectations of how well those children will perform both in school and in future occupations.

When we discuss the stratification of the curriculum, we are also talking about a hierarchy of power. Underlying this stratification is the notion that some types of knowledge and some types of instructional practices are considered superior to others. Similarly, some curricular programs are more valued than others. For example, a college preparatory program is considered superior to a vocational program, both because the former is believed to lead to more desirable occupations and because the children assigned to them tend to be more valued and have more social power in school. These placements are often based on perceived levels of ability, but, as we indicate in Chapters 7 and 8, they also are based on teachers' expectations of the children's academic performance, as mediated by the teacher's knowledge of their socioeconomic backgrounds, effective interaction with teachers and other students, behavior, appearance, use of language, and other markers of cultural capital.

In the next section we will discuss how stratification of the curriculum affects the school life of children. Questions to be considered include the following:

1. Which kinds of knowledge have more prestige in the school curriculum and why?
2. Who is eligible for inclusion in these programs?
3. Who is eligible to teach in the more prestigious courses and programs?

Choose a textbook in your field of study. Analyze the content and format of the text for the implicit messages provided to students and teachers.

Ability Grouping

Students at all levels of schooling are placed in groups according to their abilities as perceived by school personnel. This type of organization at the elementary school level is called **ability grouping.** It begins at least as early as kindergarten, but studies of nursery schools and day-care centers indicate that it may begin much earlier (Cox 1980; Woodhouse 1987). Students are most commonly grouped for instruction in reading and math. Throughout the kindergarten year classroom teachers and administrators assess their students' abilities, both formally and informally, and students begin to be identified as having different levels of ability or as being different kinds of learners. Some seem to "catch on" faster than others; some need a lot of extra individual help. Ability grouping is continued throughout the school years. Even through middle and high school children may remain in the groups that were established in their first year of school, for all subjects, as Jennifer's story documents (see box on p. 214).

Ability grouping even has echoes in higher education, as institutions themselves are stratified. The most able students are recruited for elite private schools. The next echelon consists of elite public state universities and private liberal arts colleges. Following those schools are a range of multipurpose state and private colleges and universities. At the bottom are two-year community and junior colleges, whose enrollment consists, for the most part, of less affluent or less able students who were not able to attend more prestigious institutions (Karabel and Halsey 1977).

Think back to when you were in elementary school. What reading group were you in? Were you ever changed from one to another? Why? What do you remember about learning to read in these groups? What did you think about the students in other groups?

Tracking

High school course offerings are differentiated both horizontally and vertically (Powell, Farrar, and Cohen 1985). Horizontal differentiation refers to diversity in content, or the number of disciplines in which courses are offered. The horizontal differentiation increased dramatically, for example, when vocational programs and a variety of electives were added. Vertical differentiation refers to the number of levels at which individual courses are offered. Vertical differentiation creates tracking. It occurs when, for example, senior high school physics is offered at the advanced, general, and remedial level, or when requirements for English can be met either by remedial reading classes or by advanced placement literature courses that include Chaucer and

Jennifer's Story

Hello. My name is Jennifer and I am in seventh grade, and I just turned 13 a little while ago. I have a teacher who puts us into groups, and the groups are smart group and dumb group.

She doesn't say they're smart group and dumb group, but they are the smart group and dumb group. All the smart people are in the smart group, and all the other people are in the dumb group, and I'm always in the dumb group because I always have been in the dumb group. Anyway, the other day we were all joking around because all the smart group people were downstairs doing algebra, and we were all joking around and saying, "Hey, you're the president of the dumb group," and we were just fooling around, and the teacher called me over to her desk and said, "There's no smart group or dumb group, it's all equal," and I said, "No, it's not." I said, "Listen, you don't give us any credit for what we do. We know this stuff like the back of our hand" and she said, "No, I just taught it to you today, you don't know this stuff," and I said, "Yes, we do. We learned this like a month ago." She said, "No, you didn't" and I said, "Yes, we did." She said, "When did I put you in groups? I just put you in groups today and you just learned it today." I said, "No, Ms. Jones, we did this last night in homework." I was getting really mad at her and she was like, "No, you didn't," and I was like, "Yes, I can take it out of my book right now, I did it last night for my homework." Well, to make a long story short, she was yelling at us and all, and she was telling me how I needed reinforcement or I was gonna fail, and I said, "Ms. Jones, I worked really hard this year and I got on the honor roll, and I got a B+ in math, and I don't need this reinforcement." I guess she was upset at me and I was really upset at her. She teaches us like we don't know anything and that we are really stupid. I know I'm not the smartest person in the world but I'm not the stupidest, either, and I can't believe she could say something like that, and do stuff like that, in front of the smart and dumb groups, if the groups are even equal. They're not equal. The teacher may think they're equal. They are not equal. They're smart and dumb. It may not be smart and dumb; maybe it's fast and slow. Well, that's smart and dumb. And if you're dumb, you're always dumb. I have always been put in the lower reading group and the lower math groups ever since first grade. I may not have read very well in first and second grade, but I did pretty good, and ever since then I was always put in the stupid groups and I don't think it's fair because I worked really hard this year to get a B+ in math, and I got a B+ in reading and I got on the honor roll, and I'm pretty proud of myself, I don't think it's fair at all that you should be put into groups.

Beowulf. A single high school can have as many as six or seven levels of basic academic courses. These courses share similar titles but their content and intellectual challenge differ significantly (Cusick 1983; Oakes 1985).

Vertical differentiation actually creates a vertical curriculum (Powell, Farrar, and Cohen 1985) when entire programs are created of courses at a given level. The vertical curriculum organizes students into tracks according to their perceived abilities, as determined by school personnel on the basis of standardized and nonstandardized testing and classroom performance. Allison and Bennett (1989) describe an example of a vertical curriculum in a high school. The tracking system contains five levels with admittance into each determined by the district's Language Arts supervisor and based on students' scores on the Stanford Test of Academic Skills, administered in the eighth grade. Level One, the Adaptive Program, contains those who read at a third-grade level or below, including nonreaders. Level Two, called Fundamental, was designed for those who read at fourth-, fifth-, and sixth-grade levels. Level Three, the Basic Program, is for students reading at seventh- and eighth-grade levels, and Level Four, Standard or College Preparatory, is for those reading "on grade" level. Level Five is an Honors Program to which students are invited if they scored at or above the 88th percentile on their achievement test.

This is fairly typical of the way high schools are organized, although some schools may be more explicit about the tracking system than others. Students who perform well academically in elementary school generally go on to the tracks that prepare them for college. Those who are not as academically talented are scheduled for classes in the basic or adaptive tracks.

Tracking is a common management strategy for organizing students in secondary schools. However, a growing body of literature as well as public concern raises questions about the practice (cf. Oakes 1985), because it labels children so early in their academic career as a success or a failure, and it contributes to the underachieving of students in what Jennifer describes as the "dumb group."

Analyze your high school experience in relation to the discussion on tracking systems. Which track were you in? How did this track differ from others? Did you have friends from other tracks? Were students from different tracks labeled with distinctive names? How many of the members of your track did the same things you did after high school?

Research on Ability Grouping and Tracking

Much current research indicates that ability grouping and tracking have detrimental effects on students. Studies about reading instruction report substantive differences in the content, delivery, and amount of instruction in reading in ability-grouped classes. Higher-level groups read more actual text than the lower-ability groups and also receive more direct instructional time. They are provided with more opportunities for independent silent reading, in contrast to the public oral reading required of the lower-level groups, a practice that limits the amount of actual reading practice

---

Rachel's Story

My most vivid experiences with ability grouping and tracking occurred in high school. There were three levels of all academic classes: low (remedial), average, and advanced. Some people had all their classes in one level, such as all low, or all advanced, but the majority of the people were mixed between the levels. I, for instance, had one of the lowest-level math classes, but I also took AP [Advanced Placement] English, AP Chemistry II, and AP American History. Many of my friends who took the highest math classes available were in the average English classes. One girl I knew who took four hours of cosmetology, which was considered by all students—the ones who took it and the ones who didn't—to be something you took if you weren't smart enough to go to college, also took advanced English and math. In spite of all this mixing, teachers and other students carried specific opinions about students. I think this had to do more with the lifestyle and social class background of the student rather than the classes they managed to get into. I lived in a small town; my teachers saw my mom and dad at City Council and Chamber of Commerce meetings. I came from a "good family," so they didn't think too much about the fact that I was extremely slow in math. Becky, who in spite of her four hours of cosmetology, and fighting her way into advanced English and math, was still a "redneck." Teachers knew where Becky lived, and they knew where she hung out on weekends. So, even though Becky could greatly outscore me on any math test around, I was "a good, smart girl," while Becky was just "one of those vo-tech kids."

---

received. Lower-ability groups are provided with fewer opportunities to read text (Allington 1977, 1980a, 1980b, 1983, 1984; Barr 1974, 1975, 1982; K. P. Bennett 1986; Borko and Eisenhart 1986; Borman and Mueninghoff 1982, 1983; Dreeben 1984; Featherstone 1987; Gambrell, Wilson, and Gantt 1981; McDermott 1976, 1977; Shavelson and Stern 1981). According to the *Harvard Education Letter*, "there is no persuasive evidence that ordinary elementary schoolers benefit from tracking" (July 1987, p. 1). In fact, some evidence (Barr 1982) indicates that tracking creates an achievement gap between children who had begun first grade with similar initial capabilities.

Interview a teacher (supervisor, principal, school board member, parent, student) about ability grouping and tracking practices. How do they support their views on these practices?

Research findings are much the same for tracking at the high school level. Oakes's *Keeping Track* (1985, and Page 1987) found that students' school experiences in more academic tracks were far different from those in lower tracks. There were significant differences in teacher expectations, academic content, and student achievement based on the level of the class. High-track classes involved more complex concepts, critical thinking, and discussion. Higher expectations were placed on these students because teachers understood that they were "college bound." Notwithstanding this evidence, many middle- and upper-class parents assume the high performance of their children and favor tracking for them. They argue that heterogeneous grouping with slower students, who also are more likely to be disadvantaged or minority students, will retard the learning of their ostensibly more advanced offspring.

Present a case for or against ability grouping and tracking. Support your arguments with evidence from scholarly journals.

The "Catholic School Effect"

In the 1980s attention was focused on the impact of Catholic schools on disadvantaged students. Studies indicated that Catholic schooling seemed to "push" achievement in these students, regardless of their social class standing (Coleman, Hoffer, and Kilgore 1982; Greeley 1982). However, Lee and Bryk (1988) have demonstrated that the supposed "Catholic School Effect" is a consequence of the less differentiated curricula in Catholic schools. Because they usually are smaller and have fewer resources than public schools, Catholic schools are unable to support the number of tracks commonly found in public school. Their students are therefore forced to enroll in the only classes available: solid academically oriented courses. As a consequence, most receive a more rigorous instructional program than public school students. Catholic school students were twice as likely as public school students to be assigned to an academic track, and a far greater proportion of Catholic school students who *wanted* to go to college were enrolled in the requisite preparatory program. Even general-track students in Catholic schools took more academic courses than similar students in the public schools.

Lee and Bryk repeat the findings that disadvantaged students in public schools are more often found in nonacademic tracks (Bowles and Gintis 1976; Cicourel and Kitsuse 1963; Oakes 1985). They also point out that the differentiated curriculum was initially developed as an equitable means to serve the presumed needs of a highly diverse public school enrollment (Cicourel and Kitsuse 1963; Heyns 1974; Powell, Farrar, and Cohen 1985). However, because the public schools offer so many nuances in courses, they amplify the initial differences in socioeconomic status and achievement that students bring with them to school. The reverse seems to be true for Catholic schools. The more constrained the curriculum, the greater is the academic rigor for all students. Hence student achievement is higher and the effects of poor background tend to wash out.

We believe that these findings demonstrate that activities initiated under the aegis of an ideology of democracy and egalitarianism can actually have the unintended effect of reducing equality. We will discuss these implications in Chapter 9.

SUMMARY

In this chapter we have looked at the ideologies underlying the formal and hidden curriculum of public schooling. We have also looked at the ways in which schools stratify this curriculum. We hope that you have begun to examine your own beliefs and values regarding what is taught in school. On the basis of this critique of current school practices, you may now be wondering what alternatives there are to the way we "do school" now. Chapter 9 will explore various possibilities for alternative, more appropriate ways to organize school curricula for both teachers and students.

chapter 7

Ethnic Minorities: Equality of Educational Opportunity

Chapter Overview

INTRODUCTION

In previous chapters we defined culture as a way of life shared by a group of people. In this chapter we are concerned with those cultural groups perceived in this society to be different from the "mainstream" dominant European American culture — ethnic minorities. Although membership in ethnic minority groups cannot really be considered apart from social class status (see Chapter 5), for our purposes here we will focus on group membership based on racial and ethnic identification. However, we urge you to keep in mind that one's identification is not related solely to ethnic group but is complicated by gender and social class. Each of us has multiple identities based on our gender, social class, ethnicity, sexual orientation, abilities, and other features. These identities play crucial roles in our interactions with individuals and institutions, and we continually reinterpret them on the basis of our interactions with others. For example, experiences of a working-class African-American female are profoundly different from those of an upper-middle-class African-American male, and the experiences of a white working-class Appalachian male are quite different from those of a middle-class Chinese-American female.

After an initial discussion about the labels given to or chosen by groups of people, we will define the terms *race, ethnicity, ethnic minority, prejudice,* and *discrimination.* We will then summarize the federal legislation related to equal educational opportunities for minorities. Next we will identify how social scientists have explained the question of school success and failure in minority student populations over the past two decades. Finally, we will address a question we consider to be the core issue in our discussion of equality of educational opportunity for minorities: What is the purpose of schooling for minorities, anyway?

What are your ethnic backgrounds? Many of us can trace our roots from several ethnic backgrounds. What values, beliefs, and behaviors have you learned as part of your cultural backgrounds? What biases do you think you would bring to the classroom as a teacher?

A Note about Labels

Terms used to refer to groups of people are constantly changing in response to political, economic, and social realities. For example, the term *African Americans* is currently used to describe people who have been labeled *Black, Afro-American,* and *Negro* during different historical periods. Often labels are ascribed by the dominant group in society but, particularly in recent decades, ethnic groups have selected their preferred labels. We have tried to use terms currently preferred or accepted by the particular groups we are discussing. In this chapter we use the terms *Anglo* and *European American* to describe people commonly referred to as "whites" in the United States. You may be more familiar and comfortable with the term *white* as a category to describe people from European backgrounds. We believe it is important to deconstruct this term. In her article, "White Is a Color! White Defensiveness, Postmodernism, and Anti-racist Pedagogy," Leslie Roman (1993a) reminds us that being white is not "colorless" and that people who are considered white in this society have their own racial subjectivities, interests, and privileges. She argues that the term *people of color,* which has been used as an alternative to more pejorative labels and as a celebration of multicultural diversity, "still implies that white culture is the hidden norm against which all other racially subordinate groups' so-called 'differences' are measured" (1993a, p. 71). By using the terms *Anglo* and *European American,* we emphasize that all people have ethnic backgrounds. *Anglo* or *Anglo American* is generally used to describe people from English heritage. *European American* refers to people from one or more European cultures. Since many "white" Americans can trace their roots to several European cultures, this is a broader term.

Considering themselves "American," European Americans in this society often do not self-identify as having ethnic backgrounds. We challenge the European American readers of this book to think about their beliefs, values, and behaviors as culturally based. As Nieto notes, "because whites in U.S. society tend to think of themselves as the 'norm,' they often view other groups as 'ethnic' and therefore somewhat exotic and colorful" (1992, p. 16).

Labels change frequently and not all labels are universally accepted by all members in a particular group. For example, we know people of African descent who prefer the descriptor *Black* to *African American.* We need to recognize that people may have multiple ethnic backgrounds and that they may or may not choose to be identified by one or all of these backgrounds. As we will see in this chapter, ethnicity is not static but quite complicated and always evolving—and so are the labels used to describe it.

What Is Race?

Race was the earliest term used by social scientists to address differences in group membership. Early anthropologists and some sociologists have used the term to describe a group of people with common ancestry and genetically transmitted physical characteristics. Although many complicated classification systems were developed in the nineteenth century to categorize different races, three racial groups traditionally were recognized in early anthropological writings: Caucasian, Mongoloid, and Negroid (Ember and Ember 1985). These classifications, based on traits such as amount and texture of hair, skin color, and other physical attributes believed to characterize each group, are no longer accepted in the scientific community. However, people in the United States today continue to have labels imposed on them or to identify themselves as members of a racial group primarily on the basis of skin color, even though many people do not fit easily into these rigid categories.

The term *race* is too vague to have much meaning for contemporary scientists, since biologists have found few genetic or real differences between members of so-called racial groups. Nevertheless the term *race* has social meaning in that what people *believe* about race determines how they relate to other groups of people. Often mistaken beliefs about racial and ethnic identities serve as the basis for prejudice, discrimination, and racist behavior.

Vivian's Story

My mother tells this story all the time . . . [about] when I first realized there was black and white. I had a very good [white] friend named Mary Adams. This was at the Christian school when this happened. . . . One day she [my friend Mary] came to school and told me she couldn't play with me any longer. I was in about the first grade, and I said, "Well why can't you play with me?" So she took me by my hand and she told me, "It's because you're black." . . . I said, "Oh, I'll fix that." I said, "When I go home, I'll tell my mother to wash me real clean."

SOURCE: Quoted in Etter-Lewis, 1993, p. 106.

In summary, *race,* a term with no scientific meaning, is a concept that has been used historically to categorize people in the ethnocentric belief that one race is superior to others. Cashmore and Troyna explain:

> . . . race is arbitrary. It's a convenient label applied to some groups to legitimate, justify or explain treating them unequally. And, while it refers, often explicitly, to biological differences, our interpretation of race is as something quite independent of physical phenomena. Race exists in the mind of the believer only. . . . Humans possess a striking faculty for defining not only their confederates, but also those who clearly don't belong. Physical characteristics are as reliable indicators of "them" as they are of "us." This is a worldwide, historical pattern: it seems to recognize no boundaries nor time limits. Human beings simply have this proclivity for dividing up the world in this way. (1990, p. 20)

What Is Ethnicity?

Ethnicity involves "ways of thinking, feeling, and acting that constitute the essence of culture" (Steinberg 1989). In other words, ethnicity is composed of shared values, cultural traits, behavior patterns, and a sense of peoplehood (Banks 1979; Spradley and McCurdy 1972). Smith defines ethnicity as being characteristic of people who "conceive of themselves as being alike, by virtue of their common ancestry and . . . are so regarded by others" (M. G. Smith 1982, p. 4). Irish Americans, Jewish Americans, Polish Americans, African Americans, Mexican Americans—all can be identified as distinct ethnic groups.

Ethnic identity is particularly useful in facilitating our understanding of who we are as people. There is an element of choice to ethnicity in that we can choose to identify ourselves according to particular groups. For example, an individual of Irish heritage may or may not choose to self-identify as Irish American. It is important to remember that ethnicity is not fixed but may change within the larger cultural context. It is also important to remember that people commonly have their cultural roots in several different ethnic backgrounds.

However, the term *ethnicity* is insufficient for our purposes because it is too broad and inclusive and does not address the question of the group's relative power in the society. It simply refers to common cultural ties. Each of us can claim ties to a particular ethnic group or groups, but not all of us experience discrimination on that basis. Cohen's definition of ethnicity as "fundamentally a political phenomenon as the symbols of the traditional culture are used as mechanisms for the articulation of political alignments" (1974, p. 97) comes closer to addressing power issues in society. In other words, people, including the dominant group, use cultural symbols, language, and behaviors to identify who is affiliated with the group and who is not.

What Is an Ethnic Minority?

The term *ethnic minority* is a more precise way to describe groups of people of concern in this chapter. What does the term mean? We already have defined what an ethnic group is, so we just need to look at the word *minority*. If our only concern is comparative numbers, all of us could be considered part of a minority group, given a particular set of circumstances. For example, a few Republicans at a national Democratic convention is a minority group. Because they are a small percentage within the total, women engineering professors or women high school principals can be considered minority groups. Male teachers in elementary schools could be considered a minority group for the same reason.

Christina's Story

I have always felt American, and learning about my Japanese background would not hinder me from being "American." However, part of who I am is partly Japanese. This doesn't make me less American. My mother brought me up with some different ideals because that is all she knew, but that doesn't make me an inferior American. It simply allows me the luxury of knowing two ways of thinking. In school I did feel some apprehension about telling anyone I was half Japanese, because it made me feel different and that is the last thing I wanted. When a child is that age, they simply want to blend in, not stick out. It is funny when I remember back because when I would have trouble pronouncing a certain word, I thought it was because I was half Japanese and therefore couldn't pronounce it correctly. It did not occur to me that it might have been a hard word for me or that other children may have the same problem. In the beginning I was very quiet about my background and sometimes felt angry at my mother for making me different. I guess I was afraid that everyone would treat me differently if they knew. It is completely different now. I appreciate my differences and appreciate my mother much more. It also has made me very open-minded and I hope to encourage this in my own classroom. If I can model an appreciation for diversity, hopefully my students will be more tolerant and open-minded about other cultures.

However, for our purposes we use the terms *minority* or *ethnic minority* to denote groups whose common characteristics go beyond mere numbers. Sociologists continue to struggle to find a definition for the term *minority* precise enough to be used by social scientists. Dworkin and Dworkin offer four qualities that characterize a minority group: (1) identifiability, (2) differential power, (3) differential and pejorative treatment, and (4) group awareness (1982, p. 16).

Identifiable characteristics of minority groups include patterns of language or dialect, religion, behavior or dress, and such physical characteristics as gender, complexion, or eye shape. In Western societies, despite scientific rejection of biologically determined racial characteristics, people continue to use complexion shade as the most crucial factor in group identification. The social and political power of ethnic minorities often depends upon how identifiably different they are from the dominant groups. The degree of difference generally determines where they are placed in the social class structure, how much prestige, power, and respect they are accorded, and how they are treated. For example, African Americans, Hispanics, and American Indians may be identifiable by distinctive physical characteristics, language, and cultural practices. On this basis, they are often subjected to discriminatory treatment. They occupy less powerful positions than do European Americans. Their subordinate position is reflected in their relative lack of educational attainment, less prestigious occupational placement, and lower level of participation in social and political life. Much of this is a product of discriminatory patterns of exclusion.

Discriminatory treatment by others often acts as a catalyst for the development of increased awareness, a sense of group identification, and solidarity among group members. In recent years we have seen some movement of oppressed groups into fuller participation in our society, but certainly not to an extent equitable with that of the dominant group.

Banks (1979) affirms these four qualities of minority groups. He defines ethnic minorities as those groups that often are a numerical minority, constituting a small part of the total population, but that also are easily distinguished physically and/or culturally from "white" Americans and are treated in a discriminatory way. Today in the United States the ethnic minority groups most likely to be defined in these terms are Latinos, African Americans, Asians, and American Indian/Alaskan Natives. These groups can be subdivided further. For example, Japanese, Filipinos, Chinese, Vietnamese, Hmong, and Asian-Indian Americans are all subsumed by the larger category of Asian Americans.

Identification of ethnic minorities is contextual: Whether a group is labeled by itself or others as an ethnic minority depends on the historical period and geographic location. For example, Irish immigrants in Boston in the nineteenth century were a distinct ethnic minority group, but today they tend to be assimilated into mainstream European-American culture. Although they can still be considered an ethnic group, Irish Americans cannot be considered an *ethnic minority*. Many Irish, Italians, Greek, Germans, and other European immigrant minorities have adopted much of the culture of mainstream Americans and blend into the majority population (Dworkin and Dworkin 1982). We need to remember, however, that many people from these ethnic groups became bicultural by maintaining their cultural beliefs and practices while participating in mainstream culture.

Pilar's Story

I was born in Colombia, South America, which is where all of my family is from. I lived in Colombia until I was one and then my family and I moved to the United States. Even though I have lived in the United States all of my life, my parents have instilled in me many Latin customs and have raised me with various Latin values and traditions. Although now I am extremely proud of my heritage and my family background, I can remember times when I was in grade school when being Latin was a hindrance. Even though my Latin-American background has enabled me to be bilingual, which is a very big asset to me now, it was something I avoided. I can remember wanting to be just like everyone else in my class, "American," and I wanted to ignore the fact that I was Colombian. At times I did not appreciate my culture because it was different from everyone else's, but now I realize how fortunate I am to have grown up exposed to two such rich cultures and I am so thankful for this experience.

I think that if my elementary school classroom would have been more multiculturally centered, I would have been able to feel more comfortable expressing my culture. If my peers and I would have been positively introduced to other cultures outside our own, they would have been intrigued by my culture and the culture of others, enabling them to be more accepting.

Ethnic minority status also depends upon where one lives. The impact of geographic location is illustrated by the experience of approximately 3 million Appalachians from the mountains in West Virginia, Kentucky, and Tennessee, who moved to northern cities in the Midwest between 1940 and 1970 in search of employment. Appalachians were viewed socially as ethnic minorities despite their Anglo ancestry in England, Scotland, and Wales. They were subjected to considerable discrimination and prejudice (Obermiller 1981), even though they had no physical characteristics that would distinguish them from other white Americans. This lack of physical distinctiveness also precluded them from being categorized politically as an ethnic minority group, so they were not eligible for federally funded programs for minorities. In the 1970s Appalachians began a movement to identify themselves politically as a minority group in order to qualify for certain governmental funding (Obermiller 1981; Zigli 1981).

Prejudice and Discrimination

Humans tend to categorize people into racial, ethnic, and minority groups and evaluate them using their own groups as the norm. This type of evaluation is known as *ethnocentrism* when it results in seeing other groups of people as inferior to one's own. Ethnocentric attitudes toward other groups of people are the basis for prejudice. Banks defines prejudice as a set of rigid and unfavorable attitudes toward a particular group or groups that is formed in disregard of facts. Prejudiced individuals respond to members of these groups on the basis of preconceptions, tending to disregard behavior or personal characteristics that are inconsistent with their biases. (1988, p. 223)

Prejudice usually results in two forms of behavior: stereotyping and the establishment of social distance.

Stereotyping. Stereotyping is depicting people on the basis of preconceptions and limited information. When stereotyping, we create caricatures, exaggerations of beliefs about the characteristics of a group, and then apply them unquestioningly to all members of that group. Hence all Chinese women are described as shy, all Italians are expected to be excitable, and all feminists are man-haters.

While Banks defines stereotypes only as negative, Dworkin and Dworkin (1982) assert that stereotypes can be both negative and positive. They also become part of the dominant ideology, serving to justify patterns of oppression and social differentiation, as well as differences in treatment. People use stereotypes to explain why some groups are greedier or lazier, more prone to irreligious or immoral behavior, more honest or sneakier, better lovers or more adept at mathematics than others. Stereotypes are the basis for and reinforce patterns of prejudice and are difficult to dislodge by logic or new information.

Social Distance. Stereotypes help to define how people relate to others because they determine the amount of social distance groups require from each other. Social distancing describes the degree of intimate interaction people can maintain without discomfort or repugnance. People feel little need to avoid those whose stereotype is positive. In fact, such a stereotype encourages social interactions. By contrast, a negative stereotype fosters social avoidance and even the desire for physical distance. If you agree with stereotyping that characterizes a particular group as intelligent, hard-working, and interesting, you are likely to want to become socially involved with its members. In contrast, if you view a group of people as lazy, dirty, lacking in intelligence, and untrustworthy, you probably would prefer to avoid them.

In 1993 in a rural, predominantly white school in Indiana, girls wearing clothes associated with young blacks—baggy clothes, braids, and other "hip-hop" fashions—have been harassed since mid-November by boys accusing them of "acting black." At least five of the girls have withdrawn from school. "It's gotten to the point where you can't think in your classes because all you can think about is what they are going to do to you in the halls" said one of the girls.

SOURCE: *New York Times*, December 8, 1993, p. B8.

One of our European-American middle-class female students was placed, as part of her teacher education program, in an inner-city school with a predominantly African-American student population. Her stereotypes about African-American young men became evident when she became frightened while walking by two young men smoking in an empty corridor between school buildings. The incident frightened her so much that she asked to be moved to a school she considered "safer." Like this young woman, we are unlikely to be easily convinced that members of groups can behave in ways that do not fit our stereotypes of them.

Racism

Race is the root word for the term *racism.* Racism in the United States refers primarily to ethnocentric beliefs and behaviors based on the notion that European Americans are superior to African Americans, Asians, Latinos, and other ethnic groups. Categorization according to race and other ethnic identification has provided a means for

---

Theresa's Favorite Breakfast

Having breakfast before going to school was a promise my mom never broke. Every morning she would get up at five and begin the day cooking. She would make tortillas and potatoes which filled the house with a delicious aroma. She would also make avena for me and my brothers. This was a favorite of ours and we ate it often with buttered toast and orange juice.

We had just moved to Michigan from New Mexico and my parents enrolled my brothers and me in a local elementary school. Even though our routine was somewhat altered, we still had our breakfasts before going to school. Since my parents are bilingual, my mother coded some words in Spanish. So when my teacher asked the class what we had for breakfast that morning, I didn't hesitate to raise my hand and say *"avena."*

However, after I said "oatmeal" in Spanish, there was silence. My teacher looked at me with a puzzled expression and asked me to repeat my answer. I did and there was even more silence. Then she said, "I've never heard of that." I believe my expression was more puzzling than hers because I just ate it that morning. Only, I did not know how to say *avena* in English. Not probing my mind any further, she went on to another child and I was left confused and wondered why she didn't understand what I was saying.

Being a first grader, this had an impact on me. It pointed out that I was different. This is perhaps the first time where I absolutely felt like I did not belong. We eventually moved back to New Mexico and I was happy to be back in our home state where just about everyone knows what *avena* is.

setting up a hierarchy in which some groups are relegated to social and economic positions dominated by others.

We can distinguish between the *individual racism* of people in their daily lives and *institutional racism*, which is so deeply embedded in the curriculum, policies, and practices in schools and other institutions that it often goes unrecognized. Institutional racism may be seen in the form of ability grouping and tracking, differential disciplinary practices, uneven representation in special education classes, and the like. This institutional racism perpetuates the differential educational and economic achievement of many minority people.

Think of examples of individual and institutional racism you have experienced or witnessed in your own life.

THE FEDERAL GOVERNMENT AND EQUALITY OF EDUCATIONAL OPPORTUNITY

A primary concern among sociologists of education is the impact of individual and institutional prejudice and racism on the schooling experiences and achievement of ethnic minority students. At first sociologists simply noted that minorities seemed to be less successful in school than other students. Then they began to ask *why* minority students fared so poorly. Was it because, in a land of supposedly equal opportunity, these children somehow were treated unequally?

Equality of Educational Opportunity

Equality of educational opportunity requires giving everyone the same initial opportunity to receive an education (Spring 1989). The history of U.S. social reform is replete with attempts by European-American policy makers to direct attention away from inequities in the economy by reforming the educational system rather than by redistributing wealth and eliminating oppression. Rather than creating policies ensuring that everyone had an equal chance to compete for jobs, policy makers have concentrated on equality of educational opportunity. Addressing this problem has proven to be very complicated. First, even if everyone had the chance to receive an equal education, societal discrimination on the basis of race precludes equality in the job market. Second, the roots of racism and unequal treatment in schools are so deep, and the practices so subtle, that it has been difficult to identify them, much less change their course.

In the next few pages we will discuss how policy makers have tried to manipulate the educational system to ameliorate racial inequality. We will present a short history of the pertinent major federal legislation and court cases over the last century. This discussion sets the stage for our later examination of minority student failure in schools.

Equal Access

American schools foster a powerful ideology about the existence of individual freedom and opportunity. Young children are indoctrinated in the belief that anyone can
be successful, given enough ambition and hard work. These myths are belied, however, by reality. Equal opportunity requires and begins with equal access to the same
facilities, and historically ethnic minority groups have less access to economic and
social opportunities (LeCompte and Dworkin 1988).

Ask your local board of education for its most recent figures on minority
student enrollment, achievement, and dropout rates. Do some schools in
the district have higher proportions of minority students than others? Do
some schools have higher dropout rates than others? How do you account
for the differences? Compile your findings and present them to your class.

The Role of the Federal Courts

In 1895 the U.S. Supreme Court heard a case, *Plessy* v. *Ferguson,* in which Homer
Plessy (one-eighth black and seven-eighths white) refused to ride in a separate "col-
ored coach" of a train in Louisiana as required by law and was arrested. The Supreme
Court decided that as long as the facilities were equal, they could be separate. This
decision came to be known as the "separate but equal doctrine" and was used until
1954 to justify segregated facilities for African Americans and whites. Then a landmark Supreme Court decision, *Brown* v. *Board of Education of Topeka, Kansas*
(1954), overturned *Plessy* v. *Ferguson,* stating that separate facilities are inherently
unequal and therefore illegal under the Fourteenth Amendment of the U.S. Constitution. The Brown ruling states in part:

in the field of public education the doctrine of "separate but equal" has no
place. Separate educational facilities are inherently unequal. . . . We hold
that the plaintiffs and others similarly situated . . . are, by reason of the segregation complained of, deprived of equal protection of the laws guaranteed
by the Fourteenth Amendment.

In *Brown* v. *Board of Education* sociological data were used by the Supreme
Court for the first time as the basis for its decision. This research demonstrated to the
satisfaction of the justices that separate treatment is inherently unequal treatment.
This 1954 decision began the desegregation process of American schools, justified on
the basis of providing *access* to equality of educational opportunity. Minority students
would have to attend the same schools as European Americans in order to have equal
access. Despite the Enforcement Decree of 1955, which required that federal district
courts be used to end segregation of public schools at the local level, the process was
and continues to be painfully slow.

One Lonsdale man recalls that opportunities were often closed to black students. In the days before integration, this young man wanted to attend summer school. But he could not go because there was no summer school for blacks.

"I received a letter from the Superintendent of the Knoxville public schools. He had written me this nice form letter, the superintendent of public schools, explaining why I couldn't go. That I couldn't go because I was black."

SOURCE: The Lonsdale Improvement Organization 1992.

After the 1950s African Americans finally obtained legal access to equal schooling. Additional court cases, often on a district-by-district basis, began to ensure that a legal right became an educational reality. While African Americans no longer were legally segregated, the fact of residential segregation often meant that most children still attended racially isolated schools. The emphasis of subsequent legislation was on providing *equal access* for all children. Soon, however, research results began to show that even after segregated schools were legally banned, equal access did not necessarily guarantee equal outcomes for minority children (Hess 1989; Metz 1978; Murnane 1975). Equal treatment for people who started out unequal did not permit disadvantaged people to "catch up." Subsequent legislation then began to provide *unequal* or *compensatory education* in order to offset the effects of economic and educational disadvantage. We will discuss these programs later in this chapter.

This legislation has been part of a continuing struggle to ensure the civil rights of all U.S. citizens, regardless of ethnic affiliation. *Civil rights* refers to the rights of individuals by the fact of their status as citizens. These rights are guaranteed by the Fourteenth Amendment, which provides "equal protection under law" for all citizens. This means that all citizens are to have equal access to opportunities for economic and social gain despite their racial or ethnic background, gender, age, sexual orientation, or disabling condition. Civil rights are guaranteed by the Constitution — the right to an education is not. Since education was a responsibility left to state governments, opportunities for schooling, particularly for ethnic minorities, varied from state to state.

Create an ethnic map of your neighborhood. First define the neighborhood and list all institutions—churches, stores, schools, places of entertainment—and classify them according to their ethnic group of origin. Were they initially begun or once used by a specific ethnic group? Determine if the clients who use them live in the neighborhood or elsewhere. Then try to determine the ethnic breakdown of the residences in your area.

The 1964 Civil Rights Act was passed by Congress to speed up the desegregation of public schools. Title IV of the Civil Rights Act gave the U.S. Commissioner of Education the power to help desegregate schools and the U.S. Attorney General the power to initiate lawsuits to force school desegregation. This power was enforced by Title VI, which denied federal funds to schools with racially discriminatory programs. For many school districts, this threat was effective.

School districts were given a clear message from the federal government that they must take steps to provide equal educational opportunities for minority students through both desegregation and compensatory education programs. These were closely linked, because schools were required to desegregate in order to receive federal funds for the compensatory programs.

Using a map of your school district, code the schools according to the ethnic composition of their students. What are your findings?

Desegregation and the Coleman Report

The unequal performance of minority students indirectly gave impetus to school desegregation. Conventional wisdom argued that inequalities of performance must be a consequence of inequalities in the schools, and therefore schools with high-achieving students must be spending more money on them than those whose students did poorly. To test that theory, Section 402 of the 1964 Civil Rights Act authorized the Commissioner of Education to examine "the lack of availability of equal educational opportunities for individuals by reason of race, color, religion, or national origin in public educational institutions at all levels in the United States." A survey, conducted by James Coleman and his associates, was entitled *Equality of Educational Opportunity* (1966). It looked at material differences between districts, comparing such things as school and class size, the background and level of training of teachers, provision of facilities such as libraries and laboratories, and per-pupil expenditure. These data were aggregated at the district level; Coleman did not look at differences among schools *within* districts.

Coleman expected to find that poor schools produced poor students. What he found out was surprising. First of all, the differences between school districts were not large enough to explain the differences in student performance among the six racial groups in the study. Second, he found that differences between minority and majority students' test scores greatly increased from the first to the twelfth grade. Third, minority and majority children did not differ in the value they attached to school and academic achievement (Borman and Spring 1984, p. 204). What he did find was that minority students who attended school with European-American students seemed to have higher levels of academic achievement than those who attended all-minority schools.

This research finding was a catalyst to mix students racially to improve the performance of minorities. And, while the impetus for desegregation certainly was congruent with American social ideology, it unfortunately was based upon a misinterpretation of Coleman's research; subsequent reanalyses showed that the real effect was not racial, but socioeconomic. What really seemed to have an effect on students was the peer group. Students whose classmates were from a higher socioeconomic group did better in school. Since minority students usually were poorer than their majority classmates, it appeared that going to European-American schools made the difference.

Different methods have been used to desegregate American schools in response to the 1954 Supreme Court decision, the 1964 Civil Rights Act, and the Coleman Report. U.S. schools have tried to comply in a variety of ways, some more effective than others. A few complied only under court order. A few refused to disband racially segregated systems and closed down the public schools until ordered to reopen by the courts. Many schools postponed compliance. Some districts still are fighting court battles over desegregation, under continued threats from the government to cut off federal funding and institute lawsuits (Borman and Spring 1984; Hughes, Gordon, and Hillman 1980; Kirby, Harris, and Crain 1973; P. E. Peterson 1976; Rogers 1968; Tatel, Lanigan, and Sneed 1986).

Bussing was one of the most widely used and controversial plans for achieving racial balance. Students from one neighborhood school—usually minority dominated—would be bussed to another, usually in European-American neighborhoods. Where this method is enforced by law, it is referred to as *involuntary desegregation* and has been met with resistance and hostility by both African-American and European-American parents. It has been argued that forced bussing encourages European Americans to flee from the districts affected, that it destroys neighborhoods and disrupts parents' involvement with their children's schooling. Parents objected to the long bus rides to which their children were subjected, especially since the majority bussed were minority children (Borman and Spring 1984; Crain 1977; Pettigrew and Green 1976; Reynolds 1986; Rist 1973).

A recent example of community tensions over bussing occurred in Wausau, Wisconsin, during the 1993–1994 school year. In accordance with a bussing program to distribute poor and/or Southeast Asian children across the district, 600 children were bussed up to 2.2 miles so that no school would have more than a 32 percent minority enrollment. This plan was in response to concern by teachers and principals overwhelmed by the needs of immigrant children, mostly from Hmong refugee families that settled in the area with the help of church groups. The group made up 16 percent of the district's enrollment and were concentrated in just a few schools, which also had disproportionate numbers of low-income European-American children. Parents rebelled against the bussing and collected 10,000 signatures to hold a recall election for the local school board. In December five school board members who had helped to implement the bussing program were voted out of office. At this writing the community continues to be in controversy over the bussing plan (Schmidt 1994).

In another district the school board used a lottery to institute a policy of involuntary transfers of teachers in an attempt to provide a racially balanced faculty. The names of European-American teachers and the names of African-American teachers in schools with predominantly African-American student populations were placed in separate sets of containers grouped according to grade level. At a public meeting the names of African-American teachers and corresponding European-American teachers were drawn, according to grade level. These teachers switched places for the next three years. Little in the way of in-service training was provided for these transferred teachers. The program was somewhat effective in desegregating faculties but caused major upheaval for the teachers and children whose lives were changed by the move. Four years after the transfer, one teacher captured her experience: "I've never been so angry in my entire career. I felt so powerless."

Voluntary desegregation plans use programs such as magnet schools, minority-to-majority transfers, metropolitan redistricting, and school pairing to improve ethnic balance. Magnet schools, usually inner-city schools with a history of minority enroll-ment, historically are transformed into centers offering programs designed to attract students from all over the district. In many cities ordered to desegregate, these mag-net schools have been developed as an alternative to bussing. Schools specializing in arts, languages, computer science, applied arts, medicine, math and sciences, physi-cal education, and programs for the gifted have replaced inner-city segregated schools. Students voluntarily apply to these schools and may even be required to audi-tion, as in Cincinnati and Houston, where inner-city high schools were transformed into schools for the creative and performing arts or programs for the gifted and tal-ented. The assumption is that if the school, despite its location, can offer an excellent program, students from outside the immediate neighborhood will be attracted to it, thus reducing the effects of de facto or residential segregation (Borman and Spring 1984; Ferrell and Compton 1986). However, magnet schools have been criticized for drawing away the best students and resources from other schools. Some magnet schools housed within larger schools have been criticized for "in-school segrega-tion," since locating the program in one portion of the building discourages interac-tions between students within and outside of the program.

The impact of social life on children in desegregated schools also has been dis-puted. The organization in some of these schools facilitates the development of cross-racial friendships (Damico, Bell, and Green 1980; Schofield 1982). All of them have made the development of such friendships more possible. However, desegregation has not always meant social integration, especially since the bussed children usually arrive and leave in intact groups on a scheduled bus and have little time to socialize with others. Sometimes the children even remain segregated in distinct classrooms. Especially where ability grouping and tracking reinforce racial differences, students tend to remain in racially segregated groups in the lunchroom, on the playground, in classes, and on the bus. Differences in cultural styles also impede the formation of friendships. European-American children tend to be intimidated by African Americans and to feel threatened by the noise and movement natural among African Americans (Clement, Harding, and Eisenhart 1979; Hanna 1987; St. John 1975; Schofield 1982; Wax 1980).

Despite the Supreme Court rulings requiring the desegregation of schools and federal legislation denying funding to racially discriminatory districts, the majority of American schools today continue to be relatively segregated, in large part because of persistent racial and economic residential segregation. Enforcement is a problem. In many cases federal funding has not been withheld despite serious, continuing viola-tions of the Civil Rights Act. Giving control over federal funds to state and local authorities, as happened in the early 1980s with the "block grant" program, has affected the dispersion of funds. Fred Hess, executive director of the Chicago Panel on Public School Policy and Finance, explained that "more than 80 percent of all minority students in Chicago continue to attend segregated schools and receive no significant compensatory education to offset the effects of this segregation" (1989). In fact, the neediest schools in Chicago often get fewer funds than those in more affluent neighborhoods. (See also Knapp and Cooperstein 1986; Lecompte and Dworkin 1988.) Hess and his associates called for shifting more resources from wealthier schools to deal with this problem.

In large part these inequities exist because the ethnic composition of schools parallels the ethnic composition of neighborhoods. Most of the major cities in the United States have racially and economically segregated patterns of residence which have been enforced by custom and legal statute, a situation that is becoming worse rather than better—despite Civil Rights legislation (W. J. Wilson 1987).

A recent study by the Harvard Project on School Desegregation (Orfield 1993) describes the increased segregation of African-American students across the United States. The study found that, after a rather dramatic decline of segregation in the South from the mid-1960s through the early 1970s and a period of stability until 1988, segregation significantly increased from 1988 to 1991. In addition the study reports the following findings:

- The proportion of black students in schools with more than 50% minority students increased from 1986 to 1991, reaching the level that had existed before the Supreme Court's first busing decision in 1971. The share of black students in intensely segregated (90–100% minority) schools— which had actually declined during the 1980s—rose. (Orfield 1993, p. 7)

- During the 1991 school year, Latino students were more likely than African American students to be in predominantly minority schools and slightly more likely to be in intensely segregated schools. (Orfield 1993, p. 7)

- African American and Latino students are much more likely than white students to find themselves in schools of concentrated poverty. Segregation by race is strongly related to segregation by poverty. (Orfield 1993, p. 7).

- Minority students are much more likely to be in high poverty schools. They face not only discrimination and stereotypes about minority schools but schools struggling with the much greater concentration of health, social, and neighborhood problems that are found in high poverty schools. (Orfield 1993, p. 1)

Forty years after the *Brown* v. *Board of Education* ruling called for the abolition of school segregation, communities and school districts continue to struggle over the issue of desegregation as large numbers of poor and minority children continue to attend schools that offer separate and unequal educational opportunities.

Compensatory Legislation

As we have described, the findings of the Coleman Report contradicted policy makers' expectations. Differential student achievement was strongly related, not to school characteristics, but to family background of students and aspirations of peers. Coleman's work led to theories linking poor academic achievement to the "cultural deprivation" of poor families. It gave scientific credence to the popular belief that children from ghetto families live in a "culture of poverty" (Valentine 1968) which puts them at a disadvantage in school. Federal policy makers used this argument to implement programs that would compensate for the home environment and facilitate equality of *results* rather than just equality of *access* (Baratz and Baratz 1970; Karabel and Halsey 1977). Initiated in the 1960s as part of the federally funded War on Poverty, these programs became known as "compensatory education." The Elementary and Secondary Education Act (ESEA), passed in 1965 as part of President Lyndon B. Johnson's "War on Poverty," provided approximately $1 billion in federal funding for programs and services beyond the regular school offerings (Ballantine 1983). These programs targeted preschool and elementary school children from poor and minority families and were predicated upon the assumption that early intervention would compensate for the disadvantages resulting from their family background. While the various titles of the ESEA provided funds for a wide variety of programs, the most important for instructional programs was Title I. It provided programs such as Head Start for preschoolers and remedial reading and math programs for school-aged children considered to be educationally deprived.

The importance of the ESEA to the issue of equality was that it improved opportunities for children by improving their education. It also reinforced the Civil Rights Act by linking federal funding for Title I programs to compliance with desegregation requirements.

These programs still exist under the 1981 Education and Consolidation and Improvement Act (ECIA); however, lumping federal funds into state-disseminated "block grants" gives control of the program and its funding to local districts. These Chapter I federal funds can be used for a wide variety of programs, not just those aimed at poor children. As Hess (1989) pointed out, local districts can structure programs so as to divert funds from those most in need, thereby weakening their impact. In 1994 congressional debates over federal funds for education, Senator Edward M. Kennedy called this block grant funding program "a slush fund for states" (Pitsch 1994).

Currently as of this second edition, the Clinton administration is working toward congressional reauthorization of the Elementary and Secondary Act. The Democratic administration has pushed Congress to eliminate the block grant funding of the 1980s and replace it with categorical aid directly to school districts serving the poorest children. Clinton's controversial plan would increase funds for the neediest districts through "concentration grants" for counties with high concentrations of poor students. His proposal also calls for increasing from 15 percent to 18 percent the proportion of poor students needed for a county to qualify for the grants. Clinton's proposal requires states to set standards for student performance and curriculum content in order to participate in Chapter I (Pitsch 1994). This change in the funding of compensatory education will require more accountability from school districts on their use of federal funding and is a step toward a national system of standards for performance in academic areas.

Special Needs Legislation

In the late 1960s and early 1970s lawmakers continued attempts to provide federal funding for specific student populations that had not yet received special educational services. The 1966 Education of Handicapped Children (Title VI) and the 1967 Bilingual Education Programs (Title VII) were added to the Elementary and Secondary Act. The Education of Handicapped Children Act provided for free public education for all handicapped children. It provided at public expense services previously available only in the private sector and too costly for poor families. The purpose of the Bilingual Act was to meet "the special educational needs of the large number of children of limited English speaking ability in the United States." An Indian Education Act of 1972 provided funds for health and nutrition programs for American Indians as well as innovative and bilingual programs. The Ethnic Heritage Act was passed in 1972 to assist in the establishment of ethnic studies programs. All of these programs were aimed at providing poor and minority students with the same educational opportunities that middle-class white students had.

Nura's Story

I still try to improve my reading ability, but since I came to this country and started learning English I have a hard time differentiating between the rules of reading the two languages. I keep getting mixed up by the rules of reading and writing Oromo versus English. English is a difficult language to learn. The other students use dictionaries to translate new words but there is no Oromo/English dictionary. If my husband doesn't know the words, then I will never find out. And sometimes even after they are translated they don't make much sense. Even worse, some words in English don't even exist in the Oromo language and vice versa.

My teacher says that we should be in contact with Americans to practice our English, but I hardly come in contact with Americans. There aren't any in my neighborhood. The only time I see them is when I watch television or go to the store. But at the store they have no time for discussions. My husband and I were advised to talk to one another in English, which we tried for a while. But since we kept running out of English words, we cut down on communicating with one another. That made us feel even worse, so we gave up on the idea of communicating with one another in English.

SOURCE: Center for Literary Studies 1992.

Underlying these programs was the assumption that if minority students could acquire the same cultural capital that mainstream European Americans had, they would have the same opportunities for economic success as whites. In other words, if you could teach them to "act white" (Fordham and Ogbu 1986), they would be equal. This is, however, an individualistic solution to what really is a problem generated by structural inequities in the society. It ignores the reality of how unequally distributed economic resources are in this country and how difficult it is for minority groups to gain access to them.

RESEARCH ON SCHOOLING FOR MINORITY STUDENTS

Research on the performance of minority students over the last three decades has attempted to explain why these children do not succeed in school in the same way that European-American children do. Three distinct theories have been developed: unequal resources and treatment, cultural background, and the labor market.

A Theory of Unequal Resources and Treatment

This approach to school failure examines the imbalance of financial resources available to minority students and the differential treatment they receive in school. Jencks, in his work *Inequality* (1972), examined this theory, testing it at the macro or structural level by reanalyzing Coleman's data from the mid-1960s. Since it had been determined that schools were not unequal enough to produce the observed differences in achievement, Jencks introduced what essentially was a class-conflict explanation: Poverty and poor performance were a function of social class rather than race (Scimecca 1980). He argued that family background was the most important determining factor in students' educational achievement. Students from families with higher incomes are more likely to acquire more education than those from lower-income families. According to Jencks, equalizing the resources for schools and the time spent in school would not be enough to reduce economic inequality. He argued:

> There is no evidence that school reform can substantially reduce the extent of cognitive inequality, as measured by tests of verbal fluency, reading comprehension or mathematical skill. Neither school resources nor segregation has an appreciable effect on either test scores or educational attainment. (1972, p. 8)

He argued that large-scale redistribution of wealth, not school reform, was the key to a more equitable society. He criticized the legislation of the 1960s for concentrating on children rather than directly attacking adult inequality.

Unfortunately, though economic reform is certainly a necessary strategy in reducing inequality in the society, this argument was interpreted to mean that because of the determining power of family background, schools made no difference and could be ignored as sites for social change.

Rist, by contrast, examined inequality in the treatment of children at the microlevel—inside schools and classrooms. Rist (1970) studied the school experiences of African-American primary-aged children from a poor, urban neighborhood. He found that teachers' perceptions of students' home lives made a significant difference in the way they treated students. Students perceived to come from poor homes—as determined by their appearance as well as informal knowledge of family background—were placed in lower-ability reading groups and provided with less direct instruction. Rist also observed that students in the top groups came from middle-class homes. Kindergarten teachers spent two to three times more time instructing these children than they did children in the slower, lower-class groups. Consequently, the "fast" group was able to complete the kindergarten curriculum while the "slower" groups did not. The slow group entered first grade already far behind their peers academically.

Theories of Cultural Background

Cultural Deprivation.   In the 1960s researchers began to look away from the schools and toward the home to explain why minority and poor children failed in school. Educators from this perspective argued that a "culture of poverty" (Valentine 1968) explained the poor performance of minority children. The core of this explanation was the alleged "cultural disadvantage" of the children's home environment.

Children thought to be culturally deprived were described as those who lived in ghettos where they were not provided with proper nutrition or adequate health care. They attended poor schools, were not adequately prepared for jobs, and if and when they finished school, they repeated this "cycle of poverty" to the next generation. The homes in which they grew up—primarily the ethnic minorities—did not provide them with the tools they needed to succeed in school. It was believed that their parents did not read to them, did not encourage the kinds of home learning activities used by middle-class parents, and generally did not provide an intellectually stimulating environment. Minority children often came to school with a language or dialect different from middle-class or standard English (Bernstein 1977). Commonly referred to during the 1960s—and even sometimes today—as "culturally deprived" or "socially disadvantaged," these children were believed to be deprived of the cultural or social advantages necessary to succeed in school (Baratz and Baratz 1970; Erickson 1987).

Cultural deprivation theory was in large part responsible for the development of the compensatory education program. Schools were called upon to break this "cycle of poverty" through Head Start and the other preschool programs described above, including bilingual education and health and nutrition programs. Politicians and educators believed that if schools could intervene prior to entry into kindergarten, some of the effects of the home environment could be alleviated and the students would have a better chance to succeed in school.

The use of the term *culture* in this theory is misused in the anthropological sense. What was documented was not so much a culture per se, but a response to oppressive conditions of racial isolation, powerlessness, and poverty. Anthropologists argue that growing up in one culture does not mean being deprived of another and that the children described as "culturally deprived" actually functioned quite well in their own milieu. European-American middle-class youngsters in a barrio setting would be found similarly "culturally deprived."

The cultural deprivation theory was strongly criticized by scholars in the mid-1960s as ethnocentric. Rather than looking to the structure of schools or societal forces, blame was placed on the victims: individual children or minority groups (Ryan 1976). Educators, "frustrated by their difficulties in working with minority children, [were able] to place the responsibility for school failure outside the school" (Erickson 1987, p. 336).

Cultural Differences. To counter cultural deprivation theory, social scientists began to look at differences or discontinuities between the cultures of the school and the home, particularly in communication and other interactions. Researchers working with Appalachian, African-American, Hawaiian, and American Indian students found that interactional difficulty in schools can be related to cultural differences in communication styles (Au and Mason 1981; Cazden, John, and Hymes 1974; D'Amato 1988; Erickson and Mohatt 1982; Heath 1983; Jordan 1984; Labov 1972; S. U. Phillips 1972; Piestrup 1973; Rist 1973).

According to the cultural difference explanation, school failure is a result of differences between the culturally derived white-middle-class communication patterns of the school and those of the students' home culture. Dissonance can be reduced if teachers are familiar with the verbal and nonverbal communication patterns of both the school and home culture. If educators can enhance classroom interaction and communication by adapting to and respecting the culture of minority students, they may be able to increase feelings of comfort and communicative competence in these students. As Erickson suggests:

> it may be that culturally congruent instruction depoliticizes cultural difference in the classroom, and that such depoliticization has important positive influences on the teacher–student relationship. Such a situation in the classroom might prevent the emergence of student resistance. (1984, p. 543)

These researchers believe that if classroom settings were structured so that cultural differences in communication patterns were reduced, achievement of minority students might be improved (Au and Mason 1981). Several examples of this type of research are presented here to give us a better understanding of this theory.

The work at the Kamehameha Early Education Program (KEEP) in Hawaii is a primary example of this research. On the basis of research in the local community, a team of teachers and researchers developed a way of teaching reading based on the communication style of the Hawaiian "talk story," in which conversational exchanges overlap rapidly in the cooperative building of a story. The basal reading program was reorganized so the everyday pattern of communication used by Hawaiian children replaced the Western structure in which children wait to be called on and speak one at a time. Researchers at the KEEP center documented increased academic achievement in reading through this more culturally congruent style (Au and Mason 1981).

The structures used in the KEEP program were then transplanted to a school with a Navajo population. Vogt (1985) reports that although the increased cultural congruency led to increased effectiveness in the reading programs for both groups of students, the original KEEP program had to be rather dramatically changed because participation structures were different for each group. What was culturally congruent

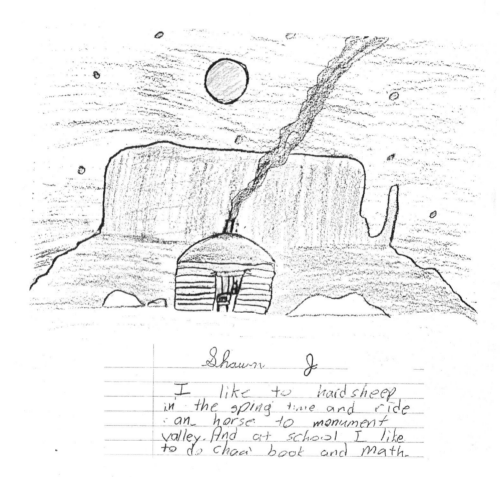

Shawn J

I like to haid sheep in the sping time and ride an horse to monument valley. And at school I like to do chaa' book and math.

FIGURE 7.1   The Navajo student refers to his chaa' book, the Navajo equivalent of an English language vocabulary workbook. The chaa' book was introduced as a means of revitalizing and incorporating the Navajo language and culture in the Kayenta Intermediate School.

SOURCE: Shawn Johnson, Third Grade, Kayenta Intermediate School, Kayenta, AZ. (Teachers: Sylvia Dugi, Ruth Bradley; Principal: Debbie Braff; Superintendent: Joe Martin)

Jenny's Story

It's hard not knowin' how to read. A lot of these women, you know, they think it ain't that hard to read. Just sit down and read. . . . It's not easy. . . . That's why it was a little hard for me startin' to like . . . sound my words out . . . 'cause I talk different . . . 'cause I'm, you know . . . countrified. And my words don't come out the way they're supposed to.

SOURCE: Jenny is an urban Appalachian woman whose story of learning to read is beautifully portrayed by Victoria Purcell-Gates (1993).

---

for Hawaiian students didn't fit the cultural patterns of the Navajo students. (Figure 7.1 shows a drawing with a brief story by a Navajo student.)

In a study of Native Alaskan schools, Van Ness (1981) found that the interactional smoothness of lessons taught by a native teacher could be attributed to the teacher's cultural knowledge of the social situation. He argued that since social behavior is culturally organized, cultural congruency between the teacher and students allowed for smooth interactions even at the kindergarten level.

In a study of African-American children in two first-grade reading programs, Piestrup (1973) reported differences in reading achievement which she attributed to the way in which each teacher responded to the use of Black English Vernacular (BEV). The children whose use of dialect was often corrected during lessons obtained lower scores on reading tests and actually used more BEV than children who were permitted to use BEV in reading groups without correction. The uncorrected children actually scored higher in standardized reading tests, many above the national norms. Piestrup argued that when the dialect was treated as a barrier to communication, more time was spent in correcting the dialect than in actual reading.

Theories about cultural differences call for educators to understand the differences of minority students so as to establish a more culturally congruent classroom situation. However, critical theorists argue that doing this might be viewed as co-optation. Under the guise of cultural appropriateness, teachers can use a culturally congruent curriculum taught in culturally sensitive ways to lead students gradually into adopting the ideology of the dominant class. This is a less painful or coercive way to colonize the minds of students (McLaren 1989) and, for this reason, may be even more effective than force.

It is important to realize that its developers did not intend the cultural differences theory to be seen as the only way to view the problem or as a means to co-opt minority students. This explanation is restricted to the microlevel: a classroom view of factors in schooling that lead to minority student failure. It does not address the political and economic societal forces at the macrolevel which influence these students outside the structure of schools.

Examine a textbook in your subject area. Analyze the treatment of minority groups by examining the number of minority group members depicted in the text, the way in which they are described, and the extent to which they are integrated into the text rather than "highlighted" in a special section.

Labor Market Theory

A macrolevel or societal view of minority student failure is central to the work of John Ogbu. A core element in his theory is student perception of their chances in the labor market. Ogbu argues that the school performance of minority students is rooted in the connection they see between schooling and how successful they will be in the job market. If they see school as a means to become economically mobile, they are more likely to participate in the schooling process. If they do not consider school a viable avenue to employment, they will resist the experience.

Ogbu argues that minority students vary in their reactions to school according to their status as subordinated or migrant groups. Ogbu (1987) categorizes minority students into three groups: (1) autonomous minorities, (2) voluntary or immigrant minorities, and (3) involuntary or castelike minorities. *Autonomous minorities* are those who are born in the United States and who do not (or no longer) experience systematic discrimination, despite cultural differences from the mainstream such as religion or culture. Examples of autonomous minorities are Jews and Mormons.

Voluntary or immigrant minorities are groups who voluntarily moved to the United States from all parts of the globe for economic, political, or religious opportunities. They exhibit *primary cultural differences* from mainstream groups, including differences in language use, dress, food preferences, child-rearing, marital practices, and patterns of socializing and leisure. Despite these primary cultural differences, they view schooling as a way to advance socially and economically in this society, and they internalize "folk theories of success" congruent with those of dominant groups. These include viewing hard work and success in school as primary

---

Oliver's Story

Oliver, a 17-year-old from Nicaragua, describes his first day in a California school:

> That first day I went to Westmont, I didn't know what to do because everybody was speaking English and I didn't saw no one or I didn't heard no one speaking Spanish. . . . I saw a teacher, he looked to me Spanish. So I talked to him. I told him that I was looking for my classroom and he took me to my classroom and everything. He helped me a lot.

SOURCE: Center for Literary Studies 1992.

means for getting ahead economically. In addition, the immigrants' faith in "the system" is bolstered by the fact that most immigrants can favorably compare their present status in America with their past. No matter how bad their present situation here, life in the United States offers significantly more hope than life in their country of origin. These beliefs are fostered and reinforced among immigrant children by their families and communities.

Involuntary or castelike minorities were incorporated into the society forcibly either through conquest or colonization. African Americans who were enslaved and brought to this country, Mexican Americans who were conquered, American Indians who were conquered and forced onto reservations, and Puerto Rican Americans who were colonized in their own country are all examples of castelike minority groups. Involuntary or castelike minority groups exhibit *secondary cultural differences* from dominant groups. These are not as visible as primary differences; they developed *after* the castelike minority was forced into a subordinate status and can be thought of as coping mechanisms developed to address the psychological, political, economic, and social conflict inherent in interaction with the dominant culture.

Groups such as American Indians and African Americans have a long history of subordination and oppression in this society. They have had few opportunities to develop the favorable comparisons with U.S. society that immigrants construct; already at the bottom of the socioeconomic ladder, they can only compare up, to the unattainable status of more favored ethnic groups. Even though they may pay lip service to American myths about the efficacy of hard work and success in school, their actual experience of racism and oppression prevents them from believing that these efforts lead to socioeconomic success.

Their schooling experiences have involved deculturalization and forced assimilation, including stripping away of their primary language and culture. In place of indigenous ethnic identities, Ogbu suggests that castelike minorities

> appear to develop a new sense of social identity in opposition to the social identity of the dominant group after they have become subordinated, and they do so in reaction to the way that dominant-group members treat them in social, political, economic, and psychological domains. (1987, p. 323)

Fordham and Ogbu (1986; Fordham 1991) argue that involuntary minority students may engage in "cultural inversion," or resistance to the cultural behaviors and language forms of the dominant culture. They adopt cultural behaviors that specifically differentiate them from the dominant group. Getting good grades, speaking standard English, and listening to "white" music may be construed by their peers as "acting white"; speaking Black vernacular English, listening to rap music, being truant, and failing classes are oppositional behaviors which could be classified as secondary cultural differences. They also constitute a form of habitus (Bourdieu and Passeron 1977), or way of justifying why they do or do not succeed in the white man's world.

Fordham and Ogbu state that involuntary minority groups face a "job ceiling" constructed by a racist American society, which puts a limit on their economic opportunities, even if they are academically successful. In her ethnographic study of "Capital High School," located in a predominantly African-American section of Washington,

D.C., Fordham (1991) found that many students did poorly because they had difficulty reconciling school achievement and maintenance of African-American cultural identity. She found that the "fictive kinship" or sense of peoplehood of the African-American students she studied was a compelling reason for them to assign more importance to success with their peers and community than to success in the school community. Fordham said she was "flabbergasted" by the amount of resistance to "acting white" she found among the African-American students in her study. "I never believed it would be so pervasive, and so pronounced, and so academically stifling," she said in an interview (Schmidt 1993).

Although some researchers believe that Ogbu's typology does not fully characterize all minority groups (Deyhle 1991), his categorization nonetheless is useful because it provides a viable explanation why some groups succeed in school despite vast differences in language patterns and cultural understandings and why others with languages and cultures closer to those of European Americans fail. Also it is important to recognize that the negative responses of some minority students do not necessarily apply to all individuals. We would be stereotyping if we thought that all African Americans resisted schooling because it could be considered "acting white," or if we expected all immigrant minority students to succeed in school. These theories merely provide us with a way to consider the sociocultural and historical background students bring to school.

School Success through Accommodation

Some minority students succeed in school through *accommodation,* a process by which they maintain their ethnic identity while at the same time adopting whatever behaviors of the mainstream society they see as appropriate.

This process is illustrated in Gibson's (1988) study of a California high school where the Punjabi Sikh immigrant students were more serious about school and attained higher academic achievement than their European-American classmates. Gibson attributes their success to parental expectations as well as to cultural values that placed respect for family and authority at a premium. Punjabi parents urged their children to do well in school so they could compete in American society, but at the same time insisted that they maintain the home cultural values. Maintaining Punjabi cultural traditions earned them ridicule and harassment from non-Punjabi school peers, but family life provided a meaningful haven which not only buffered the prejudice at school but offered a viable cultural alternative to mainstream American life. Thus they were able to be accepted in their home milieu while accommodating to school life.

Student Resistance to School

In Chapter 3 we discussed resistance as a way for students to oppose the culture of the school. Resistance, in the form of acting out, tuning out, or dropping out of school, can be a way for minority students to reject degrading and racist experiences in school. Kunisawa (1988, pp. 62–63) found that the ten states with the highest

Jean's Story

People of rural Appalachia have been discriminated against for decades. I am one of these people. There is a distance between the poor whites and upper-class whites that exists even today. As a child I knew these differences existed, but it was not until I started to school that I learned I was different. I lived in a rural area with no other children to identify with. Going to school in town, the only school in town, was a big step for me. There I learned about culture. Culture, I gathered, was something only the rich could attain or had a right to. I had a culture all my own but did not know this. My culture was not respected by my teachers or peers. Maybe they did not know that I lived in abject poverty not more than ten miles from the school. Maybe they did, but instead of bringing my family's lifestyle to light, I believe now that I was deculturalized. Soon I began to fit the mold, or tried to, although I never did. I had very few friends throughout school who understood my way of life. I could not have friends home from school to sleep over. I could not ask them to sleep in a cold house or to eat what food we had—food they were not used to like fried potatoes, gravy, and biscuits, when we were out of other staples such as beans and meal. I cannot deny that living in poverty has left its scars on me. Had I lived in Kentucky near the Appalachian coal mines, I would have fared better, no doubt, but living in rural Appalachia in east Tennessee, I was a fish out of water.

dropout rates all had minority enrollment exceeding 25 percent, six of them greater than 35 percent. A labor market explanation of these figures would be that these are students from castelike minority groups who do not see school as a viable avenue to economic success.

Resistance is also a way in which minority youth establish their own cultural identity while rejecting dominant-class ideologies embedded in schooling. Social scientists have documented resistance to school through the establishment of peer group cultures in working-class Caribbean, European-American, and African-American communities (e.g., McLaren 1980; McLeod 1987; Willis 1977). Deyhle's (1986) work with Navajo youth illustrates how minority youth resist the imposition of the dominant culture on their lives by forming a peer group centered on break dancing. This group became successful break dancers in an

indifferent or negative school and community environment. As one young breaker explained with a smile, "It used to be cowboys and Indians. Now it is breakers and cowboys." With break dancing they had the motivation to assert themselves and prove to themselves and their peers that they were successful individuals. They worked hard, performed to the delight of many peers, and created a "space," even though it placed them on the fringe. (Deyhle 1986, p. 11)

Through this clique, Navajo youth were able to build self-confidence, achieve success through dancing, and establish an identity that challenged the type encouraged by school personnel.

Critical theorists view this active refusal to adopt the dominant group's beliefs as culture, class, and race resistance to a school-imposed culture which is contrary to their lives (McLaren 1989). They explain school failure of minority students, then, not from the standpoint of individual incompetencies, but from the perspective of a school system that attempts to impose on youth a culture they do not accept as a viable alternative to their own way of life. McLaren argues:

> Teachers must be aware of how school failure is structurally located and culturally mediated, so they can work both inside and outside of schools in the struggle for social and economic justice. Teachers must engage unyieldingly in their attempt to empower students both as individuals and as potential agents of social change by establishing a critical pedagogy that students can use in the classroom and in the streets. (1989, p. 221)

CONFLICTING PURPOSES OF SCHOOLING FOR MINORITY STUDENTS: CULTURAL ASSIMILATION OR CULTURAL PLURALISM?

Throughout the history of American schooling there has been a constant tension between those who believe in schooling for *assimilation* and those who believe in *cultural pluralism.*

Assimilationists believe that schools should teach all groups a common language, cultural heritage, and set of values that are distinctly American. In most cases the notion of the "melting pot" means following a European-American middle-class and upper-class model. As different cultural groups relinquish their ethnic identity, they are assimilated into American culture. The Americanization programs at the turn of the century tried to teach new immigrants the language, customs, and skills needed to fit into mainstream society. That notion is still current, evidenced in the "English only" legislation and the debate over the ongoing Anglocentric versus multicultural curricula.

Those who value cultural pluralism believe that minority groups can maintain their cultural identity while at the same time developing an allegiance to the nation. For example, a cultural pluralist believes that African Americans, Vietnamese, Irish, and Mexicans can retain the supporting benefits of their cultural groups while considering themselves part of a larger American culture. Rather than a "melting pot," one might envision this process as a "stew pot" or a "salad bowl" in which each ingredient maintains its own distinctive characteristics but enriches the final product. Cultural pluralists believe in affirming and celebrating diverse cultures in school policies, practices, and the curriculum. The whole issue of multiculturalism is one that challenges the definition of what it means to be an "American." Schools have long been the contested sites where people struggle with notions of ethnic and national identi-

> Did you ever think of what it feels like choosing a Barbie doll at Toys 'R Us? You know, white girls can choose from thirty Barbie models and black girls have only one.
>
> SOURCE: Teacher education student in children's literature class, quoted by her instructor.

ties. In the final chapter we will explore the issue of multicultural education more fully as we consider alternatives to the way we "do school."

These tensions between assimilationist and pluralist purposes of schooling are crucial to understanding minority student failure. Those who espouse assimilationist views explain this failure in terms of individual incompetency or a failure to take advantage of the educational system. They fail to recognize the limitations of schooling for minority students and end up "blaming the victim." Consequently, they do not question the structure and practices of schooling. Cultural pluralists, on the other hand, attempt to understand minority student culture and alter school practices to meet the needs of all students. Their goals are equality of educational opportunity as well as of economic opportunity. There are also those extremists who believe in neither cultural pluralism nor assimilation. These groups believe that there is no accommodation or compromise possible between their beliefs and those of other groups. They remain a challenge to societies which, however poorly, retain an ideology of tolerance (Burtonwood 1986).

SUMMARY

In this chapter we discussed key terms: race, ethnicity, ethnic minority group, racism, prejudice, and stereotyping. We then traced the development of the role of the federal government in schooling for minority students. In a discussion of research on schooling for minority children, we examined a theory of unequal resources and treatment, a cultural deprivation theory, a cultural differences theory, and a labor market explanation. Recent research illustrates how minority students respond to their schooling experiences through assimilation, accommodation, or resistance.

As you continue your explorations into cultures — your own as well as those of others — you might want to immerse yourself in the literature of various groups. There are wonderful novels and films available that can engage you in the lives of others, portraying the complexities of race/ethnicity, social class, gender, and sexual orientation. You may want to use the lists of multicultural books for children and adults available in current journals (cf., *Democracy and Education*, Winter 1991).

chapter **8**

Gender Equity in Schooling

Chapter Overview

INTRODUCTION

Children's identity as well as their school experiences are shaped by their membership in socioeconomic and/or ethnic minority groups. In Chapters 5 and 7 we demonstrated that students from ethnic minority or low socioeconomic groups have less access to equal educational opportunities than whites and/or students from more privileged social classes. Professionals concerned with equity in education generally direct their attention to the ways in which race, ethnicity, and socioeconomic class affect access and treatment. However, gender also directly affects the experiences children have in schools.

It has been common for researchers to investigate only the separate effects of race, class, and gender on children. More recently, scholars have called for examinations of the ways in which these three categories combine to affect school experiences. While it is impossible to separate out the effects of any of these three factors with real people in real schools, we have organized this book to examine each category separately. It is essential, therefore, to remember as you read that each student comes to school *both* as an engendered person *and* with membership in a particular ethnic and social class group.

Equality of Educational Opportunity or Gender Equity?

When we talk about equality of educational opportunity for girls and boys, women and men, we are referring to providing the same educational opportunities, support, and expectations regardless of gender. The implication that school programs will provide for females what they have been providing for males means that women's progress and the excellence of programs for them has been judged in terms of what has been thought standard and good practice for men. It does not examine the unique experiences of boys and girls in order to provide programs, structures, and practices that are geared toward the differing needs of both genders but that are nevertheless fair. This is certainly a beginning, but not nearly enough. The term *gender equity* goes beyond equality of educational opportunity. Maxine Greene argues:

> To work for sex equity in education and the social order as a whole is to move to alter the oppressiveness that makes individual autonomy antithetical to social concern. It is to rediscover what it signifies to be a person and a woman, while discovering what it signifies to transform. (1985, p. 42)

Understanding the Terms *Sex* and *Gender*

As a prelude to our discussions of school experiences based on gender, we need to clarify some terms. **Sex** and **gender** do not carry the same meaning and therefore are not interchangeable. *Sex,* a visible and usually permanent identifying attribute which is acquired at birth, refers to the physical characteristics associated with being male or female. *Gender* is a more inclusive term which refers not only to physiological characteristics but to learned cultural behaviors and understandings. Historian Joan Wallach Scott reminds us that usage of the word *gender*

> seems to have first appeared among American feminists who wanted to insist on the fundamentally social quality of distinctions based on sex. The word denoted a rejection of the biological determinism implicit in the use of such terms as "sex" or "sexual difference." . . . Instead, gender becomes a way of denoting "cultural constructions"—the entirely social creation of ideas about appropriate roles for women and men. It is a way of referring to the exclusively social origins of the subjective identities of men and women. Gender is, in this definition, a social category imposed on a sexed body. (1988, pp. 31–32)

Another useful perspective on the differences between sex and gender is quoted in *A Feminist Dictionary:*

> Gender is often used as a synonym for *sex,* i.e. biological male or femaleness. However, it is also used, particularly by contemporary writers, to refer to the socially imposed dichotomy of masculine and feminine roles and character traits. Sex is physiological, while gender, in the latter usage, is cultural. The distinction is a crucial one, and one which is ignored by unreflective supporters of the status quo who assume that cultural norms of masculinity and femininity are "natural," i.e. directly and preponderantly determined by biology. (Warren 1980, p. 181, quoted in Kramarae and Treichler 1985, pp. 173–174)

Recent scholarship has used *gender* as a synonym for "women" (Scott 1988). The title of this chapter, "Gender Equity in Schooling," may be seen as an example of this use. Though much of our discussion here is centered on the experiences of girls and women, we need to remember that these experiences are in relation to those of boys and men, so as you read the chapter, be sure to consider what the research shows for *all* children in school settings.

Gender Socialization and Differential Treatment

Children's gender determines the ways in which they are socialized, first by their families and later by school personnel, to learn what are considered to be appropriate male and female roles. Different patterns of behavior are learned by boys and girls through interaction with their primary caretakers and peers. Sex role stereotyping occurs when children are socialized to behave primarily in ways that are considered to be gender appropriate. For example, girls may be encouraged to be nurturing and cooperative, while boys may be encouraged to be aggressive and competitive. These socialization patterns lead to different and unequal expectations for males and females in this society.

The differential patterns of socialization and treatment in schools puts females in a position very similar to that of disadvantaged minority groups. Although females constitute 51 percent of the U.S. population, they do fit our definition of minority status. You will recall that attributes of minority group status were identifiability, differential power, differential treatment, and group awareness (Dworkin and Dworkin 1982). Hacker (1951), one of the first sociologists to utilize an understanding of race relations to create a theoretical framework for examining gender relationships, argued for the inclusion of women in minority group studies. Similarities between women and ethnic minorities in terms of group visibility, discrimination in the labor market, stereotypes attributed to them by majority members, and their accommodation to such treatment suggest that knowledge from other minority groups could be helpful in understanding women (Dworkin and Dworkin 1982).

Research data clearly illustrate that the treatment females receive in schools is neither the same as nor equal to that given males, just as other categories considered to be minorities—the socioeconomically disadvantaged, handicapped, and culturally different—also receive unequal treatment from members of the mainstream, able-bodied middle class. Despite a growing body of literature detailing sexist practices in schools, gender is a sorely neglected category in recent reform literature calling for equity and excellence in schooling. Tetreault and Schmuck (1985) report that gender is virtually ignored as an equity issue in schooling by at least eight of the major commission reports. They argue:

> Gender is not a relevant category in the analysis of excellence in schools. When gender was considered, it appears to merely embellish the traditional—and male—portrait of the school. The proposed vision for excellence in the schools is of education for the male student in the public and productive sphere. Because gender, as a relevant concept, is absent, even Title IX is ignored. Issues of gender in relation to policy, students, curricula, and faculty are not identified nor treated as educational problems to be solved. The goal of excellence does not even have the female student in mind. (1985, p. 63)

An analysis of 35 reports issued by commissions and special task forces regarding education reform revealed that 60 percent had a female membership of less than 30 percent. In addition, few of the reports defined educational issues in terms of gender or suggested recommendations for changes regarding women's issues (AAUW 1992).

This chapter focuses on gender issues related to equality of educational opportunity, gender equity, and differential outcomes in academic achievement and economic opportunities for men and women. We will first discuss how the socialization process acts to construct gender roles in American society. Next is a discussion of sexism and the legislation designed to fight sexist practices in educational institutions. We will then provide an overview of how sexist practices are still evident in both the formal and hidden curricula of schooling. Finally we will discuss how sexism makes the outcomes of schooling—academic achievement and occupational placement—different for males and females. Despite two decades of feminist activism, research detailing discriminatory practices in schools, and legislation designed to ensure equality of access and treatment, females in this society do *not* have equal access to educational and economic opportunities because of their status as women. The chapter ends with a discussion of feminism and the ways we can use feminist theories to understand schooling.

THE DEVELOPMENT OF GENDER ROLES — *Sources of "sex-role socialization"?*

Children learn what it means to belong to any society through a socialization process which begins in infancy. Interacting verbally and nonverbally with family members and other caretakers, they learn behavior appropriate to the cultural norms. As part of this process, they learn how to be males and females (Maccoby 1966; Maccoby and Jacklin 1974).

In a summary of research on sex role differences, Lee and Gropper (1974) report that males and females are socialized to different lifestyles through child-rearing practices which entail differential expectations. Despite learning a common language, they differ in their verbal and nonverbal expressions. They are socialized to belong to sex-segregated social groups, wear gender-appropriate clothing, prefer activities and toys associated with one sex or another, and develop different competencies based on those activities. As we see from Lisa's story (see box on p. 254), by the age of 4, children see the sexes as opposite and understand concepts of "girls' things" and "boys' things." In preschool and kindergarten, even in the 1980s, girls are more likely to be found playing in the doll corner while boys spend their time with the building blocks and trucks. By 6 or 7, children have a clear idea about gender roles, prefer sex-segregated play, and tend to strive to conform with stereotypic gender roles. In children between 8 and 10, researchers have found more flexibility in notions about occupational roles for men and women. There is somewhat less sex segregation in their play during this period, but they still tend to prefer same-sex play. In early adolescence girls and boys tend to adhere more rigidly to stereotypic gender roles (AAUW 1992).

Television and other media play a crucial role in transmitting the culture's sex role behaviors and values. Children watch television and movies, listen to popular music, and are confronted daily with advertisements—in magazines, in newspapers, on TV, on buses. Popular culture transmits messages about the values, behaviors, and communication styles of men and women, generally in stereotyped and often derogatory forms. We need only flip through the pages of popular magazines to see the gender models offered to young people.

Find images of gender roles in current examples of popular culture. Compare them to examples found in media from the 1940s, 1950s, and 1960s.

Lisa's Story

I overhead the following conversation between two four-year-old male children at the local child development center. The first child has very liberal parents and they allow him to dress himself in the morning for school. This child has an older female sibling and decided to wear one of her pink shirts. The second child looked at the first child's shirt and said, "You have on a pink shirt and I know that is a girl color. You look like a girl! Boys wear blue." The first child argued, "No, I am not a girl." At this point I casually mentioned that all different kinds of people like different colors. I added, "Look, my shirt is blue and I'm a girl, and Joey (my husband) has a pink shirt that is one of his favorites." The children listened to what I had to say and then decided to play in a different area of the classroom.

Children's literature has always played a crucial role in the socialization process as well. Those of us who grew up in the 1950s and 1960s vividly remember the Nancy Drew mysteries, with Nancy fearlessly stepping into dangerous situations. Nancy provided a courageous, intelligent female role model for young women. In contrast, in a recent study about a current series of children's books, The Baby-sitters Club Books, Jill Goodman (1993) found that the girls there were depicted as selfless, capable of balancing untold family burdens and responsibilities, and constantly nagged by guilt. Since the series was first printed in 1986, over 78 million Baby-sitters Club Books have been printed, most sold to girls between 8 and 12. Goodman captures the main message of the series: "Life's work is assigned according to gender, and women's work is caring, nurturing, worrying about relations, making things right, and feeling guilty" (p. 10). In addition to reading the books, children caught up in the world of the Baby-sitters Club can watch Baby-sitters Club videos, play with Baby-sitters Club dolls, and use Baby-sitters Club cosmetics, backpacks, and sleeping bags (Goodman 1993). This bombardment of values is a powerful socializer for young women.

How were you socialized to become a man or woman? What toys did you play with as a child? What books did you read? Were there gender messages in these? What messages about gender roles were you given from parents, teachers, and other adults as you were growing up? What messages do you receive today from the media and popular culture about men's and women's roles in society?

Lyn Mikel Brown and Carol Gilligan (1992), along with colleagues at the Harvard Project on the Psychology of Women and the Development of Girls, have made major contributions to our understanding of ways girls are socialized from childhood through adolescence. In *Meeting at the Crossroads: Women's Psychology and Girls' Development*, Brown and Gilligan explore the lives of young girls through extensive interviews, documenting a silencing of their voices as they move through adolescence:

> For girls at adolescence to say what they are feeling and thinking often means to risk, in the words of many girls, losing their relationships and finding themselves powerless and all alone. Over the years of our study, even as they became more sophisticated cognitively and emotionally, young girls who had been outspoken and courageous in both an ordinary and a heroic sense became increasingly reluctant to say what they were feeling and thinking or to speak from their own experience about what they knew. Honesty in relationships began to seem "stupid"—it was called "selfish" or "rude" or "mean." (1992, p. 217)

The researchers found that as young girls begin to understand the relational cost of expressing real thoughts and feelings, they respond by silencing themselves and behaving in ways considered more appropriate for "good little girls." They may hide their thoughts or feelings so as to avoid hurting people or risking relationships.

> [As] girls mature and enter mid-adolescence, their voices become more tentative and conflicted. Their responses reveal a sometimes debilitating tension between caring for themselves and caring for others, between their understanding of the world and their awareness that it is not appropriate to speak or act on this understanding. (AAUW 1992, p. 12)

What are the implications of the Brown and Gilligan study for girls in middle and high schools? How can this information about girls' development influence classroom interactions and expectations of young women?

A national survey by the AAUW in 1990 addressed the issue of self-esteem in children and adolescents and found that 69 percent of males and 60 percent of girls in elementary schools reported being "happy the way I am." The same question given to high school students produced a significant drop in the positive response—46 percent of males and 29 percent of females. These data varied across ethnic lines at both elementary and high school levels. In the elementary group 55 percent of white girls, 65 percent of African-American girls, and 68 percent of Hispanic girls reported being "happy the way I am." In high school the numbers declined, with 22 percent of white girls, 30 percent of Hispanic girls, and 58 percent of African-American girls agreeing with the statement. The authors are quick to point out that the African-American girls did not have high levels of self-confidence when it came to academics (AAUW 1992).

EQUALITY OF EDUCATIONAL OPPORTUNITIES FOR WOMEN

Differential socialization patterns in the society lead to differences in the goals of schooling for males and females. Men and women are expected to play different roles and are trained to fulfill these roles. These roles change with social and economic changes in society. One way to examine changes in the purposes of schooling for women is to look at the dramatic changes that have taken place in educational practices since the turn of the century. The following fictional vignettes, based on actual experiences, provide a sense of what schools were like for American women since the early part of the twentieth century. The stories, which span three generations of one family, describe school experiences for white, working-class women and consequently do not capture the experiences of women from other social class or cultural backgrounds.

Changes in Twentieth-Century American Schools for Women

Time: *1912*

Place: *A Small Rural High School in East Tennessee.*   Emily, the 15-year-old daughter of a farmer, attends a school which was established in 1903 as a "model" rural school. The school was funded with the help of northern philanthropists for the purpose of training young men in the art of agriculture. The school is expected "to make better and wiser husbandmen of the country boys and more economical and skillful housewives of the farmers' daughters" (local newspaper, July 24, 1903). Emily is very happy attending this school, which offers the skills she will need later in her role as a housewife. There is a department of domestic economy for the girls "consisting of a cooking school and instruction in good substantial and fancy needlework," and in the second-year sewing classes the girls learn "the use of the needle, the highest of the feminine arts."

A U.S. Bulletin report about this school states that "if the subject to be discussed deals with technical phases of agriculture in which they are not interested, the women will meet in another room and discuss some problem of housekeeping. The discussions are made as practical as possible" (Allison 1989). Emily attends many classes in the department of domestic economy with her female classmates. They are becoming proficient in sewing, cooking, and the general management of the household. Emily hopes that soon she will meet a man who will make a good husband and provide a comfortable life for her in this community. She wants her life to revolve around the farm, the home, and the children.

Time: *1956*

Place: *A Neighborhood Elementary School in a Small New Jersey Town.* Emily's granddaughter, Jennifer, lives in a small New Jersey town across the river from Philadelphia. Emily's daughter had moved from East Tennessee with her husband looking for work in the 1940s and settled here. Jennifer is in the third grade at the elementary school just three blocks away from her home. Each day she walks back and forth from school to home twice. Like the rest of the children, she goes home at noon to eat lunch. When she arrives at the school yard in the morning and again after lunch, she uses the entry on the girl's side. The girls' playground is separate from the boys' and about one third the size. The boys usually play football and baseball on their side and the girls jump rope and play hopscotch on theirs. When the bell rings, announcing the time for classes to begin, the girls line up according to class in front of the door on their side of the school yard. The first-grade girls are on the far right and sixth-grade girls on the far left. The boys do the same on the other side of the building.

Jennifer is in the top reading group. She knows this because her group is always called to read first and reads more stories than the other groups. Like everyone who lives in this town, all the characters in Jennifer's reading books have white skin. The boys in the stories play outside, running, playing, and building things. They often help the girls when they get in trouble. The girls tend to play inside quietly with their dolls. Jennifer and her brothers and sisters tend to play much like this at home. She likes to play school and fantasizes about being a teacher when she grows up.

Time: *1962*

Place: *A Junior High School in a Small New Jersey Town.* Jennifer is now in eighth grade at the local junior high school, which is about a mile from her home. In addition to her "regular" school subjects such as English, math, history and science, she takes home economics and physical education. These subjects she takes with other girls. In seventh grade the girls take cooking and in eighth grade they take sewing. The boys take "shop" or industrial arts at this time. The males and females are separated for their gym classes, with girls engaged in such activities as field hockey, lacrosse, and tennis and the boys engaged in football, baseball, and track. Jennifer has joined an after-school club in industrial arts for girls. She has enjoyed making several projects from plastic and wood using the tools and machinery available in the shop. She feels that it isn't fair for the girls in the school to be excluded from the regular shop classes during the school day and petitions the administration to open these classes to both sexes. Unfortunately, despite the support of other students and the shop teacher, Jennifer's request is denied on the basis that females do not need to learn the skills offered in the industrial arts program.

Time: *1966*

Place: *A High School in the Same Town of New Jersey.* Jennifer dreams of becoming an elementary school teacher. She believes that teaching and nursing are the occupations open to her. In teaching, she would be able to have a career and still marry and raise a family. Jennifer's parents, who did not attend college, have never talked with her about going on for further educational or career pursuits. They expect that she will marry and raise a family as her mother did. Jennifer would like to go to a state teacher's college but doesn't know how to begin the process. She talks with the guidance counselor at her school, Mr. Jones, who is surprised at her interest in college. He discourages her from this pursuit, knowing that her parents do not have the money to support a college education. Jennifer is surprised and hurt that Mr. Jones does not seem willing to help her. She knows that her grades are good; she has earned high scores on her SATs and has been a member of the National Honor Society. She has not been involved in school activities because she worked four hours every day after school and six hours each Saturday. She remembers last year when her sewing teacher gave her a "D" one grading period for not modeling a knitted sweater she made in the school fashion show. It was an evening she was committed to work.

Jennifer decides to apply to college without help from the counselor. She uses the money she has saved for the five applications she sends and is pleased that spring to receive acceptances from those colleges.

Time: *1988*

Place: *A Large Suburban High School in East Tennessee.* Jennifer's daughter, Susan, is now a senior at a sprawling suburban high school in East Tennessee, the home of her maternal grandmother. Jennifer decided to move the family back to Tennessee following her divorce. Her love of the family's original home place precipitated this move. Susan attends the same school that her great-grandmother attended in the early part of the century, but there is now a newly built, consolidated high school in its place. Much has changed since her great-grandmother attended classes here. Susan is offered the same choices as the male students. All students are able to take whatever subjects they choose and join whatever clubs and sports they want. Susan is the editor of the school newspaper and is also involved with a variety of school activities. She intends to go on to college but has not decided on a field of study. She was encouraged by the recruiters on College Night to pursue studies in law, medicine, computers, veterinary science, and engineering. Whatever she decides, she looks forward to a profession that will be challenging and rewarding.

Time: *1994*

Place: *A Large University in the Southeast.* Last year Susan completed a B.A. degree in Liberal Arts. She began college with a major in the sciences, hoping to go to veterinary school after completing her undergraduate degree. After the first two years she took courses in several different programs and finally switched her major to anthropology. She felt that she didn't belong in the sciences. She enjoyed some of the coursework but seemed to have difficulty making connections with her teachers. She met with her professors only when it was time to get advice on her schedule. Susan had little contact with the one woman professor in the program. In anthropology she was excited about the courses and felt that the professors were supportive and interested in her.

Now Susan is in a Master's program in anthropology, but doesn't really know what she wants to do with this degree. She has been toying with the idea of going into education. She has always liked working with young children and believes that her anthropology and sociology courses have helped her become interested in people who come from a wide variety of backgrounds. She thinks she would like to try teaching in an inner-city school but hasn't had much experience working with kids from the city. Since she relied on her mother's support all through college, she feels increased pressure to be financially independent. She has heard that teachers don't make much money, but teaching would be a challenge.

What do you think Susan will decide to do about her career? What are some possible explanations for Susan's change in major in undergraduate school? How do your experiences compare with Susan's?

These short vignettes illustrate some of the changes that have taken place for women. Does this mean that discrimination based on gender differences no longer exists? Unfortunately, although sexism is less explicitly practiced, it is still evident in American society. Female students like Susan often *believe* that they will have complete and equal access to educational and economic opportunities. Expectations about the role of men and women have changed considerably since the turn of the century. Particularly as a result of the feminist movement of the 1970s and 1980s, there is greater consciousness about gender-based inequity and subsequent expansion of opportunities for women. However, sexism is still evident in this society; it has just become more subtle.

What Is Sexism?

cf. other defs. we've used— "system of advantage" base on se

Sexism refers to "a social relationship in which males denigrate females" (Humm 1990, pg. 202) or to "discrimination against women, as in restricted career choices, job opportunities, etc." (Webster's New Universal Unabridged Dictionary 1992). Sexism, analogous to racism, is the belief that women are inferior to men and justifies discrimination based on gender. Sexism is generally used to describe prejudice against females, although it "indicates any arbitrary stereotyping of males and females on the basis of their gender" (Guidelines . . . in McGraw-Hill . . . Publications 1980, p. 346).

It is important for us as educators to understand and confront sexism in the structures, practices, and curricula of schooling. Researchers in the past three decades have examined how sexist practices affect girls' and women's experiences in school settings. We explore this research in more detail through the chapter.

Think about your own schooling experiences. How did being a female or male play a role in these experiences? Have you had experiences in which you felt sexism was involved? You might want to share some of these experiences with classmates.

Federal Legislation Related to Gender Discrimination

In 1972 Congress passed Title IX of the Education Amendments to the Civil Rights Act to address issues of sex discrimination in educational programs that received federal funding. This legislation begins by stating:

> [N]o person in the United States shall, on the basis of sex, be excluded from participation in, be denied the benefits of, or be subjected to discrimination under any education program or activity receiving federal financial assistance.

In other words, any educational institution receiving federal funds must provide equal opportunity for both sexes to participate in all programs and activities of that institution. According to Title IX, practices once common in schools, such as subject area segregation based on gender, are no longer legal. In our story above, the policy that excluded Jennifer from participating in "male" classes such as industrial arts was prohibited by federal legislation after 1972. This legislation was an important force in changing explicit sexist practices in public schools. It has given students like Susan more freedom of choice in their academic and extracurricular programs than their mothers and grandmothers had. Susan's male colleagues likewise are able to enroll in once "female" courses such as cooking.

Despite Title IX, researchers have found that sexist practices still exist in schools. Tetreault (1986) noted that research on sex-role biases in schools in combination with the movement for gender equity in the 1970s and 1980s have resulted in significant changes in the past fifteen years. These changes include increased enrollment of women in science and mathematics, increased expenditures for women's athletic programs, and a higher number of female elementary principals. The use of gender-inclusive language (see Appendix) and inclusion of women in textbooks are also a result of a movement toward sex equity. However, Tetreault argues that despite equal access, separate provisions for male activities continue to be the norm. The different educational needs of men and women are ignored and women are implicitly socialized into "the behaviors of men in the public sphere" (Tetreault 1986). Shakeshaft supports this view:

> [U]nfortunately, few schools provide an equitable culture in which all students and faculty members can grow. Most offer white males more options in an environment that is hospitable to their needs. Females and members of minority groups, on the other hand, must obtain their education in systems

that are at best indifferent and at worst hostile to them. Women and members of minority groups learn that their concerns, their lives, their cultures are not the stuff of schooling. They discover that school is not a psychologically or physically safe environment for them and that they are valued neither by the system nor by society. (Shakeshaft 1986, p. 500)

Women's athletics was particularly affected by Title IX, since it required the funding of athletics programs to be changed significantly. Acosta and Carpenter (1990) reported that the number of sports programs had increased over the intervening eighteen years, enabling more women to participate at all levels. The number of young women participating in high school athletics rose from 4 percent in 1972 to 26 percent in 1987 (AAUW 1992).

However at the collegiate level women's programs consistently receive less funding and have less adequate facilities than those of men. There has also been a significant decrease in the number of women coaches. Prior to Title IX 90 to 100 percent of coaches on women's teams were female, but by 1990 the percentage had dropped to 47.3 percent. In 1972, 90 percent of women's intercollegiate sports programs were under the directorship of a female athletic director; in 1990 this percentage had dropped to 5.9 percent. Women today hold only about 32 percent of the administrative positions in women's collegiate sports programs (Acosta and Carpenter 1990). Veri argues:

This decrease was marked by the removal of previously established female coaches and administrators and fewer opportunities for women to enter the field in those capacities. These opportunities decreased because colleges and universities chose to instead place men in those positions. In essence, it was male sports leaders' reactions to women's increased athletic participation that caused women to become victims of yet another backlash. (1993, p. 15)

GENDER DIFFERENCES IN THE FORMAL CURRICULUM

The formal school curriculum serves as the core for the daily activities of teachers and students. Earlier in this chapter we described a school in 1903 which proudly prescribed a separate curriculum for males and females so that they could be prepared for the work they would be doing after high school. Girls were taught homemaking and needlecrafts and boys were schooled in the science of agriculture. This separate curriculum reflected the supposed needs and values of the community at that time. Today, because of changed perceptions of gender roles, Title IX of the Elementary and Secondary Education Act mandates that schools must permit males and females to study the same curriculum. However, in reality, gender-based differential patterns of enrollment in courses, different patterns of treatment for men and women in classes, and inequities in how women are portrayed in the formal curricular content still exist.

Banks & Banks
ch 6 ?
"Girls are the only
group that starts
out ahead + ends
up behind" i.e.

Gender-Identified Subject Matter

Tradition categorizes curricular content areas by gender. Math, science, and many of the vocational areas (auto shop, woodworking, drafting) historically have been considered by educators, parents, and students as more appropriate for males. The humanities and a few vocational courses (bookkeeping, typing, shorthand, cosmetology) are perceived to be more relevant for females. Gender differences according to subject matter continue, particularly in math and the sciences.

Although there is little gender difference in enrollment in beginning science and math, these differences do emerge at the more advanced levels. More men than women take higher-level courses (AAUW 1992). Fewer women enroll in the most advanced math courses in secondary schools (Fennema and Leder 1990). A 1991 survey by the Council of Chief State School Officers reported that 60 percent of the high school students enrolled in first-year physics and 70 percent of the second-year students are male. A 1987 report prepared for the Committee on Research in Mathematics, Science, and Technology Education reports that males spend more time on microcomputers and are more likely to participate in after-school computer-related activities. More males than females take computer programming courses and go on to high-paying positions in the computer industry. The authors of this report attribute these inequalities to a belief that quantitative fields are a male domain.

Sorensen and Hallinan (1987) studied 1,477 students in 48 fourth- to sixth-grade classes in ten public schools to determine the effects of gender on ability-grouped math classes. Analyzing standardized achievement test scores, the researchers found that females are more likely to be assigned to the wrong ability group than males. Girls with high aptitude in math were less likely to be assigned to high-ability math groups than boys with similar aptitudes. Sorensen and Hallinan suggest that the teachers' placement decisions "may reveal" discrimination based on gender expectations. This study supports the notion that quantitative subjects "belong" to males.

Girls tend to have less confidence in their math abilities than do boys (AAUW 1992). Fennema and Sherman (1977) found a drop in girl's confidence in math during middle elementary school, preceding a decrease in their academic achievement. It is not difficult to understand how lack of confidence would be a serious obstacle to continued pursuit of a subject.

In a Michigan study on physical education, students reported gender bias in their perceptions of sports activities. All sports were seen as male domains with the exception of gymnastics, jumping rope, figure skating, and cheerleading. Despite legal requirements for gender equity in programs, this study found that 70 percent of the school districts surveyed did not provide girls with athletic opportunities comparable to those available for boys (AAUW 1992).

Gender-Based Staffing

Segregation of the curriculum along gender lines is evident in the staffing of these courses. Since more men than women go into areas of quantitative subject matter, more men teach in these areas. Kelly and Nihlen (1982) report that teaching staffs are segregated by subject matter, with women predominant in language arts, foreign languages, and to some extent social sciences, while men dominate the math, science, computer, and engineering courses. Gender differences by subject matter reinforce to students the already clear message about what is "appropriate" knowledge for males and females.

In higher education, college classrooms are still predominantly taught by men, particularly at the senior ranks. Recent figures show that 90 percent of the full professors on U.S. campuses are male, compared with 91 percent a decade ago (Sadker, Sadker, and Klein 1986). Women at the post-secondary level find fewer female role models in the college classroom or curriculum.

Portrayal of Women in Curricular Materials

The way in which females have been depicted in textbooks has changed since the early 1970s. Feminist criticism of curricular materials has pushed publishers to portray female characters in more diverse roles. Whereas Jennifer was provided with a limited number of female role models in her texts—teachers, nurses, and housewives—her daughter Susan was more likely to read texts depicting women as doc-

---

Ten Quick Ways to Analyze Children's Books for Sexism and Racism

1. *Check the illustrations.* Look for stereotypes. Look for tokenism. Who's doing what (active, leadership roles versus passive, subservient roles)?
2. *Check the story line.* Standard for success (via "white" behavior or extraordinary abilities). Resolution of problems (are minorities the "problem" or are problems solved by Anglos)?
3. *Look at the lifestyles.* Check for inaccuracies, inappropriate or oversimplified depictions of other cultures such as American Indians.
4. *Consider the relationships between people.* Who has power, exhibits leadership, and solves problems, and how are families depicted?
5. *Note the heroes.* Whose interest is a particular hero serving?
6. *Consider the effects on a child's self-image.*
7. *Consider the author's or illustrator's background.* Assess his or her qualification to write about the topic.
8. *Examine the author's perspective.* Look for a particular ethnocentric perspective.
9. *Watch for loaded words.* Look for words with offensive overtones.
10. *Look at the copyright date.* Older books are often more laden with racism than those published more recently.

SOURCE: Council on Interracial Books for Children 1980.   *cf. pp. 14–16 in ROC*

tors, telephone repair personnel, and scientists. However, although change in the portrayal of women in textbooks can be observed, "rarely is there dual and balanced treatment of women and men, and seldom are women's perspectives and cultures presented on their own terms" (AAUW 1992, p. 62).

In an evaluation of recent editions of six popular basal reading texts, Hitchcock and Tompkins (1987) determined the number of male and female main characters as well as the range and frequency of occupations for female characters. Out of 1,121 stories, females were portrayed in 37 occupations, compared with 5 occupations in 1961–1963 readers and 23 occupations in 1969–1971 readers. In the recent editions males were main characters in 18 percent of the stories; females, in 17 percent. Surprisingly, the main characters in three times as many stories were now categorized as "other"—neutral characters such as talking trees or neutered characters such as animals. Although there has been some effort to portray women in a variety of occupational roles, Hitchcock and Tompkins argue that textbook publishers appear to be avoiding questions of sexism by creating neutral characters.

A 1989 national study of book-length works used in high school English courses found only one woman author and no minority authors in the ten most frequently assigned books. Applebee (1989) argues that there has been little change from similar lists in 1907 and 1963, on which required books were dominated by white, male authors.

Tetreault (1986) reported that although publishers have responded to pressure to include women in textbooks, they depict "outstanding women who contributed in areas or movements traditionally dominated by men" (p. 230). She argues that women have been tacked on to a history which continues to be dominated by men's values and perspectives. She calls for a gender-balanced curriculum which also looks at ordinary women's everyday lives in traditional roles as well as their efforts to move beyond these boundaries.

Peggy McIntosh (1983) provides the following curricular typology that we can use to analyze the treatment of women and minorities in texts:

Phase I: Womanless and All-White History

Phase II: Exceptional Women and Persons of Color in History

Phase III: Women and People of Color as Problems, Anomalies, Absences, or Victims in History

Phase IV: Women's Lives or the Lives of People of Color *as* History

Phase V: History Redefined and Reconstructed to Include Us All

Gretchen Wilbur (1991) gives us another way to think about curricula that are gender fair. She argues that a gender-fair curriculum has the following six attributes:

1. It *acknowledges* and affirms variation within and across groups of people.
2. It is *inclusive* in that both females and males can find and identify positive messages about themselves.
3. It is *accurate,* presenting data-based, verifiable information.

4. It is *affirmative* in that it values the worth of individuals and groups.
5. It is *representative* with a balance of multiple perspectives.
6. It is *integrated* in that the experiences, needs, and interests of men and women are woven together. (AAUW 1992)

Using these approaches as well as others may help you analyze your own work as a teacher in providing equitable school experiences for your students.

Choose several 1990s texts at different levels—elementary, middle school, high school, and college. Analyze these texts using McIntosh's typology or Wilbur's list of attributes for gender-fair curricula. You may want to compare them with earlier editions of the texts.

Silences in the Curriculum

"OTHER – ING"

In an examination of the formal curriculum, the most important aspect is not what is *presented* about women, but what is omitted. Curricular silences, that is, what is left out of the text, sends a clear message to students about what is important and what is peripheral knowledge. Research on the portrayal of women in texts indicates that females, rather than sharing central roles with men, are either ignored or relegated to domestic roles (Kelly and Nihlen 1982). A view of women as home workers profoundly affects what is taught, since the focus of the curriculum is to prepare students for future work roles. Schools will never be able to broaden instructional opportunities for women as long as cultural beliefs that men work and women stay at home prevail.

An example of how women are portrayed is found in an analysis of social studies texts for courses such as World and American History. Males dominate these texts. Women's contributions to the labor union or suffrage movement are minimized. Females are portrayed as wives, social workers, nurses, and helpmates to men (Kelly and Nihlen 1982; Treckler 1973), despite the long history of female participation in the professions and even the industrial labor force, especially in wartime. Men are *never* portrayed as caretakers or seen in traditionally female roles, such as secretaries, nurses, or day-care workers. Feminists sardonically note that the word used to describe the course is *his*-tory rather than *her*-story. They call for a rewriting of such courses to include the roles women have played (Scott 1987).

Although more recent textbooks have made efforts to incorporate women's roles, history remains the study of male military matters. Students learn American political history as a chronology of the various wars that were waged from the American Revolution through the Vietnam War. The "failure to integrate female experiences into general curriculum drives home the message that girls and their experiences are somehow 'other,' that they are not part of general literature and history" (Shakeshaft 1986, p. 501).

Select a new social studies textbook at any grade level. Analyze the content of the text for gender differences. How is the text organized? What are the major topics covered? How does the text portray women and women's issues? Compare your findings to a social studies text that is ten or twenty years old.

GENDER IN THE IMPLICIT CURRICULUM

The question of gender equity in the curriculum goes beyond the formal curriculum to incorporate implicit or hidden messages given to students (see Chapter 6 for discussion on the hidden curriculum). This section examines how ideas about sex roles are transmitted every day in schools.

Implicit Messages in the Patriarchy of Schooling

The structure of schooling has been described by educational historians as an "educational harem" (Tyack 1974) because it relies heavily on a hierarchical system in which male administrators manage female teachers and support staff. This harem-like structure remains the norm today, as we have noted in earlier chapters. Principals dominate the policy decisions that affect the daily running of the school, and women often find themselves in subordinate positions. This administrative structure clearly tells students that men hold positions of authority and power in society while women play subordinate roles, having control only over the children in their classrooms.

Implicit Messages in Classroom Organization

The sex of students is often used as an organizational tool for structuring activities. In elementary schools boys and girls are lined up separately to walk to lunch or to the restrooms. Some teachers ask children to read aloud in groups according to gender. Classroom and playground games pit the girls against the boys. Although this practice may seem innocuous, separation by gender as an organizational strategy is unnecessary and results in differential treatment based on gender.

Classroom jobs may be distributed on the basis of teachers' perceptions of appropriate sex roles. In one first-grade classroom (K. P. Bennett 1986) male students were asked to perform the tasks that would take them out of the room, such as delivering messages to the principal's office. These jobs were highly valued by the children and were considered by the teacher to require a higher level of responsibility. Female students were asked to perform chores inside the classroom such as picking up papers, straightening library books, or erasing the blackboard—traditional roles for women. A principal who comes into a classroom asking for "four strong boys" to carry some books is providing a message that boys play active roles and can handle chores that require physical strength, while girls do not.

Shakeshaft reports that research on gender and schooling provides us with two messages: "First, what is good for males is not necessarily good for females. Second, if a choice must be made, the education establishment will base policy and instruction on that which is good for males" (Shakeshaft 1986, p. 500). She argues that the school organization would better fit the needs of females if single-sex rather than coeducational schools were available. This argument is based on research findings that females perform better in single-sex schools than in coeducational ones. They exhibit higher self-esteem, are more involved in the academic life of the school, and have greater involvement in a broad range of social and leadership activities. Males do well in both single-sex and coeducational schooling (Shakeshaft 1986).

Shakeshaft argues that both the structure and curriculum of schools mirror male rather than female development. Although females mature earlier, are ready for verbal and math skills at a younger age, and have control of small motor skills sooner, classrooms are structured to meet the needs of males, who tend to develop at a slower pace. This pattern, coupled with research that shows that male students get a larger proportion of attention from and interaction with the teacher (Sadker and Sadker 1985; Shakeshaft 1986), puts female students in a difficult position. "Some grow bored, others give up, but most learn to hold back, be quiet, and smile" (Shakeshaft 1986, p. 500).

Implicit Messages in Instructional Techniques

Schools rely on what Goldman and McDermott (1987) refer to as a "culture of competition." This competition can be in the form of grades, classroom games and activities, or simply the amount of time it takes to finish a task. Despite a recent emphasis on peer tutoring and cooperative learning techniques, classrooms are usually structured so that children work individually. The stress on individual accomplishment sets up a culture of competition in which there is constant comparison of students' abilities by teachers and by students themselves. A hierarchy based upon achievement is established as classmates interact with each other and develop an understanding of others' work habits, skills, and abilities. If you were to ask first graders to name the best and worst readers in their classroom, they would have little difficulty in so doing. As we have indicated earlier, this hierarchy is duplicated in friendship groups and the organization of high school peer structures. The use of competition in schools is taken for granted by educators as the way to "do school." — *Business as usual*

In a study of high school extracurricular activities, Eder and Parker (1987) found that athletic programs encouraged males to be aggressive, achievement oriented, and competitive. Cheerleading, which was more highly valued for women than athletics, served to remind girls of the importance of being attractive. Traditional male and female roles—competition for men and emotional management (caretaking) for women—were the values integral to these activities.

Competition as an instructional strategy is problematic for female students, who tend to prefer connection and collaboration and to value relationships with others as central to their activities (Shakeshaft 1986). Competition is a threat to these relationships. Since so much of what is done in schools is based on competition, females often find themselves in an uncomfortable or alienating environment. Belenky et al. (1986) emphasize the need for building patterns of connection and collaboration into learning environments in order to facilitate women's development.

Implicit Messages in Classroom Interactions

Research on gender differences in classroom interaction demonstrates that males verbally dominate classrooms at all levels of schooling, despite the gender of the teacher (Brophy and Good 1970; Martin 1972; Sikes 1971). In a study by Sadker and Sadker (1985) a team of researchers observed more than a hundred fourth-, sixth-, and eighth-grade classes in four states and Washington, D.C. Half of these classes were in English and language arts and the other half were in science and math. The researchers found that teachers, regardless of gender and ethnic background, asked more questions of white males, and male students talked more than female students at a ratio of three to one. The Sadkers found that as the school year progressed, the participation and assertiveness of the males in the classrooms increased. Boys would "grab teachers' attention" by calling out answers, which then were accepted by teachers. When girls called out answers, they were more likely to be reprimanded for inappropriate behavior. As a consequence, girls sat patiently with their hands raised waiting to be called on. The study reports that males were eight times more likely to call out answers to teachers' questions. The Sadkers argue that through this type of interaction, teachers socialize males to be academically assertive and girls to assume a more traditional role of sitting quietly.

The Sadkers use the term "mind sex" (as opposed to "mind *set*") to describe the pattern of teachers' repeatedly calling on students of the same sex. For example, if the teacher asks a question of a male student, the next several questions will be likely to be addressed to male students. They found this serial pattern to be more pronounced for male students and suggested that this practice may be influenced by the self-selected sex segregation in seating patterns in more than half the classes they observed.

Male students receive more attention of all kinds by teachers—more praise, more time, but also more reprimands and harsher discipline (LaFrance 1985; Lippitt and Gold 1959; Sikes 1971). The attention given to males is much different from that given to females. For example, the Sadkers found that teachers were more likely to assist boys performing a difficult task, but more likely to do the entire task for the girls. As a consequence, girls learn not to confront challenging work. Also teachers give more criticism to males, so they learn to handle it better.

Female students are neither reprimanded nor praised but tend to be ignored in classrooms. This is particularly true of high-achieving females, who receive the least attention of all students. As both majority and minority females learn that their opinions are not valued and their answers are not worthy of attention, they come to believe they are not smart or important (Grant 1984; Hall and Sandler 1982; LaFrance 1985). If they do well in school, they attribute their success to luck or hard work rather than to their own abilities. School interactions "reinforce societal messages that females are inferior" (Shakeshaft 1986, p. 501).

Bonnie's Observations

During a classroom curriculum development class, we were shown a video meant to display a particular method of teaching. In one of the segments a female teacher was presenting a lesson to elementary school students. The teacher called on three boys in a row. My interest was piqued and I began to take a tally of how many times the female teacher called on male versus female students—things I've begun doing since I started your class! The results amazed and saddened me. Boys and girls alike raised their hands to all questions. A total of fourteen boys were called on, versus four girls. To make matters worse, the boys were encouraged and asked multiple questions; girls were not. I know this has been discussed in class and I have always agreed with the findings of teacher preference toward male students. However, I have never observed this behavior. Seeing this did make a strong impression on me. I am sure the teacher was completely unaware of her favoritism. The class viewing the video was oblivious to this behavior.

Observe a classroom. Count the number of males and females, and note the gender of the teacher. Keep track of the number of times the teacher calls on males and females. Note the types of questions asked of male and female students. Try to document how much time is provided to students according to gender. What are some of the gender-related patterns you see in this classroom?

Gender differences also exist in the ways men and women interact in social settings outside the academic world. Men speak more often than women and frequently interrupt them. Women are less active verbal participants in conversations, but they provide supportive and passive nonverbal cues by smiling and gazing at the speaker (Duncan and Fiske 1977; LaFrance and Mayo 1978). Researchers found that listeners recall more from male speakers than from females even when the content is identical and the style is similar.

Women may seem unsure or less competent in their comments because they often transform a declarative statement into a tentative comment by adding a tag question such as "isn't it" or qualifiers such as "I guess." To listeners this habit signals lack of power and influence (Sadker and Sadker 1985). Another interesting interpretation of this practice was provided by McIntosh (1988), who argues that such qualifiers serve to signal equality or the lack of a power differential between the speaker and the listener. By not appearing to be an all-knowing authority, the woman can encourage an equal exchange of information between the listener and the speaker.

Sociolinguist Deborah Tannen argues that conversation between men and women is cross-cultural communication. In her book, *You Just Don't Understand* (1990), she provides detailed accounts of the ways we miscommunicate or misunderstand one another because men and women live in two different worlds. Tannen differentiates between the "report talk" of men and the "rapport talk" of women. In report talk, the purpose of the conversation is to maintain independence, to establish social status, and to convey information directly and concisely. In the rapport talk of women, the purpose of the conversation is to build rapport, develop relationships, and establish connections, with little emphasis on status.

Read Tannen's book. How do the communication style differences she describes help you understand your own communication across gender lines?

Sexist Language in Schools

Sexist language is one way in which gender stereotypes continue to affect beliefs and attitudes about women. Although educators have become more aware of sexist language, it persists in many American schools. It is not uncommon for elementary bulletin boards to portray community helpers as "firemen" and "policemen." Social studies and science courses refer to "mankind" or "man's contributions to science." LaFrance argues:

> [O]ne of the more subtle ways teachers contribute to female invisibility in classrooms is by reliance on the generic "he" to refer to both men and women. . . . Theoretically, the generic "he" includes females as well as males, but recent studies show its exclusionary properties. (1985, p. 43)

Many institutions have implemented policies that discourage the use of sexist language, but these guidelines are often ignored. The use of sexist language in schools at any level is unnecessary and potentially debilitating to females. It is another way in which women are socialized to see themselves as subordinate to males.

> When a sexist word is scrawled across the lockers or when a male student uses sexist language, the silence can be deafening. Few teachers even code it as a problem, and many of the insults and put-downs of girls come from teachers and administrators themselves. After all, boys will be boys and girls will continue to receive their schooling in a hostile environment. (Shakeshaft 1986, p. 502)

Sexual Harassment in Schools

The pervasiveness of sexual harassment was dramatically highlighted in the televised hearings over Judge Clarence Thomas's fitness for confirmation as a Supreme Court Justice. His former associate, Professor Anita Hill, accused him of sexual harassment and the Senate Judiciary Committee held hearings on the matter. Attention to the issue has continued, particularly in relation to schools and the work place. Sexual harassment is defined by the Equal Employment Opportunity Commission as:

> Unwelcome sexual advances, request for sexual favors, and other verbal or physical conduct of a sexual nature constitute sexual harassment when (1) submission to such conduct is made either explicitly or implicitly a term or condition of an individual's employment, (2) submission to, or rejection of such conduct by an individual is used as the basis for employment decisions affecting such individual or (3) such conduct has the purpose or effect of unreasonably interfering with an individual's work performance or creating an intimidating, hostile, or offensive working environment. (Eskenazi and Gallen 1992, p. 63)

Sexual harassment, or unwelcome sexual attention, is a form of discrimination that violates Title VII of the 1964 Civil Rights Act, Title IX of the 1972 Education Amendments, and the Civil Rights Act of 1991 (Eskenazi and Gallen 1992). Sexual harassment in school creates an adverse environment for students and can result in embarrassment, fear, inability to concentrate on studies, poor grades, absenteeism, and physical symptoms (Bogart and Stein 1987; Bogart et al. 1992). Researchers Bogart and Stein provide us with several examples of teacher/student sexual harassment:

> A science teacher measured the craniums of the boys in the class, and the chests of the girls. This lesson in skeletal frame measurements was conducted one by one, at the front of the class, by the teacher.
>
> A classroom teacher asked one junior high school girl, in front of the whole class, how far she had gone with her boyfriend, specifically if she had gone to "second" or "third" base with him, and if they had "French kissed."
>
> A group of teachers suspected that one of their younger colleagues had been displaying excessive and inappropriate affection toward some of his students. Included among the behaviors they were concerned about was driving the students in his car, inviting them to his apartment on weekends, and generally doing a lot of touching and group hugging. Although no one had complained, they requested that the headmaster provide some staff training and discussion on appropriate and inappropriate behaviors between staff and students. (Bogart and Stein 1987, p. 151)

In June 1993 the Educational Foundation of the American Association of University Women (AAUW) released a groundbreaking study, *Hostile Hallways: The AAUW Survey on Sexual Harassment in America's Schools*. The study, conducted in February and March of 1993, surveyed representative samples of Hispanic, white, and African-American students in grades 8 through 11 from 79 schools across the United States. One of the primary questions asked is instructive for this discussion because it provides a listing of the types of behaviors considered to be sexual harassment.

During your whole school life, how often, if at all, has anyone (this includes students, teachers, other school employees, or anyone else) done the following things to you *when you did not want them to?*

- Made sexual comments, jokes, gestures, or looks in your presence.
- Showed, gave, or left you sexual pictures, photographs, illustrations, messages, or notes.
- Wrote sexual messages/graffiti about you on bathroom walls, in locker rooms, etc.
- Spread sexual rumors about you.
- Said you were gay or lesbian.
- Spied on you as you dressed or showered at school.
- Flashed or "mooned" you.
- Touched, grabbed, or pinched you in a sexual way.
- Pulled at your clothing in a sexual way.
- Intentionally brushed against you in a sexual way.
- Pulled your clothing off or down.
- Blocked your way or cornered you in a sexual way.
- Forced you to kiss him/her.
- Forced you to do something sexual, other than kissing. (AAUW 1993, p. 5)

AAUW researchers found that sexual harassment is widespread in schools, with *four* out of *five* of the students surveyed reporting some form of sexual harassment experience in school. Reports of harassment by girls across ethnic groups was similar: 82 percent of Hispanics, 84 percent of African Americans, and 87 percent of whites. The percentage of African-American boys (81%) reporting harassment was higher than of whites (75%) and Hispanics (69%). Sexual comments, jokes, gestures, or looks were the most common forms of sexual harassment reported. Touching, grabbing, and/or pinching in a sexual way were the second most common forms. Fifty-seven percent of girls as compared with 36 percent of boys reported having been intentionally brushed up against in a sexual way.

According to the survey, peer harassment is much more common than harassment by adults in school settings. Of the students who reported harassment incidents, only 18 percent were harassed by a school employee, one in four girls (25%) and one in ten boys (10%). More African-American girls (33%) reported being sexually harassed by an adult school employee than Hispanics (17%) or whites (25%). One interesting finding concerned students that were perpetrators of sexual harassment. Thirty-seven percent of them reasoned: "It's just part of school life/A lot of people do it/It's no big deal." Very few of the students had reported any incidents of harassment to adults. Only 7 percent said they told a teacher about the experience. Students were far more likely to confide in their peers—63 percent of sexually harassed students told a friend (49% boys and 77% girls).

Nan Stein argues that peer harassment in schools is often overlooked by teachers and administrators, who view it as "flirting" or as a normal stage of adolescent development. She explains:

> Sexual harassment in schools operates in full and plain view of others. Boys harass girls with impunity while people watch. Examples of sexual harassment that happen in public include attempts to snap bras, grope at girls' bodies, pull down gym shorts, or flip up skirts; circulating "summa cum slutty" or "piece of ass of the week" lists; designating special weeks for "grabbing the private parts of girls"; nasty, personalized graffiti written on bathroom walls; sexualized jokes, taunts, and skits that mock girls' bodies performed at school sponsored pep rallies, assemblies, or half-time performances during sporting events; and outright physical assault and even rape in schools. (Stein 1994, p. 2)

Stein argues that teasing and bullying behaviors learned and practiced in elementary school are antecedents to peer harassment in high school. She is currently developing a bullying and teasing curriculum for elementary schools that will help teachers engage students in confronting the problem by developing a vocabulary to talk about what are appropriate and inappropriate or hurtful behaviors. These discussions can serve as springboards for later understanding about sexual harassment in middle and high school (Stein 1994).

Sexual harassment in school seems to take a greater toll on girls than on boys. The AAUW survey indicated that 33 percent of the girls reported that they did not want to attend school after an experience of harassment. The finding varied by ethnicity; more African-American girls (39%) than Hispanics (29%) or whites (33%) responded in this way. Only 12 percent of the boys surveyed responded that a harassment incident made them want to stay away from school. Authors of the study conclude that "parents, teachers, and administrators must acknowledge that sexual

---

Sexual Harassment by Peers in a Public High School

It came to the point where I was skipping almost all of my classes, therefore getting kicked out of the honors program. It was *very* painful for me. I dreaded school each morning, I started to wear clothes that wouldn't flatter my figure, and I kept to myself. I never had a boyfriend that year. I'd cry every night I got home, and I thought I was a total loser. . . . Sometimes the teachers were right there when it was going on. They did nothing. . . . I felt very angry that these arrogant, narrow-minded people never took the time to see who really was inside. . . . I'm also very angry that they took away my self-esteem, my social life, and kept me from getting a good education.

SOURCE: 16-year-old from mid-sized city in Illinois, quoted in Stein 1994, p. 1.

harassment in school is creating a hostile environment that compromises the education of America's children" (AAUW 1993).

Sexual Orientation in Schools

Since our last edition of this book (1990) educational researchers have been giving more attention to gay and lesbian teachers and students. What once was a subject of little research has now become an area with a considerably larger knowledge base. However, many educators continue to avoid the issue of sexual orientation as it relates to schooling because it is such a volatile societal issue. As an example of how fearful heterosexual people are of homosexuality, note that in the previous section being called gay or lesbian was listed as a form of sexual harassment. Of those who responded in that survey that they had experienced sexual harassment, 17 percent said they were called gay or lesbian when they didn't want to be. Boys were more likely than girls to report this form of harassment. Open discussion in classrooms regarding homosexuality or gay and lesbian concerns continues to be met with resistance and homophobia. By homophobia we mean the "irrational fear of sexual expression between people of the same gender" (Steinem, in Kramarae and Treichler 1985, p. 195). This section will explore literature on homosexuality as related to school settings.

In a thorough and timely overview of the equity issues of homosexuality in relation to education in *Sex Equity and Sexuality in Education* (Klein 1992), Delores Grayson quotes Audre Lorde, saying, "if we truly intend to eliminate oppression, heterosexism and homophobia must be addressed" (Grayson 1992, p. 172). It helps to understand the scope of sexual orientation issues if we realize that there are an estimated 150,000 gay and lesbian teenagers in the New York city metropolitan area, 10,000 in Philadelphia public high schools, 24,000 in Washington, D.C., and between 50,000 and 70,000 in Los Angeles. In Los Angeles and San Francisco, where school dropout rates exceed 40 percent, a disproportionate number of dropouts are gay or lesbian youth. In Los Angeles an estimated one-third of the homeless youth are those with a gay or lesbian orientation who have left home voluntarily or have been thrown out (Grayson 1992). Although these data are from urban centers only, we need to remember that what we will term sexual minority youth—as well as teachers, administrators, and counselors—live in communities of all sizes and descriptions.

The invisibility of this minority group is a central issue for gays and lesbians, as well as for those who are concerned with justice for oppressed groups. Where the culture is rigidly heterosexual, it often is not safe for gay and lesbian students or teachers to be open about their sexuality. As we saw, sexual harassment of students includes being labeled gay or lesbian (usually in more derogatory forms like dyke, faggot, wimp, sissy), whether or not the students actually are homosexual. Any behavior that may be perceived as a departure from the traditional male and female roles can set students up for this type of harassment. Grayson explains:

> Schools have depended on rigid sex-role definition to control their students. Homophobia helps keep boys and girls "in their place" better than any written rule. The fear of being accused of being gay or lesbian influences deci-

sions to stay in traditional shop and home economics classes, avoid inappropriate sport teams and student activities, and hide "too exclusive" same-sex relationships. (1992, p. 173)

In this oppressive culture, sexual minority youth, as well as their lesbian and gay teachers, remain "in the closet," where they are excluded but perhaps are safer from discrimination and abuse. As long as homosexuals are invisible, heterosexual educators are able to deny the contributions of this group of people.

Researchers have demonstrated that the personal cost for gay and lesbian educators can be high, particularly when they must adopt a "dual identity." In fear that they will damage themselves personally or professionally, homosexual educators change names of partners to the opposite gender or engage in so-called gender-appropriate behaviors to "pass" as heterosexual. For example, a single young female teacher might endure other teachers' well-intentioned efforts to arrange dates with eligible males. There are many documented incidents of harassing phone calls and letters, threats of violence, and violent actions against gays and lesbians whose sexual orientation becomes known in a community (Grayson 1992). We do not mean to imply here that all gay and lesbian educators respond to their school contexts in this way; some settings are more accepting than others of a range of lifestyles.

Assumed heterosexuality is a norm which pervades school practices. For example, on a form requiring the names of the father and mother, lesbian mothers crossed out "father" and wrote in "co-mother" (Casper, Schultz, and Wickens 1992). Virtually nothing in the curriculum deals with homosexuality as an alternative lifestyle. Children with gay parents do not see their type of family represented in any way in their schools because the heterosexual family is held up as the norm. In 1993 the Rainbow Curriculum, a multicultural curriculum introduced in New York City, created a controversy by its portrayal of gay families. After heated debate and the removal of the school superintendent, the controversial curriculum was removed as a district-wide mandate.

Given the climate of homophobia in society today, many gay parents are hesitant to discuss their personal life with teachers or school administrators for fear of repercussions for their children. A lesbian raising a six-year-old son explained:

No, there's no way I would come out. If you tell them, they might . . . change their attitude against you, and you're gonna feel, like rejected. So let them find out on their own. (Casper, Schultz, and Wickens 1992, p. 118)

Researchers Casper, Schultz, and Wickens (1992) call for educators to engage in open discussion in their teacher preparation programs and in their schools about lesbian and gay families. They argue that it is essential for educators to become more comfortable with the words *lesbian* and *gay*. They remind us that "clear and nonbiased understandings of family, gender, and culture will require the actions of teachers, parents, administrators, and activists (1992, p. 134).

Think about the content of popular songs, advertisements, and leisure activities. What are some messages gay and lesbian youth get about homosexuality from popular culture, media, and school experiences? How can teachers provide equitable school experiences for sexual minority youth?

GENDER-BASED DIFFERENTIAL OUTCOMES IN SCHOOLING

We have presented data about the different treatment of males and females particularly as related to the structure, curriculum, instructional strategies, and interactions in schools. The differential treatment young men and women receive in elementary and secondary school leads to differential academic and occupational outcomes based on gender. This section will present data showing the clear differences in these outcomes. Culturally induced differences also exist. Carol Tavris (1992) summarizes some of what she believes are the "real" differences between male and female behavior; "real" differences tend to focus on the different experiences men and women have rather than on allegedly innate sex-linked characteristics.

Differences in Academic Performance

What gender differences exist in student performance on academic tasks? Female students achieve higher grades throughout public school and do better on language-related courses such as reading, writing, and literature, while males do better in math and science. Although high school girls make better grades than boys, males tend to take more computer science and science courses involving math which would prepare them for careers in science-related areas (Ballantine 1989). Males are more likely to take physics and calculus courses than females (AAUW 1992). Females are less likely to participate in special or gifted programs and less likely to take math and science courses—even if they are academically talented—because they are less likely to believe themselves capable of pursuing these fields in college.

Females tend to attribute their failures to internal factors, such as lack of intellectual ability, while attributing successes to external factors such as luck (Sadker and Sadker 1985). In a study of college retention and attrition in mathematics and science courses, McDade (1988) found differences in how men and women dealt with their failures in these fields. Men were more able to disengage their self-image from their academic performance; rather than question their own abilities, they viewed their failure as a lack of fit with the field of study. Women internalized their failures, questioning their competence as learners not only in the specific area, but in general. Holland and Eisenhart's work with African-American and white college women (1988) corroborates McDade's findings. When confronted by teachers, parents, or boyfriends who told them they lacked the drive or ability to pursue "hard" subjects, they tended to give up or lower their career aspirations rather than to question the validity of negative judgments.

An interesting longitudinal study, the Illinois Valedictorian Project, issued a first-

Do Men and Women Differ?

Where the differences aren't	*Where the differences are*
Attachment, connection	Care-taking
Cognitive abilities	Communication
Verbal, mathematical,[a] reasoning,	▪ interaction styles
rote memory, vocabulary,	▪ uses of talk
reading,[b] etc.	▪ power differences
Dependency	Emotions
Emotions	▪ Contexts that produce them
▪ Likelihood of feeling them	▪ Forms of expression
Empathy	▪ "Feminization of love"
Moods and "moodiness"	▪ "Feminization of distress"
Moral reasoning	Employment, work opportunities
Need for achievement	Health and medicine
Need for love and attachment	▪ medication and treatment
Need for power	▪ longevity differences
Nurturance[c]	Income
Pacifism, belligerence	Life-span development
(e.g., depersonalizing enemies)	▪ effects of children
Sexual capacity, desire, interest	▪ work and family sequence
Verbal aggressiveness, hostility	Life narratives
	Power and status at work, in
	relationships, in society
	Reproductive experiences
	Reproductive technology and its
	social/legal consequences
	"Second shift": housework, child
	care, family obligations
	Sexual experiences and concerns
	Violence, public and intimate
	Weight and body image

[a]Males excel at highest levels of math performance; in general population, females have slight advantage.
[b]Males are more susceptible to some verbal problems. However, many alleged sex differences seem to be an artifact of referral bias: More boys are *reported* for help than girls, but there are no sex differences in the *actual* prevalence of dyslexia and other reading disabilities (see Shaywitz et al., 1990).
[c]As a capacity; in practice, women do more of the actual care and feeding of children, parents, relatives, friends.
SOURCE: Tavris 1992.

decade report documenting the academic and nonacademic lives of 82 valedictorians and salutatorians graduating from Illinois schools in 1981. The group, predominantly white, includes five African-American students, three Hispanic students, and one Asian-American student. The study found that although the men and women received equally high college entrance examination scores and grade point averages, the women had lowered estimates of their intelligence over the course of their college years. Attrition of women from math and science started in college and continued through graduate school and postdoctoral training. The researchers found that as college seniors, women's professional expectations were less well-defined than those of the men. The men's occupational levels were slightly higher than those of the women. The study reported that females were "well represented at the highest career levels among the group, with half of the female participants working in traditionally male-dominated career fields such as law, medicine, science, engineering, accounting, and computer science" (North Central Regional Educational Laboratory [NCREL] 1993, pp. 1–2). However, the remaining female valedictorians were disproportionately employed in clerical work and jobs that did not require a college degree (NCREL 1993).

What factors might account for the differences in self-perceptions, expectations, and occupational outcomes for these Illinois valedictorians?

Gender Differences in the SAT. The Scholastic Aptitude Test (SAT) published by the Educational Testing Service (ETS) serves as a major measure of student achievement in the United States. The Project on Equal Education Rights (PEER) of the National Organization for Women, an advocacy program for equal educational opportunities for women, monitors the progress of females in schools. In their 1986 Report Card PEER found that in 1985 male SAT scores were 59 points higher than females'. The national average (of a possible 1600) was 936 for males and 877 for females, the largest gap in twenty years. Women scored lower than men on both verbal and math sections. The 1985 national average math score was 499 for men and 452 for women; the verbal score was 437 for men, 425 for women. Although the Educational Testing Service was unable to explain this discrepancy, it reported that SAT scores underpredict the grades women can expect to earn in college. The test is not an accurate predictor of women's college performance as based on grades.

Researchers suggest that there is sex bias in both the construction and the content of the SAT test. More of the test questions are set in a science context than in the humanities, where women traditionally have been encouraged to excel. The Educational Testing Service also removed both the essay writing portion of the verbal test and the data sufficiency question on the math test—items on which female students had excelled. A new version of the SAT was recently developed in an attempt to rectify the gender bias in the test. While there is some evidence that the "gender gap" in achievement test scores is diminishing on tests other than the SAT (the College Board achievement tests, the National Assessment of Educational Progress, graduate school admissions tests, the Armed Forces Qualification Tests, and the College

Boards), the reason may be that while women are improving their performance in math, their verbal performance is slipping, given the change in the test (Kolata 1989).

Studies by the College Board, by ETS, and by independent research consistently report that women "receive higher grades than men in every subject in high school and college, but lower average SAT scores by approximately 60 points" (Rosser, in Kelly-Benjamin 1990). Rosser reports that in 1989 women's average scores were 13 points lower on the verbal portion and 46 points lower on the math portion of the test. Women at all social class levels, as measured by parental income and education, scored lower than men in their groups. She argues that the test, which is designed to predict students' grades in their first year of college, *underpredicts* the performance of 780,000 young women every year. If the SATs were actually predictive, women would receive higher average scores than men by 10 or 20 points.

Women of color are especially disadvantaged in the SAT process; their average scores are lower than those of both white men and men in their own ethnic group. For example, combined verbal and math scores of high school seniors in 1989 indicated that Latin-American females averaged 63 points lower than Latin-American men and 172 points lower than white men; African-American women averaged 27 points lower than African-American men and 243 points lower than white men (Rosser, in Kelly-Benjamin 1990).

Underpredicting of their ability limits the chances of young women to get into the colleges that require SAT scores. In addition, women are disadvantaged in the competition for merit scholarships offered by corporations, foundations, professional organizations, unions, and governmental agencies because those scholarships are based largely on SAT scores. In 1989, for example, only 32 percent of the National Merit Semifinalists were women. Since the SAT scores of women of color are consistently lower, they are even less likely to be selected for these SAT-based scholarships.

In February 1994 the American Civil Liberties Union filed a federal civil rights complaint charging bias against women in the use of SAT tests to award the $25 million per year National Merit Scholarships. The ACLU argued that 60 percent of the semifinalists and finalists are boys despite the fact that only 45 percent of those who take the test are male. A spokesperson for the College Board denied any gender bias in the test, explaining that the difference reflects differential academic preparation, including the fact that women take fewer high school math courses (*Education Week* 1994).

The American Association of University Women's (AAUW) 1992 study, *How Schools Shortchange Girls: A Study of Major Findings on Girls and Education*, reports that women perform better on the verbal portion of the SAT when the material is abstract and general rather than concrete and specific. They also tend to do better when asked to deal with concepts and ideas rather than facts and things. On mathematics items, women generally do more poorly than men on word problems, even when the problems relate to stereotypic female contexts such as food preparation. Females answer fewer test items than males. They tend to score higher on open-ended or essay type items, whereas boys tend to score higher on multiple choice items (AAUW 1992).

The Educational Testing Service requests that students supply information about

My daughter had straight As in high school and my son's record was indifferent. Then they took their SATs. My daughter's four years of achievement were wiped out by her low SAT score and my son's high score suddenly made him a brain. It had a tremendous psychological impact. My daughter began to set up barriers. She couldn't apply to certain places because her scores were not as good as the books say they should be. When she entered college she didn't study hard enough at first because she thought she couldn't get As. [Eventually she realized she could and brought her grades up to her previous standards.]

SOURCE: Prominent feminist leader quoted by Phyllis Rosser in Kelly-Benjamin 1990, p. 1.

their academic goals when they take the SAT. PEER found that in 1985, 10.6 percent of the high school senior women taking the SAT reported that their goal was to major in physical sciences, compared with 34 percent of the male seniors. In 1980–1981 only 3 percent of the women graduates received a Bachelor's degree in physical sciences, mathematics, or engineering, while 23 percent of them earned degrees in education and 11 percent graduated in nursing and health-related professions—both traditionally female.

Differences in Educational Attainment

Since the 1960s women have made significant gains in education. We owe much of this progress to the work of feminist women and men. Currently over half of under-graduate college students are women. The student population also has become in-creasingly diverse, with nearly one out of every five students a person of color in 1988. In 1989, women earned the majority of college degrees at all levels except doctorate. Although they have continued to concentrate in traditional undergraduate majors such as social sciences, the arts, and education, in 1988 one out of every five women college graduates majored in business. Women have earned increasing num-bers of undergraduate degrees in science and engineering since 1960. In fact, one-half of the biological science degrees in 1989 were earned by women—almost double the 1970 percentage. In 1989 women earned more than one-fourth of the dentistry de-grees, one-third of the medical degrees, one-half of the veterinary degrees, and two-fifths of the law degrees (Ries and Stone 1992).

Despite these gains, problem areas persist. Although women *have* moved into traditionally male-dominated fields such as science and engineering, Randour, Stras-burg, and Lipman-Blumen (1982) found that at the Bachelor's degree level they con-tinue to be concentrated in education, fine and applied arts, foreign languages, health professions, home economics, and library science—all traditionally female profes-sions. In addition, although greater numbers of women are now earning Master's de-grees and doctorates, over half of the women at the Master's level and over one-third of those at the doctoral level are earning degrees in education. In traditionally male-dominated fields women are still the minority. For example, in 1989 only 15 percent of Bachelor's degrees in engineering were earned by women, and women earned only 36 percent of the doctorates awarded in that year (Ries and Stone 1992). Women continue to outnumber men significantly in undergraduate education programs. Goldin reported in 1990 that 76 percent of all education majors are women. You need only look around your class to confirm this figure.

Women have made striking advances in educational attainment since the early 1960s, when most women had two basic options—teaching and nursing. As we have seen, many more options are open to today's young women. In the next section we will examine both women's progress in occupational attainment and the subtle and not-so-subtle glass ceiling.

Occupational Attainment, Economic Rewards, and the Glass Ceiling

The existence of a "glass ceiling"—analogous to the "job ceiling" for ethnic minorities—in the labor market means that despite being highly educated, well-qualified, and extremely motivated, women still may rise only so far in their career hierarchies.

Many women who have worked their way into professional positions across a range of fields find themselves hitting their heads against the "glass ceiling." This means that despite appropriate and even exceptional qualifications, they are not promoted to the highest levels possible. Women high school principals and school superintendents are few. As we have seen, women are not well represented on the faculties or in administrative posts of colleges and universities. Women attorneys are often prevented from rising to the top of the legal profession. The Honorable William S. Russell, a Tennessee judge, using data from the Harvard Law School Class of 1974, reported that "ten years after graduation, 59 percent of the male graduates were full partners in law firms, but only 23 percent of the female graduates had obtained that status" (Fretz 1990).

Some encouraging trends are that from 1975 to 1987 the number of higher education institutions headed by women increased 100 percent, and the number of businesses owned by women also increased. By 1987, 30 percent of U.S. companies were owned by females.

However, in 1982 Kelly and Nihlen reported:

[W]omen earn less than 56 percent of male income, regardless of job categories; they are concentrated in the lowest-paying jobs in both service and industrial sectors of the economy; they are segregated into occupations which permit very little upward mobility; and they are concentrated in the "marginal" areas of the workforce. (1982, p. 165)

This statement still holds true today. Women continue to be concentrated in the traditional service industries. In 1990 more than two-thirds of working women were in service sector industries, in wholesale and retail trade, and in protective service fields such as teaching and nursing (Ries and Stone 1992). In the same year 46 percent of

> "Construction of the glass ceiling begins not in the executive suite but in the classroom."
>
> SOURCE: Alice McKee, president of the American Association of University Women, 1992.

female workers were in low-paying service and administrative-support occupations such as health aides, secretaries, and waitresses. African-American women were more likely than white women to work in these service jobs. Overall, most jobs tend to be gender segregated along traditional lines. For example, only 19.3 percent of physicians, 8 percent of engineers, 13.9 percent of police and detectives, and 36 percent of computer programmers were women in 1990. According to a 1989 survey the Fortune 500 companies continue to be male dominated; only one out of eight of their board members was a woman.

In higher education, as in the corporate world, women are depressingly underrepresented. They comprised only 28 percent of college faculty in 1985, up from 20 percent in 1910. In 1985 only 3 percent of the college faculty were women of color. Current women faculty tend to be clustered at the bottom ranks in assistant or associate professorships rather than at the full professor rank. Only one of ten top executive posts in colleges and universities were held by women in 1989 (Ries and Stone 1992).

Women also continue to lag behind men in earnings. In 1980 females earned 64 cents for every dollar earned by men. By 1990 they were earning 72 cents to a man's dollar, but African-American women continued to earn 62 cents for every dollar earned by white men (Ries and Stone 1992).

Thus we can see that unequal educational treatment in schools coupled with culturally determined notions of what constitutes appropriate women's work continue to produce inequities in the economic structure.

Think about the reasons for the glass ceiling. Why is it that women are not promoted to the highest positions in their fields or do not serve on corporate boards? Talk to some women professionals about their experiences with the glass ceiling.

We have discussed equality of educational opportunities in two ways: equal access to education and equal treatment of students in schools. By law, women, like minority groups, have achieved equal access to educational opportunities through Title IX. However, equitable treatment of women in schools is not a reality. Differences in the treatment of men and women in schools mirror cultural beliefs about appropriate roles for males and females. In the United States, as in Western countries, men are politically, economically, and socially dominant. Although there have been significant improvements in both educational and economic opportunities for women, the work force continues to be sex-segregated so that women hold subordinate positions in the economy.

> I myself have never been able to find out precisely what feminism is; I only know that people call me a feminist whenever I express sentiments that differentiate me from a doormat.
>
> SOURCE: Rebecca West, 1913, *The Clarion*, Nov. 14, quoted in Kramarae & Treichler, 1985.

I'M NOT A FEMINIST, BUT . . .

When we talk in our classes about women's issues, our students often will preface their comments with the phrase, "I'm not a feminist, but. . . ." If you recall our earlier discussion of stereotypes, it is clear that such students may be harboring a stereotype about feminists. Feminists are often portrayed in the media as man haters, aggressive bitches, as well as aging and bitter leftovers from the 1960s. Feminists also are never portrayed as male. Rush Limbaugh is currently building his career by bashing feminists with his label "feminazi." Given this backdrop, it isn't surprising that some students try to establish some distance from such a label. However, we believe it is important for both women and men in education to consider themselves feminists so they can provide equitable and appropriate practice for all children and young adults.

In this section we will consider what it means to be a feminist. There is no *one* feminism, but a range of political and theoretical feminist positions. Our discussion here is merely a cursory introduction to several of the major feminist positions in current writing and debate, rather than a detailed analysis of each position. We will briefly discuss liberal feminism, radical feminism, socialist feminism, poststructural feminism, and black feminism or womanism and the perspectives of these positions on gender and schooling. You will see a common thread throughout these discussions which serves as a backdrop for our subsequent discussions of girls' and women's experiences in school settings. As you read, consider where you stand on these issues. What do you agree with? What makes you uncomfortable? Why?

In your view, what is feminism? Do you consider yourself a feminist? Why or why not?

What Is Feminism?

Feminism is both a theory of women's position in society and a political statement focused on gaining equal rights and opportunities for women and changing existing power relations between men and women. Feminism by definition implies social action, as we see in the following. A feminist is

a person, female or male, whose worldview places the female in the center of life and society, and/or who is not prejudiced based on gender or sexual preference. Also, anyone in a male-dominated or patriarchal society who works toward the political, economic, spiritual, sexual, and social equality of women. (*The Wise Woman* 1982, p. 7)

And another framing of the definition of feminism:

Feminism is the political theory and practice to free all women: women of color, working-class women, poor women, physically challenged women, lesbians, old women, as well as white economically privileged heterosexual women. Anything less than this is not feminism, but merely self-aggrandizement. (B. Smith 1979, quoted in Morage and Anzaldua 1981, p. 61)

Although we often think of the feminist movement of the 1960s as the beginning of contemporary feminism, the roots of feminist thinking go back centuries to individual men and women and groups of women and men who worked to free women from the oppression of patriarchy.

Feminist Theories

The way in which people understand feminism depends on their view of the larger society. *Liberal feminists* focus on the *rights* of individual women; they work to transform traditional beliefs about femininity and masculinity as well as to achieve full equality of opportunity in all spheres of life. Liberal feminists do not criticize the basic structure of the nuclear family but place stress on an individual woman's right to decide how she wants to participate in that family. Liberal feminists work to transform understandings of male and female roles at home and in the workplace; they advocate individual choice rather than biological sex differences as the factor that determines what men and women do in their families and in the work place (Weedon 1987). The liberal feminist position has been crucial in achieving equality of educational opportunities for women; it opened doors for young women to careers that were once the exclusive domain of white males. Much of the research cited in the sections about gender differences in the formal and hidden curriculum was done by liberal feminists who believed that traditional or stereotypic notions of male and female roles were debilitating for all people.

Radical feminists argue that the roots of women's oppression lie in the biological differences between men and women; the patriarchal family is seen to be the primary means by which women have been controlled by men. Radical feminists work to reclaim women's bodies from male control and to celebrate their life-giving abilities. Rather than attempting to transform patriarchy, they argue for women's separation from men in order to assert autonomy and develop a women's culture independent of men (Weedon 1987). Hawthorne explains that "separatism is a politically motivated strategy for empowering women and undermining patriarchy. It varies in its manifestations within women's lives" (1991, p. 312). She argues that separatism is a feminist strategy that challenges the oppressive societal structures, providing a continuum of choices whereby women can establish separate spheres from men. Her choices begin with participating in dialogue with other women in a variety of groups (such as consciousness-raising groups, study groups, or political action groups), to working in an all-female environment, to becoming woman-identified in emotional and sexual ways, or at the end of the continuum, to living in an all-woman environment (Hawthorne 1991). Radical feminists would view single-sex schools as a way to begin to develop an empowering woman's culture.

The *socialist feminist* position also criticizes the dominant structures of Western society. Socialist feminists view family as historically constructed. They believe race, social class, and gender oppression to be the interrelated consequence of a patriarchal, capitalist system. Socialist feminists call for total transformation of the social system to emphasize the following:

> . . . full participation of men in childrearing; reproductive freedom for women, that is, the right to decide if and when to have children and under what conditions, together with the provision of the conditions necessary for the realization of the right of women to make these choices; the abolition of the privileging of heterosexuality, freedom to define one's own sexuality and the right of lesbians to raise children; the eventual abolition of the categories "woman" and "man," and the opening up of all social ways of being to all people. (Weedon 1987, p. 18)

Social feminists would challenge the historically constructed patriarchy in today's schools, calling for total transformation in the structures, policies, and practices for women and men.

Recent writings by *feminist poststructuralists* play a key role in discussions of feminism. Weedon (1987) explains that poststructuralism isn't just one theory but rather a range of positions developed in the work of Derrida, Lacan, Dristeva, Althusser, and Foucault. Language is the common element in the analysis of our individual consciousness, power, and social organizations. Through language we are able to think, speak, and attach meaning to the world around us. All social meaning is constructed within, not apart from, language. Feminist poststructuralists examine the ways competing language patterns produce our notions of gender. Rather than having a static understanding of ourselves in the world, we are constantly engaged in constructing and deconstructing, interpreting and reinterpreting ourselves and the way we understand our worlds through language (Weedon 1987). Since language is the principal focus of the poststructuralists, they would deconstruct the competing discourses found in school settings—including the policies, practices, and interactions among those who participate in school life. The feminist poststructuralist would attempt to examine schools through social, cultural, and historical lenses, analyzing the relations of knowledge and power. By understanding whose interests are served in the language of schools, they would discover whose interests are marginalized, silenced, or excluded, so they could begin work toward changes and transformations in those settings.

Black feminism or *womanism* defines African-American women's struggles around the issues of race, social class, and gender. For African-American women, the feminist movement has symbolized a struggle for equity based on a universal notion of women, with little recognition of the distinction of race. Alice Walker captures the relationship of black women to the white feminist movement: "Womanist is to feminist as purple is to lavender" (Walker 1983, p. xi). The history of African Americans in the United States has been a history of oppression. For black women, sexual abuse and harassment began with the institution of slavery, so it is impossible to separate the experience of being a woman from the experience of being an African-American woman (Brown 1994). In *Black Feminist Thought* (1990) P. H. Collins describes the grounding of black feminism in the experience of African-American women: "all African American women share the common experience of being Black women in a society that denigrates women of African descent" (Collins 1990, p. 22). The struggle against both racism and sexism is a core theme for womanists. Through their efforts, black feminists work to replace denigrated images of black women with self-defined images, to give voice to the experiences of black women, and to take action in the struggle for human freedom. Collins argues that black feminist thought "cannot flourish isolated from the experiences and ideas of other groups" (1990, p. 35); she describes the necessity of forming coalitions with others whose goals are to challenge relations of domination in the society. The Combahee River Collective characterizes this struggle:

> We are actively committed to struggling against racial, sexual, heterosexual, and class oppression and see as our particular task the development of integrated analysis and practice based upon the fact that the major systems of oppression are interlocking. The synthesis of these oppressions creates the conditions of our lives. As Black women we see Black feminism as the logical political movement to combat the manifold and simultaneous oppressions that all women of color face. (Combahee River Collective, 1977, in Morage and Anzaldua 1981, p. 210)

We have provided a brief taste of several of the primary feminist theories currently used to explain and transform societal institutions and practices. Although these theories have different key points or elements, all are concerned with equal rights for women and a transformation in the ways both women and men experience their lives. We urge you to read about each of these feminist theories in more depth.

Which of the feminist theories expresses views most like yours? Why?

SUMMARY

In this chapter, we've addressed the major issues related to gender equity in schools. It is clear, a few decades after the passage of Title IX, that women have more alternatives in schools and more equitable access to educational opportunities. The gender differences are no longer as explicit as they were in the school that Emily attended in 1903. Emily's granddaughter, Susan, has been given access to many educational alternatives and career options. However, schools continue to reproduce a patriarchal society through subtle (and often not-so-subtle) messages embedded in their organizational structure, curriculum, and social interaction patterns. "The achievement of sex-and-gender-equitable education remains an elusive dream. The time to turn dreams to reality is now" (AAUW 1992, p. 84). The following AAUW recommendations for action were proposed to address the critical gender equity issues in schools:

1. Strengthening and reinforcement of Title IX is essential.
2. Teachers, administrators, and counselors must be prepared and encouraged to bring gender equity and awareness to every aspect of schooling.
3. The formal school curriculum must include the experiences of women and men from all walks of life. Girls and boys must see women and girls reflected and valued in the materials they study.
4. Girls must be educated and encouraged to understand that mathematics and the sciences are important and relevant to their lives. Girls must be actively supported in pursuing education and employment in these areas.
5. Continued attention to gender equity in vocational education programs must be a high priority at every level of educational governance and administration.
6. Testing and assessment must serve as stepping-stones, not stop signs. New tests and testing techniques must accurately reflect the abilities of both girls and boys.
7. Girls and women must play a central role in educational reform. The experiences, strengths, and needs of girls from every race and social class must be considered in order to provide excellence and equity for all our nation's students.
8. A critical goal of education reform must be to enable students to deal effectively with the realities of their lives, particularly in areas such as sexuality and health. (AAUW 1992, pp. 84–88)

Up to this point in the book we have tried to paint a realistic picture of the way schools work—at times a rather gloomy picture. It is important for you to understand the realities of schooling so you can help transform schools into better places for teachers and children. In the next chapter we will describe some of the ways schools are currently trying to address the problems and issues raised here.

chapter 9

Alternatives to the Way We "Do School": A Critical Perspective

Chapter Overview

INTRODUCTION

CHANGING THE BALANCE OF POWER
Alternative Possibilities for School Structures
Alternative Ideologies of Schooling: Transformative Pedagogies
Alternative Possibilites for Teacher Education and Practice

A CLOSING NOTE

INTRODUCTION

What have we learned about schooling from sociology? We have attempted to provide an overview of how sociologists look at students and teachers. We have presented the major sociological interpretations used to explain the purposes of school and the experiences of students in schools. Using these interpretations, particularly a critical/feminist framework, we have examined the complex nature of work within educational institutions and the ways social class, ethnicity, and gender impact the experiences of students.

You might wonder, since we know so much about schooling from a sociological perspective, why we still "do school" in ways that clearly contradict our research findings. Why are so many schools still organized and operated in much the same manner they were a hundred years ago? Why do we ignore research on individual differences and continue to educate children in batches, like cookies? Why do we say we venerate and respect teachers and then refuse to pay them well or trust their judgment about what they teach? Why do we still believe that education is necessary in order to get ahead economically? Why—when it is clear that benefits from schooling are directly proportional to how close one is to being white, male, and middle class—do we continue to urge children who differ from white males by race, class, and gender to believe that "education pays off"? Given demographic shifts so that by the year 2000 the majority of public school students will come from non-European (African, Asian, or Latin-American) backgrounds (Hodgkinson 1985), why do those who plan and administer educational programs ignore the needs of a growing multicultural student population?

Part of the answer can be found in Tom Robbins's delightful novel *Jitterbug Perfume*. Robbins writes: "The Universe does not have laws. It has habits. And habits can be broken" (1984, p. 283). Schools, like Robbins's universe, run on old habits. For example, when you ask teachers why they put children into three groups for reading, they may tell you that they've always done it that way. The practice is reinforced and legitimated by district supervisors who require such a structure, as well as by the teachers' guides for basal readers. Much of what happens in and to schools is done because of habit.

Another part of the answer lies in the expectations that parents and communities hold for schooling and their resistance to new systems. Almost everyone has attended school for some long period of time. Almost everyone feels that she or he "knows about" schools and what they are like. Parents who benefited from school tend to want schools to be run in much the same way as when *they* were children, and to have the same supposed effects. You might hear them say, "It was good enough for me; it ought to be good enough for my kids, too." Disadvantaged parents express the same kind of conservatism, but for different reasons: They have observed the benefits that schooling seems to have provided for the children of the middle and upper classes and fear that innovative programs will be inferior. They want their children to have the same advantages—hence the same kinds of schooling—that traditionally have benefited the dominant groups in society.

Imagine what would happen if all schools suddenly were to discontinue compensatory education, ability grouping, and academic tracking. Many administrators and some teachers would be up in arms, ignoring research findings that tracking widens the differences between children and benefits only those in the highest tracks. They would feel overwhelmed with the wide range of ability in their classrooms. Middle-class parents would storm the barricades, protesting that their children's life chances had been impaired because teachers would be spending all their time on "slow" learners at the expense of the more able. Despite evidence that many so-called compensatory education programs are not targeted to instruction, that the programs often don't raise achievement, and that often they actually benefit students other than the target populations, disadvantaged parents would complain that without this special treatment their children would slide even farther behind.

Imagine further that all standardized testing was eliminated and that schools were no larger than 400 students, as has been recommended by us (Dworkin and LeCompte 1989; LeCompte and Dworkin 1988; LeCompte and Goebel 1987) and by a Carnegie Commission Report (1989). Imagine that the requirements for employment were a demonstrated background in the arts, humanities, literature, and mathematics, not a diploma. Imagine that it would be impossible to find an all-European-American classroom.

If people, particularly teachers and administrators, were able to distance themselves from their long-cherished notions about schools and take a moment to contemplate the adverse consequences that their activities have for poor and minority children, they most likely would ask: "How else can you do it? What are the alternatives?" In this final chapter we will engage in some intellectual play with these questions. On the basis of what we have learned from the sociologists of education, we will present a few alternatives to the way we "do school."

At this point in our courses our students are usually ready for action. You may be frustrated that we haven't answered certain questions: What can we as teachers and administrators do about the issues and problems you've raised here? How can we do schools better? Many sociologists, anthropologists, and educators are now addressing these questions. In this last chapter we cannot provide you with a "cookbook" for ways to improve school experiences, but we can introduce you to views of educators concerned with alternatives to traditional school structures, policies, and practices. We must remember that each context is different and what works in one setting may not be appropriate in another. We present these alternatives in three separate but interrelated categories: (1) the structure of schools, (2) alternative ideologies of schooling with an emphasis on transformative pedagogies, and (3) teacher education and classroom practice. We offer these suggestions as a mere beginning—a way for students and teachers to think in new ways about schooling and to raise questions about their own teaching and learning practices, as well as about policies that have been implemented in their own school districts.

We have tried not to be Utopian. We have restricted our own suggestions to things that are now in practice in innovative schools or that we feel current school districts might be able to accomplish. We hope your thinking and questioning will not end with the suggestions in this chapter. We challenge you to use the knowledge you have gained in this text to examine critically your own beliefs, practices, policies, and structures throughout your professional life. We hope you will work to transform your own setting into one that is culturally affirming, developmentally appropriate, intellectually challenging, and socially just.

CHANGING THE BALANCE OF POWER

Sociologists have been criticized for the terribly gloomy portrait they paint of the role of schools in social transformation. This is particularly true of reproduction theorists. In suggesting that schools have no power to act upon the source of the problems that they are called upon to solve, sociologists seem to have left educators with little to do but wish for a more humane society. While it is true that schools more reflect than shape the economic and social foundations of society—to a greater extent than educators or reformers would like to believe—there is nevertheless much that schools can do.

Since the first edition of this book, educators have challenged the traditional structures of schooling whereby classrooms are organized by age, subjects are taught in segregated units in 50-minute periods, and teachers work in isolation. Today we can find many examples of multi-age grouping, integrated curricula, changes in the scheduling of classes, and teachers immersed in transformative practice. Educators have proposed and implemented alternative and transformative pedagogies. The educational community has called for a reconceptualization of teachers' work and the way teachers are educated.

What is at the core of all these changes is a change in power relationships. Traditional hierarchies of power have come under serious critique. The traditional role of teachers and students is in question. School administrators are being asked to participate in very different ways. The whole notion of the construction of knowledge and whose knowledge is taught in schools, as well as whose knowledge is omitted, continues to be debated by educators and policy makers. Educators have formed powerful networks across schools, districts, and states to share knowledge and to support transformative projects. As critical/feminist theorists, we are excited about the critique of these traditional structures and practices and the ways in which power is currently shifting to those who have long been on the bottom of the hierarchy—women, minority groups, teachers, and students. In this next portion of the chapter we will examine the ways the balance of power is changing in (1) school structures, (2) pedagogies, and (3) teacher education.

Alternative Possibilities for School Structures

How could schools be organized to better meet the needs of a diverse population? What issues of power in schools need to be addressed? Who should determine how schools are structured? In this section we examine some of these questions and offer several suggestions.

Visit a school (or classroom) where alternative practices and structures are the norm. How does this school compare with a more traditionally organized school? Talk with some of the students and teachers about their experiences in this setting.

Keeping Schools Small.   As was described in Chapter 2, schools and school districts are currently organized into large, consolidated bureaucratic organizations, having replaced the smaller community schools which were the norm until the early twentieth century. With more students, consolidated schools could offer more curricular and extracurricular options. However, in schooling, big is not necessarily better. Increased size has come at the expense of the sense of community and belonging which schools often created. Schools also have lost the capacity for flexibility, a characteristic that enables them to accommodate to the varied needs and capabilities of students. In our opinion, schools have become so big and complex that teachers, students, and administrators can no longer perform in them the work that large schools were designed to do. Recent research indicates that the bigger the school, the higher the dropout rates, especially for minority students (R. Turner 1989). Sociological analyses consistently show that students are happier and have a higher level of participation in smaller schools.

Regardless of their size, schools that can conform to overall structural rules while still bending them enough to engage their students socially and academically tend to have lower dropout rates, even among students who are learning disabled and from minority backgrounds (Miller, Leinhardt, and Zigmond 1988). Similarly, teachers feel more competent and satisfied when they feel that they have some control over their work. They feel more alienated and less in control when they do not feel that they have supportive administrators and when they work in impersonal, highly bureaucratized school districts (Dworkin 1986; Dworkin, Lorence, and LeCompte 1989). Schools must be small enough to enable teachers, administrators, and other school staff to build strong, lasting relationships with their students. Teachers in smaller schools working with children over longer periods of time can get to know their students and respond to their needs more quickly. It is much more difficult to lose students in the bureaucracy when the bureaucracy is small.

Teaching and learning are not only *social* acts, but *intimate* social acts, facilitated by the close personal attention of the participants. Intimacy and large contemporary schools are virtually mutually exclusive, but one structural variable over which schools *do* have control is size. We propose that the school consolidation clock be rolled back so that the optimum size for elementary schools be about 300 students, and for secondary schools, 200 per grade level with a maximum of 600 students. This means that a school with four grades would have a grade level limit of 150. With innovative scheduling, these configurations can be accomplished within existing buildings. Any existing old buildings can be reopened or new ones can be constructed on a much smaller scale.

Some experiments in reducing school size, particularly at the secondary level, are being attempted. For example, the Coalition Campus Schools Project in New York City, a three-year initiative, is implementing twelve new, small high schools in an "effort to humanize urban school education and transform large failing inner-city schools into successful learning environments for all students" (National Center for Restructuring Education, Schools, and Teaching [NCREST] 1994, p. 1). The plan is to phase out two large, comprehensive high schools and replace them with twelve smaller schools on the same campuses, consisting of approximately 400 students each. The schools will emphasize personalized instruction, close school–family communications, rigorous intellectual standards for all children, and shared decision making. Deborah Meier, co-director of Central Park East Secondary School, explains: "Most human beings need to be known, and it is more critical when other things are also fragile. Kids are dying in these large schools" (NCREST 1994, p. 4). This type of innovation illustrates the potential for large urban and suburban school districts to reorganize into smaller communities or units to meet the needs of students while staying within budget constraints and maintaining the size necessary to provide the educational alternatives offered by a consolidated high school.

Flexible Groupings of Students.   Even more critical to overall school organization would be a radical departure from age-grading. We now "batch-process" children. From the elementary school level on, children are categorized by age and locked into movement through the grades one year at a time, with complete disregard for what we have learned from sociologists and psychologists about the most appropriate ways to organize learning for children.

The National Association for the Education of Young Children has consistently urged districts to adopt "developmentally appropriate practice," which gears schools to the developmental rather than the chronological age of children. This structuring permits children to learn through activities appropriate for their developmental stage and to move through the curriculum in accordance with their readiness. This type of teaching and learning has been termed a *multi-graded unit* or *multi-aged grouping.* The emphasis shifts from didactic teaching of content to providing appropriate learning activities through which children acquire content. Not only does this arrangement change the way children learn, it drastically alters the role of the teacher. They can no longer "rule" from the top down but must preside over a multitude of activities, using their expertise to work with students in a wide range of ways. You can find schools that use multi-age groupings in most communities in the United States today.

Changing the School Schedule.   Perhaps the most important act schools might perform is to take a serious look at school conditions and to arrange the school day, the types of training, and the services available so that they more closely correspond to what students need. One consideration might be the recognition that the 12-year limit on elementary and high school attendance—reinforced by state funding formulas—is unrealistic. Some students are slower learners, some must work for a living, and some just need extra time for a particularly difficult program. Students who are gifted in music, the performing arts, or athletics may need time off for competitions or for extra practice; they lose out when they must choose between missing class work or giving up their competitions. Often these are the students who are pushed out of school. Precedent for changing this arrangement exists; "special" or handicapped students can take additional years to finish their program, to age 21.

There also exist precedents for arranging the school year to correspond with labor needs of society. The long public school summer vacations are a relic from an agricultural past, when student labor was needed on the farms during the growing season. Changes in the school calendar according to the needs of the community could promote better working relationships with parents and could provide for continuous educational services for that community's students.

School schedules can be transformed to recognize that most parents or guardians work and can neither come to school during the day for conferences nor be at home after school to baby-sit or help with homework. With these accommodations, parent involvement programs would be less of an excuse for teachers to pass on blame and less of a source of guilt for parents.

Further, day care needs to be found for the *children* of schoolchildren, the babies of teenagers who must otherwise drop out of school. Most teenage mothers choose to keep their babies, and most find few incentives and little assistance to remain in school (Hess and Green 1988). Infant care programs established on public school campuses have been notably helpful in ensuring continued school attendance as well as better child care. Funds for these programs might come from redirection of vocational education monies, about which we comment below.

Schools schedules can be designed around students' learning rather than around a factory model of discreet 50-minute periods. Humans simply don't learn in neatly organized 50-minute blocks with bells ringing to signal movement to the next subject. Some schools currently provide expanded periods so teachers can work in teams with groups of students over longer time blocks, thus allowing for thematic organization and integration of subject matter. At the elementary level students are being kept together in a classroom for the entire day, so the schedule is more flexible. In his book *Schools that Work* (1992) George Wood describes how progressive schools have restructured their schedules to provide a better learning environment for children and more time for teachers to work in teams. For example, in one school Wood visited, the staff shared a 75-minute lunch period during which they planned curriculum and worked on collaborative projects. Another school staff arranged to work together one morning a week while their students were involved in community service projects.

Schools and the Labor Market.   We need to look more closely at the skills needed in the labor market, particularly those related to vocational training. Most public schools cannot afford to offer the state-of-the-art training required for technical and industrial jobs. Employers often prefer to find literate job candidates and do their own training. Vocational students, then, find themselves doubly short-changed; not only are they insufficiently trained in the basic cognitive skills, but they have spent years in training that is outdated and leads only to dead-end jobs. We have argued elsewhere that the best vocational training possible is a good liberal arts education (LeCompte 1987a, 1987b; LeCompte and Dworkin 1988). We recommend eliminating the vocational track altogether and having *all* students study health, nutrition, personal finance, automobile mechanics, carpentry, data processing, and small engine repair as everyday living skills—in addition to reading, mathematics, science, the arts, and social studies.

School Governance and Leadership.   Whereas sociologists have been criticized for being too gloomy about the prospects for reform of schooling, educational researchers have been criticized for being naive or Utopian. Regardless of how insightful their work has been, much of it remains unused. Ernest Boyer of the Carnegie Foundation for the Advancement of Teaching says:

> We've made remarkable breakthroughs in understanding the development of children, the development of learning, and the climate that enhances [them, but too often] what we know in theory and what we're doing in the classroom are very different. (Quoted in Kantrowitz and Wingert 1989, p. 51)

The issue is, how does what we know get translated into what we do? How does our sociological knowledge of schooling help us to bring about change?

A key element is an understanding of how power affects processes of change in organizations. Sociological insights have made clear that schools are not apolitical institutions in which the exercise of power is irrelevant. People who have power are not interested in giving it away, whether they are school administrators, government bureaucrats, or old-line teachers. Many people prefer to work in hierarchical structures where roles are governed by traditional habits. However, despite the deeply entrenched nature of conventional practice, we believe that redistribution of power is necessary for teachers to gain control over their work and their work place. Implicit in our thinking, and that of critical theorists, is that change needs to begin at the bottom of the hierarchy. Confrontation also needs to occur at the level of policy and power as well.

In the past several years educators have moved into the era of school restructuring. As Darling-Hammond reminds us, "over the last decade the rhetoric of school improvement has changed from a language of school reform to a language of school restructuring" with the aims of fundamentally redesigning schools and approaches to teaching and learning (1993, p. 753). At all levels of education, faculties and administrators have been called on to restructure their schools and programs to create places where people learn at a high level, develop their talents, evaluate and develop alternatives to complex problems, and construct their own knowledge (Darling-Hammond 1993). This form of restructuring demands input from teachers and communities about programs and policies. Site-based management and local community school boards have been instituted in many districts, changing more traditional hierarchical and patriarchal forms of financial and curricular control.

Perhaps the best known example of such restructuring is in Chicago, where in December 1988 the Illinois State Legislature passed the Chicago School Reform Act which fundamentally changed the governance structure of Chicago's public schools. The law created Local School Councils consisting of two community representatives, six parents, two teachers, and the principal. For high schools a nonvoting student sat on the board. With the establishment of these Local Schools Councils, principals, rather than being responsible to the central office, are chief executive officers responsible to and working with a managing board, which oversees the total running of the school and which has the power to hire and fire the principal, regardless of tenure. These councils construct school budgets, evaluate existing staff, and select new personnel. After consultation with members of the Council and the Professional Personnel Advisory Committee (PPAC) made up of school faculty, principals develop school improvement plans. The PPAC creates a mechanism where shared decision making can take place and teachers' voices are heard regarding issues that affect them. The Chicago Reform Act significantly changed the involvement and power of teachers and community members in the governance of the city's schools (Hess 1991).

Explore the Chicago school reform or current statewide reforms such as that begun by the Kentucky Education Reform Act (KERA). What changes are being made in these reform movements? How have the governance and structure of schooling changed?

While some decentralization and site-based management are touted as important reform efforts, they can also sabotage innovations, lead to fragmentation in educational policy, and create conflict between different levels of governance

(Goldwasser 1994). A number of years ago New York City, the largest school district in the United States, decentralized into a number of subdistricts, several of which have become notorious for poor student achievement and corruption in both financial and personnel matters. In one of the poorest districts, number 9, at least nine school board members were arrested within five years. Its students have repeatedly scored lower than any other district on citywide tests. In 1994 District 9 became a test case for the power of the city superintendent to enforce improvement upon a local school board. Under its new superintendent, Felton Johnson, District 9 became a model for corporate involvement in public schools. Johnson persuaded local foundations and corporations to buy computers, provide tutors, increase parent involvement, and engage in a number of other charitable projects. However, the local board decided not to renew Mr. Johnson's contract, whereupon the private-sector benefactors announced that they were ending their support, citing the district's instability and lack of commitment to reform. New York City Superintendent, Mr. Cortines countered by ordering the local board to reinstate Mr. Johnson in the interests of consistent reform and educational stability. The local district sued Cortines, stating that he had no legal right to overrule the decisions of locally elected school officials. The state courts upheld the firing of Johnson, a ruling that considerably weakened the city superintendent's power to root out corruption and institute districtwide reform (Dillon 1994).

At the same time that restructuring efforts have decentralized power, the increased standardization in statewide testing, standardized teacher evaluation, and standardized curricula have worked against restructuring efforts. The tensions between decentralization and standardization set up situations where two very different types of teachers are desired. On one hand, restructuring efforts call for teachers who share in decision making, collaborate with colleagues, develop challenging curricula to meet the developmental and intellectual needs of their students, and evaluate student outcomes through measures such as portfolio assessment. This view of teaching/learning requires teachers who have extensive professional expertise and are empowered to engage in policy decisions. On the other hand, standardized tests and curriculum, as well as more sanctions and rewards, require teachers who can work within a top-down hierarchy where decisions are made above the classroom level.

Empowered teachers working within these competing ideologies may find such conditions difficult at best. These are the teachers who have constructed classrooms where they engage children in meaningful learning activities but who must subvert the required curriculum to fit into what they know is best for their students or must interrupt their programs to administer state-mandated tests. Many examples of these competing ideologies can be found in schools today. Perhaps they occur most commonly where ability grouping is required for basal reading instruction but teachers implement the remainder of their programs through a whole language/integrated curricular approach.

School Choice.   The term *choice* has been applied to a number of approaches to school governance and structure. *Choice* is a word that has positive ideological power in the United States. As a consequence, it has been appropriated by political action groups, especially in education, from a variety of quite different and often conflicting perspectives (Lawrence 1994). In contemporary educational debates, *choice* has become a synonym for providing alternatives to the neighborhood public schools to which children ordinarily would be assigned.

The simplest way to give parents choices about the schools their children attend has been to relax the requirements that students attend the school closest to their home, that is, to eliminate attendance zones. Magnet schools have used this strategy, as have open-enrollment policies. Open enrollment plans have been criticized as advantaging only those children whose families have the ability to evaluate schools and transport their children to often distant campuses.

A rather restricted use of the term *choice* has been applied to giving teachers considerable autonomy in selecting curricular materials and instructional strategies. This approach changes governance only insofar as centralized curriculum directives are localized to the classroom and teachers are empowered to become more forceful decision makers in their own classrooms.

Another alternative to existing schools is to set up new ones at public expense. We have already discussed the multiple constituencies whose agendas compete for control of public schools. Over the years some of these constituencies have set up schools of their own. In the 1960s proponents of progressive "free" schools established a number of these institutions as private, tuition-charging alternatives. Private schools were also set up as "segregation academies" to avoid court-ordered desegregation of schools. The 1980s saw a tremendous increase in the number of Christian academies.

Current moves toward privatization differ in that they advocate the use of publicly funded alternative schools which, unlike magnet schools, do not further a socially mandated public policy. These plans exist under several rubrics. The first is a kind of fiscal reform that permits the allocation of school tax monies to parents in the form of vouchers. Advocates of this form of choice argue that if parents are allowed to use their vouchers to pay for at least part of their children's education, inferior schools would go bankrupt because no children would be sent to them. Critics argue that only the more affluent parents would have the means to provide transportation to out-of-neighborhood schools, which would persist despite their shortcomings because impoverished parents would have no choice at all. Furthermore, affluent parents could personally subsidize their voucher amount, thereby enhancing the quality of their children's schools in a way less affluent parents would be unable to do.

Choice can also encompass "charter schools," which have been established in limited numbers in several states. Charter schools resemble the magnet schools which were established to help maintain racially integrated schools, but they focus on a particular approach, theme, or curriculum, such as schools for outdoor experiences, music and the arts, and science and mathematics. They are financed by public funds, just as the magnet schools are, but they are established and governed by interested groups of parents and educators, who are given considerable autonomy. Although parents do not pay tuition, enrollment can be limited to students with certain qualifications.

A final form of privatization is allowing corporations and other institutions to set up schools which would run for profit—ostensibly more efficiently and effectively than the public schools. You may recall the arguments by the Scientific Management movement about making schools more effective by applying the tenets of corporate practice. The Whittle Corporation's Edison Project is an example. Some advocates of privatization argue that this alternative is the best one, just as they also argue for privatization of the penal system. However, as of this writing, several very ambitious attempts by well-funded corporate entities, such as Whittle Enterprises, have had second thoughts about their ability to run schools more cheaply and better than the public schools and have scaled back their efforts considerably. No examples of these efforts are currently available for assessment.

Alternative Ideologies of Schooling: Transformative Pedagogies

In this section we will examine four major approaches to transformative pedagogy currently being debated in educational literature: democratic education, critical pedagogy, multicultural education, and feminist pedagogy. These approaches in many ways encompass or overlap one another. For example, democratic educators would see multicultural education as an important part of their work. Multicultural educators would view democratic education and often critical and feminist pedagogies as processes for working with students. We have presented them separately here so as to explain briefly the main focus of each approach in the hope that you will explore them all in more detail.

All four approaches use similar specific pedagogical strategies. They all engage students in the construction of their own knowledge through methods such as whole language, an integrated curriculum, project-centered learning, Foxfire, process approaches to math and science, the use of student narratives, manipulatives, collaborative learning, peer tutoring, and authentic assessments. (See Table 9.1 for a summary of the four transformative pedagogies.)

Democratic Education.   A primary theme of democratic education is the belief that children develop democratic ideals of equality, liberty, and community by living them in their daily lives. Proponents of democratic education use John Dewey's works as a theoretical base. Writing in the late nineteenth and early twentieth centuries with a concern for the negative effects of urbanization and industrialization, Dewey believed schools could serve as social centers where people could build a spirit of cooperation and community as well as a sense of interdependence as they learned the critical thinking skills necessary for a democratic society. Heavily reliant on Dewey's notion of building community, democratic educators are concerned with constructing learning environments where children can participate in the democratic process. Lehman (Lappe and DuBois 1993) reminds us that "a sense of community is at the heart of any democratically run organization" (p. 9). There are many ways teachers and administrators can work toward democratic education. Table 9.1 gives a sense of democratic education in a real school setting.

For this example we have relied heavily on Dave Lehman (1993), principal of

TABLE 9.1   Transformative Pedagogies

Pedagogy	Focus
Democratic Education	Democratic education is concerned with constructing learning communities where children can participate actively and fully in the democratic process. Students learn democratic ideals of equality, liberty, and community by living them in their daily lives.
Critical Pedagogy	Language of critique challenges the economic and political power structures in society and the ways people are exploited and oppressed. It asks questions about whose interests are served. Through democratic classroom processes, curriculum relies on sociocultural/political analysis challenges. Through language of possibilities, it empowers students to work toward social transformation.
Multicultural Education	Focus is on knowledge and affirmation of pluralism in all forms (ethnic, linguistic, gender, religious, sexual orientation, abilities). Centering the experiences of marginalized groups in society provides a more holistic, multidimensional perspective of society as a replacement for the Western curriculum usually privileged in schools. Openly challenges and rejects racism, sexism, and other forms of discrimination and oppression through critical pedagogy; works toward social justice.
Feminist Pedagogy	Focus is on the experiences of women, particularly as related to patriarchal structures and language. Notions of student voice, alternatives to hierarchical classroom structures, and emotional connectedness to each other and to the course content are important aspects of this pedagogy. Central strategies emphasizing personal experiences are journals, narratives, and autobiography. It works toward social action and transformation.

Ithaca's Alternative Community School, a public school housing 230 students and governed through a participatory democracy that includes all students. The school community is built on Family Groups consisting of approximately ten students and a teacher who meet together at least twice a week. Four separate but interrelated governing bodies provide the mechanisms through which the democracy works: (1) An Advisory Board consisting of student, staff, parent, and community representatives meets once monthly. (2) There are 15 to 20 staff-facilitated Committees—concerned with much of the business of the school such as curriculum, discipline, appeals, school lunch, agenda for the All School Meeting, and so on—which meet twice weekly for two class periods. (3) The Staff Meeting, held weekly for at least two hours, is a collaborative effort of the school's professional staff. (4) A weekly All School Meeting attended by students and staff work through school decisions. All decisions and policies are discussed and decided in the governing bodies. Extensive in-service training for staff helps them develop skills in group processes. A democratic process also takes place in classrooms, where the teacher presents a course plan and students participate in setting the course goals and designing the structure and means to evaluate their learning.

As can be seen from this limited description, democracy is accomplished by full participation of students and staff.

Think of your own classroom, school, or college setting. Is it a participatory democracy? What would you need to do to transform it into one?

Critical Pedagogy. Critical pedagogy has grown out of the work of the critical theorists writing in the 1980s and 1990s. You may want to refer back to the discussion of critical theory in Chapter 1. Critical pedagogy is concerned, on one hand, with a critique of the society, particularly around issues of power, and on the other hand with developing students' critical abilities in order to work toward the transformation of society. This pedagogy involves a "language of critique" as well as a "language of possibilities." Teachers using this approach engage students in critical questioning of their own beliefs and assumptions, as well as the assumptions in their text materials. By *text* we mean anything used in the education process: textbooks, original source materials, popular culture, and so on. The deconstruction of textual language is especially important for critical pedagogy. What are the underlying assumptions, for example, in the phrase *manifest destiny?* Critical pedagogy attends to the question: "Whose interests are served?"

Student voice and resistance are central components of critical pedagogy. In these classrooms all students are encouraged to explore and express their own positions. Through active questioning and critique, students develop the ability to understand how people are manipulated by the economic and political power structures in society and can become empowered to work toward social change for a more democratic society in which human oppression and exploitation are not tolerated. Henry Giroux (1988) sees both teachers and students as transformative intellectuals who are able to engage in these critical dialogues of the ways power is

> understood as an embodied and fractured set of experiences that are lived and suffered by individuals and groups within specific contexts and settings. . . . First they need to analyze how cultural production is organized within asymmetrical relations of power in schools. Second, they need to construct political strategies for participating in social struggles and designed to fight for schools as democratic public spheres. (1988, pp. 101–102)

Think about a class in which you are either a teacher or a student. How could that class be transformed into one that uses critical pedagogy? What changes would be made in the way the class is structured, in the curriculum, or in the way the teacher(s) and students interact?

Multicultural Education. Multicultural education has been woven through discussions in the professional education literature since the 1960s, when social activists struggled against racial and gendered oppression. Multicultural education means quite different things to different people. Some educators have chosen the "tacos on Tuesday" approach, which is limited to celebrating the foods and customs of "ethnically different" groups. At the other end of the continuum, educators view multicultural education as anti-racist, anti-sexist education that critiques both individual and structural forms of racism, sexism, and other forms of discrimination and that works toward social transformation. Suzuki explains the consequence of this variation:

> [M]any widely differing conceptualizations of multicultural education have been formulated. As a consequence, the various programs in the field often appear to have conflicting purposes and priorities. Many educators have come to view multicultural education as ill defined, lacking in substance, and just another educational fad. (1984, p. 294)

In *Empowerment through Multicultural Education* Christine Sleeter (1991) gives a concise history of multicultural education in the United States, explaining five approaches that had been used in school pedagogy over the previous three decades:

1. A *human relations approach* is aimed toward sensitivity training, with people's interpersonal relationships and attitudes being central. A key understanding is that "we are all the same because we are all different." People are taught that through the power of love and harmony we can change insensitive or prejudiced attitudes. The human relations approach does not attend to oppression at the structural level.
2. *Teaching the culturally different* has grown out of research we reviewed in Chapter 7, which examined culturally congruent approaches to schooling. It argues that learning environments must be constructed so that culturally different children can use their abilities and knowledge for educational success.
3. *Cultural democracy* is a form of multicultural education whereby classrooms model an equal and unoppressive society that is culturally diverse. The notion here is that by experiencing this democratic, pluralistic setting, students can be empowered to work for social change in a society that does not practice these values. This approach uses an implicit rather than explicit approach to teach about oppression.
4. *Single group studies,* such as African-American studies, Chicano studies, or Women's studies, emphasize the history of the target group and the way the group's culture has formed and changed within oppressive circumstances. This form of multicultural education emphasizes group solidarity and identification for target members.
5. Education that is multicultural and *social reconstructionist* explicitly teaches about oppression and discrimination of historically marginalized groups and promotes social action to fight oppression through a coalition of oppressed and dominant groups. (1991)

Current educational literature continues to provide us with examples of all these approaches to multicultural education. We believe multicultural educators *cannot* stop at the individual or group level but must teach explicitly about ways in which racist and sexist practices are permeated through our institutions. A social action

> ### Seven Basic Characteristics of Multicultural Education
>
> Multicultural education is anti-racist education.
>
> Multicultural education is basic education.
>
> Multicultural education is important for all students.
>
> Multicultural education is pervasive.
>
> Multicultural education is education for social justice.
>
> Multicultural education is a process.
>
> Multicultural education is critical pedagogy.
>
> SOURCE: Nieto 1992, p. 208.

component is a critical one for multicultural education. We support multicultural education as described by Nieto:

> Multicultural education is a process of comprehensive school reform and basic education for all students. It challenges and rejects racism and other forms of discrimination in schools and society and accepts and affirms the pluralism (ethnic, racial, linguistic, religious, economic, and gender, among others) that students, their communities, and teachers represent. Multicultural education permeates the curriculum and instructional strategies used in schools, as well as the interactions among teachers, students and parents, and the very way that schools conceptualize the nature of teaching and learning. Because it uses critical pedagogy as its underlying philosophy and focuses on knowledge, reflection, and action (praxis) as the basis for social change, multicultural education furthers the democratic principles of social justice. (1992, p. 208)

Think of teachers you know who are multicultural educators. What approach does each take to this form of pedagogy?

Carefully examine your own knowledge of the history of oppressed groups. Do you need to expand your knowledge in order to be able to infuse your curriculum with multicultural content?

Feminist Pedagogies.   As Chapter 8 noted, there is not just one feminism or one feminist theory. Similarly, there are many forms of feminist pedagogies. This section will provide a brief overview of the central components of feminist pedagogies; we urge you to explore this literature. Consistent with feminism and feminist theory, feminist pedagogies are concerned with the experiences of women in societies, particularly as related to differential power structures. Feminist teachers critique the cultural patriarchal structures and language which continue to place women in oppressive, exploited positions. Shrewsbury explains:

> At its simplest level, feminist pedagogy is concerned with gender justice and overcoming oppressions. It recognizes the genderedness of all social relations and consequently of all societal institutions and structures. (1987, p. 7)

Using bell hooks's (1989) notions, this pedagogy moves traditional curricular content to the margins, as that which has been silenced or marginalized is moved to the center of exploration. The experiences of women and marginalized groups are the focus of class readings and discussion. Feminist teaching

> moves people and topics ordinarily defined as "marginal" into focus in the classroom and it invites people who ordinarily occupy the center of attention (i.e. white males) to notice what it's like to not be the center of attention. Students then have the opportunity to examine how power and status are used among them. (Thompson and Disch 1992, p. 5)

Concerned with hierarchical relations in their schools, feminist teachers interrupt these relations by using strategies to share the power with students. Teachers collaborate with other teachers and students in the construction of the structure, content, and interactions in the class. Therefore, like other forms of transformative pedagogies, feminists rely on democratic decision-making processes and community building. Thompson and Disch explain:

> We continually think about how our classes are going as communities. Other teachers obsess about their lectures; we obsess about both the content we teach as well as the relationships among students and our relationships with both individuals and the group as a whole. We think carefully about how to express our anger when the class isn't taking responsibility to carry on meaningful discussion of the readings. We think carefully about how to address or resolve conflicts among particular pairs or groups of students. No two semesters are alike. The results of this kind of teaching cannot be predicted because the students have power, and we never know how they're going to use it, how they're going to challenge us, or how they're going to challenge each other. (1992, p. 9)

Teachers assume roles of co-learner and facilitator rather than authority. However, because of institutional structures, feminist teachers are positioned in the role of those who have ultimate authority for student evaluation, and they struggle to find ways to engage students in making decisions about their own evaluations and grades.

Clearly, student voice is central to the feminist classroom, as are the personal experiences of teachers and students. Feminist teachers believe that students construct their own knowledge by using their personal experiences to connect with the course content. The use of journals, biography, autobiography, and narratives enhances this process. Berry and Black explain:

> We encourage them [students] to look for connections between their personal experience and the theoretical and historical concerns addressed in class; we push them to examine their own lives in the context of larger cultural, social and economic issues relating to women. (1987, p. 59)

Because of the emotional nature of sharing personal experiences in the classroom, there is often a sense of emotional connectedness among participants. These emotions are not always positive, but rather they reflect the struggle among participants as they make sense of their differing views and experiences. Feminist teachers expect a range of emotions because of both the content and the pedagogical strategies used in the teaching/learning process. Feminist pedagogy requires us to accept and explore these emotions as part of classroom life. Teachers understand that in order to really struggle with the knowledge, students must feel this emotional connectedness to the experience:

> We assume that learning needs to be close to the heart, meaning that the course must move the learner and make a lasting impact on her or his life. (Thompson and Disch 1992, p. 4)

Have you ever participated in feminist pedagogy? Share your experiences with others in the class.

A Note about Networks.   Since the last edition of this book, networks of individuals, schools, and colleges have proliferated and serve to share knowledge, support one another's efforts, and discuss their issues and concerns. These networks are coalitions of individuals and institutions, variously supported by public and foundational monies, that work to support transformative educational projects. As we end this section, we urge you to explore the work of these networks.

Just a few of the many examples are the Coalition for Essential Schools, the Institute of Democracy in Education, the Foxfire Network, Rethinking Schools, the San Diego State Multicultural Infusion Center (MEIC), the Urban Network for the Improvement of Teacher Education (UNITE), the Center for Collaborative Education (CCE), the National Coalition of Education Activists, and the National Center for Restructuring Education, Schools, and Teaching (NCREST). In addition, many local and state teachers' support groups are actively engaged in exploring new forms of teaching and learning. Some of these networks have established electronic mail discussion groups that are usually open to anyone interested in participating. We invite you to explore these networks of innovative educators.

Select a network whose efforts are centered on a project that interests you, and become part of its electronic mail discussion group. Write for the network's literature, find out about its funding agencies, and explore its purposes and activities. Write to us, through Longman, Inc., to share your findings. Maybe for our next edition we will compile a list of these networks.

Alternative Possibilities for Teacher Education and Practice

What types of teachers are needed to provide quality schooling in a multicultural world? How should these teachers be educated? What is the role of teachers in schools today? The 1980s brought a new reform movement in teacher education calling for complete restructuring of the profession. One set of critics was based in universities and colleges of education; the other found its impetus in school districts and state legislatures. The former provided their central arguments in two documents: The Holmes Group's *Tomorrow's Teachers* (1986), and *A Nation Prepared: Teachers for the 21st Century* by the Carnegie Task Force on Teaching as a Profession (1986). Both call for a more highly educated professional teaching force.

The Holmes Group proposed a five-year program, with students pursuing a fifth year of teacher education after completing a Liberal Arts degree. The underlying assumption is that a Liberal Arts degree in a specific academic field would provide preservice teachers with the necessary knowledge base and then the fifth year would furnish the pedagogical knowledge and experience for teaching of that subject matter. These reforms leave control of entrance to the teaching profession in the hands of the university teacher training programs.

A counterproposal, calling for a different route to certification, has been spearheaded largely by school district personnel who feel that college teaching is out of touch with the realities of public school life and who resent the poor preparation given to many teachers. While the content of such routes to certification does not differ from that proposed by the Holmes Group, the control mechanisms do. They seek to weaken or even eliminate the role of colleges of education in teacher preparation. One approach places teacher certification in the hands of school districts. It calls for the establishment of district-level "teacher centers," where methods courses and other requirements would be provided. People who already have degrees would enter a teacher center and, while taking courses, would begin an apprenticeship under the supervision of the school district. A variation calls for the teacher center to be located in a local teachers' college but for all other activities to be carried out by the district. Other proposals call for centers to be established and examinations to be given under state supervision, with districts providing the supervised apprenticeships.

These plans differ substantially from traditional teacher training programs which have been in place in colleges of education throughout most of the twentieth century. The extreme case is in elementary education, where in some programs a teacher trainee is limited to two years of academic training, a year and a half of methods—or "Mickey Mouse"—courses, and student teaching, leaving college with no real specialization whatsoever. Currently teacher training often does not prepare students for the political arena, either on the microlevel or on the macrolevel. By retaining what we call a "psychocentric" focus on individual differences and cognition, teacher training has avoided confronting the social and political context of schooling altogether. This gap makes new teachers exceedingly vulnerable to pressure, prone to sliding into teaching at the lowest common denominator for survival and to accepting the conventional wisdom of senior teachers about "how it's always been." This is why we have advocated explicit training and practice in the critical and political for pre-service teachers. In-service activities for practicing teachers could also make good use of such instruction.

The demand for a more rigorously educated teaching force has gained support from both the radical left and neoconservative right. The call for raising entrance standards, increasing the number and rigor of classes, and establishing tests for exit-level competencies conforms to the neoconservative "back to the classics" excellence movement propounded by William Bennett, Secretary of Education under President Reagan. These proposals argue from the "top down" for more centralized state control over the training and evaluation of students and teachers. They are based upon a deep suspicion that teachers cannot be trusted to work competently and the belief that only a program of tight, centralized control will put things right.

Teachers as Intellectuals.   On the left, critical theorists such as Henry Giroux (1988) argue for the concept of "teachers as intellectuals." Contrary to the neoconservatives, critical theorists argue for less rather than more control over teachers. In fact, they wish to shift the locus of power from state, university, and district administrators to the classroom teacher.

Giroux argues that current demands for reform in teacher education are at variance with the democratically informed schooling needed in a pluralistic society. Giroux states that these proposals lead to de-skilling of teachers—the process by which teachers lose the ability to utilize professional training, judgment, and autonomy. He argues that a "teacher-proof" standardized curriculum, uniform text adoptions, centralized and test-driven systems of student evaluation and placement, routinized classroom management systems, and reduction in decision-making power all act to reduce teachers to mere technicians. He further calls for a complete restructuring of teachers' work so that they are viewed as valued intellectuals, not barely competent, mindless technicians. The first step in this process would be to transfer instructional control from administrators, state bureaucrats, and textbook publishers to teachers. As intellectual leaders, teachers would be responsible for determining the goals of schooling—what should be taught, how these goals would be translated into curricular materials, and how the materials should be presented.

Central to Giroux's argument is the concept of the teacher as a critical pedagogue or transformative intellectual. To be intellectually critical educators, teachers must not only be intellectuals in the sense that they reflect seriously on the meaning and consequences of their practice, but be critical in the sense that they question the taken-for-granted assumptions—the "that's the way it's always been"—of school practice and societal organization. Critical pedagogues have the *responsibility* to question political motives and social inequities with their students in an ongoing effort to create a more democratic and equitable society. Giroux is worth quoting at length on the role of teachers as transformative intellectuals:

> Transformative intellectuals need to develop a discourse that unites the language of critique with the language of possibility, so that social educators recognize that they can make changes. In doing so, they must speak out against economic, political and social injustices, both within and outside of schools. At the same time, they must work to create the conditions that give students the opportunity to become citizens who have the knowledge and courage to struggle in order to make despair unconvincing and hope practical. As difficult as this task may seem to social educators, it is a struggle worth waging. To do otherwise is to deny social educators the opportunity to assume the role of transformative intellectuals. (1988, p. 128)

There are limitations in Giroux's critique. First, neither neoconservatives nor critical theorists have addressed the impact of their proposals on the participation of minorities in the teaching profession. On the one hand is a concern that raising standards and increasing the length—and cost—of teacher training would make it more difficult for minority individuals to become teachers (Halcon and Reyes 1989). On the other is a concern that minority teachers who advocate radical change would threaten their legitimacy and acceptance. Standing too far from conventional practice might well place such teachers, already in the minority on most faculties, in danger of being fired—or at least ostracized professionally—as troublemakers.

Another concern is that it is difficult to imagine how today's teachers could be critical, intellectual pedagogues given the limits of their preparation, the structural constraints on their activities, and their largely oppressive working environments. Implicit in Giroux's notion of the teacher as transformative intellectual is a critique of the entire system of schooling. Clearly, a complete restructuring is required if teachers are to be reflective, to have their skills, expertise, and creativity celebrated, and to work in situations that do not denigrate their sense of professionalism.

Unfortunately, both the neoconservative right and the radical left calls for reform focused primarily on teachers. This may be so because blaming teachers is relatively easy. This stance may be due to an optimistic hope that only through a "grass roots" community-based organization of teachers will significant changes be accomplished. Much more difficult is addressing the structural and political constraints which have created the radically alienating conditions prevalent in many schools. However, as we've described above, present alternatives for the structure of public schools empower teachers to begin to function in the ways prescribed by critical theorists.

Teachers as Feminists.   We have earlier discussed how hegemony consists of the practices and thinking that justify existing patterns of domination and subordination in society. In this section we look at ways in which the educational system might begin to question these patterns.

We demonstrated in Chapter 4 that teaching is a predominantly female activity, that schools resemble "pedagogical harems" where women teach and men supervise and administrate. Increasing the professional status of teaching—in our view as well as that of scholars like Apple, Blau, Kelly, Lortie, Simeone, Weiler, Weis, and others cited in previous chapters—cannot be discussed without a consideration of the engendered nature and patriarchal structure of schooling. The unequal distribution of power among men and women is one of the most salient features of the profession, one that undermines its status. As long as teaching is considered to be "women's work," neither it nor its participants (male and female) will enjoy the power and prestige they seek.

Through feminist critiques, teachers can question the legitimacy of the male-dominated hierarchy of schools in order to gain a voice in the decision-making process. Feminist teachers are those who are sensitive to and directly address issues of gender inequality in the curricular content, instructional methods, and organization of schools. Their knowledge of gender and power issues enables them to assess their own and their students' experiences in schools, question the oppressive aspects of these experiences, and provide more democratic alternatives. Weiler (1988) suggests that feminist teachers, both male and female, are more sensitive to and respectful of the racial, cultural, and class identities of their students because they have been made sharply aware of patterns of gender discrimination.

Recruitment to Teacher Education.   What would teacher education look like from critical theoretical and feminist perspectives? If you were to walk through the halls of most colleges of education in the United States today, you would find a fairly homogeneous population of white, middle-class, female students being taught by a fairly homogeneous population of white, middle-class, male professors—despite an increasing number of young female and minority assistant professors. A salutary change would occur if the ranks of both professors and students in these colleges more closely resembled the general population of public schools.

Although minority recruitment programs have been in place in most colleges for some years, the number of actual recruits is small and decreasing, especially in colleges of education. The continued low status and salary of teachers as well as the lack of scholarship funds limit the number of minority students interested in pursuing teaching as a career. In addition, as colleges move toward five-year degree plans, tuition costs soar, and financial aid continues to diminish, the hardships of attendance as well as the opportunity costs of becoming a teacher become overwhelming to minority students.

Despite these barriers, it is essential for colleges of education to be sensitive to the type of students they are admitting. With the current reform movement's emphasis on "excellence," concerns about race, ethnicity, class, and gender balance may be obscured by concerns over "quality." It will be easy for insensitive teacher educators to mistake being white, middle-class, and comfortable with school culture for academic quality. A college of education committed to preparing intellectual teachers for a multicultural world will work to ensure the comparable diversity of the student body. These colleges must be committed to recruiting and educating a multi-ethnic, gender-balanced teaching population.

Multicultural Infusion.   A college committed to social justice and to training teachers for today's multicultural schools will place emphasis on courses and experiences that prepare students to function among those who are ethnically, culturally, and economically different from themselves. These materials should not be "ghettoized" into isolated courses or parts of courses, nor taught only by minority faculty. The multicultural emphasis achieves legitimacy only when it becomes part and parcel of everyday life in every subject—infused throughout the programs.

Teaching in teams so that faculty become familiar with each other's subject areas and work toward integrating each into their instruction—including material relevant to other ethnicities, classes, and genders—would help normalize the currently exotic nature of both the multicultural content and the faculty who teach it. We suggest also that colleges go beyond advocating and teaching sensitivity to cultural differences. Colleges should also establish a "minimum competency" for affirming diversity, such that candidates who demonstrate bigoted attitudes do not receive certification. Such a competency is no more subjective than demonstrated competence to evaluate visual art or poetry.

Watch the movie *Stand and Deliver,* an illustration of alternative teaching methods in a barrio school in Los Angeles. What worked for the teacher and students in this film? How was the teacher able to engage his students effectively? Do you think these methods would work in other settings?

An Interdisciplinary Perspective.   Teachers can be neither critical, intellectual, nor competent if they have never experienced intellectual challenges nor been exposed to the world of content and ideas. With this in mind, we conform to certain aspects of the neoconservative reform, which calls for basing the curriculum on a Liberal Arts education. At the same time, it is important to remember the multicultural curriculum. Liberal Arts does not mean a return to a traditional androcentric and ethnocentric emphasis on classics of the Western European heritage. Rather, it means that students would specialize in a particular discipline of their choice for the requisite four-year program and only then enter a teacher education program.

This preparation would be based upon an experiential study of schooling within its social context. Departing from the heavily cognitive teacher training programs, we propose to place greater emphasis on child and adolescent development, on the historical and philosophical antecedents of current practice, and on the social, political, and cultural context within and outside of the schools. These studies derive from what have come to be known as the foundations of education—history, philosophy, psychology, anthropology, and sociology.

At the present time, despite the fact that whole children are the primary focus in what teachers do, teacher trainees take only an introductory course or two in human growth and development; their study of psychology is narrowly limited to experimental and behavioral studies of cognition. Similarly, they get only the barest smattering of the other foundational studies, usually crammed into a single survey course covering the history, philosophy, sociology, anthropology, and politics of education. Graduate programs are rarely more rigorous. The program we propose would have a much stronger psychological and social foundation in order to prepare teachers to examine critically current practices and procedures, to analyze patterns of control and governance in education, and to critique text materials, instructional techniques, and classroom management strategies.

Form small groups or committees in your class to design a school based on the research knowledge presented in this text. Share your ideas in a general group discussion. How could you incorporate some of these ideas into your real world of school practice?

A CLOSING NOTE

The suggestions above are just a beginning. Professional journals as well as the popular press are full of articles calling for reform and describing successful innovative programs purporting to resolve some or all of the crisis in education. Yet the innovations, like cream, still float to the top, serving the most advantaged students; programs for the most disadvantaged seem remarkably ineffective. We believe that the insights offered in this text provide a way of beginning a new kind of thinking about schools. What *are* the purposes of schooling in contemporary society? What *should* they be? Are the two compatible? How will the characteristics of the students change in the next few years? What will the teaching force look like? How would this work force, as well as curricula, school structures, forms of control, and instructional practices, have to change to be congruent with the incoming population of children—and teachers? What can *you* do about it?

Do's and Don'ts for Non-Sexist Language

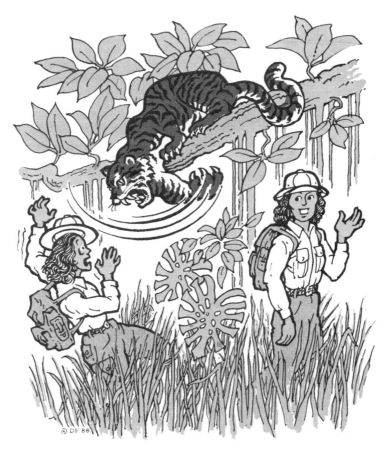

"Relax...it's only a <u>man</u>-eating tiger."

GENERAL PRINCIPLES

■ *Degender*, don't *regender* (e.g. degender *chairman* to *chair*, don't regender it to *chairwoman*).

■ Create gender-neutral terms: convert adjectives to nouns by adding *ist* (e.g. active: activist).

■ Replace occupational terms in *man* and *boy*, if possible, with terms that include members of either sex.

■ Avoid occupational designations having derogatory *-ette* and *-ess* endings.

NAMES AND TITLES

■ When Mr. is used, Ms. is the equivalent. Use Ms. to designate both a married and unmarried woman. A woman should be referred to by name in the same way that a man is. Both should be called by their full names, by first or last name only, or by title.

　⊘ Miss Lee, Ms. Chai and Mrs. Feeney ♦ Ms. Lee, Ms. Chai and Ms. Feeney or Lee, Chai and Feeney.

　⊘ Governor Burns and Anna Kahanamoku ♦ Governor Burns and Representative Kahanamoku.

■ Forms for using a woman's name before marriage should be gender-neutral.

　⊘ maiden name ♦ pre-marital name, birth name.

■ Issue invitations or notices, bills, financial statements, etc. in the name of each of the individuals concerned.

　⊘ Mr. and Mrs. John Tanaka ♦ Ellen and John Tanaka (if both names are known), or (if the name of spouse is not known) Ellen Tanaka and spouse.

SALUTATIONS IN LETTERS

■ If the name of the addressee is unknown, start the letter immediately without a salutation. Alternatively, especially in letters of recommendations or memos not addressed to a specific person, start with "To Whom It May Concern."

　⊘ Dear Sir/Madam/Gentlemen:

　　♦ Aloha: (Use only in Hawaii.)

　　♦ Dear Customer/Colleague/Subscriber:

　　♦ Dear Editor/Manager/Account Executive/(other job title):

　　♦ Dear Representative/Senator/Delegate/(other honorary title):

　　♦ Dear Friend(s):

⊘ indicates DON'T, a sexist expression to be avoided.
　♦ indicates DO, a non-sexist alternative.

PRONOUNS

■ Avoid the pronoun *he* when both sexes are meant. Alternative approaches are:

● Recast into the plural.

　⊘ Give each student *his* paper as soon as *he* is finished. ♦ Give students *their* papers as soon as *they* are finished.

● Reword to eliminate the pronoun.

　⊘ The average student is worried about *his* grades. ♦ The average student is worried about grades.

● Replace the masculine pronoun with *one, you,* or (sparingly) *he or she* as appropriate.

　⊘ If the student is dissatisfied with *his* grade, *he* can appeal to the instructor. ♦ A student who is dissatisfied with *her* or *his* grade can appeal to the instructor.

● Alternate male and female expressions.

　⊘ Let each student participate. Has *he* had a chance to talk? Did *he* feel left out? ♦ Let each student participate. Has *she* had a chance to talk? Did *he* feel left out?

● Use plural indefinite pronoun.

　⊘ Anyone who wants to go to the game should bring *his* money tomorrow. ♦ All those who want to go to the game should bring *their* money tomorrow.

● Use the double-pronoun construction.

　⊘ Every person has a right to *his* opinion. ♦ Every person has a right to *his or her* opinion.

● Use *he/she, his/her*, etc. in printed contracts and other forms so the inapplicable pronoun can be crossed out.

SPORTS

■ Let language usage reflect the fact that sports do not exclusively concern males.

■ Use gender-free terms in writing or talking about sports events.

　⊘ sportsmanship ♦ fair play, team play, sporting attitude.

　⊘ baseman (as in first baseman) ♦ base (as in first base), baseplayer.

　⊘ crewman ♦ crew, crew member.

　⊘ ironman (event and participant) ♦ (iron) triathlon, triathlete.

　⊘ tinman (event and participant) ♦ (tin) triathlon, triathlete.

actress ◆ actor.

anchorman ◆ anchor, anchorperson.

authoress ◆ author.

average or common man ◆ average person, ordinary people, typical worker.

bachelor ◆ single (or unmarried) man.

bachelorgirl, spinster ◆ single (or unmarried woman).

brotherhood (unless only men are meant) ◆ community, amity, unity.

businessman ◆ business executive, business person, business manager, manager, entrepreneur.

cameraman ◆ camera operator, photographer.

career girl ◆ professional woman.

chairman, chairwoman ◆ chair (for both sexes).

Chinamen ◆ the Chinese.

cleaning lady/woman, maid ◆ housekeeper, housecleaner, office cleaner.

clergyman ◆ clergy, minister, priest.

coed ◆ student.

congressman ◆ member of Congress, representative, legislator.

copy boy, copy girl ◆ messenger, runner.

councilman, councilwoman ◆ councilmember.

countryman, countrymen ◆ people of the country, country's citizens.

craftsman ◆ craftsperson, artisan, crafter.

draftsman ◆ drafter, drafting technician.

Dutchmen ◆ the Dutch.

early man, caveman ◆ early humans, early societies.

Esquire ◆ Attorney at law, lawyer.

executrix ◆ executor.

fellow worker ◆ colleague, co-worker, peer.

fireman ◆ firefighter.

forefathers ◆ ancestors, precursors, forebears.

foreman ◆ supervisor.

founding fathers ◆ the founders, pioneers.

gal or girl Friday ◆ assistant or secretary.

gentlemen's agreement ◆ personal agreement, informal contract.

great men in history ◆ great figures in history, people who made history, historical figures.

heroine ◆ hero.

hostess ◆ host.

hula girl ◆ hula dancer.

insurance man ◆ insurance agent.

Irishmen ◆ the Irish.

lady doctor ◆ doctor, physician.

layman ◆ layperson, lay, laity, lay people, lay member.

libber ◆ feminist, liberationist.

mailman, postman ◆ mail carrier, letter carrier, postal worker.

male nurse ◆ nurse.

(to) man ◆ to staff, run, operate.

man and his world ◆ world history, history of peoples.

manhood ◆ adulthood, maturity.

man-hours ◆ work hours, staff hours, hours worked, total hours.

manhunt ◆ a hunt for . . .

mankind ◆ humanity, human race, human beings, people, human family.

man-made ◆ artificial, hand made, of human origin, synthetic, manufactured, crafted, machine made.

manned flight ◆ piloted flight.

manned orbital flight ◆ piloted orbital flight.

manning chart ◆ staff chart.

man-on-the-street ◆ ordinary person, ordinary citizen, average voter, average person.

manpower ◆ work force, human resources, labor force, human energy, personnel, workers.

man's achievements ◆ human achievements.

man-sized job ◆ big or difficult (job), requiring exceptional abilities.

men of science ◆ scientists.

middleman ◆ go-between, liaison, agent.

Mr. Chairman! Madam Chairwoman! ◆ Chair! (for both sexes).

one-man band or show ◆ soloist, performer, artist, individual, individual show.

poetess ◆ poet.

policeman ◆ police officer.

police matron ◆ police officer.

primitive man ◆ primitive people, primitive human beings, a primitive.

repairman ◆ repairer.

right hand man ◆ assistant, helper.

rise of man ◆ rise of the human race or humanity, rise of civilization, rise of cultures.

salesman ◆ salesperson, sales representative, salesclerk, seller, agent.

salesman ◆ sales staff, sales personnel.

showman ◆ performer.

spokesman ◆ representative, spokesperson.

statesman ◆ official, diplomat.

tradesman ◆ shopkeeper, trader, merchant, entrepreneur, artisan.

tradesmen ◆ trades people, tradespersons.

weatherman ◆ forecaster, weathercaster.

woman lawyer ◆ lawyer.

working man ◆ workers, typical worker.

workman ◆ worker, laborer, employee.

workman like ◆ competent.

■ The following assumptions are obsolete and should be avoided.

- That only men hold influential jobs. E.g. ⊘Congressional representatives urged the President to find the right *man* for the job. ♦ Congressional representatives urged the President to find the right *person*.

- That children are cared for by their mothers only. E.g. ⊘*Mothers* should note that a nutritious breakfast is more important for a child than it is for an adult. ♦ A nutritious breakfast is more important for a child than . . .

- That men head all families and are the major wage earners. E.g. ⊘The average worker with a wife and two children pays 30 percent of *his* income to taxes. ♦ An average family of four pays 30 percent of *its* income . . . *or an* average worker with three dependents pays 30 percent of income . . .

- That certain professions are reserved for one sex. E.g. ⊘Sometimes a nurse must use *her* common sense. ♦ Sometimes nurses must rely on common sense . . .

- That women perform all work related to homemaking. E.g. ⊘The family grocery shopper wants to get all *her* shopping done in one stop. ♦ The family grocery shopper wants to get all the shopping done in one stop.

- Housewives are not using the new truth-in-weight information. ♦ *Homemakers (shoppers, customers)* are not using the new . . .

- That women are possessions of men and are not responsible for their actions. E.g. ⊘Henry *allows* his wife to work part time. ♦ Odette Lee works part time.

■ Describe the appearance of a woman only in circumstances in which you would describe the appearance of a man.

⊘ The *attractive well-dressed* interior minister fielded questions from reporters. ♦ The interior minister fielded . . .

■ Do not report the marital status of a woman or a man, unless marital status is the subject of the story.

⊘ Divorcee Judy Petty lost her bid to unseat Representative Wilbur Mills. ♦ Candidate Judy Petty lost her bid . . .

■ An employed person should be identified by his or her occupation, when relevant. Do not use the terms "homemaker" and "mother" unless his or her homemaking role and family relationship, respectively, are the subject of discourse.

- Mrs. Marion Chong, *wife* of Dr. Allan Chong, gave a report on recent zoning variances. ♦ Marion Chong, *member* of the Zoning Board, gave a report on . . .

■ Use title, terms and names in parallel construction, with females mentioned first sometimes to avoid stereotyping.

⊘ Man and wife ♦ Wife and husband (or husband and wife)

■ Do not suggest that women are immature, adolescent and emotional and hence inferior to men.

⊘ Sports stories and pictures that portray females merely as spectators. ♦ Sports stories and pictures that portray females as active participants

⊘ The term *girl* for a female over 18 ♦ The term *woman*

⊘ Fair sex, weaker sex ♦ Women

⊘ The little woman or better half ♦ Wife

⊘ Housewife ♦ Homemaker

⊘ ALSO AVOID: Stories that emphasize exceptions to stereotypes (examples: John Kealoha is glad his mother-in-law is visiting); and expressions that demean women (example: distaff, women's work, woman driver, weak sister, sissy, old-maidish, spinsterish, womanish).

■ Avoid stories, photographs, captions, or phrases that imply:

⊘ That the sole or primary interest of an unmarried woman is "catching a man."

⊘ That certain categories of women are shrewish or overbearing. (Examples: mothers-in-law, feminists.)

⊘ That certain categories of women are scatterbrained, incompetent, or excessively dependent upon men to manage their lives. (Example: young, pretty, or blond-haired women.)

⊘ That women are incompetent in areas once considered "man's domain." (Example: Leilani is mechanically inept.)

⊘ That career women generally lack homemaking skills, do not have children, or are not good parents if they do have children.

⊘ That all or nearly all female homemakers are unsympathetic to the objectives of the women's movement. [Surveys and articles indicate the contrary.]

⊘ That men have the active roles, women have the passive roles.

⊘ That men are brutish, violent, crude, harsh or insensitive.

⊘ That women are fearful, squeamish, passive, dependent, weepy, frivolous, weak, shrewish, nagging, easily defeated, hysterical, scatterbrained.

This material has been adapted from *Women, Men and the Changing Language,* a 13-page brochure produced by the Media Task Force of the Honolulu County Committee on the Status of Women. Produced by HCCSW. Cover art by David Friedman. Edited by John Defrancis, Laudra B. Eber, Gerald H. Ohta, Katsue Akiba Reynolds, 1988. Additional copies of the brochure are available. Send stamped, self-addressed envelope to Office of Human Resources, 650 S. King St., Honolulu, HI 96813 (phone 523-4073).

Glossary

Ability grouping is the practice, used in elementary schools, of organizing students into instructional groups according to their abilities as assessed by school personnel on the basis of classroom performance and standardized test scores. These groups are used primarily for math and reading instruction.

Adolescence refers to the transition stage in one's life which usually begins at puberty and ends when one participates in activities normally associated with adulthood: economic independence from parents, marriage, or the birth of a child.

Alienation is a sociological word for the more popularly used term *burnout*. It occurs when the social and cultural context in which individuals live changes so drastically that personal goals that were once valued and desired cannot be achieved. As a result, the individuals lose faith in the institutions that structure their lives. Alienation is manifested in six types of feelings: *powerlessness,* or the sense that people have no control over their personal or work lives; *meaninglessness,* or a sense that the world has become absurd or incomprehensible; *normlessness,* or the feeling that the rules that structure the world have disappeared or become ineffective; *personal isolation,* or feeling apart from other human beings; *cultural isolation,* or being in opposition to or isolated from values held by one's community; and *self-estrangement,* or being forced to engage in activities that are intrinsically unrewarding or counter to one's beliefs and self-definition. (LeCompte and Dworkin 1991, p. 5)

Bureaucracy is a sociological term referring to a large, hierarchically structured formal organization whose purpose is to carry out some complex task. Both work and administration in bureaucracies are rationally subdivided and supervised by career professionals specifically trained for their jobs.

Caste refers to a social group or class whose membership is fixed by hereditary rules and defined by occupational status. In societies where castes exist they are the primary means by which society is stratified.

317

Caste-like minority (Ogbu 1978) is a native-born stigmatized group whose destiny is caste-like because it has experienced so many generations of systematic economic discrimination that its poverty becomes virtually hereditary.

Civil rights refers to those rights belonging to individuals because of their status as citizens; all citizens are guaranteed equal protection under the law by the Fourteenth Amendment of the U.S. Constitution.

Class refers to a category of things grouped together because they share common characteristics.

Cohort is a demographic term identifying a category of people who share a characteristic such as age or the date of entering an institution. Sociologists frequently refer to an *educational* or *age cohort*, people who are of the same generation or who entered the educational system or other social institution at the same time.

Compensatory education refers to school programs funded by the federal government to provide additional, individualized education to compensate for disadvantages resulting from a poor environment.

Conflict theory uses the same general systems analysis as does functionalism but focuses on conflict, change, and inequality, which it views as a consequence of unequal resource distribution within society (Coser 1956; Marx 1955; Simmel 1955; J. Turner 1978). Conflict theorists believe that conflict, rather than equilibrium, is natural and inherent to social systems and that it in fact contributes to the healthy adaptations of social systems.

Correspondence refers to society's economic organization being mirrored in its institutions and vice versa. Thus if schools and churches resemble factories, this is so because the factory is the dominant form of economic organization in industrial society.

Critical theory asserts that existing societal structures derive from historically generated patterns of domination and subordination. Many critical theorists state that patterns of oppression derive from inequalities in the distribution of economic resources; others focus on the unequal distribution of knowledge and skill in society. These theorists are concerned with the power of language and control of information, and so they often give particular attention to curriculum. Still others emphasize asymmetries such as race, gender, religion, age, gender preference, and region. Critical theorists make two different critiques of the existing social order. The first views the hegemony of the existing order as inescapably rigid and inegalitarian, dooming most of the human race to slavery or rule by autocrats. The second and less pessimistic critique emphasizes human "agency" or self-determination in the face of institutional rigidity. The latter provides a basis for social transformation insofar as it uses social critique as a way to escape the control of the dominant classes (Tar 1985).

Cultural capital consists of the knowledge base possessed by individuals; it includes general cultural knowledge and preferences, patterns of language use, leisure activities, manners, and skills. Some kinds of cultural capital are more valuable than others, and people who possess valuable cultural capital have more social power.

Curriculum is what is taught to children in schools, whether or not the instruction is intended.

De-skilling refers to a process by which the level of specialized, professional knowledge and skill needed to carry out a task is progressively reduced until workers' autonomy over their work is shifted upward to supervisors.

Education broadly refers to the process of learning over the span of one's entire life. Education begins at birth and continues in a wide variety of both formal and informal settings.

Empowerment refers to the ability to become conscious of oppression and to learn to implement strategies to overcome it.

Ethnicity refers to a group of people bound by a sense of peoplehood based on shared cultural traits such as religion, ancestry, national origin, or language. All people can trace their roots to an ethnic background.

Ethnocentricity is the tendency to evaluate others using your own group as the norm or standard.

Feminism is both a theory or explanation about women's position in a society and a political statement focused on gaining equal rights and opportunities for women and on changing power relations between men and women.

Formal organization is one that has a legally established identity and is organized for some specific long-term purpose. Formal organizations are distinguished from informal friendship groups, associations, and families in that the former are governed by charters, by-laws, or rules and regulations. They exist independently of the identities of individual participants, and their life span exceeds the tenure of individual members.

Functionalism views societies as systems made up of interrelated components. It uses the analogy of the human body with its interrelated organs. Functionalism argues that all societies consist of systems which perform the basic functions necessary for the society to survive. Functionalism seeks to identify the basic functions that systems need to survive as well as the relationships between different functions within a society. Functionalists believe that a social system seeks its natural state of equilibrium. They assume that change tends to occur through growth or by stimulation from outside forces, rather than through internal conflict or contradictions. Functionalists suggest that societies must continually face and solve problems that threaten its survival. Consequently, those elements in society that persist are those that have contributed to its continued viability. Societies continue to organize formal schooling because doing so helps societies to survive (Dworkin 1989; Merton 1967; Parsons 1963; J. Turner 1978).

Gender, in addition to physiological traits, refers to the cultural understandings and behaviors associated with maleness and femaleness. Gender is learned through a process of socialization at birth.

Hegemony is a form of social control. It exists in the form of a social consensus created by dominant groups who control socializing institutions such as the media, schools, churches, and the political system; these institutions prevent alternative views from gaining an audience or establishing their legitimacy (McLaren 1989). Hegemony maintains the power of the existing social and political structure without the use of force because it creates a consensus in which all groups agree that the status quo is satisfactory, even if it is inequitable.

Hidden curriculum refers to the implicit and sometimes unintentional messages transmitted to students through the content, routines, and social relationships of schooling.

Ideology is a system of values and beliefs which provide the concepts, images, and ideas by which people interpret their world and shape their behavior toward other people. It is accepted as the natural and common-sense explanation of the way the world operates. Ideologies often act to reinforce the power of dominant groups in society.

Ideology of schooling refers to values and beliefs held by educators and students that inform and determine how we "do school."

Intensification refers to an increase in the amount and kind of work required on a job, without concomitant additional rewards or time in which to accomplish it.

Interpretive theory states that social structures are based upon webs of meaning created by individuals in their interaction with others. Meaning—and hence reality—is constructed during social interaction; because it is based upon interpretation of objects and events, it is flexible and negotiated rather than fixed. The meanings with which participants enter a setting affect the course of social interaction, but these meanings change in the course of interaction as they are negotiated and renegotiated. Among the most important contributions of interpretive researchers has been their shift of attention from systems to individuals; they also pioneered observational research in schools and classrooms.

Liminality refers to the time after leaving one clearly identified social identity and before entering another. Adolescence is a liminal state between childhood and adulthood.

Line offices are the positions in an organization located in the vertical supervisory structure. People in lower-line offices report to and are supervised by those directly above them, who in turn report to and are supervised by those above them. These workers carry out the actual tasks for which the organization exists. In schools, the teachers, principals, and superintendents hold line offices.

Loose coupling refers to the degree to which units within a school system are not closely linked to one another in the authority structure. It is a consequence of geography and training. Supervision is difficult in school systems because the units are geographically isolated and so the work—especially that of teachers—takes place out of the sight of supervisors. Supervisors also have little special claim to authority because the training they receive is similar to that undergone by teachers.

Minority refers to a group of people who comprise a small proportion of the total population and who are easily distinguished by physical or cultural characteristics; they often suffer discrimination because of their differences.

Peer group refers to people who share relationships because of special characteristics such as age, race, gender, or professional or social status.

Professional organizations and unions are established to further the status and power of a particular occupational or professional group. They are distinguished mostly by the characteristics of their members and the degree to which they see the interests of their members as opposed to the interests of management. *Professional organizations* are white-collar associations, while *unions* were established for blue-collar workers. Unions traditionally have viewed political activity and collective action, especially strikes, as legitimate ways to secure benefits for their members. Professional organizations have been more conservative and reluctant to engage in conflict with dominant groups in society.

Purposes of schooling can be viewed primarily as training in the cognitive, intellectual, political, economic, or social realms. Researchers, communities, politicians, educators, and others interested in schools differ in their beliefs of how these purposes should be carried out and how much emphasis should be accorded to each.

Race is a term with no scientic meaning that has been used historically to categorize people based on beliefs about their common ancestry and/or physical characteristics.

Racism refers to ethnocentric beliefs and behaviors based on the notion that one race is superior to others.

Rationalization or technical rationalization in the sociological sense refers not to the making of excuses but rather to the application of principles of reason to a task or course of action. In practice, technical rationalization means applying methods of efficiency to the work and organization of industrial and service institutions. Efficiency takes precedence over other factors in decision making. For example, efficiency is more important than what is morally right and wrong, what is esthetically desirable, or in the case of schoolchildren, what is developmentally appropriate. Technical rationalization places responsibility for institutional decision making in the hands of the management rather than the workers who are closest to the process.

Reconceptualist curriculum theory refers to the work of those who challenge the notions of traditional curricular theorists. Their work is informed by critical theory, phenomenology, and feminist theory.

Reproduction is a process by which existing patterns of social and cultural domination and subordination are duplicated from one generation to another. Schools are important in this process because they help to reproduce both the existing values and ideologies and the social class structure. Reproduction processes suggest that schools do not necessarily promote democracy, social mobility, and equality, as is widely believed and hoped in America. Conflict theorists state that reproduction takes place as members of disadvantaged groups resist or drop out of school, realizing that schools serve only the needs of elites. The disadvantaged come to believe that their lack of success lies in their own inadequacy rather than the system's inequity (Carnoy 1972; Giroux 1983a, 1983b; Karabel and Halsey 1977).

Resistance is behavior that takes a conscious, principled, and active stand contrary to the dictates of authority figures or social systems.

Restructuring refers to reforms involving reorganization of schools' authority and accountability systems. The term probably was coined in the 1986 report of the National Governors' Association, "A Time For Results: The Governors' 1991 Report on Education," which suggested that existing school practices and structures had to be changed fundamentally if any substantive reform of the U.S. educational system was to succeed.

Schooling is the process by which members of a society, particularly youth, acquire norms, values, and specific skills by participating in formal educational institutions.

Scientific management is a way to improve the operation of industrial organizations by analyzing how workers use time, machinery, and resources. It was invented by an industrial engineer, Frederick W. Taylor, who pioneered the use of "time and motion" studies to improve the efficiency of organizing and carrying out work.

Sex refers to the physiological traits of maleness or femaleness.

Sexism refers to prejudice and/or discrimination based on gender.

Sex role stereotyping refers to exaggerated beliefs about "appropriate" roles for males and females in a society. For example, girls are cooperative and nurturing; boys are competitive and aggressive.

Social class refers to groups of people who share certain characteristics of income, occupational status, educational levels, aspirations, behavior, and beliefs. Social classes are arranged in hierarchies based upon prestige, power and status, and how their members obtain a livelihood.

Socialization refers to the process of teaching and learning behaviors, values, roles, customs, and the like considered appropriate in a society.

Social mobility refers to the movement of people and groups from one social class to another.

Sociology of curriculum is the study of the content and organization of school knowledge with emphasis on the relationships between school curriculum, students, educators, and the political/economic structure of society.

Sociology of knowledge is the study of knowledge and how we construct and organize it through our social relationships. Power and hierarchy of knowledge are central to this study.

Staff offices occupy horizontal positions in the reporting structure; their tasks are ancillary or consultative to the overall work of the organization. In schools, counselors, secretaries, curriculum staff, and media specialists are examples of staff. While the supervisory structure of their own departments may be hierarchical, they can only assemble information and give advice to line personnel in the organization; they have no direct power to enforce their suggestions.

Stratification refers differentiation into levels, which usually are arranged into a hierarchy. Stratification of social classes refers to a class hierarchy based on the prestige or power possessed by each social class.

Stratification of the curriculum refers to the organization of curriculum according to a hierarchy of levels in which different types of knowledge are considered more or less valuable than others.

Structural functionalism is an important variant of functionalism. Based upon the assumption that human systems have an underlying but unobservable coherence based upon formal rules, signs, and arrangements, structuralists seek to understand human phenomena, such as systems of meaning, language, and culture, by identifying these underlying structures. Structuralists make inferences about underlying social structure based upon patterns observed in human life. Central to structural functionalism is the conviction that social systems are like living bodies. Structures, like bodily organs, evolve to carry out vital functions in society, and they must maintain an equilibrium with each other in order for societal health to be maintained.

Theoretical framework is a set of related theories which serve as an overall way to explain, interpret, or investigate the social world. Some major theoretical frameworks that inform sociological perspectives in education include functionalism, conflict theory, interpretive theory, symbolic interactionism, reproduction or transmission, and critical theory.

Theory is a statement of interrelated sets of assumptions and propositions which help us to explain our worlds. Theories are like mental road maps, guiding the way we perceive the world.

Tracking is the practice of categorizing students and placing them in classes at various levels of difficulty at the high school level. School personnel do this on the basis of the students' ability, as measured by classroom performance and standardized test scores. The resulting organization usually differentiates college preparatory, general, remedial, and vocational tracks. In British literature tracking is referred to as *streaming*.

Womanism or black feminism defines African-American women's struggles around the issues of race, social class, and gender. The struggle against both racism and sexism is a core theme for womanists. Through their efforts, black feminists work to replace denigrated images of black women with self-defined images, to give voice to the experiences of black women, and to take action in the struggle for human freedom.

Youth culture is a broader term than *peer group* and refers to the total way of life, the distinctive behavior patterns and beliefs of, in this case, young people.

References

Abercrombie, N., Hill, S., and Turner, B. S. (1984). *The Penguin dictionary of sociology.* Hammondsworth, Middlesex, England: Penguin Books.

Abington School District v. *Schempp,* 374 U.S. 203 (1963).

Acosta, R. V., and Carpenter, L. (1990). Women in intercollegiate sport: A longitudinal study—13-year update. Unpublished manuscript.

Adams, R. S., and Biddle, B. J. (1970). *Realities of teaching.* New York: Holt, Rinehart & Winston.

Albjerg, P. G. (1974). *Community and class in American education, 1865-1918.* New York: John Wiley.

Allington, R. L. (1977). If they don't get to read much, how they ever gonna get good? *Journal of Reading, 21*(1), 57-61.

Allington, R. L. (1980a). Poor readers don't get to read much in reading groups. *Language Arts, 57,* 872-877.

Allington, R. L. (1980b). Teacher interruption behaviors during primary grade oral reading. *Journal of Educational Psychology, 72,* 371-377.

Allington, R. L. (1983). The reading provided readers of differing abilities. *Elementary School Journal, 83,* 548-559.

Allington, R. L. (1984). Content coverage and contextual reading in reading groups. *Journal of Reading Behavior, 16*(2), 85-96.

Allison, C. B. (1989). Life history of MacArthur School. Unpublished paper, University of Tennessee-Knoxville.

Allison, C. B., and Bennett, K. P. (1989). *Life in MacArthur High School: A case study.* Paper presented at the Southwest Philosophy of Education Society Meeting, Padre Island, Texas.

American Association of University Women. (1992). How schools shortchange girls: A study of major findings on girls and education. Washington, DC: AAUW/NEA.

American Association of University Women. (1993). Hostile hallways: The AAUW survey on sexual harassment in America's schools. Washington, DC: AAUW/NEA.

American heritage dictionary. (1983). New York: Houghton Mifflin.

Anderson, B. D., and Mark, J. H. (1977). Teacher mobility and productivity in a metropolitan area: A seven-year case study. *Urban Education, 12,* 15-36.

Anderson, G. L. (1989). Critical ethnography in education: Its origins, current status and new directions. *Review of Educational Research, 59*(3), 249-270.

Anyon, J. (1983). Workers, labor and economic history, and textbook content. In M. W. Apple and L. Weis (Eds.), *Ideology and practice in schooling* (pp. 37-60). Philadelphia: Temple University Press.

Anyon, J. (1988). Schools as agencies of social legitimation. In W. F. Pinar (Ed.), *Contemporary curriculum discourses* (pp. 175-200). Scottsdale, AZ: Gorsuch Scarisbrick.

Anyon, J. (1990). Social class and the hidden curriculum of work. In F. Hammack and K. Dougherty (Eds.), *Education and society* (pp. 464-438). San Diego: Harcourt, Brace & Jovanovich.

Apple, M. W. (1978). The new sociology of education: Analyzing cultural and economic reproduction. *Harvard Educational Review, 48,* 495-503.

Apple, M. W. (1979). *Ideology and curriculum.* Boston: Routledge & Kegan Paul.

Apple, M. W. (1982). *Education and power.* Boston: Routledge & Kegan Paul.

Apple, M. W. (1986). *Teachers and texts: A political economy of class and gender relations in education.* New York: Metheun.

Apple, M. W. (1988). *Teachers and texts.* New York: Routledge & Kegan Paul.

Apple, M. W. (1992). Do the standards go far enough: Power, policy and practice in mathematics education. *Journal for Research in Mathematics Education, 23*(5), 412-431.

Apple, M. W. (1993). *Official knowledge: Democratic education in a conservative age.* New York: Routledge & Kegan Paul.

Apple, M. W., and Weis, L. (Eds.). (1983). *Ideology and practice in schooling.* Philadelphia: Temple University Press.

Applebee, A. (1989). *A study of book-length works taught in high school English courses.* Albany: Center for the Learning and Teaching of Literature, State University of New York School of Education.

Aries, P. (1962). *Centuries of childhood: A social history of family life.* New York: Vintage Books.

Armor, D. (1969). *The American high school counselor.* New York: Russell Sage Foundation.

Aronowitz, S., and Giroux, H. (1985). *Education under siege.* South Hadley, MA: Bergin & Garvey.

Ashcroft, L. (1987). Diffusing "Empowering": The what and the why. *Language Arts, 64*(2), 142-156.

Atkinson, P., Delamont, S., and Hammersley, M. (1988). Qualitative research traditions: A British response. *Review of Educational Research, 58*(2), 231-250.

Au, K. H. (1979). Using the experience-text relationship with minority children. *The Reading Teacher, 32,* 677-679.

Au, K. H. (1980). Participant structures in a reading lesson with Hawaiian children: Analysis of a culturally appropriate instructional event. *Anthropology and Education Quarterly, 11,* 91-115.

Au, K. H., and Jordan, C. (1981). Teaching reading to Hawaiian children: Finding a culturally appropriate solution. In H. Trueba, G. P. Guthrie, and K.H. Au (Eds.), *Culture and the bilingual classroom: Studies in classroom ethnography* (pp. 139-152). Rowley, MA: Newbury House.

Au, K. H., and Mason, J. (1981). Social organizational factors in learning to read: The balance of rights hypothesis. *Reading Research Quarterly, 17,* 139-152.

Ayella, M. E., and Williamson, J. B. (1976). The social mobility of women: A causal model of socioeconomic success. *The Sociological Quarterly, 17,* 334-354.

Ballantine, J. H. (1983). *The sociology of education: A systematic analysis.* Englewood Cliffs, NJ: Prentice Hall.

Ballantine, J. H. (1989). *The sociology of education: A systematic analysis* (2nd ed.). Englewood Cliffs, NJ: Prentice Hall.

Banks, J. A. (1979). *Teaching strategies for ethnic studies* (2nd ed.). Boston: Allyn & Bacon.

Banks, J. A. (1988). *Multiethnic education: Theory and practice* (2nd ed.). Boston: Allyn & Bacon.

Banks, J. A., and McGee Banks, C. A. (Eds.). (1993). *Multicultural education: Issues and perspectives* (2nd ed.). Boston: Allyn & Bacon.

Baratz, S. S., and Baratz, J. C. (1970). Early childhood intervention: The social science base of institutional racism. *Harvard Educational Review, 40,* 29–50.

Barker, R. G., and Gump, P. V. (1964). *Big school, small school.* Stanford, CA: Stanford University Press.

Barnhart, C. (1982). "Tuning-in": Athabaskan teachers and Athabaskan students. In R. Barnhardt (Ed.), *Cross-cultural issues in Alaskan education, Vol. 2* (pp. 144–164). Fairbanks, AK: University of Alaska Center for Cross-Cultural Studies.

Barr, R. C. (1974). Instructional pace differences and their effect on reading acquisition. *Reading Research Quarterly, 9,* 526–554.

Barr, R. C. (1975). How children are taught to read: Grouping and pacing. *School Review, 83,* 479–498.

Barr, R. C. (1982). Classroom reading instruction from a sociological perspective. *Journal of Reading Behavior, 14,* 375–389.

Basso, K. H. (1984). "Stalking with stories": Names, places and moral narratives among the Western Apache. In E. M. Bruner (Ed.), *Text, play and story: The construction and reconstruction of self and society* (pp. 19–56). Washington, DC: Proceedings of the American Ethnological Society.

Bastian, A., Fruchter, N., Gittell, M., Greer, C., and Haskins, K. (1985). *Choosing equality: The case for democratic schooling.* Philadelphia: Temple University Press.

Bayes, J. (1988). Labor markets and the feminization of poverty. In H. Rodgers, Jr. (Ed.), *Beyond welfare: New approaches to the problem of poverty in America* (pp. 86–114). Armonk, NY: M.E. Sharpe.

Becker, G. (1964). *Human capital: A theoretical and empirical analysis with special reference to education.* New York: Columbia University Press.

Becker, H. S. (1953). The teacher in the authority system of the public school. *Journal of Educational Sociology, 27,* 128–141.

Becker, H. S., Geer, B., Hughes, E. C., and Strauss, A. L. (1961). *Boys in white: Student culture in medical school.* Chicago: University of Chicago Press.

Belenky, M. F., Clinchy, B. M., Goldberger, N. R., and Tarule, J. M. (1986). *Women's ways of knowing: The development of self, voice, and mind.* New York: Basic Books.

Bennett, E. W. (1988). *James Madison High School.* Washington, DC: U.S. Office of Education.

Bennett, K. P. (1986). Study of reading ability grouping and its consequences for urban Appalachian first graders. Unpublished doctoral dissertation, University of Cincinnati.

Bennett, K. P. (1988). *Yup'ik women's ways of knowing.* Charleston, WV: ERIC Clearinghouse on Rural Education and Small Schools (Eric Document Reproduction Service No. ED 301 401).

Bennett, K. P. (1991). Doing school in an urban Appalachian first grade. In C. Sleeter (Ed.), *Empowerment through multicultural education* (pp. 27–47). Albany, NY: State University of New York Press.

Bennett, K. P., Nelson, P., and Baker, J. (1992). Yup'ik Eskimo storyknifing: Young girls at play. *Anthropology and Education Quarterly, 23*(2), 120–144.

Bensman, J., and Vidich, A. J. (1971). *The new American society: The revolution of the middle class.* Chicago: Quadrangle Books.

Benson, C. S. (1982). The deregulation of schools: Views from the federal, state and local levels. [Editor's introduction]. *Education and Urban Society, 14,* 395-397.

Berger, J. (1989). New York study of welfare clients: False practices of trade schools. *New York Times,* June 18, p. 14.

Berger, P. L., and Luckmann, T. (1967). *The social construction of reality: A treatise in the sociology of knowledge.* New York: Anchor Books.

Bernardi, B. (1952). The age system of the Nilotic Hamitic people. *Africa, 22,* 316-332.

Bernardi, B. (1985). *Age class systems, social institutions and policies based on age.* New York: Cambridge.

Bernstein, B. (1970). *Class, codes and control. Vol. I: Theoretical studies towards a sociology of language.* London: Routledge & Kegan Paul.

Bernstein, B. (1977). *Class, codes and control. Vol. III: Towards a theory of educational transmission.* London: Routledge & Kegan Paul.

Berry, E. and Black, E. (1987). The integrative learning journal (or, Getting beyond "True Confessions" and "Cold Knowledge"). *Women's Studies Quarterly, XV*(3-4), 59-64.

Betz, M., and Garland, J. (1974). Intergenerational mobility rates of urban school teachers. *Sociology of Education, 47,* 511-522.

Bidwell, C. E. (1965). The school as a formal organization. In J. G. March (Ed.), *The handbook of organizations* (pp. 972-1022). New York: Rand McNally.

Binder, F. H. (1974). *The age of the common school, 1830-1865.* New York: John Wiley.

Blau, P. M. (1955). *The dynamics of bureaucracy.* Chicago: University of Chicago Press.

Blau, P. M., and Duncan, O. D. (1967). *The American occupational structure.* New York: John Wiley.

Blau, P. M., and Scott, W. R. (1962). *Formal organizations: A comparative approach.* San Francisco: Chandler.

Blaug, M. (1970). *An introduction to the economics of education.* London: Allen Lane.

Blaug, M. (1976). Human capital theory: A slightly jaundiced survey. *Journal of Economic Literature, 14,* 827-856.

Bloom, A. (1987). *The closing of the American mind.* New York: Simon & Schuster.

Bluestone, B., and Bennett, H. (1982). *The de-industrialization of America.* New York: Basic Books.

Blumberg, A. (1985). *The school superintendent: Living with conflict.* New York: Teachers College Press.

Blumer, H. (1969). *Symbolic interactionism: Perspectives and method.* Englewood Cliffs, NJ: Prentice Hall.

Bobbitt, F. (1912). The elimination of waste in education. *The Elementary School Teacher, 12,* 259-271.

Boehnlein, M. M. (1985). *Children, parents, and reading: An annotated bibliography.* Newark, DE: International Reading Association.

Bogart, K., Simmons, S., Stein, N., and Tomaszewski, E. P. (1992). Breaking the silence: sexual and gender-based harassment in elementary, secondary, and postsecondary education. In S. S. Klein (Ed.), *Sex equity and sexuality in education* (pp. 192-221). Albany: State University of New York Press.

Bogart, K., and Stein, N. (1987). Breaking the silence: Sexual harassment in education. *Peabody Journal of Education, 64*(4), 146-163.

Bogdan, R. (1972). *Participant observation in organizational settings.* Syracuse University Division of Special Education and Rehabilitation and the Center on Human Policy.

Boggs, C. (1976). *Gramsci's Marxism*. London: Pluto Press.

Boocock, S. (1980). *Sociology of education: An introduction* (2nd ed.). Boston: Houghton Mifflin.

Borko, H., and Eisenhart, M. (1986). Students' conceptions of reading and their reading experience in school. *The Elementary School Journal, 86,* 589–612.

Borman, K. M. (1988). The process of becoming a worker. In J. Mortimer & K. Borman (Eds.), *Work experience and psychological development through the lifespan* (pp. 51–75). Boulder, CO: Westview Press.

Borman K. M., and Mueninghoff, E. (1982). Work roles and social roles in three elementary school settings. Paper presented at the meeting of the American Educational Research Association, New York.

Borman, K. M., and Mueninghoff, E. (1983). Lower Price Hill's children: Family, school and neighborhood. In A. Batteau (Ed.), *Appalachia and America* (pp. 210–224). Lexington: University Press of Kentucky.

Borman, K. M., and Spring, J. H. (1984). *Schools in central cities*. New York: Longman.

Bossert, S. T. (1979). *Tasks and social relationships in classrooms: A study of instructional organization and its consequences*. Cambridge, England: Cambridge University Press.

Bottomore, T. (1984). *The Frankfurt School*. New York: Tavistock.

Boudon, R. (1974). *Education, opportunity, and social inequality: Changing prospects in Western society*. New York: John Wiley.

Bourdieu, P., and Passeron, J. (1977). *Reproduction in education, society and culture*. London: Sage.

Boutwell, G. S. (1859). *Thoughts on educational topics and institutions*. Boston: Phillips, Sampson and Company.

Bowers, A. W. (1965). Hidatsa social and ceremonial organization (Bulletin 194). Washington, DC: Smithsonian Institution Bureau of American Ethnology.

Bowles, S., and Gintis, H. (1976). *Schooling in capitalist America: Educational reform and the contradictions of economic life*. New York: Basic Books.

Boyd, W. (1966). *The history of Western education* (8th ed.). New York: Barnes & Noble.

Boyd, W. L., and Crowson, R. L. (1981). The changing conception and practice of public school administration. In D. C. Berliner (Ed.), *Review of Research in Education. Vol. 9* (pp. 31–37). Washington, DC: American Educational Research Association.

Braddock, J. H., Crain, R. L., and McParland, J. M. (1984). A long-term view of school desegregation: Some recent studies of graduates as adults. *Phi Delta Kappan, 66,* 259–264.

Braroe, N. W. (1975). *Indian and white: Self-image and interaction in a Canadian plains community*. Stanford, CA: Stanford University Press.

Bredekamp, S. (Ed.). (1986). *Developmentally appropriate practice*. Washington, DC: National Association for the Education of Young Children.

Bredo, E. (1989). After positivism, what? Paper presented at the meeting of the American Educational Research Association, San Francisco.

Brenton, M. (1974). Teachers' organizations: The new militancy. In E. A. Useem and M. Useem (Eds.), *The education establishment* (pp. 60–69). Englewood Cliffs, NJ: Prentice Hall.

Britzman, D. (1991). *Practice makes practice: A critical study of learning to teach*. Albany: State University of New York Press.

Brookover, W. B., and Erickson, E. L. (1975). *Sociology of education*. Homewood, IL: The Dorsey Press.

Brophy, J. E., and Good, T. L. (1970). Teachers' communication of differential expectations for children's classroom performance: Some behavioral data. *Journal of Educational Psychology 61,* 365–374.

Brouillette, L. R. (1993). A geology of school reform: An ethnohistorical case study of the successive restructurings of a school district. Unpublished doctoral dissertation, School of Education, University of Colorado–Boulder.

Brown D. (1991). The effects of State-mandated testing on elementary classroom instruction. Unpublished doctoral dissertation, University of Tennessee–Knoxville.

Brown, L. M., and Gilligan, C. (1992). *Meeting at the crossroads: Women's psychology and girls' development.* Cambridge, MA: Harvard University Press.

Brown, R. (1986). State responsibility for at-risk youth. *Metropolitan Education, 2,* 5–12.

Brown v. *Board of Education of Topeka, KS,* 349 U.S. 294 (1955).

Brown, V. E. (1994). Unititled paper presented in session. "Sexual harassment and power politics in higher education," American Educational Research Association, New Orleans.

Burtonwood, N. (1986). *The culture concept in educational studies.* Philadelphia: Nfer-Nelson.

Butts, R. F. (1978). *Public education in the United States: From revolution to reform.* New York: Holt, Rinehart & Winston.

Butts, R. F., and Cremin, L. A. (1953). *A history of education in American culture.* New York: Holt.

Callahan, R. (1962). *Education and the cult of efficiency.* Chicago: University of Chicago Press.

Campbell, R. T. (1983). Status attainment research: End of the beginning or beginning of the end? *Sociology of Education, 56,* 47–62.

Carnegie Council of Adolescent Development. (1989). Turning points: Preparing American youth for the 21st century. New York: Carnegie Corporation.

Carnegie Task Force on Teaching as a Profession. (1986). *A nation prepared: Teachers for the 21st century.* New York: Author.

Carnoy, M. (Ed.). (1972). *Schooling in a corporate society: The political economy of education in America.* New York: McKay.

Carnoy, M., and Levin, H. M. (1976). *The limits of educational reform.* New York: McKay.

Carnoy, M., and Levin, H. M. (1985). *Schooling and work in the democratic state.* Stanford, CA: Stanford University Press.

Carroll, T. G. (1975). Transactions of cognitive equivalence in the domains of "work" and "play." *Anthropology and Education Quarterly, 6,* 17–22.

Cashmore, E., and Troyna, B. (1990). *Introduction to race relations* (2nd ed.). New York: Falmer Press.

Casper, V., Schultz, S., and Wickens, E. (1992). Breaking the silences: Lesbian and gay parents and the schools. *Teachers College Record, 94*(1), 109–137.

Cazden, C. B., John, V. P., and Hymes, D. (Eds.). (1974). *Functions of language in the classroom.* New York: Teachers College Press.

Center for Literacy Studies, University of Tennessee, Knoxville. (1992). *Life at the margins: Profiles of adults with low literacy skills.* U.S. Congress Office of Technology Assessment, Contract #H3.5365.0. Washington, DC: National Technical Information Service, March.

Chafetz, J. S., and Dworkin, A. G. (1986). *Female revolt: Women's movements in world and historical perspective.* Totowa, NJ: Rowan & Allanheld.

Chandler, J. (1981). Camping for life: Transmission of values at a girl's summer camp. In R. T. Sieber and A. J. Gordon (Eds.), *Children and their organizations: Investigations in American culture* (pp. 122–137). Boston: G. K. Hall.

Charters, W. W., Jr. (1970). Some factors affecting teacher survival in school districts. *American Educational Research Journal, 7,* 1–27.

Cherryholmes, C. H. (1988). *Power and criticism: Poststructural investigations in education.* New York: Teachers College Press.

Children's Defense Fund. (1988). *A call for action to make our nation safe for children: A briefing book on the status of American children in 1988.* Washington, DC: Author.

Chowdorow, N. (1978). *The reproduction of mothering.* Berkeley: University of California Press.

Christian-Smith, L. (1988). Romancing the girl: Adolescent novels and the construction of femininity. In L. Roman, L. Christian-Smith, and E. Ellsworth (Eds.), *Becoming feminine: The politics of popular culture* (pp. 76–102). Philadelphia: Falmer Press.

Cicourel, A. V. (1964). *Method and measurement in sociology.* New York: The Free Press.

Cicourel, A. V., and Kitsuse, J. (1963). *The educational decision makers.* Indianapolis: Bobbs-Merrill.

Cleary, E. L. (1985). *Crisis and change: The church in Latin America today.* Maryknoll, NY: Orbis Books.

Clement, D. C., Eisenhart, M. A., and Harding, J. R. (1979). The veneer of harmony: Social-race relations in a southern desegregated school. In R. C. Rist (Ed.), *Desegregated schools: Appraisals of an American experiment* (pp. 15–52). New York: Academic Press.

Cohen, A. (1974). *Two-Dimensional Man.* Berkeley: University of California Press.

Cohen, J., and Rogers, J. (1983). *On democracy: Toward a transformation of American society.* Middlesex, England: Penguin Books.

Cole, M., and Griffin, P. (Eds.). (1987). *Contextual factors in education: Improving science and mathematics for minorities and women.* Madison: Wisconsin Center for Education Research.

Coleman, J. S. (1961). *The adolescent society.* Glencoe, IL: The Free Press.

Coleman, J. S. (1965). *Adolescents and the schools.* New York: Basic Books.

Coleman, J. S. (1966). *Equality of educational opportunity.* Washington, DC: U.S. Government Printing Office.

Coleman, J. S., and Hoffer, T. (1987). *Public and private schools: The impact of communities.* New York: Basic Books.

Coleman, J. S., Hoffer, T., and Kilgore, S. (1982). *High school achievement: Public, Catholic and private schools compared.* New York: Basic Books.

Collins, G. (1987). Day care for infants: Debate turns to long term effects. *The New York Times,* November 25, p. B9.

Collins, P. H. (1990). *Black feminist thought: Knowledge, consciousness, and the politics of empowerment.* London: HarperCollins Academic.

Collins, R. (1977). Functional and conflict theories of educational stratification. In J. Karabel and A. H. Halsey (Eds.), *Power and ideology in education* (pp. 118–136). Cambridge, England: Oxford University Press.

Combahee River Collective. (1977). "A Black feminist statement." Quoted in C. Morage and G. Anzaldua (Eds.), (1981), *This bridge called my back: Writings by radical women of color* (pp. 210–218). New York: Kitchen Table: Women of Color Press.

Conant, J. (1988). Alaska's suicide epidemic. *Newsweek,* February 15, p. 61.

Connell, R. W. (1985). *Teachers' work.* North Sydney, Australia: George Allen & Unwin.

Connors, N. A., and Irvin, J. L. (1989). Is "middle-schoolness" an indicator of excellence? *Middle School Journal, 21,* 12–14.

Corwin, R. G. (1965). *Sociology of education.* New York: Appleton.

Corwin, R. G. (1970). *Militant professionalism: A study of organizational conflicts in high school.* New York: Appleton-Century-Crofts.

Coser, L. A. (1956). *The functions of social conflict.* Glencoe, IL: The Free Press.

Council on Interracial Books for Children, Inc. (1980). In M. K. Rudman (1984), *Children's literature: An issues approach* (2nd Ed.), p. 126. White Plains, NY: Longman.

Counts, G. (1932). *Dare the school build a new social order?* New York: John Day.

Cox, T. V. (1980). Kindergarten: A status passage for American children: A microethnography of an urban kindergarten classroom. Unpublished doctoral dissertation, Department of Anthropology, University of Georgia.

Crain, R. L. (1977). Racial tension in high schools: Pushing the survey method closer to reality. *Anthropology and Education Quarterly, 8,* 142–151.

Crow, M. L. (1985). The female educator at midlife. *Phi Delta Kappan, 67,* 281–284.

Cuban, L. (1984). *How teachers taught: Constancy and change in American classrooms, 1890–1980.* New York: Longman.

Cull, D. (1989). Elected officials proliferate. *New York Times,* January 14, p. 6.

Curti, M. (1971). *The social ideas of American educators.* Totowa, NJ: Littlefield, Adams & Company.

Cusick, P. A. (1983). *The egalitarian ideal and the American high school.* New York: Longman.

Dahrendorf, R. (1959). *Class and conflict in industrial society.* Stanford, CA: Stanford University Press.

Dalton, G. W., Barnes, L. B., and Zaleznik, A. (1968). *The distribution of authority in formal organizations.* Boston: Harvard University, Division of Research, Graduate School of Business Administration.

Dalton, G. W., Barnes, L. B., and Zaleznik, A. (1973). *The distribution of authority in formal organizations.* Cambridge, MA: M.I.T. Press.

D'Amato, J. D. (1987). The belly of the beast: On cultural differences, castelike status and the politics of schools. *Anthropology and Education Quarterly, 18,* 357–360.

D'Amato, J. D. (1988). "Acting": Hawaiian children's resistance to teachers. *The Elementary School Journal, 88,* 529–544.

Damico, S. B., Bell, N. A., and Green, C. (1980). Friendship in desegregated middle schools: An organizational analysis. Paper presented at the meeting of the Social Contexts of Education Conference, sponsored by Division G of the American Educational Research Association, Atlanta.

Darling-Hammond, L. (1984). *Beyond the commission reports: Coming crisis in teaching.* Santa Monica, CA: Rand Corporation.

Darling-Hammond, L. (1993). Reframing the school reform agenda: Developing capacity for school transformation. *Phi Delta Kappan, 74*(10), 752–761.

Davis, J. A. (1965). *Undergraduate career decisions.* Chicago: Aldine.

Deering, P. (1992). An ethnographic study of cooperative learning in a multiethnic working class middle school. Unpublished doctoral dissertation, School of Education, University of Colorado–Boulder.

Delamont, S. (1989). *Knowledgeable women: Structuralism and the reproduction of elites.* New York: Routledge & Kegan Paul.

Delgado-Gaitan, C. (1988). The value of conformity: Learning to stay in school. *Anthropology and Education Quarterly, 19,* 354–382.

Delgado-Gaitan, C. (1990). *Literacy for empowerment.* New York: Falmer Press.

Dellinger, D. (1991). "My Way or the Highway": The Hawkins County Textbook Controversy. Unpublished doctoral dissertation, University of Tennessee–Knoxville.

Delpit, L. D. (1988). The silenced dialogue: Power and pedagogy in educating other people's children. *Harvard Educational Review, 3,* 280–298.

Dewey, J. (1916). *Democracy and education: An introduction to the philosophy of education.* New York: Macmillan.

Dewey, J. (1929). *The quest for certainty.* New York: Putnam.

Dewey, J. (1938). *Experience and education.* New York: Macmillan.

Deyhle, D. (1986). Break dancing and breaking out: Anglos, Utes and Navajos in a border reservation high school. *Anthropology and Education Quarterly, 17*, 111-127.

Deyhle, D. (1987). Empowerment and cultural conflict: Navajo parents and the schooling of their children. Unpublished manuscript.

Deyhle, D. (1988). Dropouts cite reasons for leaving school. *Farmington (Utah) Daily Times* (American Indian News Section), October 27.

Deyhle, D. (1989). Pushouts and pullouts: Navajo and Ute school leavers. *Journal of Navajo Education, 6*, 36-51.

Deyhle, D. (1991). Empowerment and cultural conflict: Navajo parents and the schooling of their children. *International Journal of Qualitative Studies in Education, 4*(4), 277-297.

Deyhle, D. (1992). Constructing failure and maintaining cultural identity: Navajo and Ute school leavers. *Journal of American Indian Education*, January, 24-47.

Deyhle, D., and LeCompte, M. D. (in press). Cultural differences in child development: Navajo adolescents in middle schools. *Theory into Practice.*

Dillon, S. (1994). Superintendent's dismissal leads to loss of corporate grants. *The New York Times*, March 26, p. 16.

Domhoff, G. W. (1967). *Who rules America?* Englewood Cliffs, NJ: Prentice Hall.

Dreeben, R. (1968). *On what is learned in school.* Reading, MA: Addison-Wesley.

Dreeben, R. (1973). The school as a workplace. In R. M. W. Travers (Ed.), *The second handbook of research on teaching* (pp. 450-473). Chicago: Rand McNally.

Dreeben, R. (1984). First grade reading groups: Their formation and change. In P. L. Peterson, L. C. Wilkinson, and M. Hallinan (Eds.), *The social context of instruction: Group organization and group process* (pp. 69-83). New York: Academic Press.

Duncan, S., and Fiske, D. W. (1977). *Face-to-face interaction: Research, method and theory.* New York: John Wiley.

Durkheim, E. (1969). *The division of labor in society.* New York: The Free Press [first published in 1893].

Dworkin, A. G. (1974). Balance on the bayou: The impact of racial isolation and interaction on stereotyping in the Houston Independent School District. In A. G. Dworkin, R. G. Frankiewicz, and H. Copitka, *Intergroup Action Report* (pp. 7-51). Houston, TX: Houston Council on Human Relations.

Dworkin, A. G. (1980). The changing demography of public school teachers: Some implications for faculty turnover in urban areas. *Sociology of Education, 53*, 65-73.

Dworkin, A. G. (1985a). Ethnic bias in writing assignments. *American Sociological Association Teaching Newsletter, 10*, 15-16.

Dworkin, A. G. (1985b). *When teachers give up: Teacher burnout, teacher turnover and their impact on children.* Austin, TX: The Hogg Foundation for Mental Health.

Dworkin, A. G. (1986). *Teacher burnout in the public schools: structural causes and consequences for children.* Albany: State University of New York Press.

Dworkin, A. G., and Dworkin, R. J. (1982). *The minority report: An introduction to racial, ethnic, and gender relations* (2nd ed.). New York: Holt, Rinehart & Winston.

Dworkin, A. G., Frankiewicz, R. G., and Copitka, H. (1975). Impact and assessment on stereotype reduction activities in the public schools. Paper presented at the meeting of the Southwestern Sociological Association, San Antonio.

Dworkin, A. G., Haney, C. A., and Telschow, R. L. (1988). Fear, victimization and stress among urban public school teachers. *Journal of Organizational Behavior, 9*, 159-171.

Dworkin, A. G., and LeCompte, M. D. (1989). Giving up in schools: American public education in crisis. *Houston Update, 3*(12), 1, 2, 7. Houston, TX: Center for Public Policy, University of Houston.

Dworkin, A. G., Lorence, J., and LeCompte, M. D. (1989). Organizational context as determinants of teacher morale. Paper presented at the meeting of the Southwestern Social Science Association.

Ebaugh, H. R. F. (1977). *Out of the cloister: A study of organizational dilemmas.* Austin: University of Texas Press.

Eder, D. (1982). The impact of management and turn allocation activities on student performance. *Discourse Processes, 5*(2), 147–159.

Eder, D. (1985). The cycle of popularity: Interpersonal relations among female adolescents. *Sociology of Education, 58*(3), 154–165.

Eder, D., and Felmlee, D. (1984). The development of attention norms in ability groups. In P. L. Peterson, L. C. Wilkinson, and M. Hallinan (Eds.), *The social context of instruction: Group organization and group process* (pp. 189–207). New York: Academic Press.

Eder, D., and Parker, S. (1987). The cultural production and reproduction of gender: The effect of extracurricular activities on peer-group culture. *Sociology of Education, 60*(3), 200–213.

Education Week. (1988). NAEP: Results of the fourth mathematics assessment, June 15, p. 29.

Education Week, March 1, 1989, p. 7.

Education Week, February 23, 1994, p. 4.

Eisenhart, M. (1985). Women choose their careers: A study of natural decision making. *Review of Higher Education, 8*(3), 247–270.

Eisenhart, M., and Graue, E. (1990). Socially constructed readiness for school. *International Journal of Qualitative Studies in Education, 3*, 253–269.

Eisenhart, M. A., and Holland, D. C. (1988). Moments of discontent: University women and the gender status quo. *Anthropology and Education Quarterly, 19*(2), 115–138.

Eisenhart, M. A., and Holland, D. C. (1992). Gender constructs and career committment: The influence of peer culture on women in college. In T. L. Whitehead and B. Reid (Eds.), *Gender constructs and social issues.* Champaign, IL: University of Illinois Press.

Ekstrom, R. B., Goertz, M. E., Pollack, J. M., and Rock, D. A. (1986). Who drops out of school and why?: Finding from a national study. *Teachers College Record, 87*, 356–375.

Ellsworth, E. (1989). Why doesn't this feel empowering?: Working through the repressive myths of critical pedagogy. *Harvard Educational Review, 59*(3), 297–324.

Elmore, R. E., and Associates. (1990). *Restructuring schools.* San Francisco: Jossey-Bass.

Ember, C. R., and Ember, M. (1985). *Anthropology* (4th ed.). Englewood Cliffs, NJ: Prentice Hall.

Engel v. *Vitale*, 370 U.S. 421 (1962).

Epstein, J. L., and Karweit, N. (Eds.). (1983). *Friends in school: Patterns of selection and influence in secondary schools.* New York: Academic Press.

Erickson, F. (1984). School literacy, reasoning and civility: An anthropologist's perspective. *Review of Educational Research, 54*, 525–546.

Erickson, F. (1987). Transformation and school success: The politics and culture of educational achievement. *Anthropology and Education Quarterly, 18*, 335–356.

Erickson, F., and Mohatt, G. (1982). Cultural organization of participation structures in two classrooms of Indian students. In G. Spindler (Ed.), *Doing the ethnography of schooling* (pp. 132–174). New York: Holt, Rinehart & Winston.

Eskenazi, M., and Gallen, D. (1992). *Sexual harassment: Know your rights.* New York: Carroll & Graf.

Etaugh, C., & Harlow, H. (1974). The influence of sex of the teacher and student on classroom behavior. In E. Brophy & T. L. Good (Eds.), *Teacher-student relationships: Causes and consequences* (pp. 199–239). New York: Holt, Rinehart & Winston.

Etter-Lewis, G. (1993). *My soul is my own: Oral narratives of African American women in the professions.* New York: Routledge.

Etzioni, A. (Ed.). (1969). *The semi-professions and their organization: Teachers, nurses, social workers.* New York: The Free Press.

Evans-Pritchard, E. E. (1940). *The Nuer: A description of the modes of livelihood and political institution of a Nilotic people.* Oxford, England: Clarendon Press.

Falk, W. W., Grimes, M. D., and Lord, G. F. (1982). Professionalism and conflict in a bureaucratic setting: The case of a teachers' strike. *Social Problems, 29,* 551-560.

Fantini, M., Gittell, M., and Magat, R. (1974). Local school governance. In M. Useem and E. L. Useem (Eds.), *The education establishment* (pp. 86-98). Englewood Cliffs, NJ: Prentice Hall.

Fantini, M. D. (1975). The school-community power struggle. *National Elementary Principal, 54*(3), 57-61.

Farnham, C. (1987). *The impact of feminist research in the academy.* Bloomington: Indiana University Press.

Fausto-Sterling, A. (1985). *Myths of gender:* Biological theories about women and men. New York: Basic Books.

Featherstone, H. (Ed.) (1987). Organizing classes by ability. *Harvard Education Letter, 3*(4), 1-9.

Feinberg, W., and Soltis, J. F. (1985). *School and society.* New York: Teachers College Press.

Feistritzer, C. E. (1983). *The condition of teachers: A state by state analysis.* Princeton, NJ: Carnegie Foundation for the Advancement of Teaching.

Feldman, R. S. (1985). Nonverbal behavior, race, and the classroom teacher. *Theory into Practice, 24,* 45-49.

Felmlee, D., Eder, D., and Tsui, W. (1985). Peer influence on classroom attention. *Social Psychology Quarterly, 48*(3), 215-226.

Fennema, E., and Leder, G. C. (1990). *Mathematics and gender.* New York: Teachers College Press.

Fennema, E., and Sherman, J. (1977). Sex-related differences in mathematics achievement, spatial visualization and affective factors. *American Educational Research Journal, 14*(1), 51-71.

Ferrell, B., and Compton, D. (1986). The use of ethnographic techniques for evaluation in a large school district: The vanguard case. In D. Fetterman and M. A. Pitman (Eds.), *Educational evaluation: Ethnography in theory, practice and politics* (pp. 171-192). Beverly Hills, CA: Sage.

Fine, M. (1986). Why urban adolescents drop into and out of public high school. *Teachers College Record, 87,* 393-410.

Fine, M. (1987). Silencing in public schools. *Language Arts, 64*(2), 157-174.

Finn, C. E., and Ravitch, D. (1987). *What do our 17-year-olds know? A report on the first national assessment of history and literature.* New York: Harper and Row.

Firestone, W. A., and Rosenblum, S. (1988). Building commitment in urban high schools. *Educational Evaluation and Policy Analysis, 10*(4), 285-299.

Fiske, E. (1986). Student debt reshaping colleges and careers [Education Life]. *New York Times,* August 30, p. 34.

Fiske, E. (1988). American test mania [Education Life]. *New York Times,* April 10, pp. 16-20.

Fordham, S. (1991). Peer-proofing academic competition among Black adolescents: "Acting White" Black American style. In C. Sleeter (Ed.), *Empowerment through multicultural education* (pp. 69-93). New York: SUNY Press.

Fordham, S., and Ogbu, J. U. (1986). Black students' school success: Coping with the "burden" of "acting white." *The Urban Review, 18*(3), 176-206.

Fortune, R. F. (1963). *Sorcerers of Dobu.* New York: E.P. Dutton.

Foucault, M. (1980). *Power/knowledge.* New York: Pantheon Books.

Freire, P. (1970). *Pedagogy of the oppressed.* New York: Continuum.

Freire, P. (1985). *The politics of education.* South Hadley, MA: Bergin & Garvey.

Freire, P. (1987). *A pedagogy for liberation.* South Hadley, MA: Bergin & Garvey.

Fretz, C. (1990). Gender bias plagues women lawyers—judge. *The Knoxville Journal,* June 9, p. 4A.

Fuller, M. (1980). Black girls in a London comprehensive. In R. Deem (Ed.), *Schooling for women's work* (pp. 56–65). London: Routledge & Kegan Paul.

Furlong, V. J. (1985). *Deviant pupil: Sociological perspectives.* Philadelphia: Open University Press.

Gaertner, K. N. (1978). Organizational careers in public school administration. Unpublished doctoral dissertation, University of Chicago.

Gambrell, L. B., Wilson, R. M., and Gantt, W. N. (1981). Classroom observations of task attending behaviors of good and poor readers. *Journal of Educational Research, 74,* 400–404.

Gamoran, A., and Berends, M. (1987). The effects of stratification in secondary schools: A synthesis of survey and ethnographic research. *Review of Educational Research, 57,* 415–437.

Garbarino, M. S. (1983). *Sociocultural theory in anthropology.* Prospect Heights, IL: Waveland Press.

Garcia, E. (1994). *Understanding and meeting the challenge of student cultural diversity.* Boston: Houghton Mifflin.

Garfinkel, H. (1967). *Studies in ethnomethodology.* Englewood Cliffs, NJ: Prentice Hall.

Geertz, C. (1973). *The interpretation of cultures.* New York: Basic Books.

Geertz, C. (1988). *Works and lives: The anthropologist as author.* Stanford, CA: Stanford University Press.

Gennep, A. van (1960). *The rites of passage.* Chicago: Chicago University Press.

Gerth, H., and Mills, C. W. (1953). *Character and social structure.* New York: Harcourt Brace & World.

Gibson, M. A. (1987a). Punjabi immigrants in an American high school. In G. Spindler and L. Spindler (Eds.), *Interpretive ethnography of education: At home and abroad* (pp. 281–310). Hillsdale, NJ: Lawrence Erlbaum Associates.

Gibson, M. A. (1987b). The school performance of immigrant minorities: A comparative view. *Anthropology and Education Quarterly, 18,* 262–276.

Gibson, M. A. (1988). *Accommodation with assimilation: Punjabi Sikh immigrants in an American high school and community.* Ithaca, NY: Cornell University Press.

Gilligan, C. (1982). *In a different voice.* Cambridge, MA: Harvard University Press.

Ginsburg, M. B. (1979). Colleague relations among middle school teachers. In A. Hargreaves and B. Tickle (Eds.), *Middle schools: Origins, ideology and practice* (pp. 277–296). New York: Harper & Row.

Ginsburg, M. B. (1988). *Contradictions in teacher education and society: A critical analysis.* New York: Falmer Press.

Giroux, H. (1983a). Theories of reproduction and resistance in the new sociology of education. *Harvard Educational Review, 53,* 257–293.

Giroux, H. (1983b). *Theory and resistance in education: A pedagogy for the opposition.* Hadley, MA: Bergin & Garvey.

Giroux, H. (1988). *Teachers as intellectuals: Toward a critical pedagogy of learning.* Hadley, MA: Bergin & Garvey.

Gitlin, A. D., Siegel, M., and Boru, K. (1988). Purpose and method: The failure of ethnography to foster school change. Paper presented at the meeting of the American Educational Research Association, New Orleans.

Gitlin, A. D., Siegel, M., and Boru, K. (1989). The politics of method: From left ethnography to educative research. *Qualitative Studies in Education, 2*(3), 237-253.

Gitlin, A. D., and Smyth, J. (1989). *Teacher evaluation: Educative alternatives.* New York: Falmer Press.

Gleick, J. (1989). After the bomb, a mushroom cloud of metaphors. *The New York Times Book Review,* May 29, p. 1.

Glesne, C., and Peshkin, A. (1992). *Becoming qualitative researchers: An introduction.* New York: Longman.

Goetz, J. (1981). Sex-role systems in Rose Elementary School: Change and tradition in the rural transitional south. In R. T. Sieber and A. J. Gordon (Eds.), *Children and their organizations: Investigations in American culture* (pp. 58-73). Boston: G. K. Hall.

Goetz, J. P., and Breneman, E. A. (1988). Desegregation and black students' experiences in two rural southern elementary schools. *The Elementary School Journal, 88,* 503-514.

Goetz, J. P., and LeCompte, M. D. (1984). *Ethnography and qualitative design in educational research.* Orlando, FL: Academic Press.

Goffman, E. (1959). *The presentation of self in everyday life.* Garden City, NY: Doubleday.

Goldin, C. (1990). *Understanding the gender gap: An economic history of American women.* New York: Oxford University Press.

Goldman, S. V., and McDermott, R. (1987). The culture of competition in American schools. In G. Spindler (Ed.), *Education and cultural process: Anthropological approaches* (2nd ed.) (pp. 282-299). Prospect Heights, IL: Waveland Press.

Goldwasser, M. L. (1994). Restructuring schools and the gap between policy and practice. Unpublished doctoral dissertation, School of education, University of Colorado-Boulder.

Goodlad, J. I. (1984). *A place called school.* New York: McGraw-Hill.

Goodman, J. L. (1993). Reading toward womanhood: The Baby-sitters Club Books and our daughters. *Tikkun, 8*(6), 7-11.

Gordon, C. W. (1957). *The social system of the high school.* Glencoe, IL: The Free Press.

Gottlieb, D. (1964). Teaching and students: The views of Negro and white teachers. *Sociology of Education, 37,* 345-353.

Gould, S. J. (1981). *The mismeasure of man.* New York: W.W. Norton.

Graham, P. A. (1974). *Community and class in American education, 1865-1918.* New York: John Wiley.

Gramsci, A. (1971). *Selections from the prison notebooks.* Q. Hoare and G. N. Smith (Eds.) New York: International.

Grant, C. A., and Sleeter, C. E. (1986). *After the school bell rings.* Philadelphia: Falmer Press.

Grant, L. (1984). Black females' "place" in desegregated classrooms. *Sociology of Education, 57*(2), 98-110.

Grant, L., and Rothenberg, J. (1986). The social enhancement of ability differences: Teacher-student interactions in first and second grade reading groups. *Elementary School Journal, 87,* 29-50.

Graue, E. (1994). *Ready for what?* Ithaca, NY: State University of New York Press.

Grayson, D. A. (1992). Emerging equity issues related to homosexuality in education. In S. S. Klein (Ed.), *Sex equity and sexuality in education* (pp. 171-189). Albany: State University of New York Press.

Greeley, A. M. (1982). *Catholic high schools and minority students.* New Brunswick, NJ: Transaction Books.

Greene, A. D. (1989). Yates valedictorian hoping success will dispel stereotype. *The Houston Chronicle,* April 30, p. 1C.

Greene, Maxine. (1985). Sex equity as a philosophical problem. In S. Klein (Ed.), *Handbook for achieving sex equity through education.* Baltimore: The Johns Hopkins University Press.

Groce, N. (1981). Growing up rural: Children in the 4-H and the Junior Granges. In R. T. Sieber and A. J. Gordon (Eds.), *Children and their organization: Investigations in American culture* (pp. 106–122). Boston: G.K. Hall.

Grow, J. (1981). Characteristics of access to the school superintendency for men and women. Unpublished doctoral dissertation, University of Chicago.

Guidelines for equal treatment of the sexes in McGraw-Hill Book Company publications. (1980). In A. M. Eastman (Ed.), *The Norton reader* (5th ed.) (pp. 346–358). New York: W. W. Norton.

Gumbert, E., and Spring, J. H. (1974). *The superschool and the superstate: American education in the twentieth century.* New York: John Wiley.

Hacker, H. M. (1951). Women as a minority group. *Social Forces, 30,* 60–69.

Halcon, J. J., and Reyes, M. (1989). Trickle-down reform: Hispanics, higher education and the excellence movement. Unpublished manuscript, University of Colorado–Boulder.

Hall, R. M., and Sandler, B. R. (1982). *The classroom climate: A chilly one for women?* Washington, DC: Project on the Status and Education of Women, Association of American Colleges.

Hammack, F. M. (1986). Large school systems; Dropout reports: An analysis of definitions, procedures and findings. *Teachers College Record, 87,* 324–342.

Hanna, J. L. (1987). *Disruptive school behavior: In a desegregated magnet school and elsewhere.* New York: Holmes & Meier.

Hare, D. (1988). Teacher recruitment in three rural Louisiana parishes: The development of recruitment materials. Paper presented at the meeting of the American Educational Studies Association, Toronto, November.

Hargreaves, A., and Woods, P. (1984). *Classrooms and staffrooms: The sociology of teachers and teaching.* Milton Keynes, England: Open University Press.

Hargroves, J. S. (1987). The Boston compact: Facing the challenge of school dropouts. *Education and Urban Society, 19*(3), 303–311.

Harris, M. (1981). *America now: The anthropology of a changing culture.* New York: Simon & Schuster.

Hart, A. W. (1990). Impacts of the school social unit on teacher authority during work redesign. *American Educational Research Journal, 25,* 503–532.

Hawthorne, S. (1991). In defence of separatism. In S. Gunew (Ed.), *Reader in feminist knowledge* (pp. 312–318). New York: Routledge & Kegan Paul.

Heath, S. B. (1983). *Ways with words: Language, life, and work in communities and classroom.* New York: Cambridge University Press.

Held, D. (1980). *Introduction to critical theory.* Berkeley: University of California Press.

Hernstein, R. J. (1973). *IQ in the meritocracy.* Boston: Little, Brown.

Hess, G. A. (1989). Panel finds school board misuses state Chapter I funds. *Newsletter of the Chicago Panel on Public School Policy and Finance, 6*(1).

Hess, G. A. (1991). *School restructuring, Chicago style.* Newbury, CA: Corwin Press.

Hess, G. A., and Green, D. O. (1988). Invisibly pregnant: A study of teenaged mothers and urban schools. Paper presented at the meeting of the American Anthropological Association, Phoenix, AZ.

Hess, G. A., Wells, E., Prindle, C., Liffman, P., and Kaplan, B. (1985). "Where's room 185?": How schools can reduce their dropout problem. *Education and Urban Society, 19,* 320–330.

Heyns, B. J. (1974). Social selection and stratification within schools. *American Journal of Sociology, 79,* 1434–1451.

Higham, J. (1969). Origins of immigration restriction, 1882–1897: A social analysis. In S. N. Katz and S. I. Kutler (Eds.), *New perspectives on the American past: Vol. 2/1877 to the present* (pp. 82–92). Boston: Little, Brown.

Hirsch, E. D., Jr. (1987). *Cultural literacy.* Boston: Houghton Mifflin.

Hirschman, C., and Wong, M. G. (1986). The extraordinary educational attainment of Asian-Americans: A search for historical evidence and explanations. *Social Forces, 65*(1), 1–27.

Hitchcock, M. E., and Tompkins, G. E. (1987). Are basal reading textbooks still sexist? *The Reading Teacher, 41,* 288–292.

Hodge, R. W., Siegel, P. M., and Rossi, P. H. (1966). Occupational prestige in the United States: 1925–1963. In R. Bendix and S. M. Lipset (Eds.), *Class, status and power: Social stratification in comparative perspective* (pp. 322–335). New York: The Free Press.

Hodgkinson, H. L. (1985). *All one system: Demographics of education, kindergarten through graduate school.* Washington, DC: Institute for Educational Leadership.

Holland, D. C., and Eisenhart, M. A. (1988). Women's ways of going to school: Cultural reproduction of women's identities as workers. In L. Weis (Ed.), *Class, race and gender in American education* (pp. 266–302). Albany: State University of New York.

Holland, D. C., and Eisenhart, M. A. (1990). *Educated in romance: Women, achievement and college culture.* Chicago: University of Chicago Press.

Holley, F. M., and Doss, D. A. (1983). *Momma got tired of takin' care of my baby.* Publication #82.44. Austin, TX: Office of Research and Evaluation, Independent School District.

Hollingshead, A. B. (1949). *Elmtown's youth.* New York: John Wiley.

Holmes Group, The. (1983). *Tomorrow's schools.* East Lansing, MI: Author.

Holmes Group, The. (1986). *Tomorrow's teachers.* East Lansing, MI: Author.

Hooks, B. (1989). *Talking back: Thinking feminist, thinking black.* Boston: South End Press.

Hughes, L. W., Gordon, W. M., and Hillman, L. W. (1980). *Desegrating America's schools.* New York: Longman.

Humm, M. (1990). *The dictionary of feminist theory.* Columbus: Ohio State University Press.

Jackson, P. (1968). *Life in classrooms.* Chicago: University of Chicago Press.

Jacob, E. (1987). Qualitative research traditions: A review. *Review of Educational Research, 57*(1), 1–50.

Jacob, E., and Jordan, C. (Eds.). (1987). Explaining the school performance of minority students (Theme issue). *Anthropology and Education Quarterly, 18*(4).

Jacobs, G. (Ed.). (1970). *The participant observer: Encounters with social reality.* New York: Braziller.

Jencks, C. (1972). *Inequality: A reassessment of the effect of family and schooling in America.* New York: Basic Books.

Jencks, C., Crouse, J., and Mueser, P. (1983). The Wisconsin model of status attainment: A national replication with improved measures of ability and aspiration. *Sociology of Education, 56,* 3–19.

Jensen, A. (1969). How much can we boost I.Q. and scholastic achievement? *Harvard Educational Review, 39,* 1–23.

Johnson, J. (1987). Death of unattended children spurs day care bills in Congress. *The New York Times,* November 25, p. B9.

Joint Center for Housing Studies, Harvard University. (1988). Cited by Paul Reeves. (1988). *The New York Times,* March 27, p. B9.

Jordan, C. (1984). Cultural compatibility and the education of ethnic minority children. *Educational Research Quarterly, 8*(4), 59–71.

Jordan, C. (1985). Translating culture: From ethnographic information to educational program. *Anthropology and Education Quarterly, 16,* 105–123.

Kaestle, C. F. (1983). *Pillars of the Republic: Common schools and American society, 1780-1860.* New York: Hill & Wang.

Kahl, J. A. (1953). Educational and occupational aspirations of "common man" boys. *Harvard Educational Review, 23,* 186-203.

Kantrowitz, B., and Wingert, P. (1989). How kids learn: A special report. *Newsweek,* April 17, pp. 50-56.

Karabel, J., and Halsey, A. H. (Eds.). (1977). *Power and ideology in education.* New York: Oxford University Press.

Katz, M. B. (1971). *Class, bureaucracy and the schools.* New York: Praeger.

Kaufman, P. W. (1984). *Women teachers on the frontier.* New Haven, CT: Yale University Press.

Keddie, N. (1971). Classroom knowledge. In M. F. D. Young (Ed.), *Knowledge and control* (pp. 133-160). London: Collier-Macmillan.

Kelly, G. P., and Nihlen, A. S. (1982). Schooling and the reproduction of patriarchy: Unequal workloads, unequal rewards. In M. W. Apple (Ed.), *Cultural and economic reproduction in education: Essays on class, ideology and the state* (pp. 162-180). London: Routledge & Kegan Paul.

Kelly-Benjamin, K. (1990). *The young women's guide to better SAT scores: Fighting the gender gap.* New York: Bantam Books.

Keniston, K. (1968). *The young radicals.* New York: Harcourt, Brace & World.

Keniston, K. (1971). The agony of the counterculture. *Educational Record, 52,* 205-211.

Kennedy, S. (1990). *Jim Crow guide: The way it was.* Boca Raton: Florida Atlantic University.

Kerr, N. (1973). The school board as an agency of legitimation. In S. D. Sieber and D. E. Wilder (Eds.), *The school in society: Studies in the sociology of education* (pp. 380-401). New York: The Free Press.

Kilbride, P. L., Goodale, J. C., and Ameisen, E. R. (1990). *Encounters with American ethnic cultures.* Tuscaloosa: University of Alabama Press.

Kirby, D., Harris, T. R., and Crain, R. (1973). *Political strategies in northern school desegregation.* Lexington, MA: Lexington Books.

Klein, S. (Ed.). (1985). *Handbook for achieving sex equity through education.* Baltimore: Johns Hopkins University Press.

Klein, S. S. (Ed.). (1992). *Sex equity and sexuality in education.* Albany: State University of New York.

Kliebard, H. M. (1986). *The struggle for the American curriculum: 1893-1958.* Boston: Routledge & Kegan Paul.

Knapp, M. S., and Cooperstein, R. (1986). Early research on the federal block grant: Themes and unanswered questions. *Educational Evaluation and Policy Analysis, 8,* 121-138.

Kolata, G. (1989). Gender gap in aptitude tests is narrowing, experts find. *The New York Times,* July 1, p. 1.

Kozol, J. (1991). *Savage inequalities: Children in America's schools.* New York: Crown.

Kramarae, C., and Treichler, P. A. (1985). *A feminist dictionary.* London: Pandora Press.

Kunisawa, B. (1988). A nation in crisis: The dropout dilemma. *National Education Association, 6*(6), 61-65.

La Belle, T. J. (1972). An anthropological framework for studying education. *Teachers College Record, 73,* 519-538.

Labov, W. (1972). *Language in the inner city: Studies in the Black English vernacular.* Philadelphia: University of Pennsylvania Press.

LaFrance, M. (1985). The school of hard knocks: Nonverbal sexism in the classroom. *Theory Into Practice, 24,* 40-44.

LaFrance, M., and Mayo, C. (1978). *Moving bodies: Nonverbal communication in social relationships.* Monterey, CA: Brooks/Cole.

Lappe, F. M., and Du Bois, P. M. (1993). Others study democracy—We do it. *Democracy and Education,* 7(3), 9–14.

Lather, P. (1986). Research as praxis. *Harvard Educational Review, 56,* 257–277.

Lau v. Nichols, 414 U. S. 563 (1974).

Lawrence, N. R. (1994). The choice of language and the language of choice: Public/private discourse about abortion and education in the early 1990s. Doctoral dissertation, School of Education, University of Colorado-Boulder.

Leap, W. L. (1978). American Indian English and its implications of bilingual education. In J. Alatis (Ed.), *International dimensions of bilingual education* (pp. 657–669). Washington, DC: Georgetown University Press.

Leap, W. L. (1993). *American Indian English.* Salt Lake City: University of Utah Press.

LeCompte, M. D. (1969). Dilemmas in inner-city school reform. Unpublished Master's thesis, Department of Education and the Social Order, University of Chicago.

LeCompte, M. D. (1972). The uneasy alliance between community action and research. *School Review,* 79(1), 123–132.

LeCompte, M. D. (1974). Teacher styles and the development of student work norms. Unpublished doctoral dissertation, University of Chicago.

LeCompte, M. D. (1978a). Culture shock: It happens to teachers, too. In B. Dell Felder et al. (Eds.), *Focus on the future: Implications for education* (pp. 102–112). Houston, TX: University of Houston.

LeCompte, M. D. (1978b). Learning to work: The hidden curriculum of the classroom. *Anthropology and Education Quarterly,* 9, 23–37.

LeCompte, M. D. (1981). The civilizing of children: How young children learn to become students. *The Journal of Thought, 15,* 105–129.

LeCompte, M. D. (1985). Defining the differences: Cultural subgroups among mainstream children. *The Urban Review,* 17(2), 111–128.

LeCompte, M. D. (1987a). The cultural context of dropping out: Why good dropout programs don't work. Paper presented at the meeting of the American Association for the Advancement of Science, Chicago.

LeCompte, M. D. (1987b). The cultural context of dropping out: Why remedial programs don't solve the problems. *Education and Urban Society, 19,* 232–249.

LeCompte, M. D., and Bennett, K. P. (1988). Empowerment: The once and future role of the Gringo. Paper presented at the meeting of the American Anthropological Association, Phoenix, AZ.

LeCompte, M. D., and Bennett, K. P. (1990). Empowerment: The once and future role of the Bilagaana. *Navajo Education, VIII*(1), 41–46.

LeCompte, M. D., and Bennett deMarrais, K. P. (1992). The disempowerment of empowerment: Out of the revolution and into the classroom. *Educational Foundations,* 6(3), 5–31.

LeCompte, M. D., and Dworkin, A. G. (1988). Educational programs: Indirect linkages and unfulfilled expectations. In H. R. Rodgers, Jr. (Ed.), *Beyond welfare: New approaches to the problem of poverty in America* (pp. 135–167). Armonk, NY: M. E. Sharpe.

LeCompte, M. D., and Dworkin, A. G. (1991). *Giving up on school: Teacher burnout and student dropout.* Newbury Park, CA: Corwin Press.

LeCompte, M. D., and Goebel, S. G. (1985). *Issues in defining and enumerating dropouts* [HISD dropout report #1]. Houston, TX: Department of Planning, Research and Evaluation, Houston Independent School District, June 6.

LeCompte, M. D., and Goebel, S. G. (1987). Can bad data produce good program planning?:

An analysis of record-keeping on school dropouts. *Education and Urban Society, 19,* 250–268.

LeCompte, M. D., and McLaughlin, D. (forthcoming). Witchcraft and blessings, science and rationality: Discourses of power and silence in collaborative work with Navajo schools. In A. Gitlin (Ed.), *Power and method: Political activism and educational research.* New York: Routledge & Kegan Paul.

LeCompte, M. D., and Preissle, J. (1992). Toward an ethnology of student life in schools: Synthesizing the qualitative research tradition. In M. D. LeCompte, W. Millroy, and J. Preissle (Eds.), *The handbook of qualitative research in education* (pp. 815–855). San Diego: Academic Press.

LeCompte, M. D., and Preissle, J. (1993). *Ethnography and qualitative research design in educational research.* Orlando, FL: Academic Press.

LeCompte, M. D., and Wiertelak, M. E. (1992). Constructing the appearance of reform: Restructuring, site-based management and shared decision-making in a Navajo public school district. Paper presented at the American Educational Research Association Meetings, San Francisco.

Lee, E. S., and Rong, X. (1988). The educational and economic achievement of Asian-Americans. *The Elementary School Journal, 88,* 545–560.

Lee, P. C., and Gropper, N. B. (1974). Sex-role culture and educational practice. *Harvard Educational Review, 44,* 369–409.

Lee, V. E., and Bryk, A. S. (1988). Curriculum tracking as mediating the social distribution of high school achievement. *Sociology of Education, 61,* 78–94.

Lesko, N. (1988). The curriculum of the body: Lessons from a Catholic high school. In L. Roman, L. Christian-Smith, and E. Ellsworth (Eds.), *Becoming feminine: The politics of popular culture* (pp. 123–143). Philadelphia: Falmer Press.

Lever, J. (1976). Sex differences in the games children play. *Social Problems, 23,* 479–488.

Liebow, E. (1969). *Tally's corner: A study of Negro streetcorner men.* Boston: Little, Brown.

Linton, R. (1945). *The cultural background of personality.* New York: Appleton-Century.

Lippitt, R., and Gold, M. (1959). Classroom social structure as a mental health problem. *Journal of Social Issues, 15,* 40–49.

Liston, D., and Zeichner, K. (1991). *Teacher education and the social conditions of schooling.* New York: Routledge & Kegan Paul.

Littwin, J. (1987). *The postponed generation: Why America's grown-up kids are growing up later.* New York: Morrow.

Lonsdale Improvement Organization. (July, 1992). *Remembering Lonsdale: Our community, our home.* Knoxville, TN: Author.

Lortie, D. (1969). The balance of control and autonomy in elementary school teaching. In A. Etzioni (Ed.), *The semiprofessions and their organization: Teachers, nurses, social workers* (pp. 1–53). New York: The Free Press.

Lortie, D. (1973). Observations on teaching as work. In R. M. W. Travers (Ed.), *The second handbook of research on teaching* (pp. 474–496). Chicago: Rand-McNally.

Lortie, D. (1975). *Schoolteacher: A sociological study.* Chicago: University of Chicago Press.

McCarthy, C. (1988). Rethinking liberal and radical perspectives on racial inequality in schooling: Making the case for nonsynchrony. *Harvard Educational Review, 58,* 265–279.

McCarthy, C. (1990). *Race and curriculum: Social inequality and the theories and politics of difference in contemporary research on schooling.* New York: Falmer Press.

Maccoby, E. (1966). *The development of sex differences.* Stanford, CA: Stanford University Press.

Maccoby, E., and Jacklin, C. (1974). *The psychology of sex differences.* Stanford, CA: Stanford University Press.

McDade, L. (1988). Knowing the "right stuff": Attrition, gender, and scientific literacy. *Anthropology and Education Quarterly, 19*, 93–114.

McDermott, R. P. (1976). Kids make sense: An ethnographic account of the instructional management of success and failure in a first grade classroom. Unpublished doctoral dissertation, Stanford University, CA.

McDermott, R. P. (1977). Social relations as contexts for learning in school. *Harvard Educational Review, 47*, 198–213.

McDill, E. L., Pallas, A. M., and Natriello, G. (1985). Uncommon sense: School administrators, school reform, and potential dropouts. Paper presented at the meeting of the National Invitational Conference on Holding Power and Dropouts, Columbia University, February.

McGivney, J. H., and Haught, J. M. (1972). The politics of education: A view from the perspective of the central office staff. *Educational Administrative Quarterly, 8*(3), 35.

McIntosh, P. (1983). Interactive phases of curricular re-vision: A feminist perspective. Working Paper No. 124. Wellesley, MA: Wellesley College Center for Research on Women.

McIntosh, P. M. (1988). Feeling a fraud (Keynote address). American Educational Studies Association, Toronto, November.

McLaren, P. (1980). *Cries from the corridor: The new suburban ghettos.* Toronto: Metheun.

McLaren, P. (1986). *Schooling as a ritual performance.* Boston: Routledge & Kegan Paul.

McLaren, P. (1989). *Life in schools.* New York: Longman.

McLeod, J. (1987). *Ain't no makin' it: Leveled aspirations in a low-income neighborhood.* Boulder, CO: Westview Press.

McNeil, J. D. (1985). *Curriculum: A comprehensive introduction* (3rd ed.). Boston: Little, Brown.

McNeil, J. D. (1992). *Kids as customers.* New York: Lexington Books.

McNeil, L. (1983). Defensive teaching and classroom control. In M. W. Apple and L. Weis (Eds.), *Ideology and practice in schooling* (pp. 114–142). Philadelphia: Temple University Press.

McNeil, L. M. (1986). *Contradictions of control: School structure and school knowledge.* New York: Routledge & Kegan Paul.

McNeil, L. M. (1988a). Contradictions of control, Part I: Administrators and teachers. *Phi Delta Kappan, 69*(5), 333–339.

McNeil, L. M. (1988b). Contradictions of control, Part II: Teachers and students. *Phi Delta Kappan, 69*(6), 432–438.

McNeil, L. M. (1988c). Contradictions of control, Part III: Contradictions of control. *Phi Delta Kappan, 69*(7), 478–485.

McRobbie, A. (1978). Working class girls and the culture of femininity. In Women's Studies Group, Centre for Contemporary Cultural Studies (Ed.), *Women take issue: Aspects of women's subordination* (pp. 96–108). London: Hutchinson.

Main, J. T. (1966). The class structure of revolutionary America. In R. Bendix and S. M. Lipset (Eds.), *Class, status and power: Social stratification in comparative perspective* (pp. 111–121). New York: The Free Press.

Malen, B., and Hart, A. W. (1987). Career ladder reform: A multilevel analysis of initial efforts. *Educational Evaluation and Policy Analysis, 9*, 9–23.

Malen, B., Ogawa, R. and Kranz, J. (1990). What do we know about school-based management? A case study of the literature. In W. McClune & J. Witte (Eds.), *Choice and control in education: The practice of choice, decentralization and school restructuring,* Volume 2 (pp. 289–342). Bristol, PA: Falmer Press.

Malinowski, B. (1963). Quoted in Intro to *Fortune,* p. xxix.

Maloney, M. E. (1985). *School dropouts: Cincinnati's challenge in the eighties* (Working Paper #15). Cincinnati: Urban Appalachian Council.

Mann, H. (1842). *Fifth annual report of the secretary of the board.* Boston: Board of Education.

Mark, J. H., and Anderson, B. D. (1978). Teacher survival rates—A current look. *American Educational Research Journal, 15,* 379-383.

Marotto, R. A. (1986). "Posin' to be chosen": An ethnographic study of in-school truancy. In D. A. Fetterman and M. A. Pitman (Eds.), *Educational evaluation: Ethnography in theory, practice and politics* (pp. 193-214). Beverly Hills, CA: Sage Publications.

Marrou, H. I. (1956). *A history of education in antiquity.* Madison: University of Wisconsin Press.

Martin, R. (1972). Student sex and behavior as determinants of the type and frequency of teacher-student contacts. *Journal of School Psychology, 10,* 339-347.

Marx, K. (1955). *The communist manifesto.* Chicago: H. Regney.

Marx, K. (1959). *Basic writings on politics and philosophy* (L. Feuer, Ed.). Garden City, NY: Anchor Books.

Marx, K. (1971). *Economy, class and social revolution.* New York: Scribner.

Marx, K. (1973). *On society and social change.* Chicago: University of Chicago Press.

Mason, W. S. (1961). The beginning teacher: Status and career orientations. Department of Health, Education and Welfare Publication. Washington, DC: U.S. Government Printing Office.

Massachusetts teacher, The. (1851). *Immigration, 4,* 289-291.

Mechling, J. (1981). Male gender display at a Boy Scout camp. In R. T. Sieber and A. J. Gordon (Eds.), *Children and their organizations: Investigations in American culture* (pp. 138-160). Boston: G. K. Hall.

Merton, R. K. (1967). *Social theory and social structure.* New York: The Free Press.

Mertz, N. T., and McNeely, S. R. (1988). Secondary schools in transition: A study of the emerging female administrator. *American Secondary Education, 17*(2), 10-14.

Metz, M. H. (1978). *Classrooms and corridors: The crisis of authority in desegregated secondary schools.* Berkeley: University of California Press.

Miles, M. W. (1977). The student movement and the industrialization of higher education. In J. Karabel and A. H. Halsey (Eds.), *Power and ideology in education* (pp. 432-456). Cambridge, MA: Oxford University Press.

Miller, S. E., Leinhardt, G., and Zigmond, N. (1988). Influencing engagement through accommodation: An ethnographic study of at-risk students. *American Educational Research Journal, 25,* 465-489.

Millett, K. (1977). *Sexual politics.* London: Virago Press.

Mills, C. W. (1956). *The power elite.* New York: Oxford University Press.

Mohatt, G. V., and Erickson, F. (1981). Cultural differences in teaching styles in an Odawa school: A sociolinguistic approach. In H. Trueba, G. P. Guthrie, and K. H. Au (Eds.), *Culture and the bilingual classroom* (pp. 105-119). Rowley, MA: Newbury House.

Moll, L. C., and Diaz, R. (1987). Teaching writing as communication: The use of ethnographic findings in classroom practice. In D. Broome (Ed.), *Literacy and schooling* (pp. 193-221). Norwood, NJ: Ablex.

Molner, A. (1987). *Social issues and education: A challenge and responsibility.* Alexandria, VA: Association for Supervision and Curriculum Development.

Morage, C., and Anzaldua, G. (Eds.). (1981). *This bridge called my back: Writings by radical women of color.* New York: Kitchen Table: Women of Color Press.

Morgenstern, J. (1989). Can "USA Today" be saved? *New York Times Magazine,* January 1, section 6, p. 13.

Morrow, G. (1986). Standardizing practice in analysis of school dropouts. *Teachers College Record, 87,* 342-356.

Murnane, R. J. (1975). *The impact of school resources on the learning of inner-city children.* Cambridge, MA: Ballinger.

Nadel, S. F. (1957). *The theory of social structure.* Glencoe, IL: The Free Press, pp. 35-41. Quoted in Charles E. Bidwell, The school as a formal organization. In James G. March (Ed.), *The handbook of organizations.* New York: Rand McNally, 1965.

Nash, R. (1976). Pupil expectations of their teachers. In M. Stubbs and S. Delamont (Eds.), *Explorations in classroom observation* (pp. 83-101). New York: John Wiley.

National Assessment of Educational Progress (NAEP) Report. (1988). *Science and Engineering Indicators—1987* (N.S.B. 87-1). Washington, DC: U.S. Government Printing Office.

National Center for Restructuring Education, Schools, and Teaching Newsletter (1994), p. 1.

National Commission on Excellence in Education. (1983). *A nation at risk.* Washington, DC: U.S. Government Printing Office.

National Education Association. (1963). Teachers in public schools. *NEA Research Bulletin, 41*(1), 23-26.

National Education Association. (1970). Teacher strikes. 1960-61 to 1970-71. *National Education Association Bulletin, 48*(1).

National Education Association. (1972). The American public school teacher, 1970-1971: More highlights from the preliminary report. *NEA Research Bulletin, 50*(1), 3-8.

National Institute of Education. (1978). *Violent schools—safe schools: The safe school study report to Congress* (Vol. 1). Washington, DC: Department of Health, Education & Welfare, U.S. Government Printing Office.

National School Boards Association. (1993). *Violence in the schools: How America's school boards are safeguarding your children.* Alexandria, VA: National School Boards Association.

Needle, R. H., Griffin, T., Svendsen, R., and Berney, C. (1980). Teacher stress: Sources and consequences. *The Journal of School Health,* February, pp. 96-99.

New York Times. (1993). White girls jeered for "acting black," *Education,* December 8, p. B8.

Nieto, S. (1992). *Affirming diversity: The sociopolitical context of multicultural education.* New York: Longman.

North Central Regional Educational Laboratory. (1993). Executive Summary: The Illinois Valedictorian Project. Oak Brook, IL: Author.

Oakes, J. (1985). *Keeping track: How schools structure inequality.* New Haven, CT: Yale University Press.

Obermiller, P. J. (1981). The question of urban Appalachian ethnicity. In W. W. Philliber (Ed.), *The invisible minority.* Lexington: University of Kentucky Press.

Ogbu, J. U. (1978). *Minority education and caste: The American system in cross-cultural perspective.* New York: Academic Press.

Ogbu, J. U. (1983). Minority status and schooling in plural societies. *Comparative Education Review, 27*(2), 168-190.

Ogbu, J. U. (1987). Variability in minority school performance: A problem in search of an explanation. *Anthropology and Educational Quarterly, 18,* 312-335.

O'Neill, D. M., and Sepielli, P. (1985). *Education in the United States: 1940-1983* [CDS-85-1]. Washington, DC: U.S. Department of Commerce, Bureau of the Census.

Orfield, G. (1993). *The growth of segregation in American schools: Changing patterns of separation and poverty since 1968.* Alexandria, VA: National School Boards Association Council of Urban Boards of Education.

Ortiz, F. I. (1981). *Career patterns in education: Men, women and minorities in public school administration.* New York: Praeger.

Ortiz, F. I. (1988). Hispanic-American children's experiences in classrooms: A comparison between Hispanic and non-Hispanic children. In L. Weis (Ed.), *Race, class and gender in American education* (pp. 63-87). Albany: State University of New York Press.

Orum, L. (1984). *Hispanic dropouts: Community responses.* Washington, DC: Office of Research, Advocacy and Legislation, National Council of La Raza.

Page, R. (1987). Lower-track classes at a college-preparatory high school: A caricature of educational encounters. In G. Spindler and L. Spindler (Eds.), *Interpretive ethnography of education at home and abroad.* Hillsdale, NJ: Lawrence Erlbaum.

Page, R. (1988). Interpreting curriculum differentiation. Unpublished manuscript, University of California–Riverside.

Page, R. (1989). The lower track curriculum at a "heavenly" high school: Cycles of prejudice. *Journal of Curriculum Studies, 21,* 197–221.

Parsons, T. (1951). *The social system.* Glencoe, IL: The Free Press.

Parsons, T. (1959). The school class as a social system: Some of its functions in American society. *Harvard Educational Review, 29,* 297–319.

Pavalko, R. M. (1970). Recruitment to teaching: Patterns of selection and retention. *Sociology of Education, 43,* 340–353.

Perrillo, V. (1980). *Strangers to these shores.* Boston: Houghton Mifflin.

Persell, C. H. (1977). *Education and inequality: The roots and results of stratification in America's schools.* New York: The Free Press.

Peterson, K. S. (1987). School cost can cut doubly deep: Scholarship meets hardship. *USA Today,* November 17, p. 1 [Section D].

Peterson, P. E. (1976). *School politics Chicago style.* Chicago: University of Chicago Press.

Pettigrew, T. F., and Green, R. L. (1976). School desegregation in large cities: A critique of the Coleman "white flight" thesis. *Harvard educational review report series No. 11. School desegregation: The continuing challenge* (pp. 17–69). Cambridge, MA: Harvard University Press.

Phillips, B. N., and Lee, M. (1980). The changing role of the American teacher: Current and future sources of stress. In C. L. Cooper and J. Marshall (Eds.), *White collar and professional stress* (pp. 93–111). New York: John Wiley.

Phillips, D. C. (1987). *Philosophy, science and social inquiry.* New York: Pergamon Press.

Phillips, S. U. (1972). Participant structures and communicative competence: Warm Springs Indian children in community and classroom. In C. B. Cazden, V. John, and D. Hymes (Eds.), *Functions of language in the classroom* (pp. 370–394). New York: Teachers College Press.

Piestrup, A. (1973). Black dialect interference and accommodation in first grade [Monograph No. 4]. Berkeley, CA: Language Behavior Research Laboratory.

Pinar, W. F. (Ed.). (1988). *Contemporary curriculum discourses.* Scottsdale, AZ: Gorsuch Scarisbrick.

Pinar, W. F. (1989). A reconceptualization of teacher education. *Journal of Teacher Education, 40*(1), 9–12.

Pitman, M. A. (1987). Compulsory education and home schooling: Truancy or prophecy? *Education and Urban Society, 19,* 280–290.

Pitman, M. A., and Eisenhardt, M. A. (Eds.). (1988). Women, culture, and education [Theme issue]. *Anthropology and Education Quarterly, 19*(2).

Pitsch, M. (1994). House poised to clear E.S.E.A. reauthorization. *Education Week,* March 9, p. 16.

Plessy v. *Ferguson,* 163 U.S. 537 (1895).

Popper, K. R. (1968). *The logic of scientific discovery.* New York: Harper & Row.

Powell, A. G., Farrar, E., and Cohen, D. K. (1985). *The shopping mall high school: Winners and losers in the educational marketplace.* Boston: Houghton Mifflin.

Project on Equal Education Rights. (1986). *1986 PEER report card: A state-by-state survey of the status of women and girls in America's schools* [PEER Policy Paper #5]. Washington, DC: Author.

Psacharaopoulos, G. (1973). *Returns to education: An international comparison.* San Francisco: Jossey-Bass.

Purcell-Gates, V. (1993). I ain't never read my own words before. *Journal of Reading, 37*(8), 210-219.

Randour, M. L., Strasburg, G. L., and Lipman-Blumen, J. (1982). Women in higher education: Trends in enrollments and degrees earned. *Harvard Educational Review, 52,* 189-202.

Reed, S., and Sautter, R. C. (1990). Children of poverty: The status of 12 million young Americans. *Phi Delta Kappan Special Report,* K1-K12.

Reeves, P. (1988). Rising rents squeeze lower-income families. *The Houston Chronicle,* March 27, p. 6.

Reisler, R., Jr., and Friedman, M. S. (1978). Radical misfits? How students from an alternative junior high school adapted to a conventional high school. *Educational Theory, 28*(1), 17-82.

Report of the Massachusetts Senate committee on establishing a reform school. (1984). Commonwealth of Massachusetts, Senate. (Doc. No. 86, 1846).

Resnick, D. P., and Resnick, L. B. (1985). Standards, curriculum and performance: A historical and comparative perspective. *Educational Researcher, 14*(4), 5-20.

Reyes, M., and Halcon, J. J. (1988). Racism in academia: The old wolf revisited. *Harvard Educational Review, 58,* 299-314.

Reyes, M., and Laliberty, A. (1992). A Teacher's "Pied Piper" Effect on Young Authors. *Education and Urban Society, 24*(2), 263-278.

Reynolds, W. B. (1986). Education alternatives to transportation failures: The desegregation response to a resegregation dilemma. *Metropolitan Education* (1), 3-15.

Richard, D. (1990). *Lesbian lists: A look at lesbian culture, history, and personalities.* New York: Alyson.

Richardson, V., Casanova, U., Placier, P., and Guilfoyle, K. (1989). *School children at-risk.* New York: Falmer Press.

Ries, P., and Stone, A. J. (1992). *The American woman 1992-93: A status report.* New York: Norton.

Rist, R. C. (1970). Student social class and teacher expectations: The self-fulfilling prophecy in ghetto education. *Harvard Educational Review, 40,* 411-451.

Rist, R. C. (1973). *The urban factory for failure.* Cambridge, MA: MIT Press.

Robbins, T. (1984). *Jitterbug perfume.* New York: Bantam.

Roberts, J. I., and Akinsanya, S. K. (1976). *Schooling in the cultural context: Anthropological studies of education.* New York: David McKay.

Robinson, V., and Pierce, C. (1985). *Making do in the classroom: A report on the misassignment of teachers.* Washington, DC: Council for Basic Education, American Federation of Teachers.

Rogers, D. (1968). *110 Livingston Street: Politics and bureaucracy in the New York City schools.* New York: Random House.

Roman, L.G. (1988). Intimacy, labor and class: Ideologies of feminine sexuality in the Punk slam dance. In L. G. Roman and L. Christian-Smith (Eds.), *Becoming Feminine: The politics of popular culture* (pp. 148-270). London: Falmer Press.

Roman L. G. (1993a). White is a color/white defensiveness, postmodernism, and anti-racist pedagogy. In C. McCarthy and W. Crichlow (Eds.), *Race, Identity, and Representation in Education.* New York: Routledge.

Roman, L. G. (1993b). Double exposure: The politics of feminist materialist ethnography. *Educational Theory, 43*(3), 278-309.

Rose, R. (1988). "Syntactic styling" as a means of linguistic empowerment: Illusion or reality? Paper presented at the meeting of the American Anthropological Association, Phoenix.

Rosenfeld, G. (1971). *Shut those thick lips.* New York: Holt, Rinehart & Winston.

Rosenfeld, R. A. (1980). Race and sex differences in career dynamics. *American Sociological Review, 45,* 583–609.

Ross, E. A. (1901). *Social control: A survey of the foundations of order.* New York: Macmillan.

Rosser, P. (1990). Introduction. In K. Kelly-Benjamin, *The young women's guide to better SAT scores: Fighting the gender gap.* New York: Bantam.

Rudolph, L., and Rudolph, S. (1967). *The modernity of tradition.* Chicago: University of Chicago Press.

Rumberger, R. W. (1987). High school dropouts: A review of issues and evidence. *Review of Educational Research, 57,* 101–122.

Ryan, W. (1976). *Blaming the victim.* New York: Random House.

Saario, T. N., Jacklin, C. N., and Tittle, C. K. (1973). Sex role stereotyping in the public schools. *Harvard Educational Review, 43,* 386–415.

Sadker, M. P., and Sadker, D. M. (1985). Sexism in the schoolroom of the '80's. *Psychology Today,* March, pp. 54–57.

Sadker, M. P., and Sadker, D. M. (1988). *Teachers, schools, and society.* New York: Random House.

Sadker, M. P., Sadker, D. M., and Klein, S. S. (1986). Abolishing misperceptions about sex equity in education. *Theory into Practice, 25,* 219–226.

St. John, N. H. (1975). *School desegregation: Outcomes for children.* New York: Wiley-Interscience.

Sanjek, R. (Ed.). (1990). *Fieldnotes: The makings of anthropology.* Ithaca, NY: Cornell University Press.

Sarason, S. B. (1971). *The culture of the school and the problem of change.* Boston: Allyn & Bacon.

Schildkrout, E. (1984). Young traders of Northern Nigeria. In J. P. Spradley and D. W. McCurdy (Eds.), *Conformity and conflicts: Readings in cultural anthropology* (pp. 246–253). Boston: Little, Brown.

Schmidt, P. (1993). *Education Week,* June 9, p. 7.

Schmidt, P. (1994). *Education Week,* January 12, p. 5.

Schmuck, P. A. (Ed.). (1987). *Women educators: Employees of schools in western countries.* Albany: State University of New York Press.

Schofield, J. (1982). *Black and white in school: Trust, tension or tolerance?* New York: Praeger.

Schultz, T. W. (1961). Investment in human capital. *American Economic Review, 51,* 1–17.

Schumacher, E. F. (1989). *Small is beautiful: Economics as if people mattered.* New York: Harper Colophon.

Schutz, A. (1972). *The phenomenology of the social world.* New York: Columbia University Press.

Scimecca, J. A. (1980). *Education and society.* New York: Holt Rinehart & Winston.

Scott, J. W. (1987). Women's history and the rewriting of history. In C. Farnham (Ed.), *The impact of feminist research in the academy* (pp. 34–50). Bloomington: Indiana Press University.

Scott, J. W. (1988). *Gender and the politics of history.* New York: Columbia University Press.

Seeman, M. (1959). On the meaning of alienation. *American Sociological Review, 24,* 783–791.

Seeman, M. (1967). On the personal consequences of alienation in work. *American Sociological Review, 32,* 273–285.

Seeman, M. (1975). Alienation studies. *Annual Review of Sociology, 1,* 91–123.

Sege, I. (1989). Children in poverty, Part Three. The inner city: Streets of children begetting children. *The Oregonian*, June 27, p. A2. Reprinted from *The Boston Globe*.

Sennett, R., and Cobb, J. (1973). *The hidden injuries of class.* New York: Vintage Books.

Sewell, W. H., Haller, A. O., and Ohlendorf, G. W. (1970). The educational and early occupational attainment process: Replication and revision. *American Sociological Review, 34,* 82–92.

Sewell, W. H., Haller, A. O., and Portes, A. (1969). The educational and early occupational attainment process. *American Sociological Review, 34,* 82–92.

Sewell, W. H., and Shah, V. P. (1967). Socioeconomic status, intelligence, and the attainment of higher education. *Sociology of Education, 40,* 1–23.

Sewell, W. H., and Shah, V. P. (1977). Socioeconomic status, intelligence and the attainment of higher education. In J. Karabel and A. H. Halsey (Eds.), *Power and ideology in education* (pp. 197–215). New York: Oxford University Press.

Shaker, P., and Kridel, C. (1989). The return to experience: A reconceptualist call. *Journal of Teacher Education, 40*(1), 2–8.

Shakeshaft, C. (1986). A gender at risk. *Phi Delta Kappan, 67,* 449–503.

Shavelson, R. J., and Stern, P. (1981). Research on teachers' pedagogical thoughts, judgments, decisions and behavior. *Review of Educational Research, 51,* 455–498.

Shepard, L. A., and Kreitzer, A. E. (1987). The Texas teacher test. *Educational Researcher,* August/September, pp. 22–31.

Shrewsbury, C. M. (1987). What is feminist pedagogy? *Women's Studies Quarterly, 25,* 6–14.

Shultz, J., and Erickson, F. (1982). *The counselor as gatekeeper.* New York: Academic Press.

Sieber, R. T. (1981). Socialization implications of school discipline, or how first-graders are taught to "listen." In R. T. Sieber and A. J. Gordon (Eds.), *Children and their organization* (pp. 18–44). Boston: G. K. Hall.

Sikes, J. (1971). Differential behavior of male and female teachers with male and female students. Unpublished doctoral dissertation, University of Texas–Austin.

Silberman, C. E. (1973). *The open classroom reader.* New York: The Free Press.

Sills, D. L. (1970). Preserving organizational goals. In O. Grusky and G. A. Miller (Eds.), *The sociology of organizations: Basic studies* (pp. 227–236). New York: The Free Press.

Simeone, A. (1986). *Academic women: Working towards equality.* South Hadley, MA: Bergin & Garvey.

Simmel, G. (1955). *Conflict.* Glencoe, IL: The Free Press.

Simmel, G. (1968). *The conflict in modern culture and other essays.* New York: Teachers College Press.

Simpson, R. L., and Simpson, I. H. (1969). Women and bureaucracy in the semi-professions. In A. Etzioni (Ed.), *The semi-professions and their organization: Teachers, nurses, social workers* (pp. 196–266). New York: The Free Press.

Sizer, T. (1984). *Horace's compromise: The dilemma of the American high school.* Boston: Houghton Mifflin.

Sleeter, C. (1991). *Empowerment through Multicultural Education.* New York: SUNY Press.

Smith, B. (1979). Quoted in C. Morage and G. Anzaldua (Eds.), (1981), *This bridge called my back: Writings by radical women of color* (p. 61). New York: Kitchen Table: Women of Color Press.

Smith, L. M., and Geoffrey, W. (1968). *The complexities of an urban classroom: An analysis toward a general theory of teaching.* New York: Holt, Rinehart & Winston.

Smith, M. G. (1982). Ethnicity and ethnic groups in America: The view from Harvard. *Ethnic and Racial Studies, 5*(1), 1–22.

Smith v. Board of School Commissioners (82-0544-BH, 82-0792-BH), 11th Cir., March 4, 1987.

Smith v. *School Commissioners of Mobile, Alabama,* 827 F.2d 684 (1987).

Sorensen, A. B., and Hallinan, M. T. (1987). Ability grouping and sex differences in mathematics achievement. *Sociology of Education, 60*(2), 63-72.

Spencer, D. (1986). *Contemporary women teachers: Balancing school and home.* New York: Longman.

Spencer, H. (1851). *Social Statistics.* London: Chapman.

Spencer, H. (1967). *The evolution of society: Selections from Herbert Spencer's principles of sociology* (R. L. Carneiro, Ed.). Chicago: University of Chicago Press. (First printed 1898 as *First Principles.* New York: Appleton.)

Spindler, G. D. (1987). Beth-Ann: A case study of culturally defined adjustment and teacher perceptions. In G. D. Spindler (Ed.), *Education and cultural process: Anthropological approaches* (2nd ed.). Prospect Heights, IL: Waveland.

Spolsky, B., and Irvine, P. (1992). Sociolinguistic aspects of the acceptance of literacy in the vernacular. In F. Barkin, E. Brandt, and J. Ornstein-Galicia (Eds.), *Bilingualism and language contact: Spanish, English, and Native American languages* (pp. 73-79). New York: Teachers College Press.

Spradley, J. P. (1980). *Participant observation.* New York: Holt, Rinehart and Winston.

Spradley, J. P., and McCurdy, D. W. (Eds.). (1972). *The cultural experience: Ethnography in complex society.* Chicago: Science Research Associates.

Spring, J. H. (1976). *The sorting machine.* New York: David McKay.

Spring, J. H. (1985). *American education* (3rd ed.). New York: Longman.

Spring, J. H. (1986). *The American school, 1642-1985.* New York: Longman.

Spring, J. H. (1988a). *Conflict of interests: The politics of American education.* New York: Longman.

Spring, J. H. (1988b). The political structure of popular culture. Paper presented at the 10th Conference on Curriculum Theory and Classroom Practice, Bergamo Conference Center, Dayton, OH.

Spring, J. H. (1989). *American education* (4th ed.). New York: Longman.

Spring, J. H. (1992). *Images of American life: A history of ideological management in schools, movies, radio, and television.* Albany: State University of New York Press.

Spring, J. H. (1994). *American education* (5th ed.). New York: McGraw-Hill.

Srinivas, M. N. (1965). *Religion and society among the Coorgs of South India.* New York: Asia.

Stein, N. (1994). Seeing is not believing: Sexual harassment in public school and the role of adults. Paper presented at the American Educational Research Association Meetings, April.

Steinberg, L., Blinde, P., and Chan, K. (1984). Dropping out among language minority youth. *Review of Educational Research, 54*(1), 113-132.

Steinberg, L. D., Greenberger, E., Garduque, L., and McAuliffe, S. (1982). High school students in the labor force: Some costs and benefits to schooling and learning. *Educational Evaluation and Policy Analysis, 4*(3), 363-372.

Steinberg, S. (1989). *The ethnic myth: Race, ethnicity, and class in America.* Boston: Beacon.

Stern, S. P. (1987). Black parents: Drop-outs or push-outs from school participation. Paper presented at the meeting of the American Anthropological Association, Chicago, November.

Stinchcombe, A. (1964). *Rebellion in a high school.* Chicago: Quadrangle Press.

Suarez-Orozco, M. M. (1987). "Becoming somebody": Central American immigrants in U.S. inner-city schools. *Anthropology and Education Quarterly, 18,* 287-300.

Sumner, W. G. (1883). *What social classes owe to each other.* New York: Harper Brothers.

Suzuki, B. H. (1984). Curriculum transformation for multicultural education. *Education and Urban Society, 15,* 294-322.

Sykes, G. (1958). *The society of captives.* Princeton, NJ: Princeton University Press.

Tannen, D. (1990). *You just don't understand.* New York: William Morrow.

Tar, Z. (1985). *The Frankfurt School.* New York: Schocken Books.

Tatel, D. S., Lanigan, K. J., and Sneed, M. F. (1986). The fourth decade of Brown: Metropolitan desegregation and quality education. *Metropolitan Education* (1), 15–36.

Tavris, C. (1992). *The mismeasure of woman: Why women are not the better sex, the inferior sex, or the opposite sex.* New York: Simon & Schuster.

Tedford, D. (1988). Making the grade at HISD: It helps being White, well-off. *The Houston Chronicle,* October 16, p. 1.

Tetreault, M. K. (1986). The journey from male-defined to gender-balanced education. *Theory into Practice, 25,* 227–234.

Tetreault, M. K., and Schmuck, P. (1985). Equity, educational reform and gender. *Issues in Education, 3*(1), 45–67.

Thomas, K. (1990). *Gender and subject in higher education.* Buckingham, England, MK: The Society for Research into Higher Education and Open University Press.

Thompson, B., and Disch, E. (1992). Feminist, anti-racist, anti-oppression teaching: Two white women's experience. *Radical Teacher, 41,* 4–10.

Tiedt, S. W. (1966). *The role of the federal government in education.* New York: Oxford University Press.

Tierney, W. G. (1992). *Official encouragement, institutional discouragement: Minorities in academe—the Native American experience.* Norwood, NJ: Ablex.

Tinker v. *Des Moines School District,* 393 U.S. 503 (1969).

Tobier, E. (1984). *The changing face of poverty: Trends in New York City's population in poverty, 1960–1990.* New York: Community Service Society.

Today's numbers, tomorrow's nation. (1986). *Education Week,* May 14, p. 14.

Tong, R. (1989). *Feminist thought: A comprehensive introduction.* Boulder, CO: Westview.

Treckler, J. L. (1973). Women in U.S. history high school textbooks. *International Review of Education, 19,* 133–139.

Turner, J. H. (1978). *The structure of sociological theory* (rev. ed.). Homewood, IL: The Dorsey Press.

Turner, R. L. (1989). Organizational size effects at different levels of schooling. Paper presented at the meeting of the American Educational Research Association, New Orleans, April.

Turner, V. (1969). *The ritual process: Structure and anti-structure.* Ithaca, NY: Cornell University Press.

Turner, V. (1974). *Dramas, fields and metaphors: Symbolic action in human society.* Ithaca, NY: Cornell University Press.

Tyack, D. (1974). *The one best system.* Cambridge, MA: Harvard University Press.

Tyack, D. (1990). Restructuring in historical perspective. *Teachers College Record, 92*(2), 170–191.

Tylor, E. B. (1958). *Primitive culture.* New York: Harper Torchbooks (orig. pub. in 1871).

U.S. Bureau of the Census. (1986). *Statistical Abstract of the United States: 1987* (107th ed.). Washington, DC: U.S. Government Printing Office.

Valentine, C. A. (1968). *Culture and poverty: Critique and counterproposals.* Chicago: University of Chicago Press.

Valli, L. (1983). Becoming clerical workers: Business education and the culture of femininity. In M. W. Apple and L. Weis (Eds.), *Ideology and practice in schooling* (pp. 213–234). Philadelphia: Temple University Press.

Valli, L. (1988). The parallel curriculum at Central Catholic High School. Paper presented at the American Educational Research Association, New Orleans.

Valverde, S. A. (1987). A comparative study of Hispanic dropouts and graduates: Why do some leave school early and some finish? *Education and Urban Society, 19,* 311-320.

Van Galen, J. (1987). Maintaining control. The Structuring of parent involvement. In. G. W. Noblit and W. T. Pink (Eds.), *Schooling in social context* (pp. 78-90). Norwood, NJ: Ablex.

Van Ness, H. (1981). Social control and social organization in an Alaskan Athabaskan classroom: A microethnography of getting ready for reading. In H. Trueba, G. P. Guthrie, and K. H. Au (Eds.), *Culture and the bilingual classroom* (pp. 120-138). Rowley, MA: Newbury House.

Velazquez, L. (1993). Migrant adults' perceptions of schooling, learning and education. Unpublished doctoral dissertation, Department of Technological and Adult Education, University of Tennessee-Knoxville.

Veri, M. (1993). The backlash against women in sports. Unpublished paper, University of Tennessee-Knoxville.

Vogt, L. (1985). Rectifying the school performance of Hawaiian and Navajo students. Paper presented at the meeting of the American Anthropological Association, Washington, DC.

Walker, A. (1983). Quoted in P. H. Collins (1990). *Black feminist thought: Knowledge, consciousness, and the politics of empowerment* (p. 37). London: HarperCollins Academic.

Walker, S., and Barton, L. (1983). *Gender class and education.* Sussex, England: Falmer Press.

Waller, W. (1932). *The sociology of teaching.* New York: John Wiley.

Warren, M. A. (1980). Quoted in C. Kramarae and P. A. Treichler (1985). *A feminist dictionary* (pp. 173-174). London: Pandora Press.

Wax, M. (Ed.). (1980). *When schools are desegregated: Problems and possibilities for students, educators, parents and the community.* New Brunswick, NJ: Transaction Books.

Weber, M. (1947). *The theory of social and economic organizations* (A. M. Henderson and T. Parsons, Trans.). New York: Oxford University Press.

Weber, M. (1958). *From Max Weber: Essays in sociology* (H. Gerth and C. W. Mills, Eds. and Trans.). New York: Oxford University Press.

Weber, M. (1962). *Basic concepts in sociology.* New York: Philosophical Library.

Weedon, C. (1987). *Feminist practice and poststructuralist theory.* Oxford: Basil Blackwell.

Wehlage, G. G., and Rutter, R. A. (1986). Dropping out: What do schools contribute to the problem? *Teachers College Record, 87,* 374-392.

Weick, K. (1976). Educational organizations as loosely coupled systems. *Administrative Science Quarterly, 21,* 1-19.

Weiler, K. (1988). *Women teaching for change.* South Hadley, MA: Bergin & Garvey.

Weis, L. (Ed.). (1988a). *Class, race and gender in American education.* Albany: State University of New York Press.

Weis, L. (1988b). High school girls in a de-industrializing society. In L. Weis (Ed.), *Class, race and gender in American education* (pp. 183-209). Albany: State University of New York Press.

Whitty, G. (1985). *Sociology and school knowledge: Curriculum theory, research and politics.* London: Metheun.

Wilbur, G. (1991). Gender-fair curriculum. Research report prepared for Wellesley College Research on Women, August.

Wiles, J., and Bondi, J. (1981). *The essential middle school.* Columbus, OH: Merrill.

Williams, S. B. (1987). A comparative study of Black dropouts and Black high school graduates in an urban public school system. *Education and Urban Society, 19,* 303-311.

Williamson, R., and Johnson, H. J. (1991). *Planning for success: Successful secondary school principals.* Reston, VA: National Association of Secondary School Principals.

Willis, P. (1977). *Learning to labour.* Lexington, MA: D. C. Heath.

Wilson, M. (1963). *Good company: A study of Nyakyusa age villages.* Boston: Beacon.

Wilson, W. J. (1987). *The truly disadvantaged.* Chicago: University of Chicago Press.

Wirt, F. M., and Kirst, M. W. (1974). State politics of education. In E. L. Useem and M. Useem (Eds.), *The education establishment* (pp. 69–86). Englewood Cliffs, NJ: Prentice Hall.

The Wise Woman. (1982). 4(2) [June 21], 7. Quoted in C. Kramarae and P. A. Treichler (1985). *A feminist dictionary.* London: Pandora Press.

Wolcott, H. (1973). *Man in the principal's office.* Prospect Heights, IL: Waveland Press.

Woo, L. C. (1985). Women administrators: Profiles of success. *Phi Delta Kappan, 67,* 285–288.

Wood, G. (1992). *Schools that work.* New York: Dutton.

Woodhouse, L. (1987). The culture of the 4-year-old in day care: Impacts on social, emotional and physical health. Unpublished doctoral dissertation, University of Cincinnati.

Wright, E. O. (1978). *Class, crisis and the state.* London: New Left Books.

Wright, E. O., and Perrone, L. (1977). Marxist class categories and income inequality. *American Sociological Review, 42,* 32–55.

Young, M. F. D. (1958). *The rise of the meritocracy.* London: Thames & Hudson.

Young, M. F. D. (1971). *Knowledge and control: New directions for the sociology of education.* London: Collier-Macmillan.

Ziegler, S., Hardwick, N., and McGreath, A. M. (1989). Academically successful inner city children: What they can tell us about effective education. Paper presented at the meeting of the American Educational Research Association, San Francisco.

Zigli, B. (1981). A distinctive culture, but an identity crisis. In G. Blake (Ed.), *The urban Appalachians.* Cincinnati: The Cincinnati Enquirer.

Index